CLINICAL
AUDIOLOGY
The
Jerger
Perspective

Singular Publishing Group, Inc.
4284 41st Street
San Diego, California 92105-1197

Copyright © 1993 by Singular Publishing Group, Inc.

Typeset in 10/12 Baskerville by CFW Graphics
Printed in the United States of America by McNaughton & Gunn

Library of Congress Cataloging-in-Publication Data

Jerger, James.
    Clinical audiology : the Jerger perspective / edited by Bobby R.
Alford and Susan Jerger.
      p. cm.
    Collection of previously published articles by James jerger.
    Includes bibliographical references and index.
    ISBN 1-56593-234-X
    1. Audiometry. 2. Hearing disorders—diagnosis.   I. Alford
Bobby R. (Bobby Ray), 1932–   . II. Jerger, Susan.   III. Title.
    [DNLM: 1. Hearing disorders—collected works. 2. Hearing Tests—
collected works.   WV 270 J55c 1993]
RF294.J46 1993
617.8—dc20
DNLM/DC
for Library of Congress

93-21475
CIP

CLINICAL
AUDIOLOGY
The
Jerger
Perspective

Edited by

Bobby R. Alford, M.D.

and

Susan Jerger, Ph.D.

SINGULAR PUBLISHING GROUP, INC.
SAN DIEGO, CALIFORNIA

Table of Contents

Preface

James Jerger's contributions to the literature in audiology span more than four decades. In this volume, celebrating the 25th year of his association with Baylor College of Medicine, we have attempted to capture and convey to readers the breadth of Jerger's research interests and the important influence that his papers have had on the historical development of the field. We have selected for this purpose 53 seminal papers focused on eight areas: diagnostic audiology, central auditory processing disorders, speech audiometry, impedance audiometry, the acoustic reflex, auditory evoked potentials, aging, and professional issues.

From a total of more than 250 papers, touching virtually every aspect of the profession, we have chosen the papers that we felt either had the most significant impact in an area or represented a new and fresh direction or approach to an old problem. The content of these 53 papers can be read at multiple levels—for their historical interest; for their varied approaches to experimentation; for their impact on clinical practice; for their new knowledge about auditory system function, behavior, and disorder; and/or for their insights into the thought processes of a prolific investigator. As such, they should be of interest to graduate students, to practicing clinicians, to fledgling researchers, and to seasoned hands, all of whom will find, from their own perspectives, something uniquely interesting in this collection of papers.

Many of the works we have chosen convey a recurrent theme, namely a commitment to the concept that auditory disorder is nature's laboratory for the study of audition. This was not always a popular view. The systematic study of patients with hearing problems was, and still is in many quarters, viewed as "clinical" and therefore somehow second-class research, to be carefully distinguished from pure studies of "normal" processes. But Jerger has persisted in his belief that clinical material had much to teach us about the auditory system. An important by-product of this approach to research was the recurrent demonstration that clinical research could pay rich dividends in the development and improvement of clinical practices. These papers testify to the impact of Jerger's vision, as it has affected, and continues to affect, the development of clinical audiological practices. The wealth of interesting patients with well-documented disorders that resonates throughout much of his work also reflects Jerger's early realization of the value of a true partnership between audiology and otorhinolaryngology—head and neck surgery.

The papers in this volume testify to the far-ranging influence of Jerger's unique approach on his students and colleagues who have gone on to make important contributions in their own right. Readers will encounter many familiar names who are well-known for their outstanding leadership in both scientific and professional arenas, for example, auditory evoked potentials (James Hall), hearing aids (Earl Harford), speech science and speech audiometry (Charles Speaks), pediatric audiology and President of the American Auditory Society (Deborah Hayes), national health care (Bill Keith), presbyacusis and Secretary-Treasurer of the American Academy of Audiology (Brad Stach), state health services for the hearing-impaired (Terrey Oliver Penn), and clinical audiological services (Bob Fifer).

In short, as we look back over the years at Jerger's body of work, we see a dedication to continued intellectual growth, an ability to integrate new and old information, and a scholarly application of knowledge to clinical problems. Also shining through these achievements is a sense of the spirit of the individuals who pioneered a partnership of respect and cooperation between audiology and otolaryngology—head and neck surgery. It is our pleasure to present this body of work, which imparts such a full-flavored sense of audiology's past and bestows such optimism for audiology's future.

Bobby R. Alford, M.D.
Susan Jerger, Ph.D.

Introduction

This book marks the 25th anniversary of my affiliation with the Baylor College of Medicine, and is coincident with the 50th anniversary of the College itself. My wife, Dr. Susan Jerger, and I came to Baylor in 1968 at the invitation of Dr. Bobby Alford, who had recently accepted the chairmanship of the Department of Otorhinolaryngology. Together, the three of us forged a unique collaboration between audiology and otorhinolaryngology, one that has been, I think, good for both fields.

I was attracted to Baylor by a number of factors. The most important was the opportunity to develop an audiology program within a medical environment. At Northwestern, in the early 1950s, I had been impressed by the collaboration between audiologists Ray Carhart and John Gaeth and otolaryngologists George Shambaugh and Gene Derlacki. Carhart and Gaeth were on the Evanston Campus in the School of Speech, whereas Shambaugh and Derlacki were on the Chicago Campus in the Medical School, some 12 miles away. But every Wednesday morning they held a joint clinic at the Medical School. Four or five patients, chosen for the variety of their problems, were examined medically by either Shambaugh or Derlacki and audiologically by students assigned to the clinic. Then each patient was jointly counseled by an audiologist and an otolaryngologist, usually Carhart and Shambaugh, while the audiology students and a few otolaryngology residents looked on.

All this was more than 40 years ago, but I still remember it as one of the most exciting and useful learning experiences of my career. It impressed two things on me: First, the importance of the medical environment: that's where the patients were (and still are). Second, the benefits accruing to both sides when health care professionals work cooperatively rather than competitively.

When I left Northwestern in 1961, I moved to Washington, D.C. and worked both at the Veteran's Administration Outpatient Clinic in the old Munitions Building near the Lincoln Memorial, and at Gallaudet College. At the VA I worked closely with Stan Zerlin and Laszlo Stein, at Gallaudet with Bob Frisina and Ray Bernero. Although I enjoyed these affiliations and the many friends I made at both institutions, it soon became clear that neither of these settings was going to provide what I was looking for. And so I moved on in 1962, this time to Houston and the now defunct Houston Speech and Hearing Center. We did a lot of interesting things there. Throughout most of the next 6 years, the research team consisted of Chuck Speaks and Susan Jerger, assisted by a number of Rice University students, including Jim Thelin, Don Golden, and George Forman and by research audiologist, Carolyn Malmquist.

But by 1968 it became clear that this was not the environment I was looking for either. The physical facilities were extensive and impressive, but there were no patients. Susan and I were on the verge of accepting a generous offer to join the faculty at the University of Texas at Austin when Bobby Alford approached us about joining the department at Baylor and developing a comprehensive program in audiology. Although we anguished a little over losing the opportunity to move to the beautiful city of Austin, there was never any doubt about what our decision would be. Baylor was where the patients were, and the opportunity to build a cooperative program within, rather than a competitive program outside of, the medical environment, was what I had long sought.

The move to Baylor did, however, take some dedication to the concept of future development. We moved into The Methodist Hospital in the fall of 1968 with few personnel, little space, and less equipment. But Texas is a wonderful place to develop things. There really is a "can-do" spirit here that favors the entrepreneur who is willing to take chances. Within a few years we had a thriving enterprise going, and we have never looked back.

With the assistance of colleagues like Rose Chmiel, Bob Fifer, Jay Hall, Deborah Hayes, Karen Johnson, Bill Keith, Henry Lew, Louise Loiselle, Larry Mauldin, Terrey Oliver-Penn, and Brad Stach, we developed what I would like to believe is a fairly respectable clinical audiological service, turned out at least a few interesting papers, and sent several graduates of the Ph.D. program out into the world to agitate the *status quo*.

But the most important achievement has been the development of a truly cooperative working arrangement between the two professions that have so much to offer each other, audiology and otolaryngology. Thanks to the good offices of many individuals, but especially to Dr. Bobby Alford, we have made it work here at Baylor.

This book is about some of the fruits of that collaboration.

James Jerger, Ph.D.

Diagnostic Audiology

In the 1950s, we were all very much influenced by two converging lines of research from Europe. In England Dix, Hallpike, and Hood had just published their important 1948 paper, in the *Proceedings of the Royal Society of Medicine* on differentiating Meniere's disease from acoustic neuroma by means of the Alternate Binaural Loudness Balance (ABLB) test. J. D. Hood followed this up shortly thereafter with a very thought-provoking monograph on the measurement of what has come to be called auditory "adaptation," which was then believed to be a progressive decline in the loudness of an auditory signal over time. During the same period in Basel, Switzerland Professor Luscher published a series of papers on what he and his co-workers (including a young engineer, Josef Zwislocki) called the "intensity different limen" (IDL). Using an amplitude modulation detection paradigm, they tested patients with cochlear and retrocochlear hearing losses and noted that, when measured at comparable sensation levels, IDLs were smaller than normal in patients with cochlear loss but normal, or even larger than normal, in patients with retrocochlear losses.

It seemed seductively appealing to relate all of this to "loudness recruitment," or abnormally rapid loudness growth with increasing sound intensity, a phenomenon that had already been described by E. P. Fowler in the 1930s. According to the popular scenario of that day, loudness recruitment was the parent phenomenon. If it were characteristic of cochlear disorders, but not of retrococh-

lear disorders, it would explain why the ABLB, a direct measure of loudness recruitment, was positive in the Meniere's disease patients of Dix, Hallpike, and Hood, but negative in their acoustic tumor patients. And, since loudness recruitment means that the function relating loudness to intensity is abnormally steep, it would follow that a just-noticeable change in loudness would be achieved by a smaller than normal increment in intensity, resulting in an abnormally small intensity difference limen. The argument was strengthened by Bekesy's report, in the late 1940s, that when he tested people with cochlear losses on his newly built automatic audiometer, the width of their threshold crossings (the "first difference limen" in contemporary parlance) was abnormally narrow compared to those of persons with normal hearing.

We now realize, of course, that most of this compelling reasoning was seriously flawed. Loudness recruitment is not the parent phenomenon and is itself not as unidimensional as had been assumed. Nor do the amplitude modulation and threshold tracking techniques bear one-to-one correspondence with intensity difference limens measured in rigorous psychophysical fashion. Finally, the phenomenon of abnormal adaptation, especially prominent in retrochochlear disorder, thickens the plot considerably.

But in the innocent '50s, we were all driven by the exciting goal of differentiating cochlear from retrocochlear hearing loss—the first step, it was hoped, in ultimately understanding the many varieties of what was then called "perceptive" and now is known as "sensorineural" hearing impairment. And, surprisingly enough, in spite of its theoretical weaknesses, the overall concept seemed to work in clinical practice.

In 1949 my mentor, Ray Carhart, had traveled to Stockholm to participate in one of the first international audiology courses. While there he saw a device, made by the Amplivox Co in England, for measuring the IDL by amplitude modulation according to the Luscher paradigm. He brought one of the units back to Chicago, plugged it into an old ADC audiometer at the audiology clinic at the Medical School, and asked for a volunteer to test some patients. Although I was still an undergraduate student, I volunteered and began to test every patient being evaluated during the Wednesday morning clinic. That experience piqued my interest in the general area of intensity difference limens, loudness recruitment, and differentiating cochlear from retrocochlear hearing loss. My doctoral dissertation investigated the effect of cochlear hearing loss on the IDL as measured by the "quantal" psychophysical method, a technique developed by Stevens and Volkman in the early 1940s, in which to-be-detected intensity increments are added to a steady-state carrier signal. Interestingly, Ray Carhart was one of my experimental subjects. He had a substantial high-frequency sensorineural hearing loss, apparently due to large doses of aspirin he was taking for relief of pain. It was during this testing that he and I both noticed the striking fact that, over the course of the presentation of 20 increments at 5 second intervals, the apparent loudness of the 4000 Hz test tone diminished substantially. It was this observation that ultimately led Carhart to the formulation of the "tone decay" test, which was, for many years, a staple in the armamentarium of diagnostic techniques.

My own interest in this observation led me to explore, in greater detail, the phenomenon of adaptation and how it might be used clinically. Using Hood's median-plane localization methodology, I studied "normal" adaptation as functions of frequency and level, culminating in the first paper in this section, "Auditory Adaptation," which appeared in the *Journal of the Acoustical Society of America* in 1957. The following year, Carhart and I pooled our observations on the very interesting phenomenon of strikingly abnormal adaptation in a small number of patients with surgically verified acoustic tumors, leading to the paper "Clinical Observations on Excessive Threshold Adaptation," which appeared in the *Archives of Otolaryngology* in 1958. Following up on my doctoral dissertation, I worked out, with my colleagues Earl Harford and Joyce Lassman (Shedd), a clinical technique, based on the quantal psychophysical method, for measuring a patient's ability to detect very small (1.0 dB), short (500 msec), intensity increments superimposed on a carrier tone presented at a sensation level of 20 dB. We devised the acronym SISI to stand for "short increment sensitivity index," and proposed it as a rapid technique for differentiating cochlear from retrocochlear hearing loss. The paper describing the technique, "On the Detection of Extremely Small Changes in Sound Intensity," appeared in the *Archives of Otolaryngology* in 1959. The

test enjoyed some popularity, especially in Europe, until it was replaced by ABR in the late 1970s.

Our first Bekesy-type audiometer at Northwestern was built for Carhart by Scott Reger of Iowa. Scott was an avowed gadgeteer who could build virtually anything out of wood and aluminum. He charged Ray the princely sum of $75 for the instrument, but gave the Northwestern accountants headaches because he never cashed the check. I used Reger's instrument to study the effect of signal duration on recovery from temporary threshold shift. When the first Grason-Stadler E-800 arrived, we took it down to the medical school and began to use it on every patient we could corner. The idea of comparing the threshold tracings for interrupted and continuous tonal sweeps came from an original suggestion by Peter Denes, when he visited Evanston in the late 1950s. The paper outlining the four Bekesy types (I, II, III, and IV), "Bekesy Audiometry in the Analysis of Auditory Disorders," appeared in the *Journal of Speech and Hearing Research* in 1960. Thanks to the kind intervention of then-editor Dorothy Sherman, we were able to color code the interrupted (green) and continuous (red) traces. This was the first use of color in an ASHA journal.

During the decade of the 1970s, I collaborated with Deborah Hayes on a number of projects. Together we collected a considerable body of data on performance-intensity (PI) functions for phonemically balanced (PB) words and synthetic sentence identification materials. In the paper "Diagnostic Speech Audiometry," which appeared in the *Archives of Otolaryngology* in 1977, we tried to emphasize the diagnostic potential of speech audiometry. We sought to show that some very important diagnostic distinctions, especially in differentiating peripheral from central problems, could be made by suitable expansion of the basic speech audiometric battery. Shortly thereafter, I was at a meeting in Sun Valley where a speaker tried to make the point that audiometric evaluation was not helpful in the diagnosis of space-occupying retrocochlear lesions. The speaker summarized a number of cases with confirmed retrocochlear disorders in which audiometric findings were "normal." This individual's definition of "audiometrically normal" was simply a pure-tone audiogram within normal limits and a "discrim score" of better than 80%. After returning to Houston I asked my associate, Connie Jordan, to work backward through our clinical files until she had found 20 patients with retrocochlear auditory disorder who met such a definition of "normalcy." In less than an hour she had accumulated 20 such cases. In every instance speech audiometry was abnormal by one or both of two simple indices, rollover of the PI function for words or a significant discrepancy between PB_{max} and SSI_{max}. We summarized results in these 20 cases in a paper entitled, "Normal Audiometric Findings," which appeared in the *American Journal of Otology* in 1980.

Perhaps the most significant change in diagnostic evaluation over the past four decades has been in the pediatric arena. In the 1950s, 1960s, and even into the early 1970s, we had to rely almost exclusively on behavioral techniques to evaluate the hearing of infants and young children. We had visual reinforcement audiometry (VRA) and the conditioned orienting response (COR), to be sure, but in the very children where we needed help most, those with multiple handicaps, behavioral methods were least satisfactory. This was the era of cults. Some venerable figure would describe his or her way of testing children and aver that it was the only sure-fire technique, but only if you did it his or her way. Then a following would develop and soon a new cult would be born. Cultists would insist, with missionary zeal, that their way was the only way to a true understanding of the hearing-impaired child. The problem was that, before immittance and auditory brain stem response (ABR) audiometry, there was little opportunity to know whether you had made a mistake. It was not difficult, therefore, to assume that you were correct in every insightful diagnosis. But the advent of ABR and immittance audiometry in the 1970s changed all that. Now, for the first time, you could get immediate and independent confirmation of your behavioral estimates. As a result, we began to see how wrong, how very wrong, you could be if you relied solely on behavioral techniques.

Deborah Hayes and I began to collect cases illustrating these points. This activity culminated in the paper, "The Cross-Check Principle in Pediatric Audiometry." Our point was simply that you could not trust behavioral testing in young children, no matter how clever you thought you were, but ABR and acoustic reflexes gave you the opportunity to cross-check your behavioral prediction. We suggested that, if behavioral and reflex predictions agreed, you were probably on safe ground. But if they did not agree, then you had better cross-check your results with ABR. Invariably, when we did this we found that the ABR results agreed better with the reflex prediction than with the behavioral results. I would like to think that this was an important contribution to the very important area of pediatric assessment.

Thanks to Dr. Victor Rivera, an outstanding neurologist here at Baylor, for many years, we have also had excellent access to a large population of patients with multiple sclerosis (MS). This has provided our research group with an unparalleled opportunity to evaluate tests of retrocochlear function in one of nature's laboratories for the study of auditory disorders in the central auditory system. My colleagues, Terrey Oliver (Penn), Henry Lew, Rose Chmiel, and I evaluated the acoustic reflex both alone and in combination with ABR, speech audiometry, and the MLD in a large series of MS patients. Two papers, "Abnormalities of the Acoustic Reflex in Multiple Sclerosis" (*American Journal of Otolaryngology*, 1986) and "Patterns of Auditory Abnormality in Multiple Sclerosis" (*Audiology*, 1986), summarize this work. In general, our findings served to re-emphasize the important role of speech audiometry in the evaluation of brainstem disease.

The discovery of otoacoustic emissions by Kemp in the 1970s added yet another weapon to our diagnostic arsenal. In the recent paper, "Otoacoustic Emissions, Audiometric Sensitivity Loss, and Speech Understanding," which appeared in the *Journal of the American Academy of Audiology* in 1992, we illustrated how effective this new tool can be in differentiating cochlear from retrocochlear site. A patient with multiple sclerosis had a very mild sensitivity loss in one ear, accompanied by extremely poor speech understanding. Because speech understanding is affected by both peripheral and central disorders, it could always be argued that the speech understanding deficit might be explained by the peripheral sensitivity loss. But the presence of robust emissions in that ear effectively ruled out a peripheral explanation for the speech understanding deficit. Thus, the combination of audiogram, otoacoustic emissions, and speech audiometric scores can make it possible to differentiate between speech understanding problems due to peripheral sensitivity loss and speech understanding problems due to central auditory processing deficits. The implications of this capability are truly profound.

The effects of auditory disorders, both peripheral and central, on binaural processing are only now being investigated. In this regard, my colleague, Henry Lew, was instrumental in the development of the concept we now call "binaural interference." In the course of topographic brain mapping studies of children and adults with central auditory disorders, he noticed that, when both ears were stimulated, the resultant brain map was sometimes worse than when only one ear was stimulated. Henry thought this suggested an auditory analog of the visual disorder known as amblyopia, where the input from one eye so interferes with the input from the other eye that the "bad" eye must be blocked or covered up. As we pursued the matter, we found that the phenomenon could also be demonstrated behaviorally in some elderly hearing aid users. When tested in the sound field, it was evident that their performance was better with only one ear aided than with both ears aided. At about the same time we had been corresponding with colleagues Shlomo Silman and Carol Silverman in Brooklyn about their observations on auditory deprivation effects when one ear was deprived of amplification for an extended period of time. As we mulled over these two phenomena, it soon became apparent that we might be talking about different manifestations of a common underlying effect. Could it be that, as the deprived ear loses its function relative to the aided ear, the growing asymmetry in performance eventually leads to binaural interference when one attempts to aid both ears. Silman and Silverman began searching for the effect, and soon we had an interesting series of patients from both laboratories illustrating the binaural interference effect both behaviorally and electrophysiologically. Our joint paper summarizing these findings, "Case Studies in Binaural Interference" recently appeared in the *Journal of the American Academy of Audiology*.

Diagnostic audiology has made great strides since our first halting steps at differentiating cochlear from retrocochlear site of lesion. With the advent of ABR, the acoustic reflex, evoked autoacoustic eissions, and especially more sophisticated speech audiometry, we are able to identify the site of auditory disorder at several levels within the peripheral and central systems. And we are pushing the frontier forward into the realm of binaural processing interactions. Our strides have been rewarding, but the future promises even more exciting challenges.

Reprinted from THE JOURNAL OF THE ACOUSTICAL SOCIETY OF AMERICA, Vol. 29, No. 3, 357–363, March, 1957

Auditory Adaptation*

JAMES F. JERGER

Audiological Laboratory, Northwestern University, Evanston, Illinois

(Received October 8, 1956)

The apparent decline in the ear's response under sustained stimulation, a phenomenon which has been variously labeled "auditory fatigue," "perstimulatory fatigue," and "auditory adaptation," was measured for pure tones over a wide range of frequencies and intensities by the median-plane-localization method.

For a given intensity, increasing the frequency from 125 to 1000 cps increased both the initial rate and maximum amount of adaptation. Above 1000 cps further increases in frequency did not appreciably change the adaptation curves.

For a given frequency, increasing the intensity of the sustained stimulus also increased both initial rate and maximum amount of adaptation. The function relating adaptation, in db; to stimulus intensity was, in general, negatively accelerated.

The duration of sustained stimulation at which adaptation reached a maximum value was related to both frequency and intensity.

INTRODUCTION

IN spite of extensive exploration in vision, the decline in response under sustained stimulation has received comparatively little attention in audition. Wood,[1] in 1930, measured the decrease in the apparent loudness of a 1000 cps tone for durations ranging from 5 sec to 2 min, but his method was somewhat too time-consuming to lend itself easily to extensive exploration.

In 1950, Hood[2] described a considerably less cumbersome technique permitting relatively rapid measurement. In Hood's method a tone is first presented to both ears for a brief period (10–20 sec). The intensity of the tone on one ear (test ear) is fixed, while the subject varies the intensity of the tone on the opposite ear (control ear), until the two tones are "equally loud."† After two or three matches have been made in this fashion, the tone of fixed intensity remains on in the test ear but the variable tone is turned off in the control ear. Then, at periodic intervals (usually 1 min), the variable tone is reapplied to the control ear for a brief period (10–20 sec) and the subject varies its intensity until another match has been made. The *difference* between the intensity level required for a match initially and the intensity level required after the test tone has been sustained on the test ear for a given period represents the amount by which the response of the test ear has declined as a result of sustained stimulation for that period.

For the sake of convenience of notation this difference will be denoted by the term "adaptation" throughout the remainder of this paper. We recognize, however, that "adaptation" is not an entirely suitable term to describe the phenomenon, and employ it with that reservation in mind.

Using the above procedure, Hood measured adaptation in four normal-hearing subjects at three frequencies: 500, 1000, and 2000 cps and at sensation levels ranging from 20 to 100 db. He concluded that adaptation reached a maximum after the third min of sustained stimulation, and that the maximum amount of adaptation increased as a function of the sensation level of the sustained stimulus. At high sensation levels, adaptation amounted to as much as 50 db.

In view of the considerable degree of adaptation reflected in Hood's results, Egan[3] attempted to determine whether the median-plane-localization process required by Hood's method was critical to the demonstration of the phenomenon. He attacked the problem by having subjects match identical frequencies, as Hood had presumably done, then having them match frequencies that differed by from 5 to 200 cy. The slight frequency difference presumably prevented the subject from making a median-plane localization and forced him to make a true loudness balance. Results showed that, if precautions were taken to minimize the subject's tendency to form an absolute loudness standard, very nearly the same amount of adaptation was measured whether the frequencies were identical or slightly different. Egan concluded, therefore, that the median-plane localization process was not critical to the occurence of the phenomenon.

Carterette[4] extended Hood's results by measuring adaptation for both continuous and interrupted white noise. Maximum adaptation increased as a function

* This study was supported by funds provided under Contract AF18(600)-630 with the U. S. Air Force School of Aviation Medicine, Randolph Field, Texas.

[1] A. G. Wood, unpublished Master's thesis, University of Virginia, 1930. [Cited in F. A. Geldard, *The Human Senses* (John Wiley and Sons, Inc., New York, 1953).]

[2] J. D. Hood, Acta-Otolaryngol., Suppl. No. 92 (1950).

† Relative to this "equal loudness" criterion, it is well known that when two tones of identical frequency are presented, in phase, to the two ears, the subject generally hears not two sounds but one sound whose apparent location in the head is determined by the relative intensities of the two tones. The effect is most prominent for low frequencies, but may be observed at high frequencies as well. Thus, the subject is forced to make, not a true equal loudness judgment, but a median-plane localization. He can only adjust the relative intensities until the phantom sound appears to be in the middle of the head.

[3] J. P. Egan, J. Acoust. Soc. Am. 27, 111–120 (1955).

[4] E. C. Carterette, J. Acoust. Soc. Am. 27, 103–111 (1955).

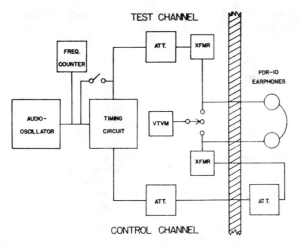

FIG. 1. Block diagram of apparatus used to measure adaptation for pure tones.

of the intensity of the sustained stimulus, a result in agreement with Hood's results for pure tones. In contrast to Hood's data, however, maximum adaptation for noise was not reached until at least the 7th min of sustained stimulation, over twice the duration reported by Hood for pure tones. Finally, for discontinuous noise, adaptation was found to increase as a function of interruption rate.

Thwing[5] measured the spread of adaptation of a pure tone to neighboring frequencies and found that the frequency gradients on either side of the stimulus frequency were approximately symmetrical, a result in sharp contrast to the markedly skewed patterns of masking audiograms and spread functions for auditory fatigue as measured by threshold shift.

These investigations have delimited the main outlines of the adaptation phenomenon. The purpose of the present study was to extend the results for pure tones to a wider range of frequencies and intensities.

APPARATUS AND PROCEDURE

Ten young adults (4 male, 6 female) with normal hearing served as subjects under a series of 42 experimental conditions. Each condition consisted of the measurement of adaptation for a given frequency and intensity at 1-min intervals over a 5-min period. Seven frequencies (125, 250, 500, 1000, 2000, 4000, and 8000 cps) and seven intensities‡ (30, 40, 50, 60, 70, 80, and 90 db) were explored. Of the 49 possible combinations of these seven frequencies and intensities, seven combination (125 cps at 30, 40 and 50 db; 250 cps at 30 and 40 db; 500 cps at 30 db; 8000 cps at 30 db) represented either inaudible or barely audible conditions and could not be used. For this reason the total number of experimental conditions was 42.

Figure 1 shows a simplified block diagram of the

experimental apparatus. The output from an audio-oscillator passed through a timing circuit in which it was split into two channels. Within this circuit a recycling timer turned the tone "on" in each channel for 15 sec, then "off" for 45 sec. A switch permitted the upper channel to by-pass the timing circuit without altering the on-off sequence in the other channel. With this switch open the temporal pattern of the signal was identical at the two earphones. With the switch closed, however, the signal in the upper channel was sustained while the signal in the lower channel continued to cycle on and off.

From the timing circuit the signal in the upper, or test, channel passed through a standard attenuator, then to a matching transformer, and finally to a PDR–10 earphone mounted in an MX41/AR cushion. The signal in the lower, or control, channel passed through another standard attenuator, then to a special attenuator operated by the subject, and finally, through a matching transformer, to another PDR-10 earphone mounted in an MX41/AR cushion. The subject-operated attenuator had a range of 60 db in 2-db steps.

Adaptation was measured according to the general method of Hood.[2] but following the specific procedure outlined by Egan[3] as his "method of fixed intensity" (i.d., maintaining the intensity of the test tone at a constant level over the entire period of sustained stimulation). Throughout an experimental run, the subject's task was simply to adjust his 2-db step attenuator until the tone was localized in the median plane. He was instructed to make this judgment as quickly as possible since only 15 sec were allowed for each match. A small pilot light, synchronized with the 15-sec "on" period of the recycling timer, signaled whenever the tone was on in the control channel and a match was to be made. When this light went on, the subjected adjusted the 2-db step attenuator until he had bracketed the point of median-plane localization as closely as possible.

At the end of the 15-sec matching period the pilot light went off. The subject then reported his attenuator setting to the experimenter and turned the knob to full attenuation. Thus, each match began by increasing the intensity of the control tone from a relatively faint level. This precaution was taken in order to minimize the effect of the slight adaptation incurred by the control tone during its 15-sec duration. Between successive matches, the experimenter varied the level of his own control-tone attenuator randomly over a 60-db range.

The experimental run always began with the test-channel by-pass switch open. In this case the tone came on in each phone simultaneously for 15 sec of each minute. During this period the subject adjusted the intensity of the signal in the control-channel phone until he judged that the tone was localized in the median plane.

After three matches had been made, the experimenter

[5] E. J. Thwing, J. Acoust. Soc. Am. **27**, 741–748 (1955).
‡ SPL in db *re* 0.0002 microbar developed in NBS No. 9A coupler.

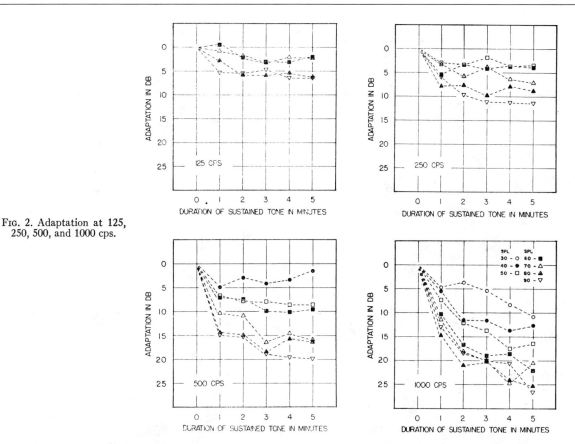

Fig. 2. Adaptation at 125, 250, 500, and 1000 cps.

closed the test-channel by-pass switch for 5 min. During this period, the fixed-intensity tone remained on continuously in the test-channel phone, but the temporal pattern of the signal in the control phone remained unchanged (on for 15 sec, off for 45 sec). Throughout the 5-min period of sustained stimulation the subject continued to execute matches at 1-min intervals.§

Prior to the first experimental run, each subject was given four practice runs at widely varying frequencies and intensities (125 cps at 90 db; 1000 cps at 50 db, 4000 cps at 30 db, 8000 cps at 70 db). He then completed the 42 experimental runs in from 9 to 21 experimental sessions. Depending on how much time the subject could contribute to a particular experimental session, he was allowed to complete anywhere from 2 to 5 experimental runs per session. A rest period of at least 5 min was interposed between adjacent runs within a given session.

In setting up the order in which a given subject would undergo the 42 experimental runs it was thought desirable to avoid the situation in which two relatively

similar conditions of frequency and intensity occurred in succession during the same experimental session. For this reason a purely random order was not employed. Instead, the random order which had been arranged for each subject was modified, throughout the course of the experiment, to avoid successions of similar frequencies or intensities within a single session.

The right ear was used as the test ear in half of the subjects, the left ear in the remaining half.

RESULTS

The amount of adaptation, in db, at each 1-min interval during the 5-min period of sustained stimulation was computed by subtracting the SPL required on the control ear for a match at each interval from the mean of the three SPL required on the control ear in the three matches made prior to sustained stimulation.

A mean adaptation curve was then derived for each experimental condition by averaging the individual curves of the 10 experimental subjects.‖

Figures 2 and 3 present the mean curves thus obtained for each of the 42 experimental conditions. Inspection of these figures suggests a number of generalizations relative to the influence of frequency, intensity, and duration on adaptation for pure tones.

---

§ At high frequencies (2000–8000 cps) a number of subjects were unable to localize the stimulus to the median plane during the period of sustained stimulation. This was apparently due to the marked difference in quality between the adapted test tone and the unadapted control tone. In this case the subject was instructed to find that level of the control tone which yielded equal loudness in the two ears.

‖ Median curves were also computed. Since they yielded virtually identical results, all subsequent discussion will be confined to mean curves.

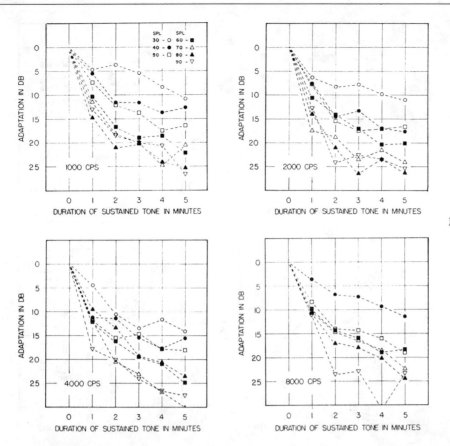

FIG. 3. Adaptation at 1000, 2000, 4000, and 8000 cps.

Adaptation as a Function of Frequency

The most obvious generalization to be drawn from Figs. 2 and 3 is the fact that high frequencies show considerably more adaptation than low frequencies. At 125 cps, adaptation after 5 min of sustained stimulation is quite negligible, even at an SPL of 90 db. At 4000 cps, however, a substantial amount of adaptation has occurred after only 1 min of sustained stimulation at levels of 50 db and above.

The relationship between adaptation and frequency is nonlinear. Adaptation shows a progressive increase as frequency is increased from 125 to 1000 cps, but remains approximately constant from 1000 through 8000 cps.

Adaptation as a Function of Sensation Level

Figures 2 and 3 show that, at each frequency, adaptation increases with intensity. In order to illustrate this relationship in a more easily interpreted manner, the basic data have been recast in Figs. 4 and 5. Here adaptation is plotted, not as a function of the SPL of the test tone, but as a function of its sensation level (db *re* threshold SPL at each frequency).

Figure 4 shows adaptation after 1 min of sustained stimulation as a function of the sensation level of the test tone with frequency as the parameter. Although there are minor variations in configurations for individual frequencies, the over-all pattern suggests a fairly linear relationship between adaptation, in db, and sensation level, in db, in the range from 10 to 80 db.

Figure 5 is analogous to Fig. 4, but shows adaptation after 5 min of sustained stimulation. Although high frequencies now show considerably more adaptation than low frequencies, the relationship between adaptation and sensation level is still roughly linear. There is, however, a suggestion of a slight negative acceleration above 60 db.

Adaptation as a Function of Duration

Hood, in his pioneer study of the phenomenon, concluded that adaptation reached a maximum after $3\frac{1}{2}$ min, irrespective of the intensity of the sustained tone. This generalization was necessarily confined to the three frequencies (500, 1000, and 2000 cps) at which his measures were obtained. Inspection of the present results suggests that Hood's conclusion oversimplified the situation somewhat. Figures 2 and 3 indicate that the duration at which maximum adaptation occurs appears to be a function of both frequency and intensity. At 125, 250, and 500 cps, a maximum seems to be reached after 3 min, but in the range from 1000 through 8000 cps, only the curves for the very low intensities show any tendency to stabilize at a maximum value. At the higher intensities the curves continue to drop even after the 5th min. In a previous report from our laboratory[6] adaptation was measured for a 4000 cps tone at an SPL of 80 db, over a 10-min period of sustained stimulation. Results indicated that, at this frequency, maximum adaptation was not reached until the 7th min, a finding in close agreement with Carterette's[4] results for adaptation to sustained thermal noise.

Between-Subject Variability of Adaptation

A salient feature of the adaptation phenomenon is the marked variability in results obtained from different subjects. In one of the present experimental conditions, (1000 cps at 70 db, SPL), for example, one subject showed adaptation of only 5 db, after the 5th min of sustained stimulation, while another subject showed a decline of 45 db. Figure 6 illustrates the effects of frequency and sensation level on the variability of adaptation after 5 min of sustained stimulation. Each point in this figure represents the standard deviation of the adaptation values in db yielded by

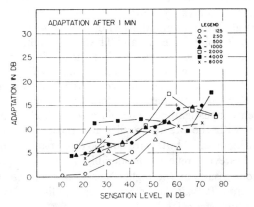

Fig. 4. Adaptation after 1 min of sustained stimulation as a function of frequency and sensation level.

the 10 subjects in each of the 42 experimental conditions. The over-all effect is a "scattergram" showing that, in general, variability increases as a function of sensation level.

Adaptation in Relation to Loudness

In all of the foregoing, care has been exercised to avoid the use of the term "loudness." Adaptation has been defined solely in terms of the measuring operation; i.e., the difference between the intensity required on the control ear to achieve median-plane localization before and after the application of a sustained tone on the test ear.

If it is assumed, however, that adaptation, as measured by the median-plane localization method, represents a decline in the *loudness* of the sustained tone over time, then one may express the db measure of adaptation (reduction in control ear intensity) as a

[6] J. F. Jerger, School of Aviation Medicine, U. S. Air Force, Project No. 7755-19, Report No. 56-9 (January, 1956).

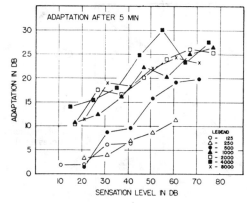

Fig. 5. Adaptation after 5 min of sustained stimulation as a function of frequency and sensation level.

loudness decline in which the unit of measure is the sone. Figure 7 plots this "adaptation in sones" as a function of the initial loudness level of the test tone. The amount of sone adaptation was computed by subtracting from the sone value corresponding to the initial intensity of the control tone, the sone value corresponding to the intensity of the control tone after 5 min of sustained stimulation on the test ear. Steven's revised loudness scale[7] was used as the basis for all sone computations. The loudness level (sensation level of equally loud 1000-cps tone) corresponding to each experimental condition was computed from the equal-loudness-level contours of Fletcher and Munson.[8]

Two interesting features emerge from this conversion. In addition to yielding a reasonably linear relationship between loudness level and log adaptation in sones, it tends to reduce the frequency differential, exemplified in Fig. 5, appreciably. The frequencies of 125 and 250 cps show the least sone adaptation at a given loudness level; 500 cps shows slightly more adaptation; 1000, 2000, 4000, and 8000 cps are essentially equivalent and

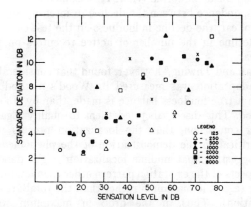

Fig. 6. Between-subject variability of adaptation as a function of frequency and sensation level.

[7] S. S. Stevens, J. Acoust. Soc. Am. 27, 815–829 (1955).
[8] H. Fletcher and W. A. Munson, J. Acoust. Soc. Am. 5, 82–108 (1933).

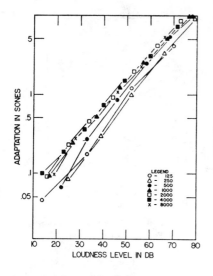

FIG. 7. Adaptation, in sones, as a function of frequency and loudness level.

lie slightly above 500 cps. In general, however, the frequency differential is not great.

A straight line visually fitted to the data at 1000, 2000, 4000, and 8000 cps gives the equation,

$$\log A = 0.03N - 1.5, \tag{1}$$

where A is adaptation in sones and N is loudness level in db. This equation is similar to Steven's fundamental loudness equation,

$$\log L = 0.03N - 1.2, \tag{2}$$

where L is loudness in sones and N is loudness level in db.

It is pertinent to ask, however, whether the progressive decline in the intensity required for a match over successive minutes of sustained stimulation is due solely to a progressive decline in the loudness of the tone on the test ear, or whether factors other than loudness, *per se*, contribute to the median plane localization of a dichotically presented stimulus.

Hood[2] held the former view. He assumed a complete correspondence between the decline in intensity on the control ear, the decline in loudness on the test ear, and the decline in the number of active receptors on the test ear.

Egan and Thwing,[9] however, found that considerably less adaptation was measured by Wood's method[1] in which a true loudness balance is made, than by Hood's method. This discrepancy led them to qualify Egan's earlier conclusion, than the localization process was not critical to the demonstration of the phenomenon, by suggesting that midline localization might depend on aspects of the excitation pattern other than loudness, *per se* (e.g., the maximum rather than the total area of excitation). Thus, if the drop in maximum were relatively greater than the decrease in the total area of excitation, a method requiring median-plane localiza-

tion would measure more adaptation than a method requiring a true loudness balance.

In view of this finding, we are inclined to suspect that the conversion from adaptation in db to adaptation in sones is somewhat misleading. Apparently the db drop on the control ear over time reflects a more complex change in the response of the test ear than simply a decline in loudness. In any event, further exploration of the relationship between equality of loudness and median-plane localization is essential to a more complete understanding of the problem.

Relation to Other Experiments

It is of some interest to compare our findings with those obtained by other investigators. Figure 8 shows how the present results at 1000 cps compare with the results of five previous investigators who obtained data at this frequency. All points represent adaptation measured after 3 min of sustained stimulation. The data for Hood are taken from his 1950 monograph,[2] the data for Palva from his 1955 paper,[10] and the data for Wright from an unpublished doctoral dissertation.[11] The single point for Egan and Thwing was taken from Fig. 1 of their recent paper,[9] while the single point for Thwing was taken from Fig. 3 of his 1955 paper.[5] When these various data are compared it is apparent that there is less than complete agreement among different investigators. The data of Wright agree closely with the present results and those of Thwing and of Egan and Thwing are not too discrepant. Hood's data, however, reflect considerably more adaptation than our results at the higher sensation levels. On the other hand, Palva's data show amazingly little adaptation at high sensation levels.

In seeking some reasonable explanation for this marked disagreement we have been stuck by one

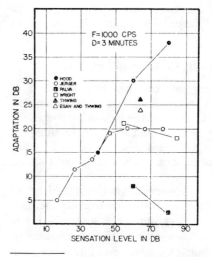

FIG. 8. Comparison of results obtained by six different investigators. All points represent adaptation for a 1000-cps tone after 3 min of sustained stimulation.

[9] J. P. Egan and E. J. Thwing, J. Acoust. Soc. Am. 27, 1225–1226 (1955).

[10] T. Palva, Laryngoscope 65, 829–847 (1955).
[11] H. N. Wright, unpublished doctoral dissertation, Northwestern University, Evanston, Illinois (1956).

salient factor, differences in experimental technique, or, more specifically, differences in the procedure used to obtain the median-plane localization. Wright's procedure was identical to our own, and it, in turn, was patterned closely after the procedure first described by Egan and later used by Thwing. This procedure has four important characteristics. First, the frequency of the tone presented to the control ear is identical to the frequency of the tone presented to the test ear. Second, the tone is on in the control ear continuously for 15 sec, then off for 45 sec. Third, the subject adjusts the intensity of the tone on the control ear by means of a 2-db step attenuator with a 60-db range. Fourth, the tester inserts an arbitrary amount of attenuation in the control channel prior to each 15-sec matching period.

The four investigators who have used this specific procedure (Jerger, Wright, Thwing, Egan, and Thwing) have obtained results in fairly good agreement with each other as shown in Fig. 8.

Hood's procedure, on the other hand, was somewhat different. The tone was presented continuously to the control ear for only 10 sec and the interval of silence between tonal presentations was only 20 sec. Furthermore, the fact that the two ears were stimulated by different audiometers would suggest that the frequencies of the tones stimulating the two ears were not identical. Finally, Hood required the subject to adjust a contin-

uously variable attenuator so as to execute a rhythmic oscillation around the point of median-plane localization. No provision was made for random variation of attenuation in the control channel. Using this procedure Hood measured considerably more adaptation than anyone else.

Palva's procedure represents still another technique. He used the 15-sec-on, 45-sec-off timing sequence, and presented identical frequencies to the two ears, but the subject's median-plane match was made by means of a Békésy-type, automatic attenuator mechanism. This method resembles Hood's more closely than that of Egan et al. but has the important difference that the subject has no direct control over his attenuator. He can only determine the direction in which it moves at constant speed. Like Hood, Palva does not report any provision for inserting random attenuation in the control channel between successive matches.

Palva's results, using this procedure, show astonishingly little adaptation, even at a sensation level of 80 db. Exactly how these procedural and instrumentation differences may be determining the discrepant results is not yet clear. It seems likely, however, that they will ultimately afford the key to this rather marked disagreement. In any event these results highlight the importance of seemingly minor procedural variables in the measurement of adaptation by the median-plane localization method.

Reprinted from the A. M. A. Archives of Otolaryngology
November 1958, Vol. 68, pp. 617-623
Copyright 1958, by American Medical Association

Clinical Observations on Excessive Threshold Adaptation

JAMES JERGER, Ph.D.; RAYMOND CARHART, Ph.D., and JOYCE LASSMAN, M.A., Evanston, Ill.

In 1955, Lierle and Reger [1] reported an unusual finding in connection with their extensive studies of threshold tracings obtained with the Békésy-type audiometer. When subjects were asked simply to trace threshold for a fixed frequency over a 20-minute period, they found that the tracings remained relatively constant in two cases of end-organ lesion, but dropped markedly in one patient with a subsequently confirmed eighth-nerve tumor. In other words, in the case of end-organ lesion, the intensity level required to maintain a threshold response did not change appreciably over the 20-minute tracing period. In the case of eighth-nerve lesion, however, the patient rapidly required more and more intensity to keep the tone at threshold. Similar results were subsequently reported by Kos. [2]

This finding is, of course, exactly opposite to the earlier observations of Dix and Hood. [3] According to these investigators, the threshold "adaptation" exemplified by the gradual decline in the threshold tracing over time characterizes and, indeed may be attributed to, certain features of cochlear as opposed to retrocochlear pathology.

In view of these seemingly conflicting reports, we think it is important to report that we have confirmed the findings of

Submitted for publication Feb. 10, 1958.

From the School of Speech and Department of Otolaryngology, Northwestern University.

This investigation was supported by research grant B-1310 from the National Institutes of Health, Public Health Service.

Lierle and Reger in two cases of acoustic neurinoma. Conversely, the threshold tracings we have obtained in presumably cochlear losses invariably fail to support the position of Dix and Hood.

We have selected, for illustrative purposes, two cases exemplifying this distinction. Figure 1a shows the preoperative audiogram of a 45-year-old white man with a unilateral loss of the sensorineural type. Speech reception threshold and discrimination of PB words were within normal limits on the right ear, but, on the left ear, the patient was unable to understand speech of any kind. Subsequent surgical intervention revealed a relatively large acoustic neurinoma in the left cerebellopontine angle, extending from the tentorium above to the

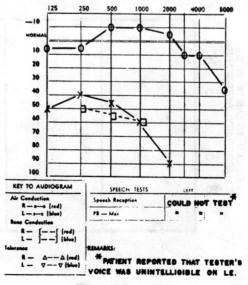

Fig. 1a.—Patient 1.

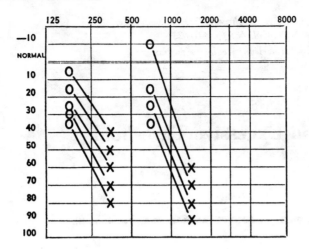

Fig. 1b.—Patient 1.

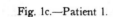

Fig. 1c.—Patient 1.

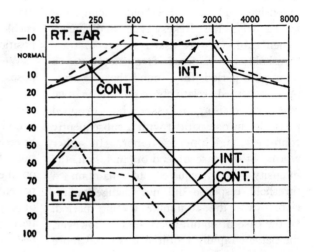

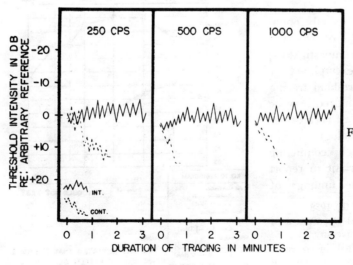

Fig. 1d.—Patient 1. Test ear: left.

foramen magnum below and extending laterally into the internal auditory meatus.

Figures 1b through 1d summarize the results of other special tests performed preoperatively. Figure 1b shows the results of alternate binaural loudness balances at 250 and 1000 cps. There is little, if any, evidence of loudness recruitment on the left ear. Figure 1c shows the hearing loss as measured with the Békésy-type audiometer (Grason-Stadler, type E-800). The solid curve represents the audiogram obtained with a pulsing stimulus which was interrupted three times per second, while the dashed curve represents the audiogram obtained with a noninterrupted, or continuous, stimulus.

On the right, or normal, ear the two kinds of tracing stimuli, continuous and interrupted, yield essentially equivalent thresholds, but on the left, or impaired, ear an interesting pattern emerges. At very low frequencies, the two thresholds overlap. At about 170 cps, however, they diverge sharply. Above this frequency, the patient requires considerably more intensity to maintain the continuous tone at threshold than to maintain the interrupted tone at threshold. At 1000 cps, the difference reaches the extreme magnitude of 40 db.

Figure 1d shows the same phenomenon in another way. Here the patient traced threshold for a tone of fixed frequency for three minutes. While he was listening to the interrupted tracing tone, the threshold remained relatively stable over the three-minute period. When the tracing tone was continuous, however, the tracings dropped rapidly, indicating that the patient required progressively more and more intensity in order to keep the continuous tone audible. Of particular interest is the rapidity and severity of this drop. At 1000 cps, for example, the tracing dropped 35 db., to the limit of the equipment, in less than 30 seconds. Even at 250 cps a drop of 35 db. occurred in less than 90 seconds.

We have observed this same pattern of results in a second case of surgically confirmed acoustic neurinoma. Again, in this case, loudness recruitment was absent on the affected ear, and, again, the patient was unable to understand any kind of speech delivered to the impaired ear.

The marked difference between the threshold tracings of continuous as opposed to interrupted stimuli observed in these two cases of acoustic neurinoma contrasts sharply with the behavior in cases of end-organ lesion. Figure 2a, for example, shows the conventional audiogram of a 34-year-old white man with a unilateral loss, clinically diagnosed as due to Ménière's disease. Figure 2b shows the result of alternate binaural loudness balances establishing the presence of loudness recruitment on the impaired right ear. Administration of a standard PB-word list by live voice at a level of 40 db. above the spondee threshold yielded a discrimination score of 54% on the right ear.

Figure 2c shows the audiogram for both interrupted and continuous stimuli as measured on the Békésy-type audiometer. Here, the two types of stimuli result in nearly identical thresholds on both the normal and the impaired ear. The continuous tone threshold drops somewhat below the interrupted tone threshold at frequencies above 1000 cps on the impaired ear, but the difference is slight in comparison with the marked disparity observed in Figure 1c.

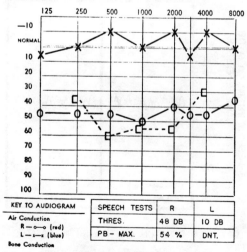

KEY TO AUDIOGRAM	SPEECH TESTS	R	L
Air Conduction	THRES.	48 DB	10 DB
R—o—o (red)	PB - MAX.	54 %	DNT.
L—x—x (blue)			
Bone Conduction			

Fig. 2a.—Patient 2.

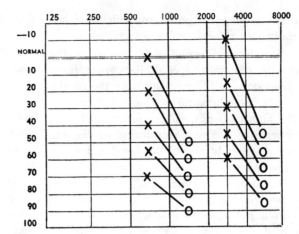

Fig. 2b.—Patient 2.

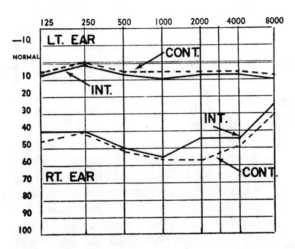

Fig. 2c.—Patient 2

Figure 2d shows three-minute threshold tracings for fixed frequencies in the patient with Ménière's disease. In contrast to Figure 1d, the continuous tone threshold remains quite stable over time. Indeed, the continuous and interrupted tracings are virtually indistinguishable.

According to our experience to date, this finding appears to be uniformly present in end-organ lesion. The threshold tracings of continuous fixed frequencies over time have all been quite stable. Figure 3, for example, summarizes tracings obtained in eight cases of sensorineural loss, in whom the clinical history, diagnosis, and presence of loudness recruitment led to the presumption that the loss was of cochlear origin. Recruitment was established by monaural, bifrequency loudness balance (Reger method) in five cases and by alternate binaural loudness balance (Fowler method) in the other three cases. The open circles in Figure 3 represent the mean interrupted-tone

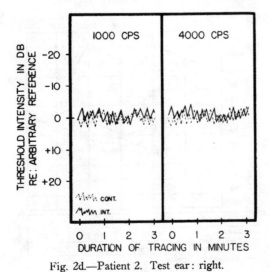

Fig. 2d.—Patient 2. Test ear: right.

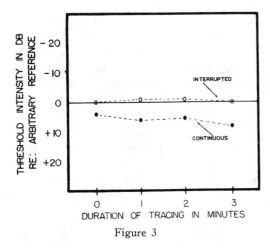

DURATION OF TRACING IN MINUTES

Figure 3

threshold tracings. Six of the eight tracings were done at 4000 cps; the remaining two at 1000 cps. Although there is an initial intensity discrepancy between the two types of thresholds of about 5 db., the mean tracing for the continuous tone drops only an additional 3 db. over a three-minute period.

We certainly do not interpret these results to mean that continuous and interrupted tone thresholds are identical in cochlear losses. The slightly poorer threshold for the continuous tone, exemplified by the fixed frequency tracings in Figure 3, appears to be fairly general at high frequencies in ears with recruitment. Our results do not deny the reality of Dix and Hood's observations in cochlear pathology, but they indicate that, under carefully controlled conditions, the magnitude of these effects is relatively slight. In contrast, when we do observe these effects in an extreme degree, we find them in cases of eighth-nerve rather than cochlear lesion.

Comment

The findings presented above are, as yet, based on an extremely limited number of observations, particularly in connection with eighth-nerve losses. In spite of this limitation, however, we believe it important to report these results because of what we feel to be their significant implications for both auditory theory and clinical practice.

The fact that confirmed cases of damage to the eighth nerve have exhibited extreme adaptation challenges one to speculate regarding the underlying mechanism. This speculation must be tentative, but it is worthy of mention because of its unique implications, provided subsequent observation and analysis confirm it.

In this connection, consider the details of these phenomena as they were manifested by the patient whose responses are summarized in Figures 1a through 1d. The following facts are the pertinent ones.

First, surgery performed subsequent to these tests revealed a large tumor in the left cerebellopontine angle. This tumor extended into the internal auditory meatus. Thus, the site of major pathology was along the trunk of the eighth nerve.

Second, the lesion had induced sufficient destruction of auditory function so that a substantial hearing loss was encountered, irrespective of the manner of testing. Presumably, some destruction of neural elements (and possible secondary degeneration of associated cochlear structures) had taken place.

Third, the lesion had not eliminated auditory responses entirely. Some neural units were still excitable, and the function of the organ of Corti was sufficiently normal to activate them.

Fourth, the lesion had induced an abnormality of such nature that somewhere within the sensorineural system sustained response could not be maintained. Thus, if either a continuous stimulus of fixed frequency or one of varying frequency was employed, the ability to respond at threshold deteriorated appreciably. Conversely, periodic interruption of the threshold-tracing stimulus eliminated any manifestation of excessive adaptation. For example, a continuous tone of 1000 cps (Fig. 1d) completely obliterated the patient's auditory response within half a minute after onset. However, no change in threshold intensity was evident throughout a full three minutes when the stimulus was interrupted three times per second.

Fifth, and this fact is particularly critical, the statements just made regarding hyper-adaptation under continuous stimulation are not applicable for frequencies below about 170 cps. As mentioned earlier, and as schematically shown in Figure 1c, the Békésy tracings for the interrupted and the continuous tones are indistinguishable below this frequency. In contrast, sharp adaptation to continuous stimulation is evident by the time the frequency has reached 250 cps.

The full implication of these results becomes apparent when one recalls that the volley phenomenon characterizes neural response at low frequencies [5,6]; that is, the neural units responding to the cochlear microphonics tend to be activated once for every cycle in the stimulus. The consequence is that a 250-cycle tone, for example, initiates twice as many volleys as a 125-cycle tone. It likewise gives the neural units only half as long to recover between excitations.

This difference is not critical in a normal auditory system, where the absolute refractory period is probably as brief as about one millisecond and where sustained responses at rates between 250 and 450 impulses per second may be inferred from observations made on animal preparations.[8] However, this difference seemed to be critical in the case we are discussing. One is encouraged to propose the hypothesis that here continuous stimulation at 250 cps induces prolongation of the refractory periods of those neurons activated by the stimulus. Under such circumstances of delayed recovery, too rapid a train of sound waves, appropriately transformed to a pattern of cochlear microphonics, might maintain desensitization of the individual neurons. It could be that this desensitization is highly localized and is limited to the site, along the eighth nerve, where the tumor is found. Again, it might be a more diffuse disturbance in function resulting from a more generalized disruption in the physiology of the neurons involved. In either event, the end-result would be inhibition of responses.

A sufficiently leisurely train of waves, i. e.. 125 cps, could allow enough recovery of function for transmission of the signal. The same could be true when short intervals of rest are allowed, as occurs when the stimulus is interrupted in the manner previously described. Thus, we may have here a practical example, in aural pathology, of the all-or-none law of neural behavior: namely, essentially unchanged response, insofar as one can judge from the end-result, until the condition is reached where transmission of impulses is obliterated.

At the clinical level, we urge that threshold tracings for continuous tones of fixed frequency over time be obtained in all cases of suspected eighth-nerve lesion, because we believe that this may ultimately be one of the few, or perhaps, the only auditory symptom that can reliably differentiate cochlear from eighth-nerve lesion. Goodman,[9] for example, has recently demonstrated, rather convincingly, that neither loudness recruitment nor speech discrimination can serve as an infallible differentiating sign. In his series of 18 cases with confirmed retrocochlear lesion, recruitment ranged from complete absence to complete presence, and discrimination loss ranged from none to total.

Such findings are discouraging to the clinician. They emphasize the urgent need for a full-scale frontal assault on the important problem of discovering a set of auditory symptoms unique to eighth-nerve lesions. Our purpose in presenting the above results is to suggest that response to sustained stimulation over time may hold promise as a fruitful avenue of attack.

Audiology Laboratory, Northwestern University.

REFERENCES

1. Lierle, D. M., and Reger, S. N.: Experimentally Induced Temporary Threshold Shifts in Ears with Impaired Hearing, Ann. Otol. Rhin. & Laryng. 64:263-277 (March) 1955.

2. Kos, C. M.: Auditory Function as Related to the Complaint of Dizziness, Laryngoscope 65: 711-721 (Aug.) 1955.

3. Dix, M. R., and Hood, J. D.: Modern Developments in Pure Tone Audiometry and Their Application to the Clinical Diagnosis of End-Organ Deafness, Proc. Roy. Soc. Med. 46:992-994 (Dec.) 1953.

4. Wever, E. G.: Theory of Hearing, New York, John Wiley & Sons, Inc., 1949, pp. 257-267.

5. Wever,[4] p. 166.

6. Davis, H.: Biophysics and Physiology of the Inner Ear, Physiol. Rev. 37:1-49, 1957.

7. Wever,[4] pp. 158-159.

8. Galambos, R., and Davis, H.: Response of Single Auditory Nerve Fibers to Acoustic Stimulation, J. Neurophysiol. 6:39-57, 1943.

9. Goodman, A.: Some Relations Between Auditory Function and Intracranial Lesions with Particular Reference to Lesions of the Cerebellopontine Angle, Laryngoscope 67:987-1010 (Oct.) 1957.

Reprinted from the A. M. A. Archives of Otolaryngology
February 1959, Vol. 69, pp. 200-211
Copyright 1959, by American Medical Association

On the Detection of Extremely Small Changes in Sound Intensity

JAMES JERGER, Ph.D.; JOYCE LASSMAN SHEDD, M.A., and EARL HARFORD, M.S., Evanston, Ill.

A number of investigators [1-19] have recently reported that certain kinds of hearing loss are apparently accompanied by unusually keen differential sensitivity to intensity. Their studies indicated that, in hearing loss due to cochlear lesion, the patient was able to discriminate smaller intensity changes than a listener with normal hearing. Furthermore, many of these investigators made the assumption that the apparent reduction of the intensity difference limen was due to the presence of loudness recruitment in the affected ear. On the basis of this assumed causal relationship, it was proposed that the measurement of the intensity difference limen afforded an indirect test for the presence of loudness recruitment. A normal-sized difference limen was thought to imply the absence of recruitment, while an abnormally small difference limen was interpreted to indicate the presence of recruitment.

Some investigators have failed to confirm these observations. Studies by Liden and Nilsson [20] and Lund-Iversen [21] suggested that the intensity difference limen was not effective in differentiating among types of hearing impairment. More recently, the well-controlled study of Hirsh, Palva, and Goodman [22] attacked both the empirical and the theoretical framework underlying the clinical utilization of the intensity difference

Submitted for publication May 15, 1958.

This study was supported by funds provided under Contract AF 18(600)-630 with the U. S. Air Force School of Aviation Medicine, Randolph Field, Texas.

limen as an indirect test of loudness recruitment.

These authors demonstrated that differential intensity sensitivity failed to distinguish patients with recruitment from patients without recruitment, or from persons with normal hearing. They went on to point out the logical fallacy inherent in the notion that the difference limen will be reduced as a consequence of an abnormally steep loudness function (recruitment) by noting that this belief rests on the now-disproved assumption that all difference limina are subjectively equal.

As a result of these conflicting reports some confusion exists relative to the clinical value of the various tests designed to assess differential intensity sensitivity.

It is our belief that much of this confusion can be clarified by the recognition of two fundamental considerations. First, it is important to distinguish carefully between the *observation* that some patients seem to be able to hear remarkably small changes in sound intensity, and the *theory* that there necessarily exists a unique relationship between the size of the intensity difference limen and the slope of the loudness function.

In other words, recognizing, with Hirsh et al., the theoretical argument that the presence of loudness recruitment does not necessarily imply a reduction in the difference limen need not materially affect the situation. The fact that early attempts to explain the observations of abnormally acute differential sensitivity in terms of the loudness recruitment phenomenon were obviously naïve does not alter the significance of the observation that certain patients (generally those with loudness recruitment) are often able to detect smaller intensity changes than normal ears at comparable levels above threshold.

The apparent correlation between loudness recruitment and abnormally keen differential intensity sensitivity is subject to many interpretations. It may be entirely fortuitous and coincidental; it may be due to an inherent relationship between the two phenomena of which we are yet only dimly aware, or, as one of us [23] has previously suggested, both phenomena may derive from some more basic parent disorder. While a final answer to this problem would be of extreme interest from the viewpoint of auditory theory, the question is largely irrelevant from the viewpoint of auditory diagnostic tests. For the present, the important question is whether the patient's ability to discriminate small changes in sound intensity is related either to site of lesion within the auditory mechanism or to any kind of meaningful pattern of diagnostic categories, not whether the measurement of differential sensitivity provides an indirect test for the presence of loudness recruitment.

A second important consideration to be borne in mind is that the observation of what looks like abnormally acute sensitivity to small changes in sound intensity may have very little to do with the difference limen for intensity in the classically defined sense. Stated differently, we may be dealing with a disorder or function which merely simulates an abnormally small difference limen, and then only under certain conditions. In view of the multiplicity of variables known to affect the conventional measurement of the difference limen in normal ears, it seems conceivable that any one of a number of changes in the functional state of the ear could bias the measurement in a particular direction in some methodologies but not in others. For example, it may be that behavior simulating abnormally acute differential sensitivity will arise only through the use of a test methodology involving relatively sustained stimulation. At the same time, the patient's intensity difference limen might be entirely normal when defined by a methodology not involving sustained stimulation (e. g., the method of constant stimulus differences).

This consideration implies that the *exact methodology* employed to assess differential sensitivity may be of more critical importance than has been heretofore assumed. In our opinion, it is highly possible, and not in the least heretical, to suppose that patients with cochlear lesion will manifest behavior simulating abnormally keen differential sensitivity only when the measurement is performed in a particular and unique manner.

With the above considerations as a frame of reference, we undertook, late in the fall of 1956, the development of a new methodology for the clinical assessment of differential intensity sensitivity. The purpose of the present report is twofold: first, to describe this new methodology; second, to present typical findings obtained through its application to patients with various types of hearing loss.

Rationale for New Methodology

The fundamental principle guiding the development of the new technique was our belief that the key to a successful method in this area lay in the use of relatively sustained rather than interrupted stimulation of the test ear.

Within this context of sustained stimulation an attempt was made to devise a method that would overcome the limitations of previous techniques. These limitations are well known to all who have attempted to measure the intensity difference limen in clinical patients. They appear to derive from two primary sources: first, extreme variability in the responses of the same patient from trial to trial; second, lack of reliability among different testers of the same patient. It is our belief that a substantial portion of these difficulties may be traced to one factor, the temporal pattern of the test stimulus.

In the DL tests originally proposed by Lüscher and Zwislocki [11-14] and Jerger,[8,9] the test stimulus was a continuous, fixed frequency tone, amplitude modulated at 50% duty cycle, at the rate of 2-3 cps. To the listener, this temporal pattern takes the form of a "wobbling" or "beating" sound, and the clinical task is to determine the degree of amplitude modulation necessary to produce the "beating" attribute in the auditory sensation. It seems likely that this aspect of the test situation poses a serious limitation for two reasons: first, determining when a tone is just perceptibly "beating" is an extremely difficult judgment even for the most sophisticated listener; second, the inclusion of this kind of judgment in a clinical test inevitably results in a response measure susceptible to the subjective interpretation of the tester.

The task of designing a new procedure was therefore approached with two goals in mind: first, to employ a stimulus whose temporal pattern would not require a "beating" judgment; second, to make the test procedure as objective as possible by limiting the number of decisions required of the tester.

To meet these goals, the basic temporal pattern used in the quantal psychophysical method [24] was adopted. In this method, short amplitude increments are superimposed on a signal of constant amplitude at relatively widely spaced intervals. The patient's task is to respond whenever he hears a momentary change in the loudness of the steady signal. The tester's task is merely to record the presence or absence of a response to the presentation of each increment. The method is thus characterized by (1) the use of relatively sustained stimulation over time; (2) a simplification of the patient's task by complete avoidance of a "beating" judgment, and (3) simplification and objectification of the tester's role in the procedure.

Apparatus

In the present test sequence an increment occurred once every five seconds. Each increment rose to maximum amplitude in 50 msec., remained at maximum amplitude for 200 msec., then decayed to the steady-state level in 50 msec. The size of each such amplitude increment was exactly 1 db.

Figure 1 shows a simplified block diagram of the apparatus originally used to produce this signal. The output from an audio-oscillator was split into two channels. In the lower channel, the signal passed through a fixed attenuator and a manual switch to a mixing network. In the upper channel, the signal passed through an electronic switch (Grason-Stadler, Type 829-S), through a variable attenuator, then to the mixing network, where it was combined with the signal from the lower channel. The combined output from the mixing network passed through a second variable attenuator to an impedance-matching transformer, then to an earphone (Permoflux, Type PDR-10) mounted in an MX41/AR cushion.

With the switch in the lower channel closed, the signal at the earphone consisted of the steady-state tone from the lower channel and the superimposed increments periodically added to the steady-state level by the electronic switch. An interval timer triggered the switch so that it passed the signal for 300 msec. (50 msec. rise-decay time, 200 msec. at maximum amplitude) once every five seconds. The variable attenuator (A_1) in the upper channel controlled the amplitude of the increment, while the variable attenuator beyond the mixing network (A_2) controlled the level of the composite signal. This apparatus was used until August, 1957. Since that time a modified commercial audiometer has been employed for all measurements.

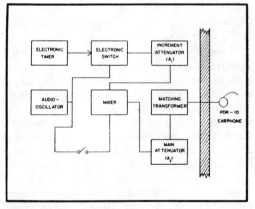

Fig. 1.—Simplified block diagram of experimental apparatus.

The initial design of the procedure was guided by the desire to construct a task so difficult that subjects with normal differential intensity sensitivity could not perform it with any degree of success. To this end, an increment magnitude of 1 db. and a presentation level 10 db. above the subject's threshold were initially chosen. Subsequent experience suggested, however, that 10 db. may have been unnecessarily low. Even at levels of 30 to 40 db., the task is sufficiently difficult, and the extreme faintness of the 10 db. tone makes the procedure somewhat frustrating for patients with a conductive loss. In view of these considerations, a sensation level of 20 db. was later adopted. The difference between results obtained at the two levels was found to be minimal. Accordingly, in the remainder of this paper, no distinction is made between results obtained at the two levels.

Test Procedure

Instructions to each patient were as follows:

"You will hear a steady sound in your ear for about two minutes. The sound will be very faint. During the time it is on you may occasionally hear a little jump in loudness. Whenever you are quite sure that you have heard one of these short loudness jumps, press the button which you have in your hand. If you *think* you heard a jump but you are not certain, then do not press the button. Only press it when you are *sure* you heard a jump in loudness."

When the patient indicated that he clearly understood these instructions, the tester adjusted the composite signal to the desired level above the patient's threshold, adjusted the increment to the desired magnitude, and turned on the signal in the patient's earphone.

A complete test run involved the presentation of 28 increments. The first five increments were each 5 db. in magnitude and served only to familiarize the patient with the task by presenting increments that could easily be heard. After this initial practice period the magnitude of the increments was reduced to 1 db., and the actual test run, consisting of the presentation of 20 one-decibel increments, commenced. In order to guard against the possibility of either false-negative or false-positive responses, three additional increment presentations were interspersed with the 20 test increments as follows. After five 1-db. increments had been presented and responses scored, the sixth increment was altered according to these rules:

1. If the subject had responded to two or less of the five increments, the sixth increment was set to 5 db.

2. If the subject had responded to three or more of the five increments, the sixth was set to 0 db.

This procedure was continued throughout the test run, i. e., after the 5th, 10th, and 15th 1-db. increments, the next increment was either increased to 5 db. or removed entirely. In other words, if the patient was not responding to the majority of 1-db. increments, a relatively large 5-db. increment was periodically introduced in order to keep his attention mobilized and to be sure that he continued to understand the test instructions.

If, on the other hand, the patient was responding to a majority of the 1-db. increments, an increment was occasionally removed in order to be sure that his responses were to the increments and not to the rhythmic five-second sequence. Responses to these three "catch" items were not included in the final score. The sensitivity index was computed solely from responses to the 20 one-decibel increments.

Method of Reporting Results

All results have been expressed in terms of the percentage of 1-db. increments to which a correct response was made. The resultant score is termed a "short-increment sensitivity index" (SISI). Thus, a patient who responded to 10 of the 20 increments received a SISI score of 50%, etc.

A convenient method for charting test results is to plot, graphically, the SISI score in per cent versus frequency, using the conventional symbols, "O" for the right ear and "X" for the left ear. It is useful to represent frequency on the abscissa and SISI on the ordinate. The resultant graphic representation is called a "SISI-gram." Examples are shown in Figures 2 through 7 of the present paper. The shaded area between 0 and 10% represents the approximate range of scores to be expected in normal ears.

Results

Administration of SISI to a wide variety of hearing-impaired subjects has revealed interesting patterns of response. In general, purely conductive losses yield very low scores, while losses presumed to be localized in the sensory structure of the inner ear

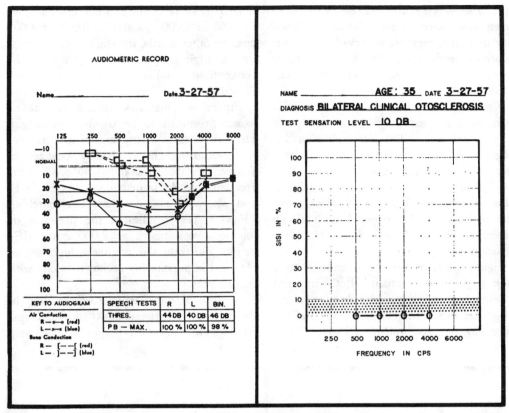

Fig. 2.—Audiogram and SISI-gram of patient with early otosclerosis.

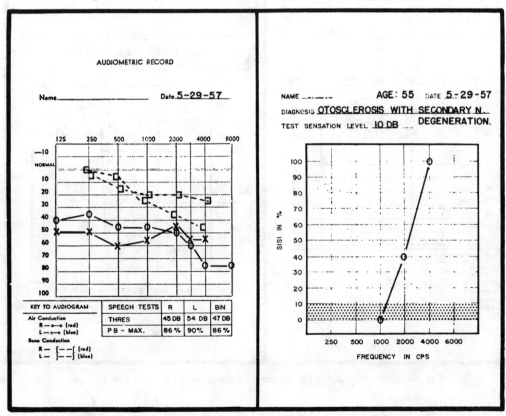

Fig. 3.—Audiogram and SISI-gram of patient with otosclerosis accompanied by secondary sensorineural loss.

tend to show very high scores. Values between these extremes are infrequent. When they do occur, they are observed most commonly in presbycusis. The following cases illustrate these generalizations more concretely.

Figure 2 shows the audiogram and SISI-gram of a 35-year-old white woman with early otosclerosis. The air-conduction audiogram shows the stiffness tilt characteristic of otosclerosis, the bone curves show the "Carhart notch" at 2,000 cps, and discrimination for PB words is unimpaired. The patient did not respond to a single increment at any of the four test frequencies.

Figure 3 illustrates typical findings in a later stage of otosclerosis. Both air- and bone-conduction thresholds show a slight fall-off at high frequencies, and the PB score shows a discrimination loss of 14%.

The SISI score is low at 1,000 cps but rises to 40% at 2,000 cps and to 100% at 4,000 cps. In other words, the slight sensorineural loss at high frequencies, suggested by the conventional audiometric findings, is reflected in the SISI-gram.

Figure 4 illustrates results typical of losses presumed to be cochlear in origin. Here the loss in acuity is due to excessive noise exposure and is sharply localized to frequencies about 3,000 cps. Monaural bi-frequency loudness matching (Reger Test) and alternate binaural loudness matching (Fowler Test) indicated the presence of loudness recruitment at 4,000 cps. SISI results illustrate the relatively high scores obtained in presumably cochlear lesions with recruitment.

Because of the sharpness of the drop in the half octave between 3,000 and 4,000 cps, SISI performance was explored at closely

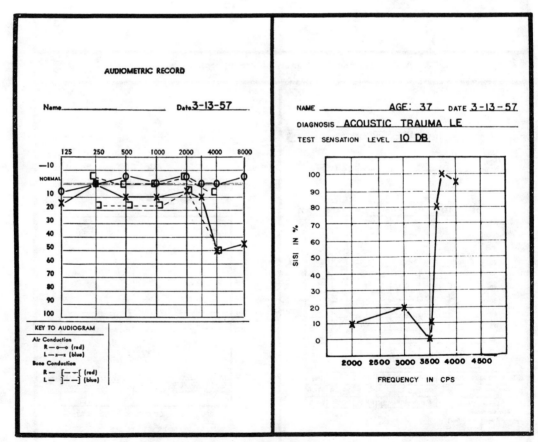

Fig. 4.—Audiogram and SISI scores of patient with noise-induced loss.

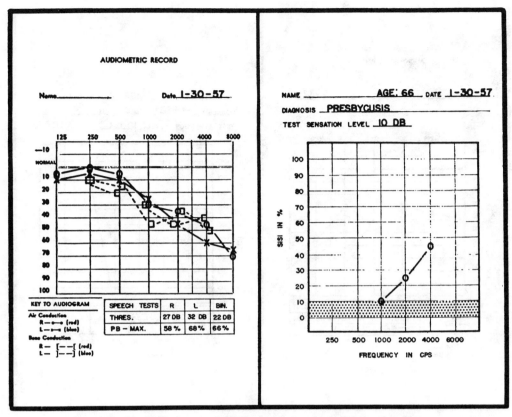

Fig. 5.—Audiogram and SISI-gram of patient with presbycusis.

spaced frequencies in this region. Note that scores are quite low out to 3,550 cps. Within the next 50 cycles, however, the score increases to 80%. Finding it difficult to accept such evidence of radically different functioning within a span of only 50 cycles, we repeated the test at each frequency and obtained virtually identical results, with a maximum variation of only 5%. This evidence of a sharp change in the SISI score within a relatively narrow span of frequencies has been observed in several subsequent cases of noise-induced loss. The break seems to occur at a frequency somewhat above the point at which the audiometric curve levels off after its descent. This would appear to be a finding worthy of further exploration in other types of loss.

Figures 5 and 6 typify findings in presbycusis. In Figure 5 the SISI score increases gradually from 1,000 to 4,000 cps, but never exceeds 45%. In Figure 6, on the other hand, the score jumps from only 10% at 2,000 cps to 90% at 4,000 cps. Presbycusis appears to be a clinical entity in which the SISI score is quite unpredictable. It is invariably low at frequencies below 1,000 cps. Above 1,000 cps, however, three distinct patterns may emerge. The SISI score may continue to be relatively low at all frequencies; it may rise gradually to an intermediate value of about 40%-50%, as illustrated in Figure 5, or it may rise sharply to a high level (90%-100%), as illustrated in Figure 6.

Figure 7 summarizes findings in a case of presbycusis with a superimposed labyrinthine hydrops on the right ear. SISI scores on the left ear are similar to those in Figure 5. On the right, or hydrops, ear, however, performance is totally different. Here, SISI scores are relatively high, even at very low frequencies.

It is worth while to pause and reflect, momentarily, on these last findings. Note that when the right, or hydrops, ear was

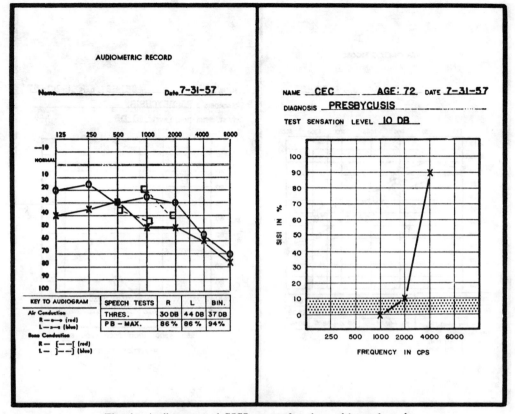

Fig. 6.—Audiogram and SISI-gram of patient with presbycusis.

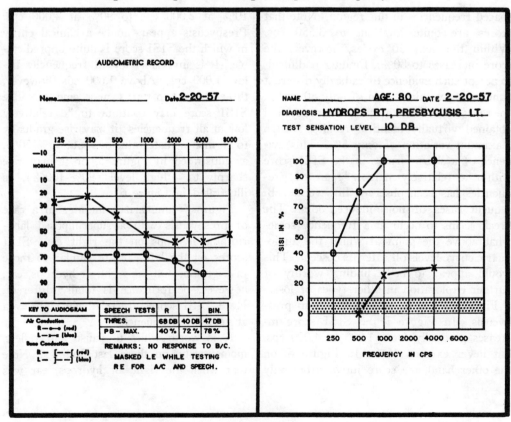

Fig. 7.—Audiogram and SISI-gram of patient with presbycusis and superimposed unilateral labyrinthine hydrops on right ear.

TABLE 1.—*Summary of SISI Results at 1,000 and 4,0000 cps in Seventy-Five Patients with Various Types of Hearing Loss*

Type of Loss	No.	Range of Hearing Loss at 1,000 Cps, Db.	Range of Hearing Loss at 4,000 Cps, Db.	Range of SISI Scores at 1,000 Cps, %	Range of SISI Scores at 4,000 Cps %
Conductive	21	5–60	15–60	0–15	0–15
Noise-induced (acoustic trauma)	9	(–10)–0	30–70	0–40	95–100
Ménière's	8	50–70	45–80	70–100	95–100
Presbycusis	34	0–65	30–75	0–100	0–100
Retrocochlear	3	(–5)–85	45–70	0	0%

tested at 1,000 cps, this patient, *a woman of 80*, was able to hear, unfailingly, a *1-db.* increment superimposed on a tone only 10 db. above her absolute threshold. The reader who has had some experience with signals of this nature will readily appreciate that 1-db. increments are not easily heard under any circumstances.

Such findings cannot be ignored. They imply that, for a reason or reasons presently unknown, certain types of hearing loss render the patient able to hear remarkably small changes in sound intensity, relative to the differential intensity sensitivity of normal listeners at equivalent sensation levels.

A number of generalizations are suggested by the above case reports. Table 1 summarizes SISI findings in 75 patients with various types of hearing loss. These 75 patients were selected from a larger pool on whom SISI scores were available, because they fitted clearly into reasonably well-defined clinical categories of loss. Patients were assigned to the pure conductive, noise-induced, Ménière, and presbycusis categories on the basis of medical diagnosis by members of the staff of the Department of Otolaryngology, Northwestern University Medical School. The three patients in the retrocochlear category were so assigned on the basis of surgical findings by members of the Staff of the Department of Neurology and Psychiatry, Northwestern University Medical School and of the Chicago Wesley Memorial Hospital. Two were cases of surgically confirmed acoustic neurinoma, and the third was a case of a surgically confirmed, relatively large space-occupying lesion of the left temporal lobe.

Inspection of Table 1 suggests several tentative conclusions. First, conductive losses found the SISI task extremely difficult. None of the 21 conductives tested achieved a SISI score higher than 15% at any test frequency.

Noise-induced losses behaved quite differently. At 1,000 cps, where hearing was still within normal limits, no subject did better than 40%. At 4,000 cps, however, in the region of the loss, the *lowest* score obtained was 75%, and the modal value was very close to 100%.

Patients with Ménière's disease demonstrated astonishing facility with the task. Again, the *lowest* score obtained by a patient in this group was 70%, and this was actually quite low for the group as a whole. The modal value was very close to 100%.

In presbycusis, any level of performance may be expected. In general, there is a tendency for the SISI score to increase with frequency, but scores may range from 0 to 100% at both 1,000 and 4,000 cps. Some patients heard none of the increments at either 1,000 or 4,000 cps; others quite effortlessly responded to all of them at either frequency.

Those with retrocochlear losses did even less well than conductives. None of the three patients in this group responded to any increment at any frequency.

Reliability

Figure 8 summarizes SISI scores obtained on a single patient on eight different occasions over a period of 10 months. The loss is primarily conductive due to a chronic otitis media, accompanied by some second-

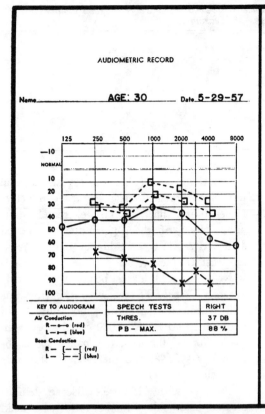

AUDIOMETRIC RECORD

Name _____ AGE: 30 _____ Date 5-29-57

KEY TO AUDIOGRAM

Air Conduction
R—o—o (red)
L—x—x (blue)

Bone Conduction
R— [——[(red)
L—]——] (blue)

SPEECH TESTS	RIGHT
THRES.	37 DB
P B – MAX.	88 %

SUMMARY OF SISI SCORES ON ONE PATIENT WITH A MIXED-TYPE HEARING LOSS

TEST DATE	TESTER	SISI SCORE	
		1000 CPS	4000 CPS
2-6-57	E R H	5 %	80 %
2-13-57	E R H	0 %	65 %
2-20-57	E R H	0 %	85 %
3-6-57	JFJ	0 %	95 %
4-17-57	E R H	0 %	80 %
4-24-57	E R H	0 %	75 %
7-10-57	E R H	0 %	95 %
12-4-57	JFL	0 %	80 %

TEST EAR: RIGHT

DIAGNOSIS: OTITIS MEDIA WITH SECONDARY NERVE DEGENERATION.

Fig. 8.—Audiogram and repeated SISI scores on a patient with chronic otitis media accompanied by secondary sensorineural involvement.

ary sensorineural loss at high frequencies. SISI scores were obtained at two frequencies, 1,000 and 4,000 cps on the right ear, by three different testers. At 1,000 cps, where the loss was purely conductive, scores ranged from 0% to 5% on eight separate tests. At 4,000 cps, where some secondary cochlear involvement was apparently present, the eight separate scores ranged from 65% to 95%. These findings typify the test-retest stability characterizing the SISI procedure.

Another aspect of test reliability is the extent to which performance on the first half of the test agrees with performance on the second half. In order to evaluate this "split-half" reliability of the total test sequence, product-moment correlation coefficients were computed between the number of responses to the first 10 increments and the number of responses to the second 10 increments of the total 20-increment sequence. This analysis was based on a total of 129 available SISI-grams. Table 2 shows the correlation coefficients thus obtained at each of three frequencies, 250, 1,000, and 4,000 cps, corrected according to the Spearman-Brown prophecy formula.

While the correlation is relatively weak (0.72) at 250 cps, it appears to be reasonably satisfactory at 1,000 cps (0.95) and at 4,000 cps (0.96). The correlations suggest that the total 20-item test sequence has relatively good internal consistency.

TABLE 2.—*Split-Half Reliability Correlation Coefficients for SISI Scores at Three Frequencies*

	Frequency in Cps		
	250	1,000	4,000
No.	46	125	129
R	0.72	0.95	0.96

Comment

In view of Dix, Hallpike, and Hood's [25,26] recommendation that continuous stimulation should be avoided in testing patients with inner-ear lesions, many investigators may question the feasibility of sustaining a tone over the two-minute period required to present 20 increments. It should be emphasized, therefore, that we have found this to be no problem whatever. There is no evidence, in the present data, that discrimination becomes progressively worse over time. Indeed, when patients failed to achieve 100% scores, analysis invariably revealed approximately equivalent performance in the two halves of the test series. We are inclined to believe that the success of the method is, in fact, closely related to the use of sustained stimulation, and suggest this as a fruitful avenue for further research.

Finally, it should be emphasized that the purpose of this paper is not to propose final answers to the problem of an adequate methodology for the clinical assessment of differential intensity sensitivity. Our sole intent is to report findings with a particular technique that we have found to be simple, easily administered, and otherwise clinically feasible, and which seems to distinguish reasonably well certain types of hearing loss.

Summary

A unique method for the clinical assessment of differential intensity discrimination is described. Short (200 msec.) 1-db. intensity increments are superimposed, at five-second intervals, on a pure tone of constant amplitude at a sensation level of 20 db. The patient responds to the momentary changes in loudness. The procedure is called SISI (short increment sensitivity index), and results are expressed in terms of the percentage of 20 increments to which a response is made.

Findings on selected individual cases are reported in order to illustrate the manner in which the SISI score varies with different kinds of hearing loss.

Results obtained in 75 patients with various types of hearing loss are reviewed. Conductive and retrocochlear losses showed very low SISI scores, never exceeding 15%. Ménière and noise-induced losses, on the other hand, yielded relatively high percentages, the lowest score obtained in any of these patients being 70%.

The School of Speech, Northwestern University.

REFERENCES

1. Bangs, J. L., and Mullins, C. J.: Recruitment Testing in Hearing and Its Implications, A. M. A. Arch. Otolaryng. 58:582-592, 1953.

2. von Békésy, G.: A New Audiometer, Acta Oto-Laryng. 35:411-422, 1947.

3. Denes, P., and Naunton, R. F.: Methods of Audiometry in a Modern Deafness Clinic, J. Laryng. & Otol. 63:251-274, 1949.

4. Denes, P., and Naunton, R. F.: The Clinical Detection of Auditory Recruitment, J. Laryng. & Otol. 64:375-398, 1950.

5. Doerfler, L. G.: Differential Sensitivity to Intensity in the Perceptively Deafened Ear, unpublished Ph.D. Dissertation, Northwestern University, 1948.

6. Halm, T.: Determination of the Difference Limen and the Latest Illustration Thereof in Audiometry, J. Laryng. & Otol. 63:464-466, 1949.

7. Harris, J. D.: A Brief Critical Review of Loudness Recruitment, Psychol. Bull. 50:190-203, 1953.

8. Jerger, J. F.: A Difference Limen Recruitment Test and Its Diagnostic Significance, Laryngoscope 62:1316-1332, 1952.

9. Jerger, J. F.: DL Difference Test, A. M. A. Arch. Otolaryng. 57:490-500, 1953.

10. Lundborg, T.: Differentiation of Hearing Impairments of Neurogenic Origin, Nord. Med. 49:714-717, 1953.

11. Lüscher, E., and Zwislocki, J.: A Simple Method of Monaural Determination of the Recruitment Phenomenon, Pract. oto-rhino-laryng. 10:521-522, 1948.

12. Lüscher, E., and Ermanni, A.: The Topical Diagnostic Significance of the Difference Limen of Sound Intensity Changes (Results of an Examination of 71 Hard of Hearing Patients), Arch. Ohren-, Nasen- u. Kehlkopfk. 157:158-216, 1950.

13. Lüscher, E.: Our Determination of the Difference Limen for Intensity Modulation of Pure Tones, Its Validity, and Its Topo-Diagnostic Efficiency, Acta oto-laryng. 45:402-415, 1955.

14. Lüscher, E., and Zwislocki, J.: Comparison of the Various Methods Employed in the Determination of the Recruitment Phenomenon, J. Laryng. & Otol. 65:187-195, 1951.

15. Lüscher, E.: The Difference Limen of Intensity Variations of Pure Tones and Its Diag-

nostic Significance, J. Laryng. & Otol. 65:486-510, 1951.

16. Miskolczy-Fodor, F., and Hajts, G.: Behavior of the Difference Limen in Otosclerosis, Magy. sebészet 3:84-90, 1950.

17. Neuberger, F.: Investigations on the Qualitative Parallelism Between Difference Limen and the Recruitment Phenomenon, Monatsschr. Ohrenh. 84:169-182, 1950.

18. Pirodda, E.: Intensity Discrimination Threshold in Bone Conduction, Oto-rino-laryng. ital. 19: 152-158, 1950.

19. Rosenberg, P. E. The Influence of Stimulus Duration upon Differential Intensity Sensitivity in Normal and Impaired Ears, unpublished Ph.D. Dissertation, Northwestern University, 1956.

20. Liden, G., and Nilsson, G.: Differential Audiometry, Acta oto-laryng. 38:521-527, 1950.

21. Lund-Iversen, L.: An Investigation on the Difference Limen Determined by the Method of Lüscher-Zwislocki in Normal Hearing and in Various Forms of Deafness, Acta oto-laryng. 42: 219, 1952.

22. Hirsh, I. J.; Palva, T., and Goodman, A.: Difference Limen and Recruitment, A. M. A. Arch. Otolaryng. 60:525-540, 1954.

23. Jerger, J. F.: Differential Intensity Sensitivity in the Ear with Loudness Recruitment, J. Speech & Hearing Disorders 20:183-191, 1955.

24. Stevens, S. S.; Morgan, C. T., and Volkmann, J.: Theory of the Neural Quantum in the Discrimination of Loudness and Pitch, Am. J. Psychol. 54: 315-335, 1941.

25. Hallpike, C. S., and Hood, J. D.: Some Recent Work on Auditory Adaptation and Its Relationship to the Loudness Recruitment Phenomenon, J. Acoust. Soc. America 23:270-274, 1951.

26. Dix, M. R., and Hood, J. D.: Modern Developments in Pure Tone Audiometry and Their Application to the Clinical Diagnosis of End Organ Deafness, J. Laryng. & Otol. 67:343-357, 1953.

Reprinted from the A. M. A. Archives of Otolaryngology
May 1960, Vol. 71, pp. 797-806
Copyright 1960, by American Medical Association

Observations on Auditory Behavior in Lesions of the Central Auditory Pathways

JAMES F. JERGER, Ph.D., Evanston, Ill.

In contrast to the extensive and systematic cortical ablation studies in animals, comparatively little is known about the effects on auditory responses of either cortical or subcortical lesions in the human auditory system.

In addition to the obvious problem of a meager supply of clinical material, the primary obstacle to experimental study in this area has, in large measure, been the extreme subtlety of the effects produced by lesions in the higher auditory pathways. They are not readily apparent in conventional audiometric tests lke the pure-tone audiogram or the conventional speech discrimination score at a substantial suprathreshold level.

Indeed, it is the thesis of the present paper that these effects can only be demonstrated by means of tasks placing relatively heavy demands on the auditory system. In Schuknecht's words,

> The auditory manifestations in patients with temporal lobe lesions, acoustic neurinoma and presbycusis, suggest that lesions involving the auditory pathways result in a system that transmits simple signals of threshold magnitude (such as pure tones) but cannot handle the complex signals of speech.[1]

Basic work in this area was pioneered by E. Bocca and his associates [2-4] at the University of Milan. These investigators explored auditory behavior in patients with intracranial tumors in the region of the

Submitted for publication June 29, 1959.

From the School of Speech and Department of Otolaryngology, Northwestern University.

This investigation was supported under Research Grant B-1310(Cl) from the National Institutes of Health, U.S. Public Health Service.

temporal lobe by means of specially devised distorted speech tests. In one of these techniques, word lists of Italian logatomes were presented under three separate conditions, namely, monaurally through a low-pass filter, monaurally unfiltered but at a relatively low intensity, and binaurally with the low-pass-filtered signal presented to one ear and the unfiltered but faint signal to the other ear.

With use of this technique, Bocca and his associates observed that patients with temporal lobe tumors manifested abnormal auditory behavior in two distinct ways. First, the discrimination score for low-pass-filtered speech was considerably poorer on the ear contralateral than on the ear ipsilateral to the affected hemisphere. Second, when speech was simultaneously presented to both ears, low-pass-filtered to one and at a very low level to the other, the discrimination score was still abnormally low, particularly when the faint unfiltered signal was delivered to the ear contralateral to the affected hemisphere. They interpreted these results to indicate that unilateral lesions of the temporal cortex impair the integrating and synthesizing functions of the central auditory system.

Analogous findings were reported by Goldstein, Goodman, and King.[5] In six cases of infantile hemiplegia, tested both before and after hemispherectomy, discrimination scores for monosyllabic test words, delivered at a level 70 db. above the spondee threshold, were an average of 25% poorer on the ear contralateral to the affected hemisphere than on the ear contralateral to the unaffected hemisphere.

Further study of simultaneous binaural stimulation has been made by Matzker and Ruckes,[6] utilizing low-pass-filtered speech to one ear and high-pass-filtered speech to the other ear. They reported a significant reduction in speech discrimination, under these circumstances, in patients with brain-stem lesions.

More recently, Sanchez Longo, Forster, and Auth [7] reported disturbance in the ability to localize the source of a sound in space in cases of temporal lobe tumor. Again, the confusion was most evident with the source placed in the field contralateral to the affected hemisphere.

In our own studies we have chosen, after some preliminary investigation, two techniques that appear to be especially useful. One is a sequence of distorted speech tests patterned after Bocca's technique but with use of English PB-50 word lists. The other is a combination of both alternate binaural loudness balancing and the median-plane-localization of a simultaneous binaural in-phase signal.

Distorted Speech Tests

The distorted speech tests involve a sequence of six PB-50 word lists presented in the following order:

1. Left ear: low-pass-filtered
2. Right ear: faint unfiltered
3. Combined (left ear: low-pass-filtered; right ear: faint unfiltered)
4. Right ear: low-pass-filtered
5. Left ear: faint unfiltered
6. Combined (right ear: low-pass-filtered; left ear: faint unfiltered)

Three NDRC PB-50 word lists (Lists 17, 18, 19) were recorded on magnetic tape by a practiced male talker with General American dialect. From this recording a master tape, containing two recordings of each list, was made. Thus, the master tape contained two identical recordings of each of three separate PB-50 lists. The two recordings of List 17 were used for the low-pass-filter condition on each ear; the two recordings of List 18 for the faint unfiltered condition on each ear; and the two recordings of List 19 for the two combined conditions. Figure 1 illustrates, in block-diagram form, the apparatus used to produce the various test conditions. The tape

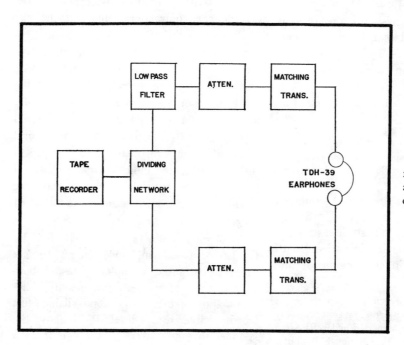

Fig. 1.—Simplified block diagram of apparatus used to deliver distorted speech tests.

recorder output was split into two channels. In the upper channel the signal passed through a low-pass filter (UTC, Type 4-C), then through a variable attenuator, and, finally, through an impedance-matching transformer to a single earphone (Telephonic, Type TDH-39). The low-pass filter was set to a cut-off frequency of 500 cps and had a rejection rate of 17 db. per octave.

In the lower channel the unfiltered signal passed through a variable attenuator, then through an impedance-matching transformer to a second TDH-39 earphone.

For each patient tested the variable attenuator in the upper channel was adjusted so that the low-pass-filtered signal was exactly 45 db. above the average of the three pure-tone thresholds for 500, 1,000, and 2,000 cps. The attenuator in the lower channel was set to a level at which the patient correctly repeated PB-words approximately 50% of the time. This level was estimated, prior to the actual test run, by administering a practice list of 25 PB-words and varying the intensity level of successive words in order to estimate the level at which 50% correct response occurred. This level necessarily varied from patient to patient. It ranged between 5 and 15 db. above the average of the pure-tone thresholds for 500, 1,000, and 2,000 cps.*

In addition to this practice at listening to faint unfiltered PB-words, the patient was also allowed to hear a list of 25 PB-words through the low-pass-filter channel, in order to acquaint him with the nature of this signal. A tape-recorded version of NDRC PB List 15 was used in all practice runs. In the actual test sequence, the entire

---

* In connection with our use of the average pure-tone threshold as a reference level for the speech material, it should be pointed out that, initially, we attempted to use the spondee threshold for this purpose. It soon became apparent, however, that, in the kind of patients we were dealing with, the spondee threshold appeared to be not only an exasperating level to estimate, but a far less stable and/or meaningful point of reference than the average pure-tone threshold for 500, 1,000, and 2,000 cps.

50 words of List 17 were presented through the low-pass filter to one ear. Then List 18 was presented, unfiltered, to the other ear. This was followed by List 19 under the combined condition. The earphones were then reversed on the subject's head, and the three-list sequence was repeated. Not only the same list of words, but the identical recording was used for each set of comparable conditions on the two ears and for the two combined conditions. This is believed to be a critical point, since the interlist equivalence previously demonstrated for the PB-50 words need not, and, in our opinion, does not, hold under conditions of gross distortion involved in the above-described procedures. The possible learning effect involved in use of the same list on both ears was felt to be slight in comparison with the problem of interlist equivalence.

Binaural Balance Tests

The alternate binaural loudness balance test (Fowler's test) is well known as a method for detecting loudness recruitment in patients with unilateral hearing loss. A pure tone at a given frequency is presented alternately to the patient's two ears. The intensity on one ear is fixed, and either the tester or the patient varies the intensity on the other ear until the alternating tones are judged to be equally loud.

A closely related procedure is to present the two stimuli not alternately but simultaneously, in-phase, to the two ears. Again, the intensity is fixed on one ear and varied on the other, but now the judgment takes the form of a median-plane-localization rather than a loudness equation. The patient now adjusts the intensity on one ear until the train of short tones appears to be in the center of the head.

The application of these two techniques, alternate binaural loudness balancing and simultaneous median-plane-localization, to patients with lesions in the higher auditory pathways represents a departure from their conventional usage, since such patients ordinarily show little hearing loss for pure

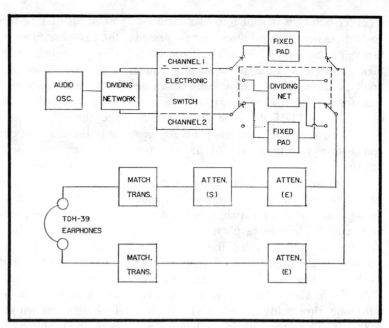

Fig. 2.—Simplified block diagram of apparatus used for binaural balance tests.

tones on either ear. Nevertheless, results have been unusually interesting.

We believe that the exact procedures used to administer these tests contribute rather more significantly to the reliability and validity of the results than has been previously supposed. Accordingly, it should be observed that our procedure is characterized by two departures from ordinary clinical practice. First, the intensity is ordinarily fixed on the ear contralateral to the affected cerebral hemisphere and varied on the ipsilateral ear. Second, whenever possible the patient makes the intensity adjustments himself by means of a 2-db. step-attenuator directly in front of him. Each match is, furthermore, defined as the average of three separate intensity adjustments, with varying arbitrary attenuation inserted by the experimenter in the variable channel between successive adjustments.

Figure 2 shows a simplified block-diagram of the apparatus essential for this technique. The output from an audio-oscillator feeds both channels of an electronic switch (Grason-Stadler, Type 829). For the alternate condition the ouput from Channel 1 passes through the experimenter's attenuator (E), then through the subject's

attenuator (S), and finally, through an impedance-matching transformer, to one of two matched dynamic earphones (Telephonic, Type TDH-39). The output from Channel 2 passes through a second experimenter's attenuator to the other earphone. Under this circumstance the pure tone generated by the oscillator alternates between the two earphones at the rate of one complete cycle each 2.5 seconds. In other words, the tone is on in one earphone for 1.25 seconds, then on in the other earphone for 1.25 seconds, etc. The rise-decay time of each such tone is 50 milliseconds.

For the simultaneous condition, the output from Channel 2 is shorted to ground and the output from Channel 1 is divided to both earphones. Now the tone is on simultaneously in both earphones for 1.25 seconds, then off in both for 1.25 seconds, etc. The two signals are always in-phase at the earphones.

Case Reports

The following three case reports illustrate preliminary findings we have obtained with these techniques.

CASE 1.—Left temporal glioblastoma. Figure 3 shows the audiologic findings in a 34-year-old

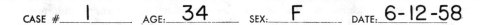

AUDIOLOGY LABORATORY — NORTHWESTERN UNIVERSITY

CASE #___1___   AGE:___34___   SEX:___F___   DATE:_6-12-58_

LEFT TEMPORAL GLIOBLASTOMA

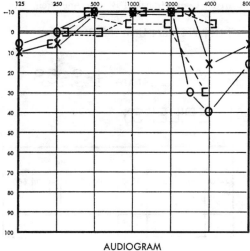

AUDIOGRAM

SISI							
FREQ.	250	500	1000	2000	3000	4000	6000
R							
L							

SPEECH TESTS			DISTORTED SPEECH TESTS		
	SRT	PB +25	LOW PASS SL=45	FAINT SL=5	COMB
R	O	88%	R-38%	L-64%	76%
L	O	92%	L-66%	R-24%	74%

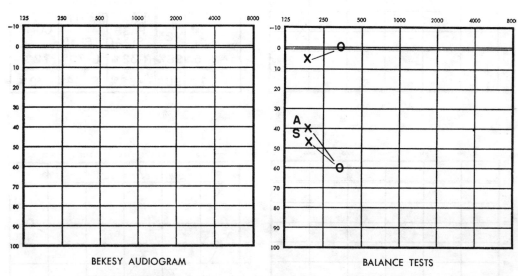

BEKESY AUDIOGRAM

BALANCE TESTS

Fig. 3.—Audiologic findings in a case of left temporal glioblastoma.

woman with a probable left temporal glioblastoma. The electroencephalogram showed a severe prominent left temporal slow-wave focus present both in the waking and sleeping state, and a left carotid angiogram indicated a space-occupying lesion lying in the posterior left temporal and inferior left parietal region.

The audiogram was relatively normal except for a bilateral notch, greater on the right ear, in the 3,000-4,000 cps region, and conventional PB scores were high on both ears.

In spite of the grossly normal picture reflected by these conventional audiometric techniques, binaural balance and distorted speech tests showed a characteristic breakdown in response to sufficiently difficult auditory tasks. Both alternate and simultaneous matches at 250 cps showed a marked departure from the intensity relations ordinarily expected to produce either equal loudness or median-plane-localization in a normal auditory mechanism. When the sensation level was 60 db. on the right ear, the patient set the tone to an average sensation level of only 33 db. on the left ear for equal loudness and to 34 db. for median-plane-localization. Furthermore, all median-plane-localization judgments were made with extreme difficulty. Indeed, one of the most striking

aspects of this patient's performance was a marked inability to appreciate any sort of unitary intra- or extracranial localization of a binaural stimulus, an observation in agreement with previous data of Sanchez Longo et al.[7]

On the distorted speech tests the characteristic pattern described by Bocca and his associates [2-4] for unilateral temporal lobe involvement emerged very clearly. Conventional PB discrimination scores

AUDIOLOGY LABORATORY — NORTHWESTERN UNIVERSITY

CASE # 2   AGE: 57   SEX: M   DATE: 4-9-58

LEFT TEMPORAL EPILEPSY

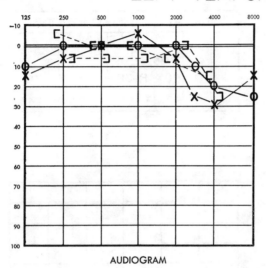

AUDIOGRAM

SISI							
FREQ.	250	500	1000	2000	3000	4000	6000
R							
L							

SPEECH TESTS			DISTORTED SPEECH TESTS		
	SRT	PB +25	LOW PASS SL=40	FAINT SL=5	COMB
R	5	98%	R-32%	L-70%	72%
L	7	90%	L-66%	R-54%	72%

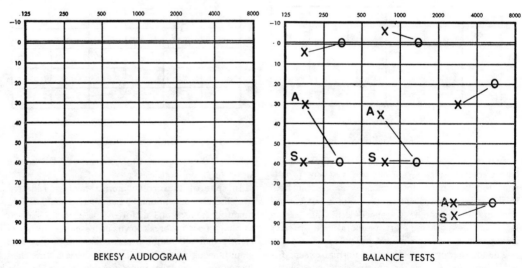

BEKESY AUDIOGRAM

BALANCE TESTS

Fig. 4.—Audiologic findings in a case of left temporal epilepsy.

were relatively good on both ears. In the low-pass-filtered condition, however, the PB score was almost 30% lower on the right ear than on the left ear. Similarly, in the faint unfiltered condition the score was 40% lower on the right ear, and in either combined condition, performance was little better than for the left ear alone.

In other words, under sufficiently difficult conditions, performance was considerably poorer on the ear contralateral than on the ear ipsilateral to the affected temporal lobe. In the balance tests this disparity was revealed as a disturbance in the intensity relations necessary to produce either equal loudness or median-plane-localization. The alternate matches suggest that stimuli delivered to the right (contralateral) ear evoked less loudness than stimuli delivered to the left (ipsilateral) ear at comparable sensation levels. Similarly, the simultaneous judgments suggest that the characteristics or parameters of the neural discharge pattern essential for median-plane-localization were, in some fashion, disturbed on the right side. One might speculate, for example, from the observed intensity relations, that intensity must be increased on the right ear in order to overcome some form of time lag introduced by the neural lesion, probably at a subcortical level.

In the distorted speech tests the interaural disparity was manifest by considerably lower PB scores on the contralateral ear under sufficiently difficult listening conditions. It is compelling to interpret these results as evidence for failure of some kind of "integrating" or "synthesizing" function ordinarily mediated by the affected temporal cortex. Whether such interpretations actually advance our thinking or not, the effect is observed consistently.

Case 2.—Left temporal epilepsy. Figure 4 shows the audiologic findings in a 57-year-old male epileptic, hospitalized after falling off a platform during an akinetic seizure. The electroencephalogram showed both spike and slow-wave foci at the left temporal pole. All areas were somewhat disrhythmic in both waking and sleeping tracings.

Again, the audiogram was relatively normal. There was a slight high-frequency loss, somewhat greater on the left ear, but a loss of this pattern and magnitude could be attributed entirely to the patient's age. Conventional PB scores were very good, 98% on the right ear and 90% on the left.

Distorted speech tests showed the familiar pattern. Low-pass filtering yielded a score of 66% on the left ear but only 32% on the right ear. When the words were unfiltered but at a sensation level of only 5 db., the right ear was 16% poorer than the left. Again, neither combined score was appreciably higher than the left ear alone.

Balance tests yielded extraordinary findings. As in the last patient, the alternate judgments re-

vealed a gross disturbance in the intensity relations producing equal loudness. At 250 cps, for example, the tone at a sensation level of 60 db. on the right ear was judged equal in loudness to the same tone only 27 db. above threshold on the left ear. In this patient, however, the simultaneous judgments were completely normal. Median-plane-localization was produced by approximately equal sensation levels in the two ears.

Further intensive exploration, in which the patient was asked to indicate the spatial localization of binaurally presented tones at various sensation levels both in and out of phase revealed that, in sharp contrast to the difficulties experienced by the previous patient, this patient exhibited no difficulty with either intra- or extracranial localization. For example, when a 500 cps tone was presented in-phase and at equal intensity in the two earphones, he reported that he heard a single sound "in the center of my head and toward the back." The precision and relative specificity of this kind of verbal report contrasted very sharply with the typical reaction of the previous patient. Under similar conditions, he heard a sound "all over the room."

Case 3.—Left frontal meningioma. Figure 5 illustrates audiologic findings in a 65-year-old man in whom diffuse CNS damage complicated an additional left cortical involvement.

All neurological findings were felt to be questionable because of the patient's lack of cooperation. However, the examination revealed signs of diffuse CNS damage as well as scattered signs, predominantly right-sided, of cortical atrophy.

The electroencephalogram showed a slow-wave focus at the left temporal pole and runs of sharp waves in the right parietal lead. Subsequent surgery revealed a left frontal meningioma in the region of the sphenoid wing.

The audiogram showed a bilateral high-frequency loss, greater on the left ear, and somewhat more precipitous than one ordinarily associates with presbycusis. Conventional PB scores were very low, 74% in the right ear and 60% in the left.

Low-pass-filtered PB scores were unusually poor on both ears, probably reflecting the rather diffuse CNS damage. Only the balance tests reflected the unilateral involvement. At both 250 and 1,000 cps, the patient required equal intensity at the two ears to place the tone in the median plane but far more intensity on the right ear than on the left to make the alternating tones equally loud. At 1,000 cps, for example, when the tone was fixed at a sensation level of 60 db. on the right ear, the patient adjusted the intensity on the left ear to a sensation level of only 29 db. and judged the two tones equally loud. As a check on the reliability of this disparity, additional judgments were made under a reversed condition, in which the intensity was fixed at a sensation level of 30

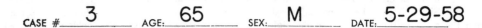

AUDIOLOGY LABORATORY — NORTHWESTERN UNIVERSITY

CASE # __3__   AGE: __65__   SEX: __M__   DATE: __5-29-58__

LEFT SPHENOID WING MENINGIOMA

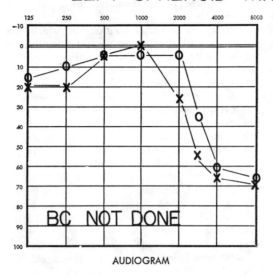

BC NOT DONE

AUDIOGRAM

SISI							
FREQ.	250	500	1000	2000	3000	4000	6000
R							
L							

SPEECH TESTS			DISTORTED SPEECH TESTS	
	SRT	PB +25	LOW PASS SL=60	
R	13	74%	R- 12%	
L	15	60%	L-14%	

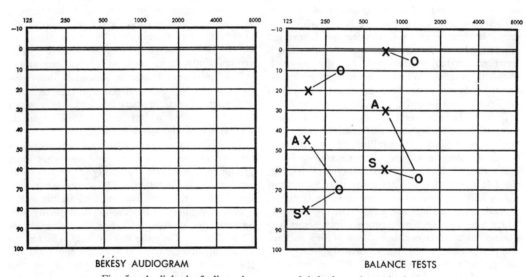

BÉKÉSY AUDIOGRAM

BALANCE TESTS

Fig. 5.—Audiologic findings in a case of left frontal meningioma.

db. on the *left* ear and the patient was required to adjust the intensity on the *right* ear until equal loudness had been achieved. Under this circumstance, he consistently set the tone on the right ear to a sensation level of 60 db., confirming the reliability of both the direction and extent of the rather marked disparity.

Comment

The extent to which the patterns of response typified by these three case reports can be generalized to all unilateral auditory pathway and temporal lobe involvement is unknown. Our purpose in presenting these findings is merely to suggest some possible avenues of attack on the problem of furthering our understanding of the mechanisms by which the central auditory system performs its unique function.

Our experience to date, however, leads us to suggest the following generalizations regarding the auditory response pattern in unilateral lesions involving the auditory pathways within the central nervous system. First, the threshold loss for pure tones is apparently very minimal, at least for frequencies below 2,000 cps. Rather sharp bilateral high-frequency losses seem to be common in these patients, but the multiplicity of possible etiologies for such losses limits the fruitfulness of further speculation. In general, it would appear, however, that there is little evidence of a hearing loss per se.

In sufficiently difficult auditory tasks, however, rather clear-cut evidence of abnormality can be demonstrated on the ear contralateral to the affected hemisphere. Scores on distorted speech tests are characteristically lower on the contralateral than on the ipsilateral ear, and there is a gross alteration in the interaural intensity relations producing equal loudness at the two ears. The intensity relations producing median-plane-localization may or may not be affected, apparently depending upon the nature and extent of the lesion.

In this connection, it is compelling to speculate on the possible relation between the evidence of strikingly dissimilar behavior in Cases 1 and 2 and the nature or extent of the brain lesion. It seems probable, particularly in view of her carotid angiogram, that in the first case there was appreciable involvement of the central auditory pathways both cortically and subcortically. The evidence pointed toward a relatively large space-occupying lesion. In the second case, however, the neurological evidence suggested a less massive lesion, perhaps involving cortical tissue alone.

This distinction suggests the hypothesis that equality of loudness depends on the integrity of the entire afferent pathways, including the temporal cortex, whereas intracranial median-plane-localization depends only on integrity of the pathways up to some critical subcortical center.

Such an hypothesis is not incompatible with Licklider's [8] "triplex theory" of hearing in which the frequency-analyzed neural signals from the two cochleas are assumed to undergo a twofold coincidence or correlation analysis at unspecified centers in the nervous system. The first analysis is presumed to correlate the signals from the two ears, thereby mediating sound localization in phenomenal space.

Of further note in this connection are the recent studies of Deatherage, Eldredge, and Davis [9] on the latency of action potentials in the guinea-pig cochlea and of Deatherage and Hirsh [10] on the localization of clicks. These studies indicate that localization is based on latencies of action potentials (AP) apparently entirely independently of their magnitudes. This suggests a reasonable physiological basis distinguishing loudness judgments from localization judgments. The present evidence indicates that these two fundamentally different physiological clues may be evaluated at different levels within the nervous system; loudness (magnitude of AP?) at a relatively high level and localization (latency of AP) at a lower level.

Whether one feels that this kind of explanation advances our thinking or not, the effect is observed very consistently. In what appear to be involvements at relatively high (cortical) levels, we have observed abnormalities in loudness without concomitant abnormalities in median-plane-localization. On the other hand, we have never observed the converse, i.e., abnormalities in median-plane-localization without concomitant abnormalities in loudness.

Relative to this generalization, it is interesting to observe that Walsh [11] found no breakdown in the horizontal localization of binaural clicks when binaural time-difference was varied or in horizontal localization of tones when phase-difference was varied in patients with varying neurological lesions. Only localization in the vertical plane was adversely affected. Walsh concluded[11] (p. 233),

It appeared likely from these studies that the auditory area of one hemisphere could be dispensed with without abolishing the ability to utilize binaural time differences.

And again (p. 246),

It should not be assumed . . . that the messages from the two ears retain their individuality in the ascending tracts and that the time intervals are judged by a cortical mechanism. It would seem that the evaluation takes place soon after the auditory impulses from the two sides meet.

Similar conclusions were reached by Teuber and Diamond.[12] These investigators presented simultaneous clicks binaurally in 10 control subjects and in 20 patients with penetrating brain wounds. Both the relative arrival time of the two clicks and their relative intensities could be varied independently. When arrival time was varied and intensity held constant, controls localized the binaural clicks with greater precision than the brain-injured, but there were no significant directional effects. When relative arrival time was held constant, however, and relative intensity was varied,

. . . There were marked directional effects: Ss with right unilateral lesions required more intensity on the left for midline judgments and conversely for men with left lesions. In this respect, judgments based on intensity behaved differently from those based on time . . . the effects are dissociable, suggesting at least partial separation of neural mechanisms underlying these two forms of localization.[12]

Summary

Two techniques, a series of distorted speech tests patterned after Bocca's methods in Italian and alternate-simultaneous binaural balancing, have been found useful in the study of unilateral lesions of the auditory pathways in the central nervous system. Three case reports illustrate distinct patterns of results. The ability to understand distorted speech is reduced on the ear contralateral to the affected hemisphere, and the interaural intensity relations producing equal loudness for pure tones under alternate presentation are grossly disturbed. The intensity relations producing median-plane-localization under simultaneous in-phase presentation may or may not be disturbed, apparently depending on the nature and extent of the brain lesion.

Drs. Benjamin Boshes, Hirsh Wachs, Joel Brumlik, Manuel Mier, and Rolando De la Torre, all of the Department of Neurology and Psychiatry, Northwestern University Medical School, supply the patients and neurological test data for our continuing study of auditory behavior in cases of brain lesion.

Audiology Laboratory, School of Speech. Northwestern University.

REFERENCES

1. Schuknecht, H. F.: Perceptive Hearing Loss, Laryngoscope 68:429-439, 1958.

2. Bocca, E.; Calearo, C.; Cassinari, V., and Miglivacca, F.: Testing Cortical Hearing in Temporal Lobe Tumors, Acta otolaryng. 45:289-304, 1955.

3. Bocca, E.: Binaural Hearing: Another Approach, Laryngoscope 65:1164-1171, 1955.

4. Bocca, E.: Clinical Aspects of Cortical Deafness, Laryngoscope 68:301-309, 1958.

5. Goldstein, R.; Goodman, A., and King, R. B.: Hearing and Speech in Infantile Hemiplegia Before and After Left Hemispherectomy, Neurology 6:869-875, 1956.

6. Matzker, J., and Ruckes, J.: Diagnosis of Morphologically Demonstrable Brain Stem Diseases by a New Hearing Test, Deutsche med. Wchnschr. 82:2187-2194, 1957; abstracted, Excerpta Med. XI 11:409, 1958.

7. Sanchez Longo, L. P.; Forster, F. M., and Auth, T. L.: A Clinical Test for Sound Localization and Its Applications, Neurology 7:655-663, 1957.

8. Licklider, J. C. R.: Three Auditory Theories, in Psychology: A Study of Science, edited by Sigmund Koch, New York, McGraw-Hill Book Company, Inc., 1959, Vol. 1.

9. Deatherage, B. H.; Eldredge, D. H., and Davis, H.: Latency of Action Potentials in the Cochlea of the Guinea Pig, J. Acoust. Soc. America 31:479-486, 1959.

10. Deatherage, B. H., and Hirsh, I. J.: Auditory Localization of Clicks, J. Acoust. Soc. America 31:486-492, 1959.

11. Walsh, E. G.: An Investigation of Sound Localization in Patients with Neurological Abnormalities, Brain 80:222-250, 1957.

12. Teuber, H. L., and Diamond, S.: Effects of Brain Injury in Man on Binaural Localization of Sounds, read at Meeting of Eastern Psychological Association, Atlantic City, N.J., March 23-24, 1956.

Bekesy Audiometry in Analysis of Auditory Disorders

JAMES JERGER

Less than 14 years has elapsed since Bekesy's original description of a self-recording audiometer (2). Within this period, however, the technique of 'Bekesy audiometry' has rapidly gained the stature of a major clinical and research tool in audiology.

Bekesy audiometry refers to a method in which the subject traces his own auditory threshold by means of a suitable self-recording audiometer. The threshold tracing signal may be either a fixed frequency or a gradually changing frequency, and the signal may be either continuous or periodically interrupted in time, but the essence of Bekesy's method is, first, that the signal intensity is always changing at a constant rate, and second, that the subject determines the direction of this change by alternately pressing and releasing a key that reverses the direction of a motor-driven attenuator. He is instructed to press this key when he just hears the tone and to release it when he just-no-longer

hears it. By connecting a pen-writing system to the attenuator a graphic representation, or tracing, of the subject's successive threshold crossings may be obtained.

The Bekesy technique is particularly useful in psychoacoustics. It lends itself admirably, for example, to the measurement of temporary threshold shift following acoustic stimulation and has been so employed by several investigators (6, 8, 10, 12, 15, 20, 31, 32, 33, 34). It finds use in the measurement of pure-tone masking (3, 5).

The present paper is concerned, however, only with Bekesy audiometry as a clinical tool in the evaluation of the hearing impaired. In the majority of papers concerned with the clinical application of Bekesy audiometry, measurement and description have been confined almost exclusively to the width or amplitude of the audiometric tracing. This distance or width may be expressed either in decibels or in number of threshold crossings over a given frequency span. In the graphic form of the Bekesy audiogram it is most easily visualized as the amplitude of the oscillating trace. Bekesy (2), in his original paper, noted that the amplitude became greatly diminished in subjects with hearing loss accompanied by loudness recruitment. He assumed that the tracing amplitude represented the first just-noticeable-difference (JND) in loudness and con-

James Jerger (Ph.D., Northwestern University, 1954) is Associate Professor of Audiology, Northwestern University. A portion of this article is based on a paper presented at the 1959 Convention of the American Speech and Hearing Association, Cleveland. This research was supported by research grant B-1310 from the National Institutes of Health, Public Health Service, and by the United States Air Force under Contract AF 41(657)-185, monitored by the School of Aviation Medicine, USAF, Brooks Air Force Base, Texas.

Reprinted from the *Journal of Speech and Hearing Research*
September 1960, Vol. 3, No. 3

cluded that a reduction in its size was compatible with the presence of an abnormally rapid rate of loudness growth with intensity (that is, loudness recruitment). However, Bekesy's assumption that the amplitude represents the first JND has been questioned by Hirsh, Palva, and Goodman (9), who feel that the amplitude actually represents the variability about the absolute threshold.

In any event, subsequent papers on Bekesy audiometry have dealt primarily with the amplitude aspect of the audiometric tracing (1, 7, 11, 17, 18, 21, 22, 23, 25, 26, 27, 28, 29, 30, 35, 36). The major point of view in this respect is best exemplified by the very thorough monograph of Lundborg (21). This investigator obtained Bekesy audiograms on 50 normals, 25 cases of acoustic trauma, 26 cases of Meniere's disease, and 21 cases of diverse retrocochlear lesion. He then classified the audiograms into four types based on the tracing amplitude. There appeared to be a rather precise relationship between type of Bekesy tracing and site of lesion. Markedly reduced amplitude was characteristically present in cases with presumably cochlear lesion (acoustic trauma and Meniere's disease) but characteristically absent in cases with retrocochlear lesion.

In recent years increasing attention has been given to another aspect of the Bekesy tracing, the change in threshold intensity over time as the subject traces threshold at a fixed frequency (4, 14, 16, 19, 26, 27, 28, 37). Kos (16), Lierle and Reger (19), Jerger, Carhart, and Lassman (14), and Yantis (37) have shown very little change over time in presumably cochlear lesion, but marked

progression toward higher and higher threshold intensity over time in retrocochlear lesion.

The present paper concerns the relationship between Bekesy audiometry and site of lesion within the auditory system. Unfortunately, almost every previous writer has confused this issue with a quite separate question, the relationship between the Bekesy tracing and the presence or absence of loudness recruitment. It must be emphasized, therefore, that the present paper is not concerned with how Bekesy audiometry relates to loudness recruitment, only with how it relates to site of lesion within the auditory system.

Procedure

Subjects. This report is based on the Bekesy audiograms of 434 subjects tested at the Hearing Clinic of the Northwestern University Medical School over a three-year period. The subjects were referred from various sources for audiological evaluation. The majority were referred by otologists, a small number by neurologists and neurosurgeons in the Chicago area. Although no formal attempt at random selection was made, the series is fairly representative of the otologic case load in a large hospital environment. In most cases Bekesy audiometry was performed as part of a larger battery of auditory tests typically administered in a three-hour test session. Although tracings were ordinarily obtained on both ears, subsequent analysis is confined to results obtained on only one ear of each subject.

Apparatus. All of the tracings on which this report is based were obtained with a single Bekesy audiometer (Grason-Stadler, Model E-800). The rate of attenuation change was always 2.5 db per second, and the rate of frequency change was always one octave per minute. The instrument offered the option of a test signal that was either continuous or periodically interrupted in time. In the latter case, the interruption rate was 2.5 ips.

The results reported below involve two kinds of tracing, subsequently referred to as 'conventional' and 'fixed-frequency' tracings. In conventional tracings, the frequency of the test signal moved gradually upward from 100 to 10 000 cps. In fixed-frequency tracings the frequency was preset and never changed as the subject traced his threshold over a three-minute period.

In either case, a complete test always consisted of two separate tracings. In one the signal was periodically interrupted, in the second it was continuous in time. Both tracings, interrupted and continuous, were always made on the same piece of graph paper with two different colors of ink. It has been found convenient to symbolize these two conditions by the letters 'I' for interrupted and 'C' for continuous in subsequent portions of this report.

Method. A relatively rigidly standardized procedure of test administration was initially designed, but could not be followed rigorously in all subjects due to the occasional subject whose ability to understand speech was extremely limited. In any event, the following instructions were used whenever verbal communication was possible:

> When I put these earphones on, you are going to hear a beeping sound in your ear. As long as you don't do anything the sound will keep getting louder. But you can make it fade away by holding down this switch. When you let up on the switch the sound will get louder again. Now, here is what I want you to do. Listen very carefully, and, as soon as you hear the beeping sound, hold this switch down until you can't hear it any more. As soon as the beeping sound is gone, let up on the switch until it comes back. Then, as soon as you hear it again, hold the switch down until it goes away again, and so forth. The idea is to keep going back and forth from where you can just hear the beeping sound to where you can just not hear it any more. Never let the sound get very loud and never let it stay away too long. Hold this switch down as soon as you hear the sound, then let it up as soon as the sound is gone.

Following these instructions a tracing was made with the periodically interrupted (I) test signal. At the termination of this tracing the subject was reinstructed as follows:

> Now we are going to do the same thing again, but this time the sound will be steady instead of beeping on and off. Your job is still the same. Hold the switch down as soon as you hear the steady sound, and let it up as soon as the steady sound goes away.

Following these instructions a tracing was made with the continuous (C) test signal. This test order, interrupted first and continuous second, was used in all subjects. Instructions were identical for either conventional or fixed-frequency tracings. When verbal communication was not possible, instructions were effected through pantomime.

Findings

An initial attempt was made to analyse and score these Bekesy audiograms quantitatively. Various indices, such as the width of the continuous tracing in db, the number of threshold crossing per quarter octave, the difference between tracing width at high and low frequencies, the difference between continuous and interrupted tracing widths, and the difference between continuous and interrupted mid-points, were evaluated, all with exceedingly discouraging results. It soon became apparent that the range of individual variability on any absolute aspect of the Bekesy audiogram could be quite substantial. A good example is the width of the continuous tracing. In most Meniere's patients it is, to be sure, quite small at high frequencies. On the other hand many young adults with otosclerosis show tracing widths considerably narrower than a large number of older Meniere's patients. There were, indeed, significant group tendencies in this quantitative analysis, but the degree of overlap among groups appeared to limit severely the use of any quantitative measure as a reliable means of differentiating site of lesion. A similar conclusion was reached by Landes (17).

On the other hand, a qualitative judgment of the patterning or relationship between the interrupted and the continuous tracings seemed to have important diagnostic value. There appeared to be a unique relationship between continuous and interrupted tracings corresponding to site of lesion within the auditory system.

One may distinguish four basic types of relationship, labelled, respectively, type I, type II, type III, and type IV. They are illustrated in Figures 1 and 2. Figure 1 shows the four types in the case of conventional tracings, Figure 2 the corresponding types in the case

of fixed-frequency tracings. Throughout these and subsequent figures, green denotes the interrupted (I) tracing and red denotes the continuous (C) tracing.

Type I. The type I relationship is characterized by an interweaving or superposition of continuous and interrupted tracings, and by a tracing width which is constant over frequency and averages about 10 db. There is, however, considerable variation about this mean value. Tracing widths as small as 3 db and as large as 20 db are not uncommon.

In the case of fixed-frequency tracings, the type I relationship is reflected in two interweaving, horizontal tracings.

Type II. Type II tracings differ from type I in two respects. First, the continuous tracing drops below the interrupted at high frequencies, but never to a substantial extent. The gap seldom exceeds 20 db and ordinarily does not appear at frequencies below 1000 cps. Second, the width or amplitude of the continuous tracing is often quite small (3 to 5 db) in these higher frequencies. This narrowing of the width or amplitude of the continuous tracing is, of course, the classical Bekesy sign thought by many to indicate the presence of loudness recruitment.

In fixed-frequency tracing the type II result is quite clear-cut. The interrupted tracing is, again, horizontal and of normal width, but the continuous trace drops from 5 to 20 db below the interrupted, *within the first minute;* thereafter, it maintains a fairly stable level. There is a reliable difference between interrupted and continuous tracings but the difference is relatively small and remains quite constant after

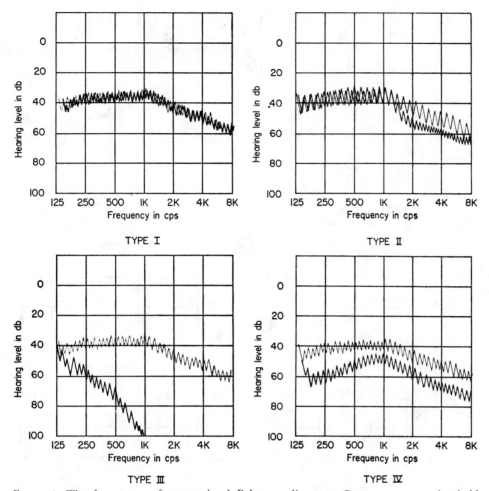

FIGURE 1. The four types of conventional Bekesy audiograms. Green represents threshold tracing for a periodically interrupted tone, red for a continuous tone.

the first 60 seconds of tracing. Furthermore, the difference appears only at mid- and high frequencies (that is, above 500 to 1000 cps).

Type III. Type III tracings are quite dramatic. The continuous tracing drops below the interrupted to a remarkable degree. Furthermore, the two curves may diverge at relatively low frequencies (100 to 500 cps). It is not uncommon to observe the continuous tracing break away at a frequency as low as

150 cps and drop to a level as much as 40 to 50 db below the interrupted tracing. The width of the continuous tracing ordinarily remains, however, quite normal.

In type III fixed-frequency tracings the interrupted tracing is horizontal but the continuous drops very rapidly and ordinarily does not stabilize at all. Typically, the continuous tracing begins at the same level as the interrupted but describes a rapidly descending trace to the limit of the equipment. A 40-to-

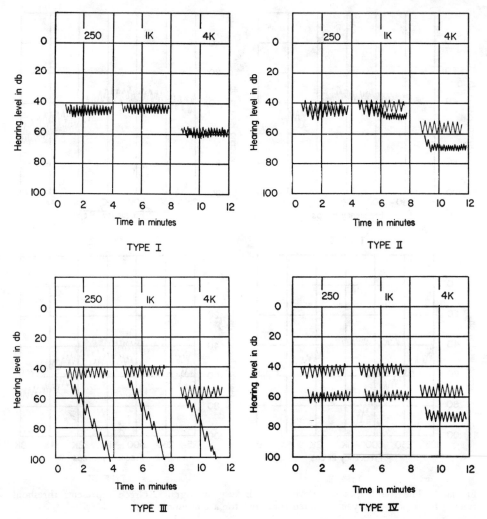

FIGURE 2. The four types of fixed-frequency Bekesy tracings. Green is interrupted; red, continuous.

50-db drop within as little as 60 seconds is not unusual.

Type IV. Type IV tracings more closely resemble type II than type III but differ in one important respect. The continuous tracing falls consistently below the interrupted at frequencies below 500 cps. At higher frequencies the continuous may fall a constant distance below the interrupted,

resembling a type II in this respect. The tracing width may or may not become abnormally small, further adding to possible confusion with type II. At mid- and high frequencies there may even be some overlap between C and I. The distinguishing feature, however, occurring in both conventional and fixed-frequency tracings, is the gap between C and I at relatively low frequencies (100 to 500 cps). Type IV tracings differ from type III tracings in that C ordinarily does not show a precipitous drop over time.

The vast majority of Bekesy tracings can be fitted into one of these four categories quite reliably. There are,

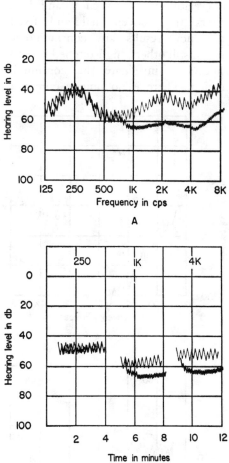

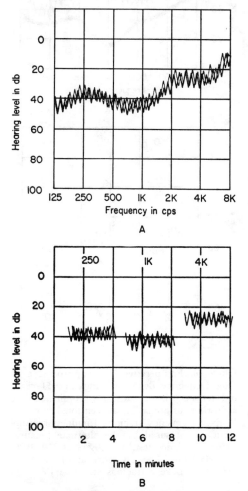

FIGURE 3. Conventional and fixed-frequency Bekesy tracings in a 31-year-old female with left otosclerosis: A, conventional tracings; B, fixed-frequency tracings. Loudness recruitment, as measured by the alternate binaural loudness balance test, was absent at 250, 1000, and 4000 cps on the test ear. The PB score at SL = 25 db was 100%. Bekesy tracings are type I.

FIGURE 4. Conventional and fixed-frequency Bekesy tracings in a 42-year-old male with left Meniere's disease: A, conventional tracings; B, fixed-frequency tracings. Loudness recruitment, as measured by the alternate binaural loudness balance test, was present at 1000 and 4000 cps but absent at 250 cps. The PB score at SL = 25 db was 24%. Bekesy tracings are type II.

however, a small number that, for one reason or another, do not appear to fit any of the four classic patterns. They may be designated by the label 'questionable.' In some of these, excessive tracing width (30 to 40 db) obscures the relationship between C and I. In others the conventional and fixed-frequency results are contradictory, and, in still others, high-pitched tinnitus appears to invalidate the continuous tracing. There is no unique common-

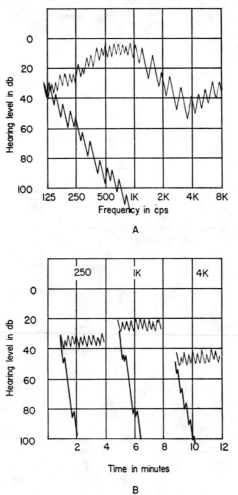

FIGURE 5. Preoperative conventional and fixed-frequency Bekesy tracings in a 47-year-old female with a surgically confirmed right acoustic neurinoma: A, conventional tracings; B, fixed-frequency tracings. Loudness recruitment, as measured by the alternate binaural loudness balance test, was absent at 4000 cps. The PB score at SL = 25 db was 26%. Bekesy tracings are type III.

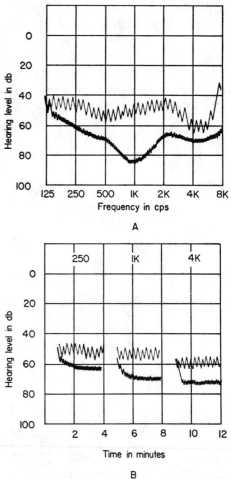

FIGURE 6. Preoperative conventional and fixed-frequency Bekesy tracings in a 51-year-old female with a surgically confirmed left acoustic neurinoma: A, conventional tracings; B, fixed-frequency tracings. Loudness recruitment, as measured by the alternate binaural loudness balance test, was absent at 250, 1000, and 4000 cps. The PB score at SL = 25 db was 58%. Bekesy tracings are type IV.

ality to these questionable tracings. They seem, instead, to reflect a general lack of validity. This category encompasses only a relatively small percentage of tracings and does not seem to be unique to any particular etiology or site of lesion.

Illustrative Cases. Figures 3, 4, 5, and 6 illustrate these four basic types of tracings as they occur in actual subjects. Figure 3 shows Bekesy tracings in a case of unilateral otosclerosis. Conventional tracings are type I. The continuous tracing and the interrupted tracing overlap, and the width or amplitude of the continuous tracing remains essentially normal (that is, about 10 db). Fixed-frequency tracings are also type I. They show essentially horizontal tracings, with the continuous and interrupted interweaving at all test frequencies.

Figure 4 shows test results in a case of unilateral Meniere's disease. Here, the Bekesy tracings are clearly type II. On the conventional tracing C breaks away from I at about 500 cps and remains 10 to 15 db below I out to 8000 cps. Throughout this range the width of the C tracing is quite small. The fixed-frequency tracing at 4000 cps shows the characteristic initial drop of 10 to 20 db in the C trace, followed by a relatively stable level. In this particular case, the width of the C tracing is relatively small, but this is not invariably the case in type II fixed-frequency tracings.

Figure 5 shows Bekesy tracings in a subject with a right acoustic neurinoma. Here, one sees a relatively extreme example of the type III Bekesy tracing. On the conventional tracings C never does overlap I. Even at 125 cps it runs about 35 db below I, and the disparity increases with frequency. At 1000 cps the C trace has dropped to the limit of the equipment, whereas the I trace is at a hearing level of about 10 db.

The fixed-frequency tracing at 250 cps is quite dramatic. On the left, or unaffected, ear, C and I are horizontal and overlap. On the right, or affected, ear, however, I is stable but C drops over 60 db to the limit of the equipment in less than 60 seconds.

The fact that such a phenomenal drop should occur at all is remarkable. That it should occur for a frequency as low as 250 cps is even more remarkable. Exploration at lower frequencies in this subject revealed the same steadily progressive drop in the C trace at 100 cps, the lowest frequency obtainable from the equipment.

Figure 6 illustrates the type IV tracing in another surgically-confirmed acoustic neurinoma. Neither conventional nor fixed-frequency tracings show the steady decline typical of a type III tracing. At the same time the relatively large gap between C and I at very low frequencies clearly differentiates this from a type II tracing pattern. In this particular case the C tracing width is relatively small, but other type IV tracings show a quite normal width.

Distribution of Patterns. In order to study the generality of this apparent relationship between type of Bekesy tracing and site of lesion within the auditory mechanism, all Bekesy audiograms obtained on subjects with hearing loss in the Northwestern University Hearing Clinics were categorized according to type.

Table 1 shows the number of subjects within each of the four categories for various etiological subgroups. In the case of the acoustic neurinoma group, classification is based on surgical confirmation. All other classification by subgroup is based on the medical

TABLE 1. Distribution of the four Bekesy types (I, II, III, IV) and of unclassifiable tracings (?) according to presumed etiology of the hearing loss in 434 subjects.

Etiology	Tracings					Total
	I	II	III	IV	?	
Normal Hearing	33	0	0	0	0	33
Otosclerosis	50	2	0	0	2	54
Otitis Media	6	0	0	0	0	6
Other Conductive Loss	9	0	0	0	0	9
Meniere's Disease	4	26	0	1	1	32
Noise Induced Loss	7	15	0	0	0	22
Acoustic Neurinoma	0	0	6	4	0	10
Unknown Sensorineural Loss	54	119	0	12	10	195
Presbycusis	24	15	0	2	3	44
Otosclerosis Plus Sensorineural Loss	2	10	0	1	0	13
Sudden Onset of Loss	1	1	10	4	0	16
Total	190	188	16	24	16	434

diagnosis supplied by staff members of the Department of Otolaryngology of the Northwestern University Medical School.

Included in this series of 434 ears are 69 presumably conductive lesions primarily due to otosclerosis and otitis media, 54 presumably cochlear lesions due to Meniere's disease and prolonged noise exposure, 10 known eighth nerve lesions due to acoustic neurinoma, and four subgroups in which the site of lesion is less well understood. One of these, the sensorineural unknown group, constitutes the largest single subgroup with 195 subjects. An additional 16 subjects from this group are treated separately because of a history of relatively sudden onset of loss in one ear, without subsequent fluctuation. Finally, there are 44 subjects with presbycusis, and 13 subjects with advanced otosclerosis accompanied by secondary sensorineural loss.

Examination of subgroups in Table 1, for which there is relatively good agreement concerning the locus of pathology, suggests a fairly strong relationship between type of Bekesy tracing and site of lesion. In lesions of the middle ear (otosclerosis, otitis media) the type I tracing predominates. In cochlear lesion (Meniere's, noise-induced) the type II tracing predominates although some fall into the type I category. No Meniere's case ever showed a type III tracing. In eighth nerve lesion (acoustic neurinoma) type III and type IV tracings predominate. No acoustic neurinoma ever gave a type II tracing.

In view of this compelling relationship, the results of the analysis in etiologic subgroups of more obscure origin are of interest. As might be expected, the majority of sensorineural unknowns are type II, suggesting cochlear lesion. This is also true of otosclerosis accompanied by secondary sensorineural loss.

Almost one-third of the sensorineural unknowns, however, show type I tracings and 12 show type IV tracings. This relatively ill-defined group may possibly include at least two and possibly three distinctly different kinds of sensorineural loss. In presbycusis the situation is even more provocative. Here, there are actually more type I than type II tracings.

Contrary to expectation, hearing loss of sudden onset is primarily type III and type IV, suggesting eighth nerve rather than, or perhaps in addition to, cochlear lesion.

Discussion

In certain respects the present results do not seem to be in very good agreement with the findings of some previous investigators. Lundborg (*21*), for example, apparently observed nothing like the present type III tracings in any of his 21 cases of retrocochlear lesion. His Bekesy thresholds were apparently in good agreement with the results of conventional threshold audiometry. Nor do Palva's (*27*) results on 39 cases agree with the present findings in fixed-frequency tracings. After four minutes of threshold tracing, there was a change of more than 10 db in only one of Palva's 33 perceptive losses. He concluded (*26*) that 'an abnormal loss in sensitivity is not common enough to give reliable clues to differential diagnosis.'

The present findings are far more encouraging. They show clear evidence of pathological adaptation (types II, III, and IV) in 226 of 332 sensorineural losses (68%). Furthermore, the manner in which pathological adaptation appears to be related to site of lesion suggests that Bekesy audiometry has the potential to become an exceedingly sharp tool in the differential diagnosis of hearing disorders.

Finally, it should be observed that the present results are in accord with the previous findings of Dix and Hood (*4*), Kos (*16*), Lierle and Reger (*19*), and Yantis (*37*).

It may be appropriate to cite two possible bases for the lack of agreement between the present results and the previous findings of Lundborg and of Palva. First, the discrepancy may be due to a simple artifact of instrumentation. Lundborg (*21*) states that, in his Bekesy audiometer, attenuation changed in 2-db steps, and Palva (*24*) states that his audiometer changed in 1-db steps. It may be that the momentary transient energy introduced by each abrupt change in level made their continuous stimuli more like the interrupted than the continuous stimulus used in the present study. In the Bekesy audiometer used in the present experiment, successive changes in level were less than 0.25 db. This distinction between virtually continuous change and change in small, discrete steps may very well be an exceedingly important variable. Jerger and Bucy (*13*) showed, for example, that only very brief silent intervals (10 to 20 msec) between successive short tones were sufficient to maintain a stable horizontal tracing in a patient who readily demonstrated a type III tracing under continuous stimulation.

Second, it should be observed that with the exception of Dix and Hood (*4*), who used different instrumentation, no previous investigator, to the author's knowledge, has compared the continuous threshold tracing with the corresponding interrupted threshold tracing. Apparently, all previous workers have employed only a continuous stimulus for either conventional or fixed-frequency tracing. The present results, however, suggest that the comparison between C and I is the key to fruitful interpretation of Bekesy tracings. Type III continuous tracings are, to be sure, so dramatic that they are easily recognized, but they are comparatively rare. In the vast majority of cases showing pathological adaptation (type II) the magnitude of the effect is not great (5 to 20 db). It occurs, furthermore, so rapidly that, if one makes measurements only at one minute intervals and seeks only a shift in the continuous threshold, he is likely to observe very little evidence of dramatic adaptation over time. When the continuous tracing is compared with its interrupted counterpart, however, the abnormality is readily recognized.

Another aspect of interpretation that deserves re-emphasis is the relationship between pathological adaptation and frequency. Again, when marked adaptation occurs (type III), it may generally be observed at almost any frequency with measurable hearing. But such tracings are, again, comparatively rare. In the more commonly encountered type II tracing, pathological adaptation is very definitely a high-frequency phenomenon. The manner in which the difference between C and I relates to frequency is, in itself, a quite stable characteristic of the over-all type II pattern.

Summary

A qualitative analysis of 434 Bekesy audiograms suggests that most tracings can be placed into one of four categories. The basis for categorization is the relationship between tracings of periodically interrupted and continuous tonal stimuli. Lesions of the middle ear are characterized by one relationship, lesions of the cochlea by a second, and lesions of the eighth nerve by a third and fourth.

Summario in Interlingua

Un analyse qualitative de quatro centos trenta-quatro audiogrammas de Bekesy suggere que le major parte del audiogrammas pote esser placiate in un de quatro categorias. Le base del categorisation es le relation inter audiogrammas de stimulos tonal que es interrupte periodicamente e stimulos tonal que es continue. Lesiones del aure medie demonstra un relation, lesiones del coclea demonstra un secunde, e lesiones del nervo octave un tertie e quarte.

Editor's note: For the interest of *Journal* readers, the author has prepared the above *Summary* in Interlingua, an international auxiliary language developed by the International Auxiliary Language Association, 420 Lexington Ave., New York 17. As of 1960, 17 American and five foreign journals are printing summaries in Interlingua; two American journals are being edited completely in Interlingua; seven international congresses thus far have furnished summaries of all papers in Interlingua. The core of this language is the vast number of internationally identical technical terms already in existence in the various national tongues of western culture. A recent UNESCO survey indicated that of all existing languages, Interlingua has the widest range of immediate intelligibility. English is second. The *Journal* will print other summaries in Interlingua when these are provided by the authors.

References

1. BANGS, J. L., and MULLINS, C. J., Recruitment testing in hearing and its implications. *Arch. Otolaryng.*, 58, 1953, 582-592.
2. BEKESY, G. v., A new audiometer. *Acta Otolaryng.*, 35, 1947, 411-422.
3. BILGER, R. C., and HIRSH, I. J., Masking of tones by bands of noise. *J. acoust. Soc. Amer.*, 28, 1956, 623-630.
4. DIX, M. R., and HOOD, J. D., Modern developments in pure tone audiometry and their application to the clinical diag-

nosis of end-organ deafness. *Proc. R. Soc. Med.*, 46, 1953, 992-994.

5. EHMER, R. H., Masking patterns of tones. *J. acoust. Soc. Amer.*, 31, 1959, 1115-1120.

6. EPSTEIN, A., and SCHUBERT, E. D., Reversible auditory fatigue resulting from exposure to a pure tone. *Arch. Otolaryng.*, 65, 1957, 174-182.

7. HEDGECOCK, L., The measurement of auditory recruitment. *Arch. Otolaryng.*, 62, 1955, 515-527.

8. HIRSH, I. J., and BILGER, R. C., Auditory-threshold recovery after exposures to pure tones. *J. acoust. Soc. Amer.*, 27, 1955, 1186-1194.

9. HIRSH, I. J., PALVA, T., and GOODMAN, A., Difference limen and recruitment. *Arch. Otolaryng.*, 60, 1954, 525-540.

10. HIRSH, I. J., and WARD, W. D., Recovery of the auditory threshold after strong acoustic stimulation. *J. acoust. Soc. Amer.*, 24, 1952, 131-141.

11. HORMIA, A. L., Difference limen of intensity in hearing impairment due to craniocerebral injury. *Laryngoscope*, 68, 1958, 808-813.

12. HUGHES, J. R., Auditory sensitization. *J. acoust. Soc. Amer.*, 26, 1954, 1064-1070.

13. JERGER, J., and BUCY, P., Audiologic findings in an unusual case of eighth nerve lesion. *J. Aud. Res.*, (in press).

14. JERGER, J., CARHART, R., and LASSMAN, JOYCE, Clinical observations on excessive threshold adaptation. *Arch. Otolaryng.*, 68, 1958, 617-623.

15. KOPRA, L. L., Threshold recoveries for continuous and interrupted pure tones following auditory fatigue. *J. acoust. Soc. Amer.*, 27, 1955, 201.

16. KOS, C. M., Auditory function as related to the complaint of dizziness. *Laryngoscope*, 65, 1955, 711-721.

17. LANDES, B. A., Recruitment measured by automatic audiometry. *Arch. Otolaryng.*, 68, 1958, 685-696.

18. LIDÉN, G., Loss of hearing following treatment with dihydrostreptomycin or streptomycin. *Acta Otolaryng.*, 43, 1953, 551-572.

19. LIERLE, D. M., and REGER, S. N., Experimentally induced temporary threshold shifts in ears with impaired hearing. *Ann. Oto. Rhino. Laryng.*, 64, 1955, 263-277.

20. LIERLE, D. M., and REGER, S. N., Further studies of threshold shifts as measured with the Békésy-type audiometer. *Ann. Oto. Rhino. Laryng.*, 63, 1954, 772-784.

21. LUNDBORG, T., Diagnostic problems concerning acoustic tumors. A study of 300 verified cases and the Békésy audiogram in the differential diagnosis. *Acta Otolaryng.*, Suppl. 99, 1952.

22. MISKOLCZY-FODOR, V. F., The Békésy difference limen in bone conduction and recruitment. (in German) *Pract. Oto. Rhino. Laryng.*, 19, 1957, 282-288.

23. MÖLLER, F., and NENZELIUS, C., An accumulation of cases of neurogenous hearing impairment. *Acta Otolaryng.*, 47, 1957, 158-166.

24. PALVA, T., Absolute thresholds for continuous and interrupted pure tones. *Acta Otolaryng.*, 46, 1956, 129-136.

25. PALVA, T., Cochlear vs. retrocochlear lesions. *Laryngoscope*, 68, 1958, 288-299.

26. PALVA, T., Recruitment testing. *Arch. Otolaryng.*, 66, 1957, 93-98.

27. PALVA, T., Recruitment tests at low sensation levels. *Laryngoscope*, 66, 1956, 1519-1540.

28. PALVA, T., Self-recording threshold audiometry and recruitment. *Arch. Otolaryng.*, 65, 1957, 591-602.

29. RANTA, L. J., Acoustic and vestibular disturbances following streptomycin-treated tuberculous meningitis in children. *Acta Otolaryng.*, Suppl. 136, 1958.

30. REGER, S. N., A clinical and research version of the Bekesy audiometer. *Laryngoscope*, 62, 1952, 1333-1351.

31. REGER, S. N., and LIERLE, D. M., Changes in auditory acuity produced by low and medium intensity level exposures. *Trans. Amer. Acad. Ophthal. Oto-laryng.*, 58, 1954, 433-438.

32. RÜEDI, L., Actions of vitamin A on the human and animal ear. *Acta Otolaryng.*, 44, 1954, 502-516.

33. SCHULTHESS, G. v., Evaluation of hearing impairment due to industrial noise. *Arch. Otolaryng.*, 65, 1957, 512-520.

34. TRITTIPOE, W. J., Temporary threshold shift as a function of noise exposure level. *J. acoust. Soc. Amer.*, 30, 1958, 250-253.

35. WEDENBERG, E., Auditory tests on newborn infants. *Acta Otolaryng.*, 46, 1956, 446-461.

36. WEDENBERG, E., Hereditary background of auditory impairment; laboratory detection of heterozygotes of deafness; a Bekesy-audiometric examination of parents with children deaf from birth. *Acta Otolaryng.*, 49, 1958, 451-452.

37. YANTIS, P. A., Clinical applications of the temporary threshold shift. *Arch. Otolaryng.*, 70, 1959, 779-787.

Reprinted from the Archives of Otolaryngology
October 1976, Volume 102
Copyright 1976, American Medical Association

The Cross-Check Principle
in Pediatric Audiometry

James F. Jerger, PhD, Deborah Hayes, MA

• We discuss a method of pediatric audiologic assessment that employs the "cross-check principle." That is, the results of a single test are cross-checked by an independent test measure. Particularly useful in pediatric evaluations as cross-checks of behavioral test results are impedance audiometry and brain-stem-evoked response audiometry (BSER). We present five cases highlighting the value of the cross-check principle in pediatric audiologic evaluation.

(*Arch Otolaryngol* 102:614-620, 1976)

Behavioral observation has been the traditional cornerstone of pediatric audiometry for many years. Some investigators enthusiastically report the success of this method for testing any child, regardless of his level of functioning:

> The trick, if there is any, is to become confidently familiar with the auditory behavior of normal-hearing children regardless of the integrity of their mental processing or central nervous system functioning. Once one knows the hearing level at which these children should respond, as well as the

Accepted for publication May 11, 1976.
From the Department of Otorhinolaryngology and Communicative Sciences, Baylor College of Medicine, Texas Medical Center, Houston.
Reprint requests to Mail Station 009, Methodist Hospital, Texas Medical Center, Houston, TX 77030 (Dr Jerger).

kind of response they will give, the deviation of the deaf child will become patently evident.[1]

We are not so sanguine. We have found that simply observing the auditory behavior of children does not always yield an accurate description of hearing loss. In our own experience, we have seen too many children at all levels of functioning who have been misdiagnosed and mismanaged on the basis of behavioral test results alone.

The mishandling of children based on the results of behavioral audiometry is an increasingly alarming problem. In our own audiology service we are evaluating children at much earlier ages than was common in the past. It is not unusual for us to evaluate infants as young as 5 weeks. Physicians and parents are becoming increasingly aware of the possibilities and implications of hearing loss in infancy. We are also seeing more multiply handicapped children. Special service agencies are requesting audiologic evaluations for these children to determine whether hearing handicap must be considered in planning the educational program. And it is just these two groups of children, very young infants and multiply handicapped children, whom we have found are most often misdiagnosed by behavioral test results alone.

During the past decade two new techniques, uniquely suited to the evaluation of young children, have been made available to clinicians. The first, impedance audiometry, is not only sensitive to middle ear disorders,[2,3] but in the case of normal middle ear function permits quantification of sensorineural level.[4,5] The second technique, brain-stem-evoked response (BSER)[6,7] audiometry, is an electrophysiologic technique that permits the clinician to estimate sensitivity above 500 hertz[8] by both air and bone conduction.

For the past three years, we have used these two techniques in combination with conventional behavioral audiometry as a pediatric test battery. Our fundamental approach has been to use either impedance audiometry or BSER audiometry as a "cross-check" of the behavioral test results.

We reasoned that, if behavioral test results obtained on a child could be confirmed by an independent test measure, then the errors made by behavioral testing alone would be substantially reduced, multiply handicapped children and very young infants could be more accurately tested, and configuration of audiometric contour could be more precisely defined. Impedance audiometry and BSER audiometry appear to be uniquely suited as cross-checks of behavioral test results. It is around these three test measures, behavioral audiometry, impedance audiometry, and BSER audiometry, then, that we have developed a test battery approach for evaluating children.

TEST BATTERY

Behavioral audiometry is used at various levels in our service—from informal observation of a child's response to sound to conditioned play audiometry. Depending on the child's age and level of functioning, we determine the most appropriate behavioral procedure. For very young children we present calibrated speech, toy noise-makers, white noise, or warble tones in the sound field and search for a behavioral response. For slightly older children, we pair the auditory signal with a visual stimulus in the performance of visual reinforcement audiometry. Finally, we use conditioned play audiometry whenever possible to test a child's hearing. Irrespective of the procedure used, however, our audiologic evaluation of the child does not stop with behavioral test results. We always insist that the behavioral result be confirmed by a cross-check.

We use impedance audiometry to confirm behavioral test results in two ways; first, to confirm middle ear disorders when behavioral test results suggest a conductive hearing loss; second, to obtain a rough prediction of the degree of sensorineural hearing loss by comparing the acoustic reflex thresholds for pure tones and for broad-band noise. We have found this prediction of sensorineural hearing loss by the acoustic reflex (SPAR) to be remarkably accurate in children. It is a powerful technique for confirming behavioral test results.

A second test method useful in confirming behavioral test results is BSER audiometry. Evoked responses to rapidly presented clicks are recorded from nontraumatic scalp electrodes and processed by an average-response computer. The latency of the brain stem response ranges from 5 to 8 milliseconds and is age- and intensity-dependent.[6] We use BSER to cross-check behavioral test results whenever impedance audiometry is

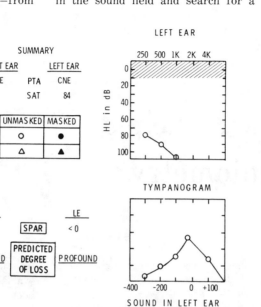

Fig 1.—Case 1—audiogram and impedance results on a 15-year-old boy diagnosed as autistic. Crossed acoustic reflexes appear under tympanograms. The following abbreviations have been used in the figures. CNE, could not evaluate; PTA, pure-tone audiogram; SAT, speech awareness threshold; AC, air conduction; BC, bone conduction; RE, right ear; LE, left ear; HTL, hearing threshold level; BBN, broad-band noise; K, kilohertz.

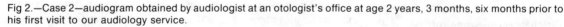

Fig 2.—Case 2—audiogram obtained by audiologist at an otologist's office at age 2 years, 3 months, six months prior to his first visit to our audiology service.

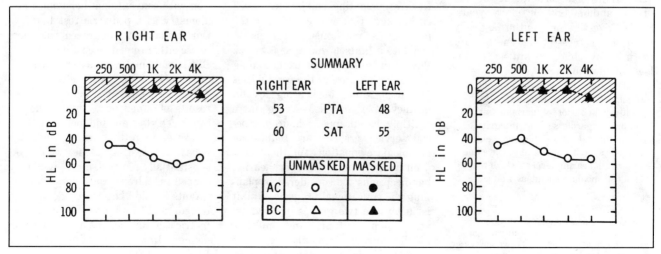

noncontributory in quantifying sensorineural level due to middle ear disorder. We also use BSER to cross-check the results of impedance audiometry when behavioral testing yields no useful information.

Irrespective of the test procedure used to gain an initial impression of a child's hearing—behavioral audiometry, impedance audiometry, or BSER audiometry—we always insist that the initial results be cross-checked by an independent measure. No one test or tester is infallible, and mistakes made with children can have devastating implications. Our experience has been that the confirmation of test results by an independent cross-check can substantially improve the audiological evaluation of children.

REPORT OF CASES

The following five cases illustrate our experience with this cross-check principle in the evaluation of children.

CASE 1.—A 15-year-old boy was referred to our audiology service by the social worker in a community home where he lived. The child had been placed in this home at the age of 8 with the diagnosis of autism. According to the child's mother, he had been identified as deaf at the age of 4. He was fitted with a body-borne hearing aid and placed in a preschool, hearing-impaired program. Noticing no improvement in the child's linguistic skills or behavior, the parents took him to a major university audiology service. The child was then 8 years old. Using psychogalvanic skin response (PGSR) audiometry, this service determined that the child had "normal hearing." Psychological evaluation following this determination of normal hearing resulted in a diagnosis of autism and the child was placed in a seemingly appropriate community center. The social worker at this center, however, did not think that this child's behavior was consistent with autism, and recommended further hearing tests.

The results of our audiologic evaluation are shown in Fig 1. The child's voluntary pure-tone audiogram, obtained by conditioned play audiometry, indicated a profound bilateral hearing loss. Speech awareness thresholds of 90 dB hearing level (HL) in the right ear, and 84 dB HL in the left ear were consistent with pure-tone results.

These behavioral test results were cross-checked by impedance audiometry. Tympanograms were type A bilaterally. Acoustic reflexes were present and elevated to pure-

tone signals of 250 and 500 Hz in both ears. No reflexes could be elicited to either broad-band noise or pure-tone signals above 500 Hz. This reflex pattern is consistent with a severe bilateral sensorineural hearing loss.

In a nonverbal child with supposedly normal hearing, a diagnosis of autism is not unlikely. For this reason, it is imperative to be certain of the hearing level in children with behavior problems. We were "confident" of the results of our behavioral

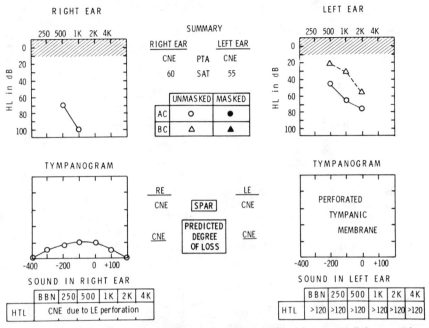

Fig 3.—Case 2—audiogram and impedance results obtained by our audiology service when child was 2 years, 9 months old. Crossed acoustic reflexes appear under tympanograms.

Fig 4.—Case 3—audiogram and impedance results on 4-year, 6-month-old boy. Crossed acoustic reflexes appear under tympanograms. Valid behavioral audiogram could not be obtained.

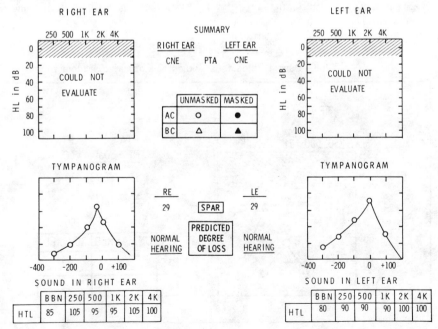

audiometry. Nonetheless, we demanded independent confirmation of these results by a cross-check. Impedance audiometry provided this confirmation.

It is unnecessary to dwell on the tragedy of this child. As long as audiologists are willing to accept the results of a single test measure they will continue to misdiagnose and mismanage some children. Perhaps this error might have been averted if the university audiologist had demanded an independent cross-check of the PGSR findings.

CASE 2.—This patient was a 2-year, 9-month-old boy. Although he had been under the care of an otologist for 18 months for recurrent ear infections, his mother thought that there was more hearing loss present than could be accounted for by simple middle ear disorder. Specifically, she did not notice any improvement in his speech or language after active medical management for middle ear disorder, including insertion of polyethylene tubes. This child's hearing had been tested three times by an audiologist at the physician's office. After each evaluation, the audiologist reported a bilateral moderate conductive hearing loss. Neither a hearing aid nor a preschool language stimulation program had been recommended. The last audiogram obtained at the otologist's office prior to evaluation by our audiology service is shown in Fig 2. These behavioral results indicate a moderate conductive hearing loss bilaterally.

Results of our audiologic evaluation are shown in Fig 3. These results indicated a severe bilateral mixed loss, greater in the right ear. Unmasked bone conduction thresholds indicated a substantial sensorineural component. Results of impedance audiometry were consistent with bilateral

middle ear disorder—a flat, type B tympanogram in the right ear and a perforation in the left ear. Because acoustic reflexes were absent, impedance audiometry could not serve as a cross-check in confirming the degree of sensorineural hearing loss. For this reason, we carried out BSER audiometry. Air-conducted clicks at 80 dB HL failed to elicit responses from either ear.

This finding was consistent with a bilateral air conduction hearing loss of at least 60 dB. Bone-conducted clicks, however, elicited slightly delayed responses at 45 and 55 dB HL. This finding was consistent with a high-frequency, sensorineural hearing loss in the better ear. Brain-stem-evoked response audiometry, therefore, confirmed the results of both behavioral

Results of Hearing Tests on Patient 3 at Four Different Audiology Centers*		
Audiology Center	Age	Result of Evaluation
1	3 yr, 6 mo	Severe hearing loss
2	3 yr, 7 mo	Normal hearing
3	4 yr	Child untestable
4	4 yr	60-dB loss in right ear; 95-dB loss in left ear

*All tests were given within the course of one year.

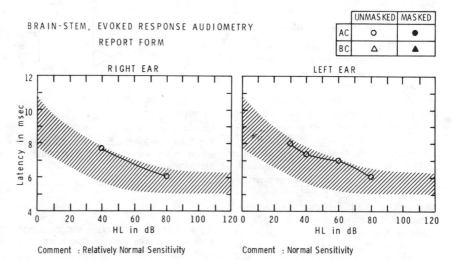

Fig 5.—Case 3—results of BSER audiometry at age 4 years, 6 months.

Fig 6.—Case 4—three serial audiograms obtained at otolaryngologist's office in South America.

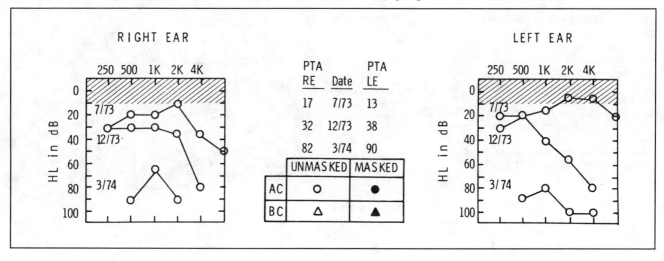

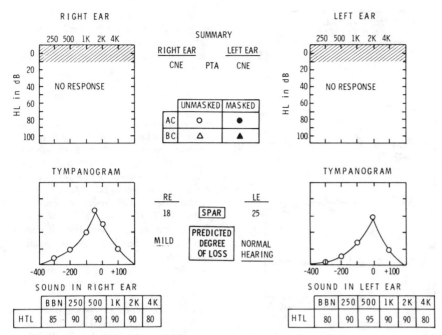

Fig 7.—Case 4—audiogram and impedance results at age 5 years, 9 months. Crossed acoustic reflexes appear under tympanograms. No behavioral responses to either puretone or speech signals at equipment limits.

Fig 8.—Case 4—results of BSER audiometry at age 5 years, 9 months.

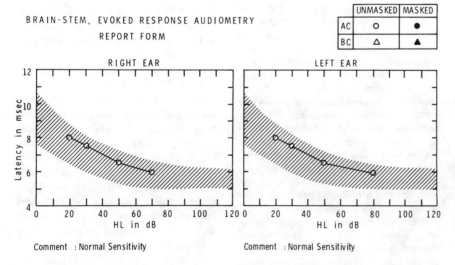

and impedance audiometry. All three measures were consistent with a bilateral, mixed hearing loss.

This case illustrates the use of BSER audiometry to confirm behavioral test results when impedance audiometry cannot contribute an effective cross-check of sensorineural level. This child's chronic middle ear disorder obscured the acoustic reflex, making prediction of sensorineural level impossible. It was essential, therefore, that the behavioral test results be confirmed by an independent procedure so that appropriate remediation could be initiated. By relying on the results of behavioral audiometry alone, the first audiologist unnecessarily delayed identification of this child's sensorineural hearing loss.

CASE 3.—A 4-year, 6-month-old boy was referred to our audiology service by an otologist. This child's hearing was first tested at the age of 3 years, 6 months. In the one year between his first hearing test and his evaluation at the Methodist Hospital, he had been tested by four different audiology facilities. The Table lists the results of these evaluations. The findings of the first evaluation suggested a severe hearing loss. The parents, seeking a second opinion, had the child tested by the second audiology service one month later. This service found normal hearing. The parents then sought a third opinion at an audiology center in another city. This group found the child "untestable" and referred him to a fourth audiological facility. This facility reported a 60-dB loss in the right ear and a 95-dB loss in the left ear. They recommended the use of an ear-level hearing aid and a preschool educational program for the hearing-impaired.

After five months in the special school program, the teacher reported that she thought the child's hearing was normal. The parents then took the child to an otologist, who referred him to our service.

The results of our behavioral and impedance audiometry are shown in Fig 4. We were unable to obtain any consistent responses to either pure tones or speech by behavioral means. Impedance audiometry indicated normal middle ear function. We were able to predict cochlear sensitivity by comparing the acoustic reflex thresholds for pure tones with the reflex threshold for broad-band noise. The SPAR results indicated normal hearing in both ears.

Because of the long history of conflicting behavioral results on this child and our inability to obtain valid behavioral results, it was necessary to cross-check this SPAR prediction of normal cochlear sensitivity by BSER.

The BSER results are shown in Fig 5. Air-conducted clicks evoked responses in the normal range of latencies at 30 dB HL in the left ear, and 40 dB HL in the right ear. These results are consistent with at most, only a mild sensorineural hearing loss. Thus, both impedance and BSER audiometry results are consistent with relatively little sensitivity loss in either ear.

This case illustrates how BSER audiometry can be used as a cross-check on impedance audiometry when behavioral audiometry fails to provide a coherent picture.

CASE 4.—A 5-year, 9-month-old girl was referred to our audiology service by a local otologist in consultation with a pediatric neurologist.

This child developed normally until age 2 years, 6 months, when she had a grand mal seizure of short duration associated with a high temperature. She had a left hemiparesis that lasted 24 hours. Seizure activity, characterized by twitching of the left side of the face, developed. The child was

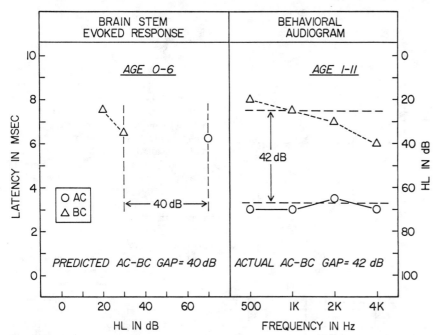

Fig 9.—Case 5—comparison of air-bone gap predicted by BSER audiometry and actual air-bone gap obtained by behavioral means 17 months later. Predicted air-bone gap based on air and bone responses at comparable latencies.

treated with phenobarbital, phenytoin, and diazepam until seizure activity subsided at age 3 years, 9 months. She was seen by an otolaryngologist at age 4 years, 6 months for possible hearing loss since she did not respond normally to verbal commands. Three audiograms, obtained in July 1973, December 1973, and March 1974 at the otolaryngologist's office are shown in Fig 6. These audiograms show a rapid progression in apparent hearing loss, from essentially normal sensitivity in July 1973, to a profound loss in March 1974.

Results of behavioral audiometry and impedance audiometry performed at our service in April 1974 are shown in Fig 7. Behavioral audiometry suggested a profound hearing loss. No consistent responses could be obtained to either pure-tone or speech signals. However, impedance audiometry suggested relatively normal hearing. Acoustic reflexes were present at normal levels to pure tones and broad-band noise in both ears. The SPAR prediction indicated normal sensitivity in the left ear, and, at most, only a mild sensitivity loss in the right ear.

In view of the discrepancy between behavioral and SPAR results, we turned to BSER audiometry as a cross-check. Results are shown in Fig 8. Well-formed responses at normal latencies were observed at 20 dB HL from both ears. This finding confirmed the overall picture of normal peripheral sensitivity predicted by SPAR.

This case again illustrates how BSER audiometry can be used as a cross-check when behavioral and impedance audiometry are discrepant. In view of this child's baffling history, appropriate diagnosis and management of the communication disorder depended on accurate estimation of auditory sensitivity. Following additional extensive testing of speech, language, and psychological and neurological behavior, a diagnosis of auditory agnosia was made, and appropriate therapy was initiated. Had this child been diagnosed as severely hearing-impaired, subsequent rehabilitation and educational management would have been inappropriate.

CASE 5.—A 6-month-old girl was referred to the audiology service by a local child care clinic. The child had first arch syndrome with bilateral atresia and left facial nerve palsy.

Behavioral audiometry suggested a severe, bilateral loss. The infant did not respond to any signal at equipment limits. In this case, impedance audiometry could not be carried out due to the absence of ear canals. However, BSER audiometry could be performed by both air and bone conduction. Air-conducted clicks elicited a response only at 70 dB HL. Bone-conducted clicks, however, elicited responses at 20 and 30 dB HL. These results suggested a large air-bone gap and were consistent with a substantial conductive hearing loss. In fact, comparison of air and bone levels yielding responses at equivalent latencies predicted an air-bone gap of approxi-

mately 40 dB. We therefore fitted the infant with a bone conduction hearing aid and recommended a parent-infant preschool program for hearing-impaired children.

In this case, BSER results could be cross-checked by neither behavioral audiometry nor impedance audiometry. For this reason, we closely monitored this child's progress with her hearing aid. At age 23 months we were able to obtain a satisfactory behavioral audiogram. Unmasked bone conduction responses were between 20 and 30 dB HL from 500 to 2,000 Hz. Air conduction, warble-tone responses were noted at 60 to 70 dB HL across this same range. Thus, behavioral audiometry ultimately confirmed the BSER results obtained at age 6 months.

Figure 9 compares the BSER responses obtained at age 6 months with the behavioral audiogram obtained at age 23 months. Note that the actual air-bone gap (average of 500, 1,000, and 2,000 Hz) is within 2 dB of the air-bone gap predicted by BSER 17 months earlier.

This case illustrates the value of BSER audiometry for early identification when neither impedance audiometry nor behavioral audiometry can be carried out.

COMMENT

What we have attempted to highlight in this article is the value of the cross-check principle in the audiological evaluation of children. Whatever technique may be used in testing a child's hearing, it is important to confirm the result with an independent cross-check. Recent developments have made this principle clinically feasible. Both impedance audiometry and BSER audiometry are viable clinical techniques for cross-checking the result of conventional behavioral audiometry. In our experience, the application of this test battery cross-check principle represents a substantial advance over reliance on a single test approach.

In most instances, behavioral test results can be cross-checked by impedance audiometry alone. In conductive hearing losses, however, the absence of the acoustic reflex prevents the use of the SPAR technique for cross-checking sensorineural level. In such cases, however, BSER can serve as the cross-check measure. In still other cases, behavioral audiometry yields no useful data at all. In these cases, impedance audiometry and BSER audiometry can serve as complementary cross-checks.

In order to implement this cross-check strategy successfully, it is important to recognize the appropriate test battery for a particular child. In so doing, however, one must understand the limitations of each test method.

Behavioral audiometry has several inherent limitations. It is least effective in testing very young children and "difficult-to-test" children. In many cases, the responses of these children are ambiguous and difficult to judge. Many do not give consistent responses to sound even though auditory sensitivity is normal. But these are the very children for whom accurate definition of peripheral sensitivity is often crucial to educational management. Since behavioral audiometry is more effective in older children, the accurate identification of hearing loss by this technique is often unnecessarily delayed.

Even under the best circumstances, mistakes are made when behavioral audiometry is the sole criterion. Observable responses often adapt quickly and are difficult to repeat. With very young infants and children, moreover, auditory signals may have to be considerably above threshold before responses are observed consistently. All of these factors increase the possibility of making a mistake in estimating auditory sensitivity by behavioral test results alone.

Impedance audiometry has its own unavoidable shortcomings. In children with conductive disorders, impedance audiometry is certainly helpful in identifying the middle ear component, but absence of the acoustic reflex prevents the use of the SPAR technique for predicting sensorineural level. Similarly, central auditory disorders due to brain damage may abolish acoustic reflexes even though peripheral sensitivity is normal. Impedance audiometry also requires a relatively quiet child. Some children resist earphones and the probe tip to such a degree that impedance audiometry is not feasible without sedation.

The major problem with BSER audiometry is the need for sedation. To obtain satisfactory BSER responses from both ears over a full range of click intensities, the child must be relatively quiescent for about one hour. Infants and very young children can usually be tested in natural sleep. Children between ages 18 months and 4 years, however, often require sedation. In our experience, chloral hydrate in the dosage 50 mg/kg of body weight is usually satisfactory. In some cases, however, more effective sedation is required.

In summary, we believe that the unique limitations of conventional behavioral audiometry dictate the need for a "test battery" approach. The key concept governing our assessment strategy is the cross-check principle. The basic operation of this principle is that no result be accepted until it is confirmed by an independent measure. In most cases, impedance audiometry serves as an effective cross-check of behavioral audiometry. If they disagree, however, BSER audiometry can serve as a further cross-check. In cases in which behavioral audiometry fails, a consistent, cross-checked picture can still emerge from the combination of impedance and BSER audiometry. We believe that the application of the cross-check principle to our clinical population has had an appreciable effect on the accuracy with which we can identify and quantify hearing loss during the critical years for language-learning.

This study was supported by National Institutes of Health program project grant NS 10940. Toni Weaver, Francis Catlin, and Gail Neely provided assistance and encouragement throughout this research.

References

1. Northern J, Downs M: *Hearing in Children.* Baltimore, Williams & Wilkins Co, 1974, p 137.
2. Jerger J: Clinical experience with impedance audiometry. *Arch Otolaryngol* 92:311-324, 1970.
3. Jerger S, Jerger J, Mauldin L, et al: Studies in impedance audiometry: II. Children less than six years old. *Arch Otolaryngol* 99:1-9, 1974.
4. Jerger J, Burney P, Mauldin L, et al: Predicting hearing loss from the acoustic reflex. *J Speech Hear Disord* 39:11-22, 1974.
5. Jerger J: Diagnostic use of impedance measures, in Jerger J (ed): *Handbook of Clinical Impedance Audiometry.* Dobbs Ferry, NY, American Electromedics Corp, 1975.
6. Hecox K, Galambos R: Brain stem auditory evoked responses in human infants and adults. *Arch Otolaryngol* 99:30-33, 1974.
7. Sohmer H, Feinmesser M, Bauberger-Tell L, et al: Routine use of cochlear audiometry in infants with uncertain diagnosis. *Ann Otol Rhinol Laryngol* 81:1-4, 1972.
8. Davis H, Hirsh S: The audiometric utility of brain stem responses to low-frequency sound. *Int Aud* 15:181-195, 1976.

Reprinted from the Archives of Otolaryngology
April 1977, Volume 103
Copyright 1977, American Medical Association

Diagnostic Speech Audiometry

James Jerger, PhD, Deborah Hayes, MA

● The scope of speech audiometry can be expanded to provide useful diagnostic information. Comparison of performance vs intensity (PI) functions for both phonemically balanced (PB) words and synthetic sentence identification (SSI) yields patterns useful in differentiating among peripheral and central sites of auditory disorder.

(Arch Otolaryngol 103:216-222, 1977)

The diagnostic value of traditional speech audiometry is extremely limited. If measurement is confined to the usual combination of spondee threshold and "PB max" at a single suprathreshold level, the performance variation within distinct diagnostic categories is so great that there is a real problem of overlapping ranges.[1,2] The difficulty is further compounded by the extreme dependence of monosyllabic word intelligibility on high-frequency sensitivity loss,[3,4] a factor which places the PB score at the mercy of audiometric configuration to an undesirable extent. For very thorough and insightful treatment of the general problem of diagnostic speech audiometry the interested reader is urged to obtain a copy of the report entitled "A Feasibility Study of Diagnostic Speech Audiometry," by P. Lyregaard, D. Robinson, and R. Hinchcliffe.[5]

During the past several years, we have experimented with a combination of speech tests designed to produce more useful diagnostic information. The test battery includes performance vs intensity (PI) functions for both conventional phonemically balanced (PB) monosyllables and for the synthetic sentence identification (SSI) task. In actual test-battery administration, blocks of 25 PB words are presented at four to six speech levels in order to define the PI-PB function, and blocks of ten sentences are presented, usually at the same levels, to define the PI-SSI function.

The importance of defining a reasonably complete PI function for each set of speech materials cannot be overemphasized. Presentation of a single block of either PB words or sentences at a single level, assumed to be at the plateau or maximum of the PI function, is almost never satisfactory for two reasons. First, in the cases of greatest interest, eighth nerve and central disorders, the exact shape of the PI function is so unpredictable that the speech level producing maximum performance can seldom be accurately estimated *a priori*. Second, the consistency of the relationship between the two complete functions, over their entire range, often reveals subtle effects not as evident or discernible from a comparison of single scores.

METHOD

Our speech audiometric materials were all recorded on magnetic tape by a single male talker. Six of the original 50-word PB lists developed by Egan[6] constitute a pool of 300 PB words from which the PI-PB functions are constructed. For the PI-SSI function, the same list of ten third-order sentences[7] has been recorded in nine different scramblings. Furthermore, sentences are always presented in the presence of competing continuous discourse recorded at the same level as the test sentences (ie, message-to-competition ratio, or MCR of 0 dB).[8] For a more complete description of the rationale and test methods for generating O-MCR, SSI functions, see "A New Approach to Speech Audiometry," by J. Jerger, C. Speaks, and J. Trammell.[8]

Each ear is tested separately, and the non test ear is always masked by white noise whenever the possibility of crossover exists. This is a particularly important consideration at the relatively high speech levels we often employ in order to define the exact shape of the PI function over its entire extent.

To date, we have carried out this complete speech audiometric testing procedure on over 3,000 patients evaluated by the Audiology Services affiliated with the Department of Otorhinolaryngology and Communicative Sciences of the Baylor College of Medicine.

In the following sections, we attempt to show how a comparison of the two PI functions, one for words, the other for sentences, can provide useful information relating both to shape of audiometric configuration and to site of auditory disorder.

RESULTS

Analysis of the relationship between the PI function for words and sentences reveals several distinct patterns. In general, we can discern cochlear, eighth nerve, and central effects. In the cochlear effect, the exact pattern depends heavily on audiometric contour. The eighth nerve effect is a characteristic modification in the shape of one or both PI functions, but is less dependent on the exact shape of the audiometric contour. The central effect is largely independent of the audiogram, but shows interesting age-related changes.

Cochlear Patterns

In patients with peripheral sensitivity loss of presumably cochlear origin, three distinct relationships between the PI-PB and the PI-SSI function emerge, depending on the audiometric contour.

Accepted for publication Dec 15, 1976.

From the Department of Otorhinolaryngology and Communicative Sciences, Baylor College of Medicine, Houston.

Presented at the 13th International Congress of Audiology, Florence, Italy, Oct 20, 1976.

Reprint requests to Department of Otorhinolaryngology and Communicative Sciences, Baylor College of Medicine, 1200 Moursund Ave, Houston, TX 77030 (Dr Jerger).

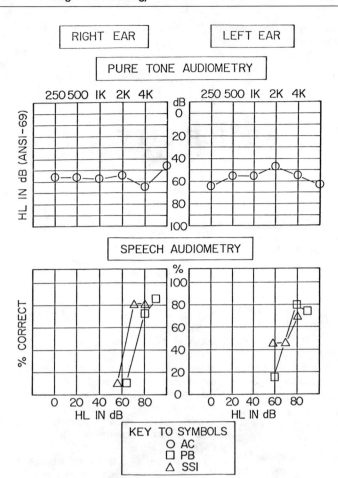

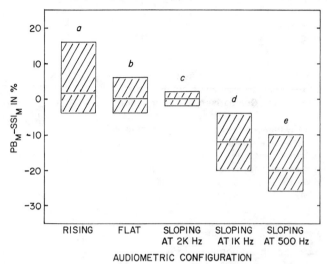

Fig 1.—Audiogram and PI functions for 51-year-old man with moderately severe flat, bilateral sensorineural loss (case 1).

Fig 2.—Median and interquartile range of the PB-SSI max difference scores for patients with rising, flat, and sloping audiometric configurations. All patients were between 10 and 59 years old.

Fig 3.—Audiogram and PI functions for 15-year-old girl with markedly sloping, high-frequency loss in left ear (case 2).

Fig 4.—Audiogram and PI functions for 39-year-old woman with rising sensorineural loss in right ear (case 3).

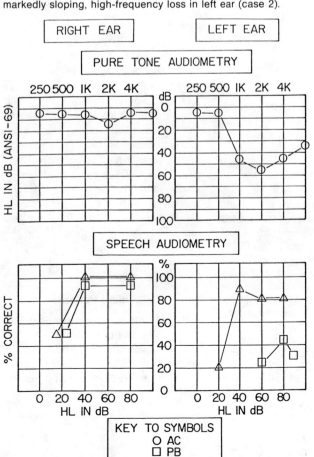

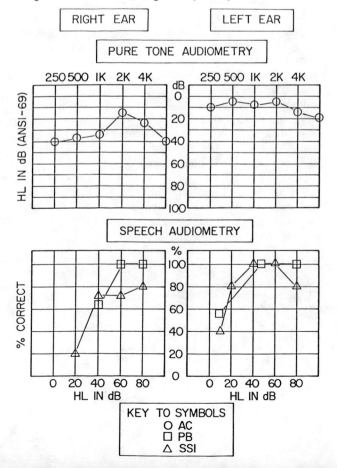

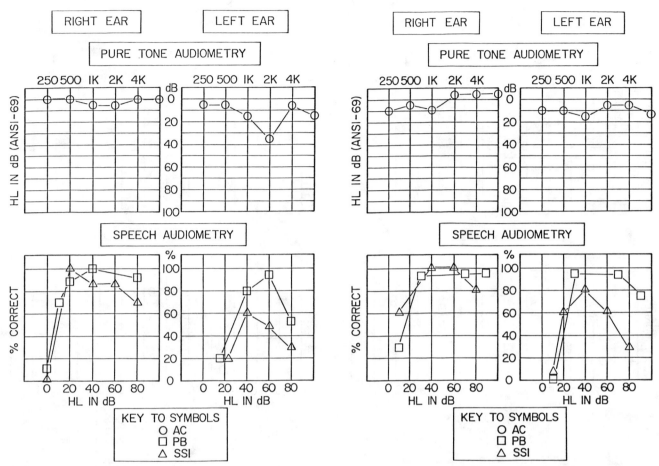

Fig 5.—Audiogram and PI functions for 53-year-old woman with left acoustic tumor. Rollover of both PI functions at high intensity levels is evident (case 4).

Fig 6.—Audiogram and PI functions for 32-year-old woman with multiple sclerosis. In spite of normal sensitivity SSI function remains consistently below PB function in left ear, and exhibits marked rollover at high intensity levels (case 5).

Patients with relatively flat sensitivity loss typically show similar, if not identical, PI functions for both words and sentences. Figure 1 (case 1) illustrates this peripheral effect in a 51-year-old man with a gradually progressive hearing loss. The pure-tone audiogram reveals a moderately severe flat bilateral sensorineural loss. Speech audiometry shows four very similar functions. On the right ear, the PB max is 84%, and the SSI max is 80%. On the left ear, the PB max is 80%, and the SSI max is 70%.

In general, whenever the audiometric contour is relatively flat the two PI functions show this close correspondence. Both shape and maxima are in good agreement.

In order to quantify the degree of this correspondence, we formed a subsample of 132 patients showing a relatively flat audiometric configuration on one ear. "Flatness" was defined as a threshold difference no greater than 20 dB over the range from 500 to 2,000 Hz. No patient in this group was over 59 years old. The pure-tone average on the test ear was always more than 20 dB, but less than 60 dB hearing level (HL). In order to ensure statistical independence of observations, data from only one ear of each patient were used. On each such test ear, we computed the difference between the maximum PB score and the maximum SSI score. The median and interquartile range of this PB-SSI difference are shown in block "b" of Fig 2. The median difference was 0%, with an interquartile range of 10% (−4% to +6%). The implication of these results is that in patients with flat audiometric configurations, the expected difference between the PB max and the SSI max is zero. Furthermore, the two maxima should agree within approximately ±10%.

In patients with sloping high-frequency loss, however, the PB function usually falls somewhat below the SSI function. Figure 3 (case 2) illustrates this relationship in a 15-year-old girl with a unilateral high-frequency loss. In the right ear, where pure-tone sensitivity is normal, the PI-PB and PI-SSI functions are in close agreement. In the left ear, however, where the audiogram shows a markedly sloping high-frequency loss, the PB function falls well below the SSI function. The SSI max is 90%, but the PB max is only 44%.

This discrepancy can be attributed largely to the penalizing effect of the audiometric contour on monosyllabic word repetition. Since the PB score depends on high-frequency consonant recognition to a much greater degree

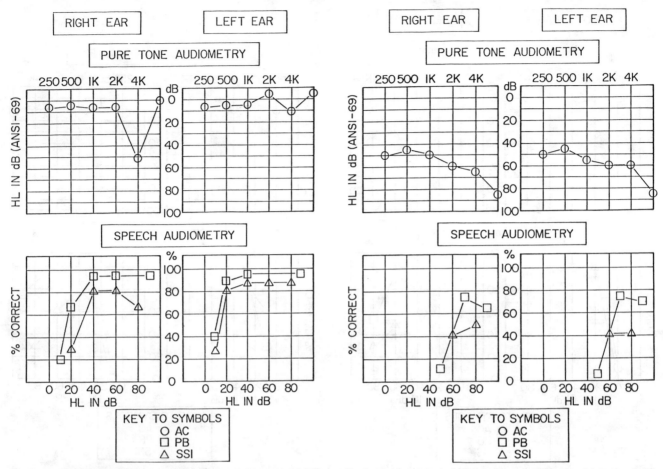

Fig 7.—Audiogram and PI functions for 30-year-old man with left temporal lobe tumor. Slight, but consistent depression of SSI max relative to PB max is evident in ear contralateral to lesion, right ear (case 6).

Fig 8.—Audiogram and PI functions for 82-year-old woman with moderate, bilateral hearing loss. Typical aging effect of SSI max substantially below PB max is seen bilaterally (case 7).

than the SSI score, the effect of this audiometric contour must inevitably be greater on the PI-PB function than on the PI-SSI function.

In general, the magnitude of the discrepancy is directly proportional to the steepness of the audiometric slope and inversely proportional to the frequency at which the slope begins. These relationships are so predictable that the PB-SSI discrepancy is virtually a cross-check on the accuracy of the pure-tone audiogram. Furthermore, the observation that PB max is below SSI max indicates that the effect is peripheral rather than central.

These relationships are quantitatively illustrated in Fig 2. Here are summarized the median and interquartile range of the PB-SSI difference in three groups of patients with sloping configurations. Block "c" sum-marizes results in 78 patients with normal sensitivity up to 2,000 Hz but with a steeply sloping drop of at least 40 dB between 2,000 and 4,000 Hz. Block "d" summarizes results for 23 patients with steeply sloping contours breaking at 1,000 Hz. Block "e" sum-marizes results for 15 patients in whom the slope begins at 500 Hz. In all cases, the slope in the octave above the cut-off frequency was more than 30 but less than 50 dB. Note how the median difference relates to cut-off frequency. When the cut-off is 2,000 Hz, the high-frequency loss has virtually no differential effect. When the cut-off is 1,000 Hz, however, the maximum PB score is 12% below the maximum SSI score. And, when the cut-off frequency is 500 Hz, the median difference is a substantial 20%. Furthermore, in the two groups of patients with sloping audiometric configurations beginning at 1,000 Hz and at 500 Hz, the expected result (ie, PB max falling below the SSI max) occurred in 92% of the cases.

In patients with rising audiometric configurations, where high-frequency sensitivity is better than low-frequency sensitivity, the SSI function typically falls somewhat below the PB function.

Figure 4 (case 3) illustrates this third peripheral effect in a 39-year-old woman with right labyrinthine hydrops. On the left ear, where the pure-tone audiogram is normal, the two PI functions interweave. On the right ear, however, where the audiometric contour rises from 40 dB at 250 Hz to 15 dB at 2,000 Hz, the SSI functions levels off at only 80%, while the PB function climbs to 100%. Again, the direction of this discrepancy is entirely predictable from the shape of the

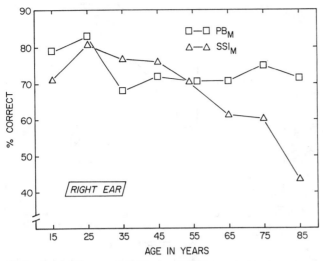
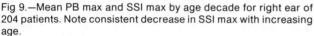

Fig 9.—Mean PB max and SSI max by age decade for right ear of 204 patients. Note consistent decrease in SSI max with increasing age.

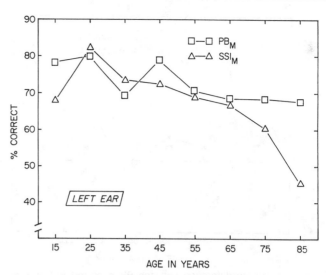

Fig 10.—Mean PB max and SSI max by age decade for left ear of 204 patients.

audiometric contour. Since the SSI score is more dependent on low-frequency information than the PB score, the effect of the rising audiometric pattern must inevitably be greater for SSI than for PB.

Figure 2 illustrates the rising peripheral effect. Block "a" of this figure shows the median and interquartile range of the PB-SSI average difference for 39 patients with rising audiometric contours. "Rise" in contour was defined as a 20-dB difference or more between 500 and 2,000 Hz. The median difference for this group was 2%, with a semiinterquartile range of 20% (−4% to +16%). Note that the rising peripheral effect is less pronounced than the sloping peripheral effect. This is not unexpected, since the sentence materials are substantially less frequency-dependent than the PB words.

These three peripheral patterns may be summarized as follows:

1. When the audiometric contour is relatively flat, the PI-PB and PI-SSI functions will be in good agreement.

2. When the audiometric contour slopes downward from low to high frequencies, the PB function will fall below the SSI function.

3. When the audiometric contour slopes upward from low to high frequencies, the SSI function will fall below the PB function.

Since these effects are determined by the nature of the audiometric contour, the PB-SSI relationship serves as a valuable cross-check on the audiogram. Whenever the expected peripheral effect does not appear, a concomitant retrocochlear or central effect must be suspected.

Eighth Nerve Patterns

In patients with eighth nerve disorder, the relationship between PB and SSI functions is less predictable from the audiometric contour. In general, the peripheral rules hold in the sense that PB max tends to be below SSI max in sloping high-frequency contours, and SSI tends to be below PB in rising low-frequency contours, but the effects are often wildly exaggerated, with differences of 50% to 60% in the two functions when the audiometric contour is only gently sloping. At other times, both functions are so depressed that little difference appears in spite of a sharply sloping audiometric contour.

To examine the eighth nerve effect more closely, we analyzed the PB max-SSI max difference in a series of 13 patients with radiographically or surgically confirmed eighth nerve tumors. The median PB-SSI difference was +2%. The interquartile range, however, was 52% (−42% to +10%), reflecting substantial variability in performance on the two speech tests. Although the peripheral-effect rules generally hold for patients with eighth nerve disorder, neither the direction nor the magnitude of the effect is usually predictable.

The distinguishing feature of eighth nerve disorders, however, is a characteristic modification in the shape of one or both PI functions.[9] At high speech intensity levels, the functions tend to show a paradoxical decrease in performance with increasing level. This "rollover" phenomenon is the signature of the eighth nerve site, although it may also appear in some cases with more central sites.

Figure 5 (case 4) illustrates this shape modification in a 53-year-old woman with a left intracannilicular acoustic tumor. The 36% difference between the PB max (96%) and the SSI max (60%) on the left ear is not particularly predicted from the left audiometric contour, but both PI functions showed marked evidence of the rollover phenomenon.

Notice, again, the importance of defining the entire PI function, especially at high levels.

Central Patterns

In patients with central auditory disorder, the SSI function typically falls well below the PB function. In contrast to the similar peripheral pattern with rising audiogram, however, the effect is not consistent with the audiometric contour. The large SSI-PB discrepancy is typically present in ears with quite normal sensitiv-

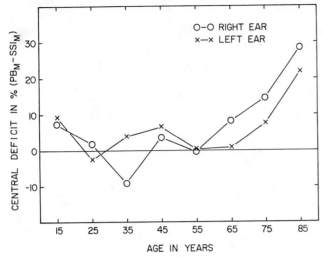

Fig 11.—Average difference between PB max and SSI max at each age decade for each ear. This central deficit (PB max-SSI max) begins at about age 60 and increases substantially thereafter. Right ear shows greater effect than left ear.

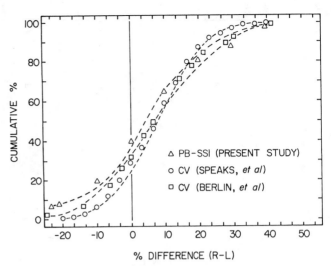

Fig 12.—Comparison of cumulative distribution function for right-left difference in PB-SSI discrepancy with analagous cumulative distribution functions for right-left difference in dichotic consonant-vowel listening task in young adults reported by Speaks et al[13] and C. Berlin (written communication, October 1976).

ity. Figure 6 (case 5) illustrates this central effect in a 32-year-old woman with multiple sclerosis. The pure-tone audiogram is relatively normal in both ears. On the right ear, the two speech functions interweave in normal fashion. On the left ear, however, the SSI function falls well below the PB function and shows the rollover effect. At 40 dB HL, the two functions are separated by less than 20%. At 80 dB HL, however, the discrepancy is almost 60%.

This case illustrates a number of important points about diagnostic speech audiometry. The patient complained of a "plugged-up" sensation in her left ear and difficulty in using the telephone on the left ear. In spite of these distinctly auditory symptoms, results of conventional speech audiometry would have looked quite normal. The PB max at 40 dB sensation level (SL) would have been 96% in each ear. These scores, coupled with virtually normal audiograms, could easily have led to the conclusion that auditory function was quite normal.

The PB-SSI discrepancy, however, demonstrated the central auditory involvement. Note, further, the importance of defining the complete PI function. Again, if words and sentences had been presented at 40 dB HL only, the presence of the central effect would not have been so obvious, since the discrepancy at this level was

only about 16%. However, when the entire PI function was defined, the presence of the central effect was demonstrated with startling clarity.

Figure 7 (case 6) illustrates the central effect in a 30-year-old man with a left temporal lobe glioblastoma. Except for a 4,000-Hz notch on the right ear, pure-tone sensitivity was well within normal limits on both ears. On the left ear, the two PI functions were normal. On the right ear, however, the SSI function is substantially below the PB function. Again we may note that the PB scores alone fail to demonstrate the central auditory involvement, and that definition of the complete PI function demonstrates the reliability of the discrepancy although the absolute size of the difference at any single level seldom exceeds 20%.

This case illustrates an additional characteristic of the central effect. The discrepancy appears on the ear contralateral to the affected side of the brain.[10] Here, the left temporal lobe is involved, and the PB-SSI discrepancy appears on the right ear.

The Aging Effect

The effect of age on speech scores may be considered a special case of the central effect. Unlike younger people with central auditory disorders, however, the elderly typically show both pure-tone sensitivity loss and de-

creased PB scores. The SSI function, however, usually falls below the PB function to a greater or lesser extent in the elderly population, a fact which we attribute to a central aging effect.

Figure 8 (case 7) illustrates this aging effect in an 82-year-old woman with a 20-year history of progressive hearing loss. The pure-tone audiograms show the typical presbycusic pattern. The PB functions show quite low maxima; 76% in the right ear and 76% in the left ear. Note, however, that the SSI maxima are even lower: 50% in the right ear and 40% in the left ear. If this patient's hearing disorder were on a purely peripheral basis, we would expect the PB functions to be either the same as the SSI functions, or perhaps slightly worse due to the sloping configuration of the audiometric contour. The fact that the SSI functions are, in fact, well below the PB functions may be attributed to the central aging effect.

In an effort to define the effect of age on the PB-SSI discrepancy more precisely, we reviewed the files of all patients tested with both speech materials at The Methodist Hospital Audiology Service for the past two years to define a subgroup of patients with sensorineural loss covering the entire range from ten to 90 years.

Excluded from consideration were all patients with conductive or mixed loss, all patients with known retro-cochlear disorders, and all patients whose PB or SSI max scores were either 0% or 100% on either ear. This rather severe selection process produced a subgroup of 204 patients with sensorineural loss, all of whose speech maxima fell within the floor and ceiling of each test on each ear. The 204 subjects were then categorized into eight age decades, beginning with the 10 to 19 year decade, and ending with the 80 to 89 year decade. The number of subjects in each age decade ranged from a low of six subjects in the 10 to 19 decade to a high of 67 subjects in the 60 to 69 decade.

Mean PB and SSI max scores were computed for each ear at each age decade. Figure 9 shows the result of this analysis for the right ear, and Fig 10 shows results for the left ear.

Performance on both sets of materials decreases with increasing age, a not unexpected finding.[11] Note, however, that SSI decreases more than PB. In the right ear, for example, the mean PB max decreases from a high of 83%, in the 20 to 29 year decade, to a low of 71% in the 60 to 69 year decade. The SSI max, however, decreases from a high of 81% in the 20 to 21 year decade to a low of only 43% in the 80 to 89 decade. The left ear shows a similar pattern. On both ears the mean PB and SSI max scores interweave up to about age 60. Above that age, however, the mean SSI max score falls dramatically below the mean PB max as the central aging effect grows ever larger.

In comparing Fig 9 and 10, we seemed to note a larger average central aging effect on the right ear than on the left ear. To examine this possibility in greater detail, we computed the average difference between PB max and SSI max at each age decade and for each ear. These mean differences are plotted in Fig 11. A positive difference indicates that SSI is below PB. Note that the two ears interweave around zero difference up to the 50 to 59 year decade. Above this age the right ear shows an increasing central deficit with increasing age. The left ear shows a similar but slightly attenuated effect. The central

effect begins, on the average, at about the age of 60 and increases substantially thereafter. A similar right ear deficit in the aged was noted by Palva and Jokinen[12] using filtered words.

The intersubject variability of this "central effect" ear difference is remarkably similar to the variability of the familiar right ear effect in dichotic listening. In Fig 12 we compare the cumulative distribution function for the right-left difference in our central effect with analogous data from dichotic CV studies of Speaks et al[13] and C. Berlin (communication, 1976). Our own curve is based on data from 96 subjects over age 60. The data of Speaks *et al* are from eight young adults, and the Berlin data are from 55 young adults.

The similarity of the distribution of the right-left difference in these various studies is certainly intriguing, especially since the type of subjects and nature of the listening tasks are so different.

COMMENT

Inevitably, some will argue that the time required to carry out all the measurements necessary for the definition of two complete PI functions on each ear is prohibitive. Actually, the total additional testing time is not all that great. Complete testing of both ears can usually be completed in less than 30 minutes. We would argue that the additional diagnostic information yielded by these functions more than justifies the time involved.

The information is useful in four ways. First, if the relationship between the two functions is consistent with audiometric contour, and significant rollover is not present in either function, then a purely peripheral cochlear site may be reasonably inferred. Second, if the difference between the two functions is out of proportion to either degree or shape of audiometric contour, and if substantial rollover is apparent in either function, an eighth nerve site must be suspected. Third, whenever the SSI function falls below the PB function, and the difference cannot be explained as a peripheral effect due to an audiometric configuration that

rises from low to high frequencies, then a central auditory site must be suspected. Fourth, in the elderly patient with presbycusis, the combination of audiometric contour and direction and magnitude of the PB-SSI discrepancy yields a rough estimate of the relative contributions of peripheral and central effects to the patients total auditory impairment. This factor, the "peripheral-central ratio," may ultimately prove useful in judging the prognosis for successful use of a hearing aid or other rehabilitative measure.

For these various reasons we suggest that the scope of speech audiometry can be expanded to truly diagnostic dimensions by measuring complete PI functions for both word recognition and sentence identification.

This research was supported in part by program project grant NS 10940 from the National Institutes of Health.

Lois Anthony, Toni Weaver, Susan Floyd, Sharron Smith, Connie Jordan, and Jay Hall assisted in the collection and analysis of data.

References

1. Jerger J, Harford E, Clemis J, et al: The acoustic reflex in eighth nerve disorders. *Arch Otolaryngol* 99:409-413, 1974.

2. Johnson E: Auditory test results in 268 cases of confirmed retro-cochlear lesions. *Audiology* 9:15-19, 1970.

3. Speaks C, Jerger J, Trammell J: Comparison of sentence identification and conventional speech discrimination scores. *J Speech Hearing Res* 13:755-767, 1970.

4. Jerger S, Jerger J: Estimating speech threshold from the PI-PB function. *Arch Otolaryngol* 102:487-496, 1976.

5. Lyregaard P, Robinson D, Hinchcliffe R: *A Feasibility Study of Diagnostic Speech Audiometry*. United Kingdom, National Physical Laboratory, Department of Industry, January 1976.

6. Egan J: Articulation testing methods. *Laryngoscope*. 58:955-991, 1948.

7. Speaks C, Jerger J: Method for the measurement of speech identification. *J Speech Hearing Res* 8:185-194, 1965.

8. Jerger J, Speaks C, Trammel J: A new approach to speech audiometry. *J Speech Hearing Dis* 33:318-328, 1968.

9. Jerger J, Jerger S: Diagnostic significance of PB word functions. *Arch Otolaryngol* 93:573-580, 1971.

10. Jerger S, Jerger J: Extra-and-intra-axial brain-stem auditory disorders. *Audiology* 14:93-117, 1975.

11. Jerger J: Audiological findings in aging. *Adv Otorhinolaryngol* 20:115-124, 1973.

12. Palva A, Jokinen J: Presbyacusis: V. Filtered speech test. *Acta Otolaryngol* 70:232-241, 1970.

13. Speaks C; Niccum N, Carney E: The bivariate normal distribution of paired responses in dichotic stimulation with speech. *J Acoust Soc Am*, to be published.

NORMAL AUDIOMETRIC FINDINGS

James Jerger, Ph.D. and Connie Jordan, M.S.

ABSTRACT

We argue that the scope of basic audiometric assessment must be broadened to include speech audiometric measures sensitive to central auditory dysfunction. Findings in twenty cases of retrocochlear disorder illustrate the fact that conventional criteria of audiometric normalcy are inadequate.

Many otologists and audiologists commonly describe as "audiometrically normal" anyone whose test results show normal sensitivity for pure tones and normal speech discrimination scores.[1-5] Commonly accepted contemporary criteria include pure-tone threshold hearing levels of less than 20 dB from 250 through 8000 Hz, and speech discrimination (PB max) scores of 86 to 100 percent. Any patient whose audiograms and PB max scores meet these criteria is said to exhibit "normal" audiometric findings.

During the past decade, however, advances in diagnostic audiometry, especially speech audiometry, have highlighted the fact that significant central auditory dysfunction can exist without substantial effect on either pure-tone sensitivity or simple monosyllabic word test scores.[6-16] Thus, many patients with brainstem and/or temporal lobe auditory disorder easily pass the traditional criteria for normalcy.

We argue that a more stringent definition of audiometric normalcy is necessary. In this discussion we present data on twenty patients with significant auditory disorder who were "normal" by conventional criteria but who were consistently abnormal on more sensitive measures of speech understanding.

Two measures, PB rollover [17-19] and PB-SSI discrepancy,[20] were selected to illustrate the point. PB rollover is defined as an excessive (20 percent or more) decline in PB performance as speech intensity is increased above the maximum of the performance vs. intensity (PI) function for PB words. PB-SSI discrepancy is a difference (20 percent or more) between the PI-PB function and the PI-SSI function which cannot be accounted for by the audiometric contour.

Table 1 summarizes pure-tone and speech audiometric data on twenty patients with well-documented auditory disorder at the eighth nerve or brainstem level. Final diagnosis was eighth nerve tumor in three cases, extra-axial brainstem tumor in three cases, intra-axial tumor in two cases, brainstem (CVA) in one case, and multiple sclerosis in eleven cases. Tumors were documented either by surgery or radiography; multiple sclerosis by McAlpines criteria.[21]

For each subject we list age, sex, PTA (average of threshold; at 500, 1000, and 2000 Hz), conventional PB max score (highest point on PI-PB function), PB rollover (difference between PB max score and poorest score above PB max), and PB-SSI discrepancy (difference between PB max and SSI max). For each subject, we present results for only one ear, the ear of interest in relation to the disorder. In all cases, the other ear showed either no abnormality whatever or a configuration of results similar to the ear of interest. Finally, in both ears of all cases, no threshold hearing level at any frequency exceeded 20 dB HL.

Table 1 shows that PTA on the ear of interest ranged from 0–20 dB, and PB max ranged from 88 to 100 percent. In fourteen of the twenty subjects, the PB max score was actually 100 percent. Yet each of the subjects showed an abnormality on one or both of the more sophisticated speech measures. There was significant rollover of the PI-PB function in eleven cases, and a significant PB-SSI discrepancy in fifteen cases. Every one of the twenty patients had a significant abnormality on at least one of these two measures.

Department of Otorhinolaryngology and Communicative Sciences, Baylor College of Medicine, Texas Medical Center, Houston, Texas.

Reprint requests: James Jerger, Ph.D., 11922 Taylorcrest, Houston, Texas 77024

TABLE 1.   AUDIOMETRIC FINDINGS IN 20 PATIENTS WITH RETROCOCHLEAR AUDITORY DYSFUNCTION

Subject No.	Age	Sex	PTA	PB Max %	PB Rollover %	PB-SSI Discrepancy %	Final Diagnosis
1	37	F	08	88	46 (+)	48 (+)	Eighth nerve tumor
2	48	F	20	100	0	30 (+)	Multiple sclerosis
3	36	M	00	100	36 (+)	0	Multiple sclerosis
4	53	F	18	96	40 (+)	46 (+)	Eighth nerve tumor
5	49	M	18	100	30 (+)	40 (+)	Multiple sclerosis
6	50	F	02	100	32 (+)	10	Extra-axial brainstem tumor
7	54	M	04	100	0	30 (+)	Multiple sclerosis
8	25	F	02	100	08	42 (+)	Extra-axial brainstem tumor
9	36	F	03	100	04	20 (+)	Multiple sclerosis
10	50	M	10	96	04	92 (+)	Multiple sclerosis
11	38	F	13	100	44 (+)	10	Extra-axial brainstem tumor
12	50	F	11	100	08	50 (+)	Multiple sclerosis
13	34	M	10	100	44 (+)	30 (+)	Multiple sclerosis
14	30	M	08	100	04	40 (+)	Multiple sclerosis
15	72	M	13	96	16	20 (+)	Brainstem CVA
16	18	F	13	92	36 (+)	46 (+)	Multiple sclerosis
17	07	F	12	96	76 (+)	CNE	Intra-axial brainstem tumor
18	55	F	01	100	0	30 (+)	Multiple sclerosis
19	33	F	07	100	28 (+)	20 (+)	Eighth nerve tumor
20	06	M	13	100	30 (+)	CNE	Intra-axial brainstem tumor

(+) Retrocochlear finding.
CNE Could not evaluate.

DISCUSSION

The twenty cases summarized in Table 1 illustrate the important point that our definition of "audiometric normalcy" must be expanded beyond the conventional criteria of pure-tone sensitivity and simple speech discrimination score. We recommend, as a minimum, the following additional criteria:

(1)   Normal performance-intensity (PI) function for PB words (i.e., absence of significant rollover); and

(2)   Satisfactory performance on at least one additional speech intelligibility test specifically sensitive to central auditory dysfunction. There are several possible tests available for this purpose:
  (a)   Synthetic Sentence Identification (SSI) test
  (b)   Staggered Spondee Word (SSW) test
  (c)   Time-Compressed Monosyllabic Words (W22 or NU-6)
  (d)   Monosyllabic Words with Competing Message (W22 or NU-6).

All of the above are commercially available in tape-recorded form.

Our argument is that unless the definition of audiometric normalcy is expanded to encompass more sensitive speech audiometric measures, a significant number of patients with retrocochlear auditory dysfunction will be incorrectly classified as "audiometrically normal."

In view of the additional testing time required for such an expanded concept, however, the issue of cost-effectiveness must be considered. Can the additional testing time be justified in terms of the number of cases likely to be identified? To a considerable extent the answer to this question will depend on the nature of the clinical population being served. In the typical nonmedical University speech and hearing clinic, for example, it may be difficult to justify the additional testing time required for sophisticated audiometric evaluation.

In the typical hospital setting, however, where referrals from otologists, neurologists, and neurosurgeons are relatively common, the increased sophistication of the basic audiometric assessment will, in our experience, more than justify the additional testing time required by the strategy proposed.

REFERENCES

1.   Dolowitz D: Basic Otolaryngology. New York: McGraw-Hill, 1952, pp 47–66
2.   Hirsh I: The Measurement of Hearing. New York: McGraw-Hill, 1952, pp 276–301
3.   Goetzinger CP: Word discrimination testing. In Katz J(Ed): Handbook of Clinical Audiology. Baltimore: Williams & Wilkins, 1972, pp 157–79
4.   DeWeese DD, Saunders W: Textbook of Otolaryngology. St. Louis: C.V.Mosby, 1977, pp 295–312
5.   Heffernan HP, Simons MR, Goodhill V: Audiologic assessment, functional hearing loss and objective audiometry. In Goodhill V(Ed): Ear Diseases, Deafness and Dizziness. New York: Harper & Row, 1979, pp 142–84
6.   Goldstein R, Goodman AC, King RB: Hearing and speech in infantile hemiplegia, before and after hemispherectomy. Neurol. 6:869, 1956
7.   Bocca E, Calearo C: Central hearing processes. In Jerger J (Ed): Modern Developments in Audiology, first ed. New York: Academic Press, 1963
8.   Katz J, Basil R, Smith J: A staggered spondaic word test for detecting central auditory lesions. Ann Otol Rhinol Laryngol 72:908–19, 1963

9. Linden A: Distorted speech and binaural speech resynthesis tests. Acta Otol Laryngol 58:32–48, 1964

10. Jerger J: Auditory tests for disorders of the central auditory mechanism. In Fields WS, Alford BR(Eds): Neurological Aspects of Auditory and Vestibular Disorders. Springfield: Charles C Thomas, 1964

11. Jerger J, Speaks C, Trammel, J. A new approach to speech audiometry. J Sp Hearng Dis 33:318–28, 1968

12. Jerger J, Frisina R: Audiology. In Ballenger JJ(Ed): Disease of the Nose, Throat, and Ear. Philadelphia: Lea and Febiger, 1969, pp 578–99

13. Antonelli A: Sensitized speech tests: results in brainstem lesions and diffusive CNS diseases. In Rojskjaer C(Ed): Speech Audiometry. Second Danavox Symposium, Odense, Denmark, 1970

14. Antonelli A: Sensitized speech tests: results in lesions of the brain. In Rojskjaer C(Ed): Speech Audiometry. Second Danavox Symposium, Odense, Denmark, 1970

15. Jerger J: Diagnostic Audiometry. In Jerger J(Ed): Modern Developments in Audiology, second ed. New York: Academic Press, 1973

16. Keith RW(Ed): Central Auditory Dysfunction. New York: Grune & Stratton, 1977

17. Jerger J, Jerger S: Diagnostic significance of PB word functions. Arch Otolaryngol, 93:573–80, 1971

18. Dirks D, Kamm C, Bower D, Betsworth A: Use of performance-intensity functions for diagnosis. J Sp Hearng Dis 42:408–15, 1977

19. Bess F, Josey AF, Humes LE: Performance intensity functions in cochlear and eighth nerve disorders. Am J Otol: 27–31, 1979

20. Jerger J, Hayes D: Diagnostic speech audiometry. Arch Otolaryngol 103:216–22, 1977

21. McAlpine D, Lumsden CE, Acheson ED: Multiple Sclerosis: A Reappraisal, second ed. Edinburgh: E & S Livingstone, 1972

DATA BANK

The corneoretinal potential on which the ENG is based varies with the amount of light striking the retina, with the minimum light-adapted potential being approximately twice that of the dark-adapted potential. Therefore, the ENG signal must be calibrated frequently, and major shifts in room lighting should be avoided.

DATA BANK

Even at its best, the sensitivity of the ENG in detecting fine eye movements (minimum about 0.5 degrees) is less than that of direct visual inspection (0.1 degree), and, therefore, direct visual inspection of small amplitude eye movements remains an important part of the vestibular examination.

Abnormalities of the Acoustic Reflex in Multiple Sclerosis

James Jerger, Ph.D., Terrey A. Oliver, M.S., Victor Rivera, M.D., and Brad A. Stach, M.A.

Acoustic reflect morphology was examined in 122 patients with a diagnosis of definite multiple sclerosis. Abnormality in some dimension of acoustic reflex morphology was observed in 75 per cent of the study population. The most commonly observed abnormality was an alteration in one or more of the three relative amplitude indices (afferent, efferent, or central pathway index). Other abnormalities included delayed onset latency, delayed offset latency, reduction in absolute amplitude, and threshold elevation.

Reflex decay and elevated reflex thresholds have long been associated with retrocochlear disorder.[1-11] Evidence is mounting, however, that the dynamic suprathreshold characteristics of the acoustic reflex may be more sensitive indicators of auditory neuropathy than either threshold or decay measures. Specifically, reflex amplitude and latency abnormalities have been suggested as early indicators of retrocochlear site.[12-23]

In the past, technological constraints have made it difficult to study and quantify patterns of abnormality of reflex morphology in a large series of patients with auditory brainstem pathway disorders. However, the recent widespread availability of microcomputers and other technologically advanced instrumentation has facilitated the precise measurement of acoustic reflex morphology. By means of signal averaging, it is now possible to achieve a satisfactory signal-to-noise ratio without the use of the narrowband analog filtering typical of commercial immittance instruments. As a result, the temporal characteristics of the reflex can be recorded and measured with accuracy and ease.

Using signal averaging techniques and computer analysis, we examined, in some detail, various suprathreshold amplitude and latency characteristics of the acoustic reflex in 122 patients with multiple sclerosis (MS) and in 37 control subjects with sensorineural hearing loss. Our goal was to determine which aspect or aspects of abnormal morphology are altered by the retrocochlear auditory disorder so frequently associated with this debilitating disease.

SUBJECTS AND METHOD

Control Group

In order to construct a set of normal boundaries for latency and amplitude measures of the acoustic reflex, it is necessary to consider the potentially contaminating effects of at least two important variables, age and degree of hearing loss. It would be inappropriate, for example, to use young adults with normal hearing as a standard against which to judge the present MS patients, a group varying with respect to both age and degree of hearing loss. We formed, therefore, a control group characterized by variation in both of these two important dimensions. We purposely sought to include in the control group subjects varying in both age and degree of hearing loss. In this way, we were able to match the distributions of these two variables in the experimental population.

The control group consisted of 37 subjects with cochlear hearing loss in one or both ears. Subjects were recruited from the routine patient load of the Methodist Hospital Audiology Service, Houston, Texas. Control subjects ranged in age from 14 to 78 years, with a mean age of 50 years. There were 22 men and 15 women.

The sensorineural loss was unilateral in 15 subjects and bilateral in the remaining 22 subjects. The loss was classified as unilateral if no threshold hearing level exceeded 20 dB hearing

Received November 12, 1985, from the Department of Otorhinolaryngology and Communicative Sciences (Dr. Jerger and Ms. Oliver), and the Department of Neurology (Dr. Rivera), Baylor College of Medicine, and Methodist Hospital (Mr. Stach), Houston, Texas. Accepted for publication January 24, 1986.

Supported in part by USPHS Grant NS-10940, NINCDS.

Address reprint requests to Dr. Jerger: 11922 Taylorcrest, Houston, TX 77024.

level (HL) at any test frequency from 250 Hz to 4,000 Hz on one ear. If this criterion was not met, then the loss was classified as bilateral.

Selection criteria to rule out the possibility of either conductive or retrocochlear disorder included the following:

1) Normal immittance findings, including normal tympanograms, normal static immittance, reflex threshold levels of 95 db HL or better at test frequencies of 500 and/or 1,000 Hz, and absence of reflex decay at either 500 or 1,000 Hz (half amplitude criterion after 10 seconds, sensation level (SL) = 10 dB), on the selected ear.

2) No rollover of either PI-PB or PI-SSI functions on either ear (20 per cent criterion).

3) Negative auditory brainstem response (ABR) in the case of unilateral loss.

4) No previous history of middle ear disease, brain disease, or retrocochlear lesion.

Experimental Group

The initial experimental group consisted of 134 consecutive patients with diagnosed "definite MS." The diagnosis was made or confirmed following the accepted modern criteria[24-26]: 1) history and neurologic findings indicating multiple lesions in central nervous system white-matter pathways scattered in time and anatomical location (clinical criteria); 2) presence of cerebrospinal fluid oligoclonal gammopathy or increased immunoglobulin G (IgG) and/or presence of enhancing lesions suggestive of acute, inflamed, demyelinating plaques, as detected by computed tomography (CT) scan of the brain, using double-dose infusion of contrast material and delayed scanning; 3) typical white-matter lesions as seen by nuclear magnetic resonance (NMR) scanning and abnormalities detected by multimodal evoked responses, visual, and somasensory potentials (laboratory criteria).

The data from 12 subjects were excluded from further analysis because of conductive hearing loss in two subjects; history of middle ear surgery in two; facial nerve involvement in one; tolerance problems at high intensities in two; hearing loss greater than 60 dB at any frequency in the 250 to 4,000 Hz range in three; and involuntary movements by patient prohibiting valid recordings in two. The remaining 122 patients, 76 women and 46 men, formed the final experimental group.

The mean age for the experimental group was 43 years, with a range from 21 to 65 years.

Average pure-tone hearing threshold levels for 500, 1,000, and 2,000 Hz (PTA_1) were determined for both the better and poorer ears for each patient. The mean PTA_1 for the poorer ear was 11 dB with a range from −2 dB to 33 dB. For the better ear, the mean was 7 dB with a range from −5 dB to 28 dB. Of these patients, 89 per cent had a PTA_1 for the poorer ear no worse than 20 dB. The average difference between ears for PTA_1 ranged from 0 to 17 dB with a mean difference of 3.6 dB. The pure-tone average of hearing levels at 1,000, 2,000, and 4,000 Hz (PTA_2) was also determined for both the better and poorer ears. The mean PTA_2 for the better ear was 10 dB, with a range from −5 dB to 47 dB. The mean PTA_2 for the poorer ear was 15 dB with a range from −1 dB to 55 dB. Of the patients, 77 per cent had a PTA_2 no worse than 20 dB on the poorer ear.

Instrumentation

The experimental instrumentation used to obtain simultaneous crossed and uncrossed reflex waveforms from both ears has been described in previous publications.[20,21] Briefly, reflex-eliciting signals are alternated between ears at the rate of one signal each 1.5 seconds. Thus, the repetition rate per ear is one signal each 3 seconds. Reflex responses are monitored bilaterally by 270 Hz probe tones. Outputs from the monitoring microphones are fed to lock-in amplifiers for amplification and rectification, then to a microcomputer for signal averaging and computational analysis. Responses to eight consecutive signals to each ear are averaged. The resulting averaged waveforms are analyzed for maximum amplitude and various onset and offset latency measures.

The time constant of the recording system is approximately 10 milliseconds. Amplitude resolution is 0.01 dB, and temporal resolution is 2 milliseconds.

Figure 1 shows the amplitude and phase transfer functions of the recording system. Included, for comparative purposes, are the analogous transfer functions for the human stapedial reflex as measured by Hung and Dallos.[27]

Procedure

Each subject was tested in a single experimental session lasting from 20 to 30 minutes. Subjects were tested while seated comfortably in a sound-treated room. After the probe assemblies had been sealed in each ear canal, air pressure was adjusted to the point of maximum immittance (peak of tympanogram). Probe-tone intensity was then adjusted in 1-dB steps, independently in each ear, to achieve an ear canal sound pressure level of 85 dB SPL (i.e., compensated for ear canal volume).

Three reflex-eliciting signals were used—tone bursts of 500 and 2,000 Hz and bursts of broadband noise. Signal duration was always 500 milliseconds with 5-millisecond rise-decay time. Testing began at signal intensities of 80 to 90 dB SPL, and was then increased in 10-dB steps up to a maximum of 110 db SPL for the tone bursts and 100 dB SPL for the noise bursts.

Threshold-seeking procedure was initiated by decreasing signal intensity, in 2-dB steps, from the level at which a reflex response was first noted. The intensity level was then increased or decreased in 2-dB steps until both crossed and uncrossed thresholds had been determined. Presence or absence of the reflex was judged by visual inspection of each averaged waveform on an oscilloscopic display.

Average reflex waveforms were stored on floppy disk and later recalled for microcomputer analysis of amplitude, latency and relative amplitude indices.

Preliminary Considerations

In order to evolve a suitable algorithm for ultimate data reduction, we first considered potential problems associated with degree of hearing loss, age, and whether results should be compared at equal sensation level (SL) or equal sound pressure level (SPL).

Effect of Degree of Hearing Loss

The possible effect of degree of hearing loss was examined by forming a subgroup, from the total control group, of 13 subjects with unilateral loss. We then compared data from the good and bad ears of this control subgroup. This analysis, which controlled for age by intrasubject comparison, revealed no statistically significant ($P > 0.05$) differences between the two ears of these subjects with respect to either onset or offset latencies or amplitude of the crossed reflex, for signals of 500 Hz, 2,000 Hz, or broadband noise (BBN).

In other words, when age was controlled, the presence of mild to moderate sensorineural hearing loss, per se, did not appear to be a problem from the standpoint of normative

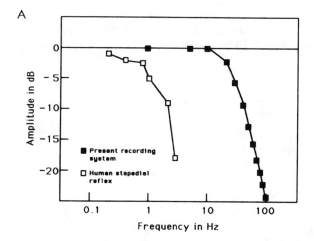

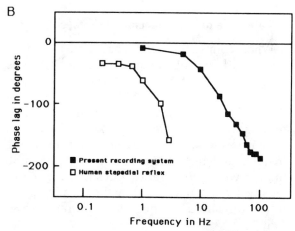

Figure 1.   Frequency transfer function of the present reflex recording system. (A, amplitude; B, phase). Included, for comparative purposes, is the transfer function of the human stapedial reflex, to broad band noise at 100 dB SPL, as estimated by Hung and Dallos (Hung IJ, Dallos P: Study of the acoustic reflex in human beings: I. Dynamic characteristics. J Acoust Soc Am 52:1168–1180, 1972).

values. To be sure, the presence of sufficiently severe cochlear hearing loss must eventually affect the acoustic reflex as it affects virtually all other indices of auditory function. In the present control group, however, degree of loss (better ear) was limited (average PTA = 16 dB, maximum PTA = 52 dB) to encompass only the distribution of hearing loss in the experimental population (average PTA = 11 dB, maximum PTA = 33 dB).

Effect of Age

All measures were affected to greater or lesser extent by age. To take this important variable into account, we plotted scattergrams of each measure as a function of age, constructed empirical boundaries encompassing 95 per cent of the

TABLE 1.   *Distributions of Crossed Reflex Thresholds in Control Subjects and in Experimental Subjects, Exclusive of Those with Elevated Reflexes*

	SIGNAL		
	500 Hz	*2,000 Hz*	*BBN*
Control group			
Mean (dB)	94	91	86
SD (dB)	7.1	8.3	8.6
Experimental group			
Mean (dB)	94	88	80
SD (dB)	5.8	6.6	8.0

control group, and referred all reflex data from the MS patients to these empirically determined, age-corrected norms. For this purpose, we used only the data from the better ear of each control subject.

Rationale for Comparison at Equal SPL

When comparing reflex characteristics of patients with peripheral hearing loss, it is customary to make comparisons at equivalent sensation level (SL), usually at SL = 10 dB. The rationale for comparison at equivalent SL is that, if reflex thresholds differ (e.g., between ears, between normal and hearing-impaired, or among frequencies), then it is necessary to compensate the ear with poorer reflex threshold for the intensity advantage enjoyed by the ear with better reflex threshold at equivalent suprathreshold SPL.

In patients with sensorineural hearing loss, the acoustic reflex threshold may be elevated for either of two reasons: 1) retrocochlear pathology or 2) cochlear pathology producing hearing loss in excess of 60 dB.[28,29] In the present study, we controlled for each of these possibilities. First, cochlear hearing loss did not exceed 60 dB in either group. Second, retrocochlear pathology was ruled out in the control group by a variety of criteria (described previously). In the experimental group, where retrocohlear pathology was expected, subjects whose reflex thresholds were, indeed, elevated were treated as a separate group, and no attempt was made to evaluate suprathreshold reflex morphology.

The actual distribution of crossed reflex thresholds in the better ear of the control group and in the better ear of subjects of the experimental group without significant reflex elevation is shown in Table 1. Intergroup comparisons of suprathreshold reflex characteristics were confined to subjects whose reflex thresholds were both theoretically and empirically within normal limits.

Equivalent distributions in the two groups seemed to justify comparison of control and experimental subjects at equivalent SPL rather than equivalent SL. Nevertheless, we carried out further analysis of this question in a subgroup of cochleas with unilateral loss. We compared interaural amplitude and latency measures first on the basis of equal SL and then on the basis of equal SPL. From the total control group, we formed a subgroup in which crossed reflex thresholds were available on both ears and a minimum reflex sensation level of 10 dB could be defined by interpolation (i.e., reflex threshold was at least 10 dB better than the highest intensity tested, 110 dB SPL for tones, and 100 dB SPL for noise). For the 2,000-Hz signal, this definition yielded subgroups of 23 subjects for the maximum amplitude measure, 19 for the onset latency measures, and 21 for the offset latency measures. In these subgroups, interaural crossed reflex threshold differences ranged from 0 to 8 dB. We computed the difference between both amplitude and latency measures (50 per cent criterion) for better ear and poorer ear, first on the basis of comparison at equal sensation level (SL = 10 dB), then on the basis of equal sound pressure level (SPL = 110 dB). Figure 2 shows the result. In the cases of both amplitude and latency, there was little systematic difference between the two methods of comparing ears, and no differences were statistically significant (P > 0.05). Similar results were found for the 500-Hz tone burst signal at 110 dB SPL and for the noise burst signal at 100 dB SPL.

We concluded, from this analysis, and the foregoing considerations, that in the present study it was irrelevant whether comparison between the control and experimental groups was made at equivalent SL or equivalent SPL. In the interest of simplicity, therefore, all comparisons were made at equivalent SPL rather than equivalent SL. In the remainder of this paper, therefore, all comparisons are made for reflex responses to tone burst signals at 110 dB SPL, or to noise burst signals at 100 dB SPL.

Amplitude

Absolute Amplitude

A presignal baseline, which reflected resting probe-tone SPL, was determined by calculating the arithmetic mean of activity during a 20-millisecond period between onset of averaging and onset of the signal. Reflex amplitude was computed by identifying the largest reflex value following signal offset and subtracting from it the presignal baseline. Reflex amplitude was calibrated and is expressed throughout this paper as the change in probe tone SPL in decibels (compensated for ear canal volume).

Relative Amplitude Indices

Rationale for the calculation of relative amplitude indices has been described previously.[20] Briefly, the index concept is used for two purposes: 1) to isolate the locus of reflex amplitude abnormality to a) the probe ear, b) the ear to which the signal is being presented, or c) the central pathway of the crossed reflexes; and 2) to reduce the considerable intersubject variability of individual measures of acoustic reflex amplitudes. These amplitude indices were derived by comparing the sums of pairs of amplitudes that reflect the afferent portion, the efferent portion, or the central pathway portion of the reflex arc. For example, to evaluate the afferent portion of the arc, the sum of the two reflex amplitudes obtained with signal to the right ear (right crossed and right uncrossed) was compared with the sum of amplitudes obtained when the signal was presented to the left ear (left crossed and left uncrossed). Theoretically, the difference between these sums should be zero under normal circumstances. If, however, the reflexes obtained with sound to one ear were substantially smaller than those obtained with sound to the other, the difference would deviate from zero accordingly.

The formulas for calculating the indices are as follows:

afferent index [AI]
$$= (RU + RC) - (LU + LC)$$
efferent index [EI]
$$= (RU + LC) - (LU + RC)$$
central pathway index [CPI]
$$= (RU + LU) - (RC + LC)$$

where RU = amplitude of the right uncrossed acoustic reflex, RC = amplitude of the right crossed acoustic reflex, LU = amplitude of the left uncrossed acoustic reflex, and LC = amplitude of the left crossed acoustic reflex. In this manner, the AI represents the difference between amplitudes obtained with signal to the right ear and those obtained with signal to the left ear. The EI represents the difference between amplitudes obtained from the right ear probe and those obtained from the left ear probe. The CPI represents the difference between uncrossed and crossed amplitudes.

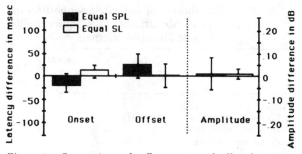

Figure 2. Comparison of reflex onset and offset latencies and reflex amplitude for 2,000 Hz signal at equal SPL (110 dB) and equal SL (10 dB) in a subgroup of patients with cochlear hearing loss (mean +1 SE). No difference was significant at the 5 per cent level.

Latency

Onset and offset latencies at 50 per cent of maximum amplitude[30] were calculated. Latency measures were expressed as the time (in milliseconds) between signal onset and the point in time at which 50 per cent of maximum amplitude was reached. These latency values were calculated for crossed onset and crossed offset conditions. The resolution with which latencies were calculated was 2 milliseconds.

RESULTS

Of the 122 subjects in the experimental group, 30 (25 per cent) showed no discernible reflex abnormality on any of the threshold, latency, or amplitude measures examined. The remainder of this section presents results on the remaining 92 subjects (75 per cent) who showed some reflex abnormality for one or more of the three test signals.

Reflex abnormalities could be classified into one or more of five general categories: 1) abnormal elevation of reflex threshold; 2) abnormal reduction in reflex amplitude; 3) abnormal relative amplitude index; 4) abnormal onset latency; and 5) abnormal offset latency.

Table 2 summarizes the number of experimental subjects who fell into each of these five categories. The totals in Table 2 do not add up to 100 per cent, since some subjects showed abnormalities in more than one category. The following sections consider each of these five abnormal categories in detail.

Elevated Thresholds

Reflex thresholds (crossed or uncrossed) were considered elevated if the threshold SPL ex-

TABLE 2.   *Distribution of Reflex Abnormalities by Signal and Type of Abnormality in 92 Patients with Definite Multiple Sclerosis*

	TOTAL*		SIGNAL		
	No.	(%)	500 Hz	2,000 Hz	BBN
Amplitude abnormalities					
Elevated threshold	28	(31)	21	16	18
Absolute amplitude	24	(26)	16	10	5
Amplitude indices	36	(39)	27	19	22
Latency Abnormalities					
Onset latency	19	(21)	16	3	9
Offset latency	26	(28)	4	25	10

* Row totals may be less than sum across signals since the same subject may appear at more than one signal. Column adds up to more than 92 subjects since the same subject may show more than one type of abnormality.

ceeded 105 dB, at 500 or 2,000 Hz, or exceeded 95 dB for broad band noise (BBN) (95 per cent boundaries of reflex thresholds in control group). Of the 92 patients with some reflex abnormality, 28 (30 per cent) showed elevated thresholds for at least one of the three signals on at least one ear. At 500 Hz, 21 subjects had elevated thresholds; at 2,000 Hz, 16 subjects and for BBN, 18 subjects.

Whenever the reflex threshold was abnormally elevated for a particular signal, no further analysis was carried out on suprathreshold amplitude or latency measures of that subject at that signal. Subsequent analyses of suprathreshold reflex characteristics for a particular signal are confined to those subjects in which reflex thresholds were within normal limits for that test signal.

Absolute Amplitude

Figure 3 shows scattergrams of the absolute amplitude of the crossed reflex, as a function of age, in the control group. In view of the considerable body of literature that has previously demonstrated an effect of age on acoustic reflex amplitude,[31-36] we thought it important to consider a possible age effect in our control data.

The problem of controlling for possible age effects on acoustic reflex measures can be approached from either an analytic or empirical point of departure. The conventional analytic approach would be either linear or curvilinear regression analysis to examine the correlation between amplitude and age, and to test for the significance of the slope coefficient of the regression line. Normal boundaries, in this approach, would be conventionally defined by the standard error of measurement, whether significant slope existed or not. A criterion such as ±2

standard errors of measurement might, for example, be used to define the 95 per cent limits of the normal amplitude range. Examination of the actual scatterplots in Figure 3 suggested to us, however, that such a conventional analytic approach would be difficult to justify for three reasons. First, we lacked reasonably equivalent sample sizes across age decades. Second, we did not feel that we could reasonably assume equivalent variability across the age range. Third, we did not feel that we could reasonably assume either normal or even symmetric distributions around the mean amplitude at a given age, especially in the older age range (above 50 years).

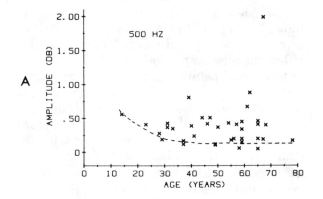

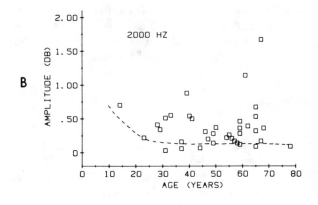

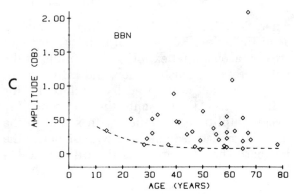

Figure 3.   Scattergrams of reflex amplitude versus age in the control group. Dashed line represents lower boundary of 95 per cent interval (A, 500 Hz; B, 2,000 Hz; C, BBN).

This assumption is particularly critical for the use of the standard error of measurement in defining the normal boundary. Because of asymmetry in the distributions of amplitudes, especially in the older age range, the use of a ± 2 standard error of measurement criterion would place the lower boundary of normalcy well below the range of actual observed scores.

For these reasons, we elected to pursue a more empirical approach to the definition of normal boundaries in the control group. Because our principal concern was the definition of a reasonable lower boundary of normal reflex amplitude, we constructed an empirical boundary by drawing a line through the scatterplot such that no more than 5 per cent of the observed data fell below this line. We make no claim that this empirically defined boundary represents a genuine age effect on acoustic reflex amplitude. The present research was not designed to evaluate this question, the data are insufficient to address this question, and we make no assertion that we have in fact answered the question. Our sole concern in this research was a reasonable definition of the lower boundary of normal acoustic reflex amplitude against which to evaluate the data obtained from the experimental subjects. We believe that we have achieved this goal by our procedure of defining a lower empirical boundary across the age range. It should be re-emphasized, however, that the purpose of this procedure was to define a boundary of the normal reflex amplitude range that would take into account any possible age effect while making no claim for the reality of such an age effect. Admittedly, the scatterplots of Figure 3 do not suggest a strong age effect on reflex amplitude in our control group of subjects with cochlear hearing loss. As subsequent sections will show, however, the age effect on measures of acoustic reflex latency was more pronounced.

Crossed reflex amplitudes from the experimental group were classified as abnormal only when they fell below the empirically defined normal boundary at the subject's age level.

Of the 92 subjects with some reflex abnormality, 24 (26 per cent) showed an abnormally small crossed reflex amplitude for one or more of the three test signals. Amplitude abnormalities were most common at 500 Hz (N = 16), relatively less common at 2,000 Hz (N = 10), and least common for BBN (N = 5).

Of the 24 subjects with some reflex amplitude abnormality, 19 showed abnormalities at one signal only, three showed abnormalities at two signals, and only two subjects were abnormal at

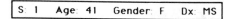

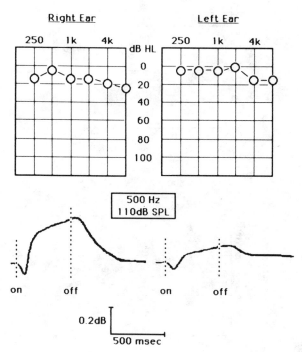

Figure 4. Unilateral reduction of absolute reflex amplitude in a 41-year-old woman with multiple sclerosis; 500 Hz signal at 110 dB SPL.

all three test signals. When only one signal was abnormal (N = 19), the abnormality was most common for the 500 Hz signal (N = 13), intermediate for the 2,000 Hz signal (N = 5), and least common for the BBN signal (N = 1).

Figure 4 shows illustrative findings in a subject with abnormally reduced absolute crossed reflex amplitude. The subject was a 41-year-old woman with a 20-year history of MS. The pure-tone audiogram shows relatively normal sensitivity on both ears. Reflex thresholds at 500 Hz were similar on the two ears (94 dB SPL on the right ear and 96 dB SPL on the left ear), but amplitudes at 110 dB were asymmetric. The response from the right ear showed a maximum amplitude of 0.34 dB, but on the left ear the crossed amplitude was only 0.12 dB, a value below the normal (95 per cent) boundary for a 41-year-old. On both ears, uncrossed amplitudes were within normal limits (0.62 dB for the right ear and 0.67 dB for the left ear). In addition, both the ABR and the masking level difference (MLD) test on this patient were within normal limits.

Amplitude Indices

Figure 5 shows scattergrams of the amplitude indices of 34 subjects of the control group. Com-

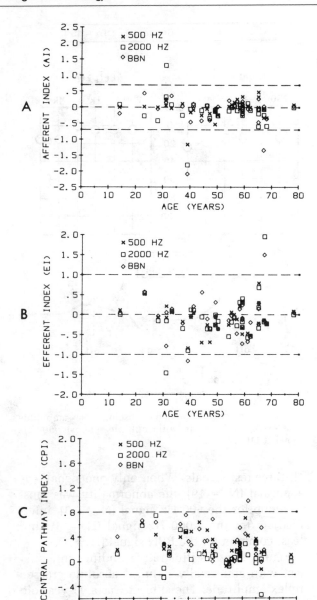

Figure 5. Scattergrams of relative amplitude indices in the control group as functions of age. Dashed lines represent boundaries of 95 per cent intervals (*A*, afferent index; *B*, efferent index; *C*, central pathway index).

plete data were not available for all signals in three of the 37 subjects of the control group. Figure 5*A* shows the distribution of afferent indices as a function of age, Figure 5*B* shows the analogous distribution for the efferent index, and Figure 5*C* shows the distribution of the central pathway index. In the case of the afferent index, the range from +0.7 to −0.7 encompasses 95 per cent of the observed indices in the control group. No consistent trends were observed either for type of signal or for age. The efferent index was somewhat more variable in the control group. The 95 per cent range ex-

tended from +1.0 to −1.0. Again, we observed no significant trends for type of signal or age. Finally, Figure 5*C* shows the distribution of central pathway indices. Boundaries of the 95 per cent range extended from +0.8 to −0.2. Again, neither type of signal nor age appeared to exert a systematic effect on the data. Indices measured from the experimental subjects were considered abnormal only if they fell outside the empirically determined 95 per cent boundaries illustrated in Figure 5.

Of the 92 subjects with some reflex abnormality, 36 subjects (39 per cent) showed some abnormality on one or more of the three amplitude indices at one or more of the three test signals. Of these 36 subjects with amplitude index abnormalities, 19 showed abnormality of CPI only, seven showed abnormality of the EI only, and three showed abnormality of AI only. Five of the 36 subjects had two abnormal indices, usually AI and CPI, and two subjects showed abnormalities on all three indices. Abnormalities of amplitude indices were most common for the 500 Hz signal (N = 27), somewhat less common for the BBN signal (N = 22), and least common for the 2,000 Hz signal (N = 19). Overall, however, differences among signals were not substantial.

Figure 6 shows an illustrative example of an abnormal afferent index. The subject was a 44-year-old woman with a ten-year history of MS.

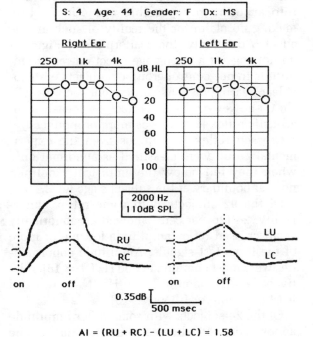

Figure 6. Abnormal afferent index in a 44-year-old woman with multiple sclerosis; 2,000 Hz signal at 110 dB SPL.

The pure-tone audiogram showed normal sensitivity in both ears. Despite these normal and symmetric audiometric levels, reflex amplitude was substantially smaller when sound was introduced to the left ear in either the crossed or uncrossed mode. Whereas the right crossed and uncrossed amplitudes were 0.85 and 1.50 dB, respectively, analogous amplitudes from left crossed and uncrossed stimulation were 0.34 and 0.43 dB, respectively. The resulting afferent index of 1.58 was well outside the normal boundary of ±0.7.

This patient's asymmetry was reflected in other audiometric measures, especially speech audiometry. Scores on the Dichotic Sentence Identification (DSI) test, for example, were 80 per cent on the right ear, but only 27 per cent on the left ear. The ABR, although showing a prolonged wave I-V interval on both ears, showed much poorer morphology on the left ear. Maximum word discrimination (PB) scores, however, were within normal limits (92 per cent right ear, 100 per cent left ear).

Figure 7 shows an illustrative example of an abnormal efferent index. The subject was a 37-year-old woman with an 11-year history of MS. The audiogram showed relatively normal sensitivity in both ears, and reflex thresholds were observed at similar levels in the two ears (84 dB SPL right ear, 80 dB SPL left ear). Nevertheless,

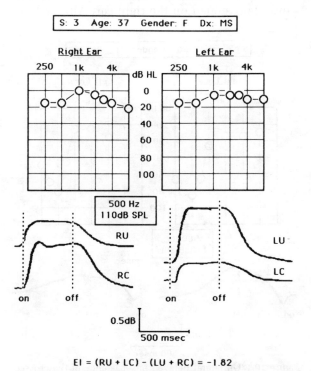

$$EI = (RU + LC) - (LU + RC) = -1.82$$

Figure 7. Abnormal efferent index in a 37-year-old woman with multiple sclerosis; 500 Hz signal at 110 dB SPL.

ABNORMAL CENTRAL PATHWAY INDEX (CPI)

ABNORMAL CENTRAL PATHWAY INDEX (CPI)

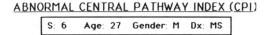

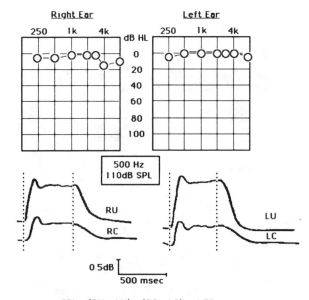

$$CPI = (RU + LU) - (RC + LC) = 1.35$$

Figure 8. Abnormal central pathway index in a 27-year-old man with multiple sclerosis; 500 Hz signal at 110 dB SPL.

the two reflexes measured with the probe in the right ear (left crossed [LC] and right uncrossed [RU]) showed substantially smaller amplitude (LC = 0.50 dB, RU = 0.51 dB) than the two reflexes (left uncrossed [LC] and right crossed [RC]) observed with probe in the left ear (LU = 1.56 dB, RC = 1.27 dB). The resulting efferent index of −1.82 is well outside the normal boundary of ±1.0. The possibility that this statistically significant efferent index might be the result of a right middle ear disorder cannot be ruled out, but is rendered unlikely by the conventional immittance battery test results, which showed normal type A tympanograms from both ears and normal and symmetric crossed and uncrossed acoustic reflex thresholds from both ears. If right middle ear disorder can be ruled out as an explanation for the abnormal efferent index, then the expected site of disorder must be either the right facial nerve itself or its motor nucleus in the brainstem.

Figure 8 shows an illustrative example of an abnormal central pathway index (CPI). The subject was a 27-year-old man with a relatively recent diagnosis of MS. The audiogram was within normal limits on both ears, and acoustic reflex thresholds were normal and symmetric. Nevertheless, examination of the four suprathreshold reflex waveforms shows that both uncrossed amplitudes were more than twice as

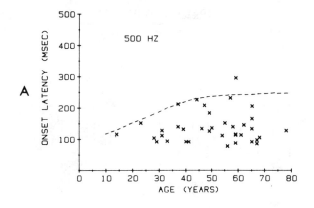

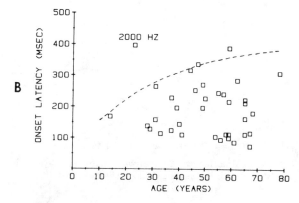

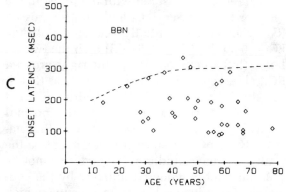

Figure 9. Scattergrams of crossed reflex onset latency as functions of age in the control group. Dashed line represents upper boundary of 95 per cent interval (A, 500 Hz; B, 2,000 Hz; C, BBN).

large as their crossed counterparts. The resulting CPI of 1.35 was well above the normal boundary of 0.8.

Onset Latency

Figure 9 shows scattergrams of the onset latency of the crossed reflex to 50 per cent of maximum amplitude in the control group. The age effect is not pronounced, except perhaps for 2,000 Hz. In any event, the empirically derived boundaries, encompassing 95 per cent of the control group data, take any possible age effect

into account. No onset latency, from an MS patient, was judged abnormal unless it exceeded this normal boundary at the experimental subject's age level.

Of the 92 subjects with some reflex abnormality, 19 subjects (21 per cent) showed some abnormality of onset latency at the 50 per cent criterion. Of the 19 subjects with onset abnormalities, 14 were abnormal at only one signal, two for two signals, and three for all three signals. Onset abnormalities were more common at 500 Hz (N = 16) and for BBN (N = 9) than for 2,000 Hz (N = 3).

Since latency characteristics of the acoustic reflex are strongly related to reflex amplitude, we considered the possibility that all of the abnormal latency results could be explained as the inevitable concomitant of abnormally reduced amplitude. In fact, however, this explanation could be invoked in only six of the 19 cases of onset latency abnormality. Five of these six cases were at 500 Hz, one was at 2,000 Hz, and none occurred for BBN.

Figure 10 shows an illustrative case of abnormally delayed onset latency. The subject was a 56-year-old man whose MS was diagnosed six years ago. The audiogram showed a severe bilateral loss above 2,000 Hz, probably related to a previous history of excessive noise exposure. At 500 Hz, however, where audiometric sensitivity was relatively normal, onset latency was significantly lengthened on the right ear. Although re-

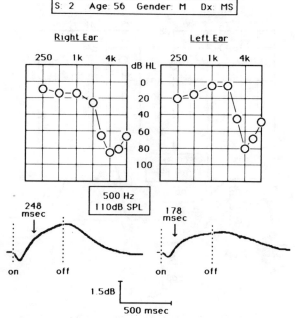

Figure 10. Unilateral delayed onset latency of the crossed reflex in a 56-year-old man with multiple sclerosis; 500 Hz signal at 110 dB SPL.

flex thresholds were symmetric at 500 Hz (90 dB on both right and left ears), latency to 50 per cent of maximum amplitude was 178 milliseconds for the left ear (within normal limits) but 248 milliseconds for the right ear (above the 95 per cent normal boundary). Reflex amplitude was actually larger on the ear with abnormal onset latency (right) than on the ear with normal latency (left). Thus, the abnormality on the right ear could not be explained as a simple amplitude effect.

Offset Latency

Figure 11 shows scattergrams of the offset latency of the crossed reflex to 50 per cent of maximum amplitude in the control group. Here, we see a pronounced age effect for all three test signals. The effect is least for BBN and greatest for 2,000 Hz. Again, as for amplitude and onset latency, the empirically derived boundaries, encompassing 95 per cent of the control group data, take the age effect into account.

Of the 92 subjects with some reflex abnormality, 26 subjects (28 per cent) showed some abnormality of offset latency at the 50 per cent criterion. Of the 26 subjects with offset abnormalities, 17 showed the abnormality at only one signal, seven for two signals, and two for all three test signals. Offset abnormalities were most common at 2,000 Hz (N = 25), next most common for BBN (N = 10), and least common at 500 Hz (N = 4).

Figure 12 shows results illustrating abnormal offset latency. The subject was a 44-year-old woman with a 19-year history of MS. Audiometric levels were within normal limits in both ears. Reflex thresholds at 2,000 Hz were 80 dB SPL for the right ear and 78 dB SPL for the left ear. The reflex waveform shows a relatively normal rise characteristic on both ears, but the offset latency of 614 milliseconds on the left ear is well above the normal boundary for a 44-year-old.

All other test results, particularly ABR, MLD, and diagnostic speech audiometric results, were well within normal limits in this patient. In addition, absolute reflex amplitude was not abnormally reduced on either ear. It is interesting, however, that the amplitude of the reflex from the left ear was actually slightly smaller than the amplitude of the reflex from the right ear. Normally, the effect of reduced amplitude is to shorten offset latency. Thus, the abnormally long offset latency from the patient's left ear

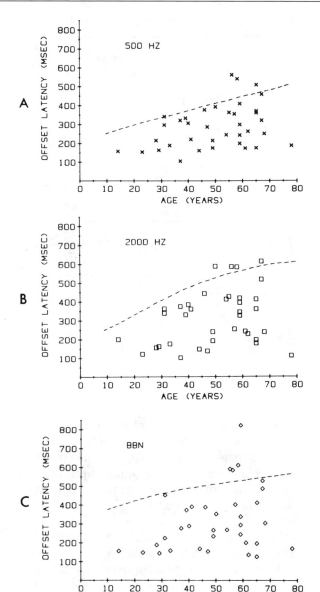

Figure 11.   Scattergrams of crossed reflex offset latency as functions of age in the control group. Dashed line represents upper boundary of 95 per cent interval (A, 500 Hz; B, 2,000 Hz; C, BBN).

cannot be explained as an artifact of the amplitude asymmetry.

Because of the high prevalence of abnormalities in offset latency of the crossed reflex at 2,000 Hz, we analyzed analogous offset data for the uncrossed reflex to determine whether the offset abnormality was unique to the crossed mode or a characteristic of both modes. Analysis showed that, of the 25 subjects who showed crossed offset abnormalities, only three showed concomitant uncrossed offset abnormalities. In the other 22 subjects, the uncrossed offset with within the normal boundary. Only the crossed offset was abnormal.

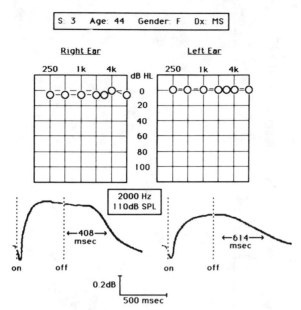

S: 3   Age: 44   Gender: F   Dx: MS

Right Ear   **Left Ear**

250   1k   4k   250   1k   4k

2000 Hz
110dB SPL

←408→
msec

←614→
msec

on   off   on   off

0.2dB

500 msec

Figure 12. Unilateral delay in offset latency in a 44-year-old woman with multiple sclerosis; 200 Hz signal at 110 dB SPL.

Multiple Abnormalities

The number of subjects showing abnormality on more than one aspect of reflex morphology for a given signal was surprisingly small. We had anticipated, for example, that the combination of abnormalities of absolute amplitude and abnormalities of amplitude indices might be a likely occurrence. But this combination occurred in only four subjects. Similarly, there was only one subject who showed abnormality of both onset and offset latencies.

The most prevalent multiple abnormality was the combination of abnormal absolute amplitude and abnormal offset latency, but this occurred in only seven subjects. Table 3 summarizes, for the three signals, the number of subjects showing abnormality on only one reflex measure and the number showing each of the various possible combinations of abnormalities. Summed across signals, the number of subjects showing abnormality on only one reflex measure and the number showing each of the various possible combinations of abnormalities. Summed across signals, a total of 66 subjects showed abnormality on only one reflex measure, 25 subjects showed abnormality on two measures, and only three subjects showed abnormality on three or more measures.

DISCUSSION

Perhaps the most significant finding of the present investigation is the relatively high pre-

valence (75 per cent) of acoustic reflex abnormalities in patients with multiple sclerosis. Previous studies of acoustic reflex abnormalities in MS primarily confined their attention to abnormal threshold elevation and reflex decay.[10–12,37] Prevalence estimates ranged from a low of 21 per cent[11] to a high of 60 per cent.[37] In general, however, these estimates are not readily comparable because, in most cases, sample sizes were small[10,12] and/or criteria for subject selection varied substantially. In the present study, abnormal threshold elevation was observed in only 23 per cent of the total group, but accounted for less than a third of the entire array of reflex abnormalities. Fully 92 of the 122 subjects of the present sample (75 per cent) showed either threshold or suprathreshold abnormality. In 69 per cent of this group of 92 subjects with reflex abnormality, reflex thresholds were actually within normal limits, but some abnormality of suprathreshold morphology was found nonetheless.

Clearly, amplitude abnormalities tended to overshadow latency abnormalities in the experimental group (Table 2). Abnormalities of relative amplitude indices, absolute amplitudes, or elevated thresholds were observed in many more individuals than abnormalities of either offset or onset latency. Interestingly, cochlear hearing loss, per se, did not seem to influence reflex amplitude, at least over the range of hearing losses contained in the present control group. It has been previously observed,[38] and the present results agree that reports of reduced reflex amplitude in patients with cochlear hearing loss are an artifact of age contamination. Unless sufficient care is taken to control for age, patients with cochlear hearing loss will appear to show reduced reflex amplitude, inasmuch as the age distribution of hearing impaired subjects is usually much higher than the age distribution of control subjects with normal hearing.

A second problem plaguing the interpretation of absolute reflex amplitude is the considerable intersubject variability that has been so consistently observed in previous studies. The present study is no notable exception. In the present data, for example, absolute reflex amplitude extended over such a great range that above about age 30 years, reflex amplitude could be considered abnormal only if it fell below 0.1 dB.

The index concept proved to be an effective method for dealing with these two perennial problems associated with reflex amplitude. We were able to demonstrate that all three of the indices were essentially independent of age and

TABLE 3. *Distribution of Single and Multiple Abnormalities of the Acoustic Reflex in 64 Subjects with Multiple Sclerosis*

	SIGNAL			
	500 Hz	2000 Hz	BBN	ACROSS ALL SIGNALS*
One abnormality (N = 66)				
Absolute amplitude	8	1	3	11
Onset latency	6	1	4	8
Offset latency	2	15	7	17
Relative amplitude indices	19	14	15	30
Two abnormalities (N = 25)				
Amplitude and onset	4	0	0	4
Amplitude and offset	0	7	1	7
Amplitude and indices	3	1	1	4
Onset and offset	1	0	0	1
Onset and indices	3	1	4	6
Offset and indices	0	2	1	3
Three or more abnormalities (N = 3)				
Amplitude, onset, and offset	0	0	0	0
Amplitude, offset, and indices	0	0	0	0
Onset, offset, and indices	1	0	1	1
Amplitude, onset, and indices	1	0	0	1
All (amplitude, onset, offset, and indices)	0	1	0	1

* Row totals may be less than sum across signals since the same subject may appear at more than one signal. Column adds up to more than 64 subjects since the same subject may show different abnormalities at different signals.

characterized by considerably less intersubject variability than absolute amplitude measures. In particular, they effectively circumvented the traditional problem of the "floor effect" in which the lower limit of normal reflex amplitude is only a short distance from essentially zero amplitude. Dramatic testimony to the viability of the index concept was the fact that, despite the persistent problem of intersubject variability of absolute amplitudes in the present study population, the amplitude indices showed the highest prevalence of reflex abnormality.

Although amplitude abnormalities dominated the present study, what appeared to be pure latency abnormalities were observed with surprising frequency. Nor could these latency abnormalities be easily explained as artifacts of reduced reflex amplitude. In contrast to eighth nerve disorder, such as acoustic tumor, where latency abnormalities have been explained as simple concomitants of reduced reflex amplitude,[23] in the present MS patients neither onset nor offset abnormalities could be so easily dismissed. In most cases, abnormally delayed onset of the latency occurred without concomitant amplitude reduction, suggesting a genuine latency abnormality. Even more interesting were offset abnormalities, which occurred in a surprising 28 per cent of the total abnormal group. In the case of offset latency, delay is actually opposite to the effect predicted by amplitude reduction. Thus, a concomitant amplitude reduc-

tion adds an even more striking dimension of abnormality to delayed offset. One would, for example, expect shortest offset latency with smallest reflex amplitude but, in the present subject group, we observed quite the opposite effect (i.e., prolonged offset latency in combination with reduced amplitude). This effect was confined primarily to the crossed mode of elicitation. It was rarely observed in the uncrossed mode. These observations lead us to suggest that offset abnormalities probably represent an alteration in central inhibitory influence on the crossed reflex rather than a more immediate afferent influence on reflex morphology.

Acknowledgment.   The authors thank Winni Breitbach for valuable contributions to the project.

References

1. Giacomelli F, Mozzo W: An experimental and clinical study on the influence of the brain stem reticular formation on the stapedial reflex. Int Audiol 3:421, 1964
2. Anderson A, Barr B, Wedenberg E: Intra-aural reflexes in retrocochlear lesions, in Hamberger CA, Wersall J (eds): Disorders of the Skull Base Region, Nobel Symposium 10. Stockholm, Almqvist and Wiksell, 1969
3. Greisen O, Rasmussen P: Stapedius muscle reflexes and otoneurological examinations in brain stem tumors. Acta Otolaryngol 70:366–370, 1970
4. Noffsinger D, Kurdziel S, Applebaum E: Value of special auditory tests in the latero-medial inferior pontine syndrome. Ann Otol Rhinol Laryngol 84:384–390, 1975
5. Liden G, Korsan-Bengtsen M: Audiometric manifestations of retrocochlear lesions. Scand Audiol 2:29–40, 1973

6. Jerger J, Harford E, Clemis J, et al: The acoustic reflex in eighth nerve disorders. Arch Otolaryngol 99:409–413, 1974

7. Johnson EW: Auditory test results in 500 cases of acoustic neuroma. Arch Otolaryngol 103:152–158, 1977

8. Jerger J, Jerger S: Diagnostic value of crossed vs uncrossed acoustic reflexes. Arch Otolaryngol 103:445–453, 1977

9. Jerger S, Jerger J, Hall H: A new acoustic reflex in eighth nerve disorders. Arch Otolaryngol 99:409–413, 1979

10. Hannley M, Jerger JF, Rivera VM: Relationships among auditory brain stem responses, masking level differences and the acoustic reflex in multiple sclerosis. Audiology 22:20–23, 1983

11. Grenman R, Lang H, Panelius M, et al: Strapedius reflex and brainstem auditory evoked responses in multiple sclerosis patients. Scand Audiol 13:109–113, 1984

12. Coletti V: Stapedius reflex abnormalities in multiple sclerosis. Audiology 14:63–71, 1975

13. Bosatra A, Russola M, Poli P: Modification of the stapedius muscle reflex under spontaneous and experimental brain stem impairment. Acta Otolaryngol 80:61–66, 1975

14. Bosatra A, Russola M, Poli P: Oscilloscopic analysis of the stapedius muscle reflex in brain stem lesions. Arch Otolaryngol 102:284–285, 1976

15. Borg E: Dynamic characteristics of the intra-aural muscle reflex, in Feldman AS, Wilbur LA (eds): Acoustic Impedance and Admittance—The Measurement of Middle Ear Function. Baltimore, Williams and Wilkins, 1976

16. Bosatra A: Pathology of the nervous arc of the acoustic reflexes. Audiology 16:307–315, 1977

17. Hess K: Stapedius reflex in multiple sclerosis. J Neurol Neurosurg Psychiatry 42:331–337, 1979

18. Mangham C, Lindeman R, Dawson W: Stapedius reflex quantification in acoustic tumor patients. Laryngoscope 90:242–250, 1980

19. Clemis JD, Sarno D: The acoustic reflex latency test: clinical application. Laryngoscope 90:601–611, 1980

20. Hayes D, Jerger J: Signal averaging of the acoustic reflex: diagnostic applications of amplitude characteristics. Scand Audiol [suppl] 17:31–36, 1982

21. Stach B, Jerger JF: Acoustic reflex averaging. Ear Hear 5:289–296, 1984

22. Bosatra A, Russolo M, Silverman CA: Acoustic reflex latency: state of the art, in Silman S (ed): The Acoustic Reflex. Orlando, Florida, Academic Press, 1984

23. Jerger J, Hayes D: Latency of the acoustic reflex in eighth nerve tumor. Arch Otolaryngol 109:1–5, 1983

24. Waksman BH, Reynolds WE: Research on multiple sclerosis. National Multiple Sclerosis Society, 1982

25. McDonald WI: The role of evoked potentials in the diagnosis of multiple sclerosis, in Bauer HJ, Poser S, Ritter G (eds): Progress in Multiple Sclerosis Research. New York, Springer-Verlag, 1980

26. Sears ES, McCammon A, Bigelow R, et al: Maximizing the harvest of contrast enhancing lesions in multiple sclerosis. Neurology 20:1–59, 1970

27. Hung IJ, Dallos P: Study of the acoustic reflex in human beings: I. Dynamic characteristics. J Acoust Soc Am 52:1168–1180, 1972

28. Gelfand S: The contralateral acoustic reflex threshold, in Silman S (ed): The Acoustic Reflex. Orlando, Florida, Academic Press, 1984

29. Jerger J, Hayes D, Anthony L, et al: Factors influencing prediction of hearing level from the acoustic reflex. Maico Monographs Contemp Audiol 1(1):1–20, 1978

30. Borg E: Time course of the human acoustic stapedius reflex. Scand Audiol 11:237–242, 1982

31. Gersdorff MCH: Modifications du reflexe acoustico-facial chez l'homme on fonction de l'age, par etude impedancemetrique. Audiology 17:260–270, 1978

32. Wilson RH: The effects of aging on the magnitude of the acoustic reflex. J Speech Hear Res 24:406–414, 1981

33. Hall JW: Acoustic reflex amplitude: I. Effect of age and sex. Audiology 21:294–309, 1982

34. Thompson DJ, Sills JA, Recke KS, et al: Acoustic reflex growth in the aging adult. J Speech Hear Res 23:405–418, 1980

35. Sieminski LR, Durrant JD, Rosenberg PE, et al: Stapedial reflexes in normal versus recruiting ears. J Auditory Res 17:251–261, 1977

36. Silman S: Magnitude and growth of the acoustic reflex, in Silman S (ed): The Acoustic Reflex. Orlando, Flordia, Academic Press, 1984

37. Kofler B, Oberascher G, Pommer B: Brain-stem involvement in multiple sclerosis: a comparison between brain-stem auditory evoked potentials and the acoustic stapedius reflex. J Neurol 231:145–147, 1984

38. Beedle RK, Harford ER: A comparison of acoustic reflex and loudness growth in normal and pathological ears. J Speech Hear Res 16:271–281, 1973

PATTERNS OF AUDITORY ABNORMALITY IN MULTIPLE SCLEROSIS*

James F. Jerger, Ph.D.,
Terrey A. Oliver, M.S.,
Rose A. Chmiel, M.S., and
Victor M. Rivera, M.D.

From Jerger et al. (1986). Patterns of auditory abnormality in multiple sclerosis. Audiology, 25, 193–209. Reprinted by permission.

Department of Otorhinolaryngology and Communicative Sciences, Department of Neurology, Baylor College of Medicine, Houston, Texas

Reprint Requests: Dr. Jerger, 11922 Taylorcrest, Houston, TX 77024

This paper stresses the relatively high prevalence of auditory abnormality in multiple sclerosis. An auditory test battery consisting of the acoustic reflex (AR), the auditory brainstem response (ABR), the masking level difference (MLD) and speech audiometry (SA) was administered to 62 patients with diagnosed definite multiple sclerosis. The AR showed the highest identification rate (71 percent). SA was next (55 percent), followed by the ABR (52 percent) and the MLD (45 percent). The combination of an abnormality on either AR, ABR, or SA yielded a 90 percent identification rate. Interestingly, the combination of AR or SA or MLD yielded an 87 percent identification rate without any contribution from ABR.

INTRODUCTION

Previous investigators have documented a number of auditory abnormalities in patients with multiple sclerosis (MS). Diminished speech understanding (Gollegly et al., 1985; Hannley et al., 1983; Jacobson et al., 1983; Olsen et al., 1975) abnormal acoustic reflex (AR) (Gollegly et al., 1985; Grenman et al., 1984; Hannley et al., 1983; Hess, 1979; Coletti, 1975), abnormal masking level difference (MLD) (Gollegly et al., 1985; Hannley et al., 1983; Noffsinger et al., 1972; Olsen et al., 1976) and abnormal auditory brainstem response (ABR) (Chiappa et al., 1980; Gollegly et al., 1985; Hannley et al., 1983; Häusler and Levine, 1980; Kjaer, 1980; Lacquaniti et al., 1979; Robinson and Rudge, 1977; Stockard et al., 1977; Tackman et al., 1980), as well as depressed audiometric thresholds (Daugherty et al., 1983; Luxon, 1980; Noffsinger et al., 1972), have all been described in the multiple sclerotic population. Few studies, however, have addressed the problem of patterns of auditory abnormality in the MS patient. Although Noffsinger et al. (1972) administered a wide variety of special auditory tests to their experimental population, neither the AR nor the ABR was included in their test battery. Hannley et al. (1983) studied patterns of abnormality associated with AR, ABR, and MLD, but their observations were confined to a relatively small sample. Only the unpublished study by Gollegly et al. (1985) included

ABR, AR, MLD, and speech audiometry (SA) in a reasonably sized sample (n = 33) of patients with definite MS.

The purpose of the present study was to examine patterns of auditory abnormality in MS in a relatively large sample of patients and to include both AR and ABR along with MLD and measures of speech understanding known to be sensitive to retrocochlear disorder. We sought to determine not only the relative prevalence of abnormality of each measure individually, but the likelihood of each possible combination of abnormal auditory test results. A secondary goal was to examine these patterns of abnormality in relation to the severity and duration of the disease.

METHOD

SUBJECTS

The subjects of this study were 41 females and 21 males with a diagnosis of definite MS. The diagnosis was made or confirmed following accepted modern clinical and laboratory criteria (McDonald, 1980; Sears et al., 1970; Waksman and Reynolds, 1982). Clinical criteria included history and neurological findings indicating multiple lesions in central nervous system, white matter pathways scattered in time and anatomical location. Laboratory criteria included presence of cerebrospinal fluid oligoclonal gammopathy or increased immunoglobulin G (IgG), presence of enhancing lesions suggestive of acute, inflamed, demyelinating plaques, by computerized axial tomographic (CT) scan of the brain, using double-dose infusion of contrast material and delayed scanning, typical white matter lesions by nuclear magnetic resonance (NMR) scanning, and abnormalities detected by visual and somatosensory evoked potentials.

Mean duration of MS symptoms in this group was 11 years with a range from 1 to 30 years. A severity rating of physical involvement for each patient was assigned based on the criteria summarized in Table 1.

No subject showed substantial periph-

TABLE 1. Basis for Rating Patients According to Severity of Symptomatology

Symptoms	Rating	Number
No visible evidence; patients need no assistance in daily function	1	10
Some visible evidence; patients need some assistance, but can function independently	2	43
Visible evidence; patients need assistance for all daily functions; cannot function independently	3	9
	Total	62

eral hearing loss on either ear, but mild or moderate loss at one or more audiometric frequencies was often observed. In 38 of the 62 subjects (61 percent), no audiometric threshold hearing level exceeded 20 dB at any test frequency over the range from 250-4000 Hz on either ear. Thus, the pure-tone audiogram was within normal limits. In 13 subjects (21 percent), the threshold exceeded 20 dB at one or more test frequencies on at least one year, but the average of the three hearing threshold levels (HTL at 1000, 2000 and 4000 Hz (PTA2) did not exceed 20 dB on either ear. Thus, the pure-tone average PTA showed no more than a relatively mild loss. In 11 subjects (18 percent), there was sufficient loss to raise the PTA2 above 20 dB on at least one ear. Thus, the pure-tone average reflected a relatively moderate loss. In all cases, the mild or moderate loss was sensorineural.

Table 2 summarizes the means and standard deviations of both PTA1 (average of pure-tone HTL at 500, 1000, and 2000 Hz) and PTA2 (average of HTL at

TABLE 2. Means, SD, and Range of HL in 62 Patients with MS

	Hearing Levels, dB		
	Mean	SD	Range
PTA1			
Right ear	8.8	5.9	−4–28
Left ear	8.1	7.0	−2–32
PTA2			
Right ear	11.0	10.0	−3–47
Left ear	11.2	11.1	−1–55

PTA1 = Pure-tone audiogram HTL at 500, 1000 and 2000 Hz; PTA2 = Pure-tone audiogram HTL at 1000, 2000 and 4000 Hz.

1000, 2000 and 4000 Hz) for both ears of the entire experimental group. In no case was the loss sufficient to compromise the interpretation of any experimental measure, with the exception of two patients whose threshold interaural asymmetry at 500 Hz precluded the interpretation of MLD test results. For this test, therefore, the total number of patients successfully tested was 60. All 62 patients demonstrated normal middle ear function based on audiologic evidence (normal, type A, tympanograms, and interweaving air and bone conduction audiometric threshold contours).

The mean age for the MS group was 42 years, with a range from 21 to 61 years.

APPARATUS AND PROCEDURE

Each patient was tested during a single 2.5- to 3-hour evaluation session. The test battery included the following procedures: (1) conventional pure-tone threshold audiometry; (2) AR thresholds, absolute amplitudes, onset and offset latency measurements, and relative amplitude indices; (3) ABR; (4) MLD; (5) SA PB words, Synthetic Sentence Identification-Ipsilateral Competing Message (SSI-ICM), and dichotic sentence identification (DSI).

Conventional Pure-Tone Audiometry

Pure-tone audiograms were obtained using a clinical audiometer (Beltone 10D) calibrated according to the ANSI-1969 standard. All threshold audiometric testing was carried out in a double-walled, sound-treated room (Industrial Acoustics Company, 1200). Audiometric thresholds were measured using a modification of the Hughson-Westlake method (Carhart and Jerger, 1959). Air and bone conduction thresholds were measured in 5 dB steps.

Acoustic Reflex

The instrumentation used to measure the AR has been described in previous publications (Hayes and Jerger, 1982; Stach

and Jerger, 1984). Briefly, a dual-probe assembly system was used to obtain, simultaneously, both the crossed and uncrossed reflex waveforms. Signals were alternated between ears at a rate of one signal each 1.5 sec. A 270 Hz probe tone was used to monitor the reflex activity. Responses to eight consecutive signal presentations to each ear were averaged. The averaged waveforms were stored on disk and later analyzed for the various suprathreshold amplitude and latency measures. The time constant of the reflex apparatus was approximately 10 msec. Amplitude resolution was 0.01 dB and temporal resolution was 2 msec.

AR testing employed three reflex-eliciting signals, tone bursts of 500 and 2000 Hz, and bursts of broad-band noise (BBN). Signal duration was 500 msec with a rise/fall time of 5 msec. The probe assemblies were sealed in each ear canal and the air pressure was adjusted to the point of maximum admittance. Probe tone intensity was adjusted in 1 dB steps, independently in each ear canal, to achieve an ear canal SPL of 85 dB. Thus, individual ear canal volume was compensated. Threshold levels for each of the three test signals were sought for all four reflex conditions (right to left crossed, left to right crossed, right uncrossed, and left uncrossed). The threshold-seeking procedure was carried out in 2 dB steps. Absolute amplitude, onset latency to 50% of maximum amplitude, offset latency to 50% of maximum amplitude, and relative amplitude indices (afferent, efferent, and central pathway) values for each signal at 110 dB SPL (100 dB SPL for BBN) were determined and compared to the empirical norms defined previously by Jerger et al. (1986). Figure 1 shows examples of the various abnormalities of AR morphology observed in the present experimental group.

Auditory Brainstem Response

To measure the ABR response, click stimuli (the haversine transformation of a single cycle of a 5000 Hz sinusoid) were generated (Wavetek, 186), amplified (Macintosh, 250), attenuated (Hewlett-Packard, 350D), and delivered to a dynamic earphone (Telephonic, TDH-39) mounted in a pair of sound-attenuating ear muffs (Mine Safety Appliances, Noisefoe Mark II). Click intensity was calibrated in dB normal hearing level (nHL) by determining the behavioral threshold on a jury of 11 adult listeners with normal hearing. Two-channel ABR recordings were obtained from scalp electrodes located at the vertex (active), each earlobe (reference) and the forehead (ground). EEG activity was preamplified (Grass P511) for a voltage gain of 200,000:1, and bandpass filtered from 30 to 3000 Hz (6 dB/octave skirt). The amplified EEG was delivered to a signal averager (Nicolet, 1174). A time base of 10 msec was used to record the ABR to rarefaction clicks. A total of 2048 sweeps was averaged. Averaged responses were plotted on an X-Y recorder (MFE).

ABR was analyzed separately for each ear. Results were considered abnormal if the absolute latency of wave V on either ear, the I-V interwave interval on either ear, or the wave V interaural difference exceeded the upper boundary of the 95 percent range of normal, or if morphology was degraded, based on an absence of one or more waves, an asymmetry between ears, or extreme difficulty in identifying peaks. The waveforms from each ear were categorized using the following criteria: type 1: normal response. All waves (I-V) are present with normal I-V interwave

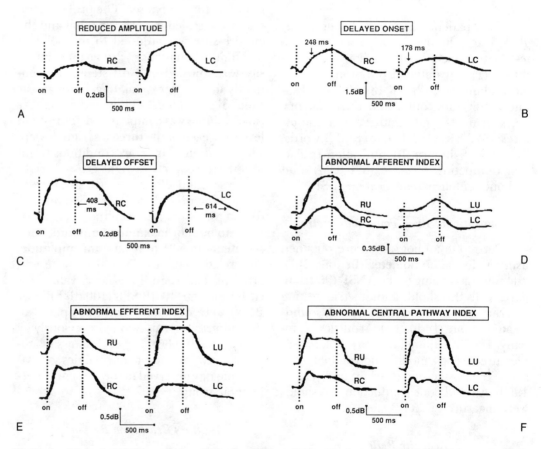

Figure 1. Examples of abnormalities of AR morphology observed in the present study. a: Abnormally small absolute amplitude of the right crossed reflex. b: Abnormally delayed onset latency of the right crossed reflex. c: Abnormally delayed offset latency of the left crossed reflex. d: Abnormal afferent index, AI=(RU+RC) − (LU+LC)=1.58. e: Abnormal efferent index, EI=(RU+LC) − (LU+RC)=−1.82. f: Abnormal central pathway index CPI=(RU+LU) − (RC+LC)=1.35.

interval; type 2: abnormality prolonged I-V interwave interval; type 3: waveform degradation. The response shows poor morphology. Landmark peaks are difficulty to identify, and/or amplitudes are reduced, and/or amplitude ratios are abnormal; type 4: selective loss of late waves. Later waves are absent, but early waves are present at appropriate latencies; type 5: extreme abnormality of the response. Only wave I is present. All later waves are absent. Figure 2 illustrates these five response types using actual waveforms gathered from this test group.

ABR testing was carried out at 80 dB nHL or at 90 dB nHL if no response was observed at 80 dB nHL. The presentation rate was 21.1/sec (or 11.1/sec if the re-

sponse was uninterpretable at 21.1/sec). In all cases, responses at the higher intensity or the slower rate were also abnormal.

Masking Level Difference

The MLD was obtained with a threshold tracking method. A 500 Hz sinusoid, pulsed on a 50 percent duty cycle, was presented binaurally along with a BBN signal at 65 dB HL. The patient tracked masked hearing threshold for the 500 Hz signal on a Békésy-type audiometer (AEC Model BA-75), first for the homophasic (SoNo) condition, second for the antiphasic (SπNo) condition. Interaural phase relations were manipulated by an MLD adapter (Calder, Model MLD-10K). The MLD was defined as the decibel difference between thresholds in the homophasic and antiphasic conditions.

The MLD was considered interpretable only if threshold HLs at 500 Hz did not exceed 20 dB HL for each ear and showed no more than a 10 dB difference between ears at 500 Hz (Jerger et al., 1984). The MLD was considered abnormal if the difference score was less than 7 dB (Jerger et al., 1984).

Speech Audiometry

Speech materials (PB words and SSI sentences) were presented via a two-channel audiometer (Tracoustics, Program III) and delivered via THD-49 earphones mounted in CZW-6 cushions. All speech audiometric materials were prerecorded on magnetic tape by the same male talker. Three speech scores were obtained: (1) PB score; (2) SSI-ICM score and (3) DSI score. NDRC Harvard Psycho-Acoustic Laboratory (PAL) PB-50 word lists were used to obtain the PB score. The patient repeated each word presented and the tester scored the response. PB word lists were presented at a sensation level (SL) of 30 dB (re: the average PTA1 for both ears). Percent correct performance was compared to scores previously determined to define the lower boundary of normalcy as a function of hearing level

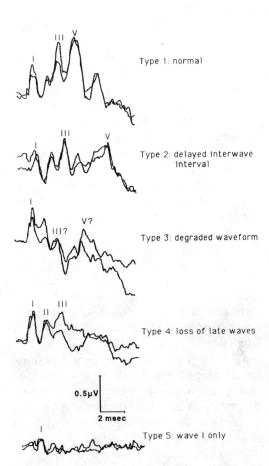

Figure 2. Examples of the five types of ABR waveforms observed in the present study. Type 1: normal; type 2: prolonged I-V interwave latency; type 3: waveform degradation; type 4: selective loss of late waves; type 5: extreme abnormality.

(PTA2) in ears with cochlear hearing loss (95 percent range). If a PB score fell below this range, it was considered abnormal. For the SSI-ICM procedure (Jerger and Jerger, 1975), a single list of 10 third-order, 7-word synthetic sentences, presented at the same 30-dB SL as the PB words, was mixed with competing continuous discourse at three message-to-competition ratios (MCR); 0, −10, and −20 dB. After each sentence had been presented, the patient identified the sentence he heard from a closed-set list and responded with the appropriate number. Abnormal SSI scores were defined as scores <30 percent for an MCR of −20 dB, <50 percent for an MCR of −10 dB and <70 percent for an MCR of 0 dB for either ear. The DSI was presented at 50 dB HL. The absolute scores for each ear were compared to the normal performance boundary (Fifer et al., 1983) based on the PTA1 for a given ear.

Definition of Abnormality

Much of the disagreement among previous investigators relative to the prevalence of a given auditory abnormality can be traced to variation in criteria of abnormality. Although many investigators have used a 95 percent criterion (i.e., a result is abnormal when it exceeds the mean ± 2 SD of the normative data), some have used a 99 percent criterion (i.e., a result is abnormal when it exceeds the mean ± 3 SD of the normative data). Such differences may have a substantial effect on estimates of prevalence of abnormality, especially in the case of ABR, where many observed absolute and relative latencies fall in the interval between 2 and 3 SD above the mean normal result.

A further complication is that the application of any criterion of abnormality based on a specified range of standard deviations assumes a symmetric distribution of normal results around their central tendency. To the extent that such distributions are skewed, estimates of prevalence of abnormality based on a standard deviation criterion can be in error. In such a circumstance, it may be more appropriate to determine the range of scores encompassing 95 percent of the normative group by empirical, rather than statistical, means.

Finally, investigators have not always considered the contaminating effects of age and hearing loss on the various auditory measures. It has been demonstrated repeatedly that both chronological age and degree of peripheral hearing loss may exert strong effects on virtually all auditory measures, but especially the AR, ABR, SA, and MLD. Since the multiple sclerotic patient population spans the entire adult age range and includes many individuals with hearing loss (39 percent in the present study), the effects of age and hearing loss on normative values must be given serious consideration.

In the present study, we have defined abnormality, as much as possible, on the basis of normative data developed in our own laboratory on the same equipment used to test the present patients. In addition, we have corrected, wherever possible, for the effects of both age and peripheral hearing loss by defining normal boundaries on the basis, not only of young adults with normal hearing, but also of patients of various age with various degrees of peripheral hearing loss. Criteria of AR abnormality, for example, are based on 95 percent boundaries empirically derived from the distributions of results on variously aged patients with cochlear hearing loss (Jerger et al., 1986). In all reflex data, therefore, both age and hearing loss effects are taken into account in the normative boundaries for both amplitude and latency.

In the case of MLD, we used a boundary developed empirically in our own laboratory to encompass exactly 95 percent of the results obtained in our normative group of young adults with normal hearing (Jerger et al., 1984). Previous research has failed to document a significant age effect on MLD. We did, however, apply stringent criteria (see above) to control for the known effects of peripheral hearing loss on MLD.

For speech audiometric data, we used

95 percent boundaries empirically determined in our own laboratories for the PAL-PB words used in the present study and for SSI-ICM. Since these materials are not substantially affected over the age range of the present MS group (21–61 years), we concentrated on the effect of degree of peripheral hearing loss on normative values. Since PB word discrimination is adversely affected by high-frequency loss, we based the PB word score boundaries on the distributions of PB_{max} scores in patients with cochlear hearing loss of varying degree. But, since SSI scores are only minimally affected by high-frequency loss, we based the SSI-ICM criteria on adults with normal hearing (Jerger and Jerger, 1975). For DSI, a test specifically designed to be relatively independent of the contaminating effects of high-frequency hearing loss, the 95 percent boundary was similarly empirically defined on young adults (Fifer et al., 1983).

In the case of ABR, we thought it advisable to use published norms, for the sake of comparability with previous investigators. We chose, for this purpose, the data of Cox (1985). Here, we defined the 95 percent boundary according to the mean + 2 SD convention. The I-V interwave interval was considered to be abnormally prolonged if it exceeded 4.5 msec on either ear. The V:I amplitude ratio was considered abnormal if it fell below 1.0.

Throughout this investigation, whether using empirically or statistically determined criteria of abnormality, we have adhered to an alpha-level, or type-I error, of 5 percent. That is, we have set the boundary of normalcy at a level where 5 percent of normal individuals would be classified as abnormal by our criteria. In so doing, we adhere to popular convention while recognizing that any prevalence estimate is a function of this alpha-level.

RESULTS

Individual Test Outcomes

In this section, we consider the outcome of each of the four test procedures individually. We ask, irrespective of the outcome on any of the other procedures, how often each of the four procedures was abnormal in the study population. Subsequent sections will consider the problem of joint outcomes of two or more procedures and the question of how often a particular procedure was the only test yielding an abnormal outcome.

Auditory Brainstem Response

Thirty-two (52 percent) of the 62 patients in the study population showed some abnormality of the ABR on one or both ears. In 10 of these patients, the abnormality was unilateral; in the remaining 22 patients, it was bilateral. This yielded a total of 54 abnormal ABR waveforms. Of these 54 waveforms, the abnormality was type 2 (delayed interwave latency) in eight ears; type 3 (poor morphology) in 10 ears; type 4 (selective loss of late waves) in 20 ears, and type 5 (loss of all waves after wave I) in 16 ears. Thus, the most commonly observed abnormality was the selective loss of late waves with preservation of early waves. Such a result is not unexpected in view of the relatively discreet nature of the typical sclerotic plaque. It is also interesting to observe that prolonged interwave latency, a commonly observed symptom of acoustic tumor, was the test least likely to be abnormal in this group.

Acoustic Reflex

Forty-four (71 percent) of the 62 patients showed some abnormality of the AR. In 13 patients, the abnormality was an elevation of one or more absolute AR thresholds beyond the criteria of 105 dB SPL for 500 or 2000 Hz, or 95 dB SPL for BBN. In the remaining 31 patients, all AR thresholds were within normal limits, but there was some abnormality in either absolute amplitude, absolute latency, or one of the relative amplitude indices. There were eight instances of absolute amplitude abnormality, eight instances of onset latency abnormality, 11 instances of offset latency abnormality, and 22 instances of relative amplitude index abnormality. Of the latter, six were abnormalities of the afferent index (AI), seven were abnormalities of the efferent index (EI) and nine were abnormalities of the central pathway index (CPI). These various abnormalities add up to more than 33, since some patients showed more than one type of AR abnormality.

It is interesting to note that, of the various possible AR abnormalities, the most common was abnormality of a relative amplitude index, and the most common of this subset was abnormality of the CPI. Such a result was not, however, unexpected, since the CPI is, in theory, maximally sensitive to lesions at the level of the caudal brainstem (Jerger et al., 1986).

Speech Audiometry

Thirty-four (55 percent) of the 62 patients showed some abnormality on one or more SA measures on one or both ears. The SSI-ICM measure was abnormal in 31 individuals. In this subgroup, the abnormality was unilateral in 12 and bilateral in 19 individuals. The PB score was abnormal in 10 patients. On this group, the abnormality was unilateral in eight patients and bilateral in two. The DSI score, based on simultaneous dichotic processing, was abnormal in seven patients.

It is not surprising that the SSI-ICM score showed the greatest prevalence of abnormality, since much previous research has documented the sensitivity of this task to retrocochlear auditory disorder, especially at the brainstem level (Jerger and Jerger, 1975; Russolo and Poli, 1983). It is interesting to note, however, that DSI, a dichotic measure designed to be specifically sensitive to disorders at the temporal lobe level, was abnormal in seven cases. Similar results with the dichotic paradigm have been reported by Jacobson et al. (1983) and by Daugherty et al. (1983).

Masking Level Difference

Twenty-seven patients (45 percent) had abnormal findings on the MLD task. This prevalence estimate is consistent with the findings of previous studies (see Table 3)

TABLE 3. Percentage of Abnormalities Reported by Different Investigators for ABR, AR, SA, and MLD in Patients with MS

| Investigator(s) | Year | No. | Percent Abnormal | | | |
			ABR	AR	SA	MLD
Present study	1986	62	52	71	55	45*
Gollegly et al.	1985	33	63	27	41	52
Kofler	1985	119	74	—	—	—
Oberascher	1985	72	—	64	—	—
Grenman et al.	1984	53	40	32	0	—
Kofler et al.	1984	47	72	64	—	—
Russolo and Poli	1983	20	80	65	55	—
Hannley et al.	1983	20	75	44	25	75
Kjaer	1983	58	78	—	—	—
Parving et al.	1981	13	0	—	—	—
Purves et al.	1981	33	45	—	—	—
Chiappa et al.	1980	81	47	—	—	—
Häusler and Levine	1980	29	62	—	3	—
Maurer et al.	1980	27	89	—	—	—
Tackmann et al.	1980	23	26	—	—	—
Hess	1979	20	—	33	—	—
Lacquaniti et al.	1979	25	64	—	—	—
Robinson and Rudge	1977	51	63	—	—	—
Stockard et al.	1977	30	93	—	—	—
Olsen et al.	1976	100	—	—	—	47
Coletti	1975	13	—	69	0	—
Olsen et al.	1975	31	—	—	19	—
Noffsinger et al.	1972	61	—	—	24	49
Dayal and Swisher	1967	14	—	—	36	—
Average (present study excluded)			61	50	23	56

*For MLD, n = 60.

and highlights the sensitivity of the MLD test to disorder at the level of the caudal brainstem.

Figure 3 (left-hand panel) compares the identification rates of the four procedures in the present study population. We may note that, while differences in identification rate among the four tests were not large, they were statistically significant (Cochran's Q = 11.98; p <0.01). The highest identification rate was observed for the AR, followed closely by the SA and ABR. Somewhat surprising was the fact that the identification rate for speech audiometry was at least as good as the identification rate for the ABR. It is commonly assumed that electrophysiological measures like the ABR are more sensitive to retrocochlear auditory disorders than speech audiometric measures. The present results demonstrate, however, that if the speech audiometric measures are carefully chosen, they are capable of demonstrating an identification rate rivaling ABR.

Table 3 compares the present identification rates for individual measures with analogous identification rates reported by various previous investigators. In general, there is relatively good agreement across the various studies. Where differences do exist, they are usually explained by differences in criteria of abnormality or differences in criteria for the establishment of the definite MS diagnosis. In the case of ABR, the identification rate has varied from 0 to 93 percent, a range due, at least in part, to wide variation in criteria used to define definite MS and/or to differences in criteria of normalcy. Our own identification rate of 52 percent is very close to the average identification rate of 16 previous studies (61 percent).

In the case of MLD, there has been less variation in identification rate. The range has been from 45 to 75 percent. Our own identification rate of 45 percent is near the lower end of this range.

In the case of SA and AR, however, the present identification rates are considerably above those observed in previous studies. In the case of SA results, for example, the present identification rate of 55 percent far exceeds the average of the nine previous studies (23 percent). Similarly, in the case of the AR, our identification rate of 71 percent is considerably greater than the average identification rate of the eight previous studies (50 percent). We believe that these differences reflect the greater attention which these measures have received in the present investigation. In the case of the AR, for example, we used signal averaging to maintain the fidelity of the waveform configuration, measured both amplitude and latency aspects of waveform morphology, and exploited the relation between crossed and uncrossed reflex waveforms to a greater degree than has been achieved in previous investigations. Similarly, in the case of SA, we employed a battery of speech audiometric measures specifically chosen for their sensitivity to retrocochlear auditory disorder.

COMBINATIONS OF TEST OUTCOMES

In this section, we consider the joint outcomes of two or more test results. We consider, first, the likelihood that results will be abnormal on specific combinations of tests (e.g., the likelihood of abnormality on ABR and MLD); second, the likelihood that results will be abnormal on at least one of a combination of tests (e.g., the likelihood of abnormality on ABR or MLD).

Table 4 summarizes the number of patients abnormal on various combina-

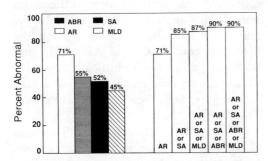

Figure 3. Comparison of individual and combined identification rates for the four tests of the present battery.

TABLE 4. Summary of Abnormalities as a Function of Joint Outcome on One or More Test ('and' Criterion)

Combination	Number of Patients	Percent of Total Group Tested
All tests normal	6	10
AR only	6	10
SA only	5	8
ABR only	2	3
MLD only	0	0
AR and SA	8	13
AR and ABR	2	3
AR and MLD	3	5
ABR and MLD	1	2
ABR and SA	1	2
SA and MLD	0	0
AR and MLD and SA	2	3
AR and ABR and SA	3	5
AR and MLD and ABR	8	13
SA and MLD and ABR	3	5
AR and ABR and SA and MLD	12	19

TABLE 5. Summary of Abnormalities as a Function of Joint Outcome on One or More Test ('or' Criterion)

Combination	Number of Patients	Percent of Total Group Tested
AR alone	44	71
SA alone	34	55
ABR alone	32	52
MLD alone	27	45
AR or SA	53	85
AR or ABR	51	82
AR or MLD	48	77
ABR or MLD	37	60
ABR or SA	47	76
SA or MLD	46	74
AR or MLD or SA	54	87
AR or ABR or SA	56	90
AR or MLD or ABR	52	84
SA or MLD or ABR	51	82
AR or ABR or SA or MLD	56	90

tions of joint outcomes (the 'and' question). The table shows that six patients (10 percent) were normal on all four tests. In the remaining 56 patients (90 percent), however, there was some combination of abnormalities. If only one test outcome was abnormal, that test was most likely to be the AR (10 percent) or SA (8 percent). ABR was the only abnormality in 3 percent of cases. There were no patients showing abnormality only on MLD. The combination of two tests most likely to show joint abnormality was AR and SA (13 percent). All other combinations of two tests showed smaller percentages. The combination of three tests most likely to show joint abnormality was AR, ABR and MLD (13 percent). Finally, every test outcome was abnormal in 19 percent of the group.

Table 5 summarizes the number of patients abnormal on at least one test in a combination of test outcomes (the 'or' question). This table shows how the identification rate may be improved by examining the outcomes of two or more test outcomes, relative to the outcome on any single test procedure. These results are further illustrated in the right-hand panel of Figure 3. We observed earlier that the best identification rate for any single test was achieved by the AR (71 percent). If the AR test result is combined with the result of SA, then the identification rate increases to 85 percent. This pair of tests, AR or SA, gave the best joint outcome for abnormality on either one of the two tests. The combination of ABR or SA (76 percent), while reflecting a substantial improvement over the 52 percent rate for ABR alone, still did not equal the 85 percent rate for the combination of AR or SA. When the joint outcome on three tests is considered, then the addition of ABR to the combination of AR or SA increases the identification rate from 85 to 90 percent. No other test triplet achieved as high an identification rate. Interestingly, however, the three-test combination of AR, SA, and MLD showed an 87 percent identification rate, a value very close to the best identification rate (90 percent) without the inclusion of ABR at all. Finally, we may observe that, since the identification rate for the three-test combination of AR, ABR, and SA was equal to the identification rate for all four tests combined, the MLD test added nothing to the efficacy of the total test battery.

The present results of combinations of test outcomes are in remarkably good agreement with the analogous data of Kofler et al. (1984) for ABR and AR. These investigators found that the combination of ABR or AR identified 91 percent of their definite MS group compared to 82 percent in the present study. Similarly, Kofler et al. (1984) found that the combination of ABR and AR abnormality occurred in 45 percent of their definite MS group compared to 40 percent in the present study.

RELATION TO SEVERITY OF MS

As noted above, each of the 62 patients was categorized, on a three-point scale, according to severity of multiple sclerotic symptoms. Figure 4 shows prevalence of abnormality, on each of the four tests, according to degree of severity. For patients with the mildest symptoms (severity rating 1; n=10), abnormality was greatest for AR, followed by SA. ABR abnormalities were relatively low in this subgroup, only 30 percent, and there were no MLD abnormalities at all. For patients with symptoms of moderate severity (severity rating 2; n=43), prevalence of abnormality was about equal for all four tests. Finally, in the category with most severe symptoms (severity rating 3; n=9), prevalence of abnormality was somewhat less for SA and MLD than for AR and ABR. These results suggest that severity of symptomatology, to some extent, at least, interacts with prevalence of abnormality across the four-test battery. The overall superiority of identification rate for AR in the entire group is largely attributable to its sensitivity in patients with relatively mild symptoms, where it enjoyed a 60 percent advantage over ABR. The overall inferiority of MLD seems, also, to derive largely from its poor sensitivity in the mild subgroup. In general, the prevalence of ABR abnormality increased with greater severity, whereas the prevalence of SA and AR abnormalities declined slightly with greater severity. Overall, however, severity did not emerge as an important factor in relation to prevalence of abnormality. In severity subgroup 1, the identification rate for abnormality on any of the four tests was 100 percent. In severity subgroup 2, it was 88 percent, and in severity subgroup 3, 89 percent.

RELATION TO DURATION OF MS

The total group of 62 patients was divided into four subgroups according to length of time since initial diagnosis. The four duration intervals were chosen to provide approximately equal numbers of patients in each of the four subgroups. Figure 5 shows how the prevalence of abnormality varied, for each of the four test procedures, as a function of disease duration. It is difficult to discern any systematic effect of duration on prevalence of abnormality for any of the four test procedures.

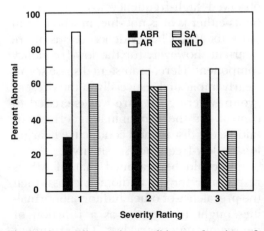

Figure 4. Auditory abnormalities as function of severity rating.

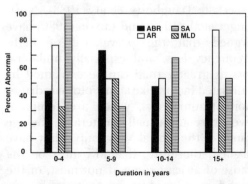

Figure 5. Auditory abnormalities as functions of duration of disease.

RELATION TO PURE-TONE AUDIOGRAM

The presence of audiometric hearing loss, in patients with MS, raises an interesting theoretical question. Does MS produce the audiometric deficit or are the observed losses due to factors such as aging, noise trauma, ototoxic drugs, etc., factors unrelated to the primary brainstem disease? The problem is complicated by the fact that the audiometric contour, in MS, may show both a low- and a high-frequency loss. Noffsinger et al. (1972) described a dome-shaped or arched contour with best hearing in the mid-frequency range in 17 of their 61 subjects. A similar pattern was observed by Cohen and Rudge (1984). In addition to the arched contour, both low-frequency "rising" and high-frequency "falling" contours have also been observed. Dayal and Swisher (1967) were among the first to compare MS patients with age- and gender-matched controls. When they compared mean audiograms of their total groups (n=22), the MS group showed greater loss than the control group and the difference was greatest at low and high frequencies, least at mid-frequencies, especially on the left ear (their Fig. 1). Interestingly, this difference varied with gender. In females, there was a larger discrepancy between MS patients and controls than in males. In general, females showed relatively flatter losses, while males showed more steeply sloping high-frequency loss. It is noteworthy to observe that a similar gender difference in audiometric contour was described by Hayes and Jerger (1979) in elderly subjects with presbyacusis.

In a number of subsequent studies, especially Daugherty et al. (1983), Noffsinger et al. (1972) and Luxon (1980) have argued that the prevalence of high-frequency loss, and especially unilateral loss, is greater than can be explained by unrelated factors like aging, ototoxic drugs, noise trauma, etc., which are comparatively rare and usually bilateral in the age range of the typical MS group. They have argued, therefore, that MS must be the cause of at least some, if not most, of the high-frequency loss so commonly observed.

But in 1984, Cohen and Rudge compared the average audiogram of 44 MS patients with the average audiogram in a control group of 44 subjects in the same age range as the MS group and recruited from the same hospital wards in which the MS patients were admitted. They did not, however, control for gender distribution. Cohen and Rudge (1984) observed the often described arched or dome-shaped pattern in both groups. Of particular interest, however, was that the two groups seemed to differ only in the low-frequency region. High-frequency loss was essentially equivalent in the MS and control groups. Cohen and Rudge (1984) concluded that only the low-frequency component could be attributed to MS. This conclusion is flawed, however, by failure to control for distribution of gender in the control group. Since the MS population contains more females than males (2:1 ratio in the present series, but see Baum and Rothschild (1981) for a more comprehensive survey), a simple 1:1 ratio in the control group would bias results in the latter group toward greater high-frequency loss for reasons unrelated to MS. Thus, a genuine high-frequency loss effect in the MS group could be obscured.

Figure 6 shows the average audiogram for the 41 females and 21 males of the present experimental group. The expected greater high-frequency loss in males is readily apparent.

It is still not possible to conclude with certainty, therefore, that the frequently observed high-frequency loss in MS patients either is or is not due, in whole or in part, to MS. The evidence seems more clear-cut, however, for the low-frequency component. Here, brainstem disease seems clearly implicated, especially in the present group, where great care was exercised to control for the contaminating effects of middle ear disease and conductive hearing loss on low-frequency sensitivity.

It could be reasoned that, if MS is responsible for the audiometric loss, then the prevalence of other auditory abnormalities ought to increase as a function of degree of audiometric loss. The argument is, unfortunately, nontransitive. The dem-

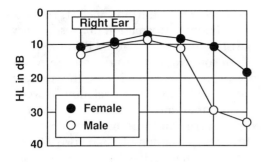

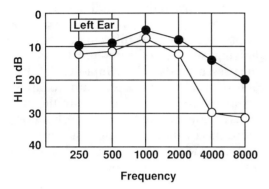

Figure 6. Average audiograms for male and female subgroups of 62 patients with MS.

TABLE 6. Percentage of Abnormalities for ABR, AR, SA, MLD, and Average Age as a Function of Pure-Tone Audiometrical Level for 62 Patients with MS

Test Procedure	Audiometric Category		
	Normal	Mild	Moderate
ABR	45	54	45
AR	68	69	54
SA	58	62	0
MLD	45	38	56
Average age, years	41	46	44

onstration of a relation would argue for such a causal effect, but failure to observe a correlation could be explained by the hypothesis that the nature of sclerotic plaque distribution within the CNS could produce relatively independent effects (i.e., some plaque locations might affect ABR only, some might affect audiometric level only). There need not necessarily be a high correlation between the various effects.

In any event, we failed in the present study to demonstrate a trend with degree of audiometric loss.

One possible explanation for such lack of association might be that the audiometric losses are due to aging, and would have occurred whether MS was present or not. Arguing against this hypothesis, however, is the fact that average chronological age (Table 6) was approximately equivalent (F=2.42; p>0.05) in the three groups.

In summary, the relation between MS and audiometric loss has still not been clearly defined. The study of Cohen and Rudge (1984) argues strongly that the high-frequency component is not uniquely related to MS, but their failure to control for gender distribution leaves us uneasy with this conclusion. The low-frequency component, however, seems more clearly related to brainstem disease.

In the present study, we observed prevalence of loss and audiometric contour entirely consistent with previous studies. We showed, furthermore, that the degree of audiometric loss was related to neither chronological age nor to prevalence of other auditory abnormalities. It was, however, strongly related to gender.

We suspect that Cohen and Rudge (1984) are probably correct in concluding that only the low-frequency component is due to MS, but would like to see their well-conceived study repeated with control of gender distribution.

DISCUSSION

One of the most significant findings of the present study is the relatively high prevalence of auditory abnormalities in patients with MS. A single procedure, the AR, yielded a 71 percent identification rate. It is important to reemphasize, however, that the present AR testing procedure included more than the analysis of reflex threshold elevation and/or reflex decay. If we had confined our attention to conventional parameters of the AR, our identification rate would have been no better than that of previous investigators. In order to achieve the substantial increase in sensitivity, it was necessary to include a considerably more sophisticated analysis of amplitude, latency, and crossed/uncrossed difference characteristics of the signal-averaged suprathreshold reflex waveforms. Consideration of the joint outcome of three procedures, AR, ABR, and SA, yielded an identification rate of 90 percent. Thus, auditory testing is shown to be extraordinarily sensitive to the presence of MS.

A second significant observation is the support that the present findings provide for the concept of a multiple test battery. Reliance on a single auditory test procedure, for example ABR, would have detected only 52 percent of the present study population, an identification rate virtually equivalent to the analogous rate for SA. Interestingly, the three-test battery consisting of AR, SA, and MLD yielded an 87 percent identification rate without any contribution from ABR. These results stand in some contrast to a popular conception of the relative superiority of the ABR in detecting brainstem lesions. The present results suggest that ABR enjoys no special advantage in this regard. Indeed, the AR demonstrated a higher identification rate. Finally, the present results indicate that, while the MLD test is attractive from the standpoint of testing time and cost of instrumentation, it did not, in fact, contribute additional information to a test battery consisting of AR, SA, and ABR.

In contrast to the findings of previous investigations (Kjaer, 1980), the present study found only a weak relation between the various auditory test abnormalities and either severity or duration of the MS symptomatology. Neither of these two factors seemed strongly related to any of the observed abnormalities in auditory function. This discrepancy may, however, be, at least in part, the result of differing criteria for judging severity of symptomatology. In the present study, for example, categorization of severity was based entirely on assessment of physical handicap. In the previous investigation of Kjaer (1980), however, more specific brainstem signs (likely to be correlated with auditory test results) played a part in the definition of severity.

ACKNOWLEDGMENT

This study was supported, in part, by NINCDS grant NS-10940 from the National Institutes of Health, US Public Health Service. We thank Winnie Breitbach for valued assistance in data collection and analysis.

REFERENCES

Baum, H.M., & Rothschild, B.B. (1981). The incidence and prevalence of reported multiple sclerosis. *Ann. Neurol. 10*, 420–428.

Carhart, R., & Jerger, J.F. (1959). Preferred method for clinical determination of pure-tone thresholds. *J. Speech and Hearing Disorders 24*, 330–345.

Chiappa, K.H., Harrison, J.L., Brooks, E.B., & Young, R.R. (1980). Brainstem auditory evoked responses in 200 patients with multiple sclerosis. *Ann. Neurol. 7*, 135–143.

Cohen, M., & Rudge, P. (1984). The effect of multiple sclerosis on pure tone thresholds. *Acta Oto-lar. 97*, 291–295.

Coletti, V. (1975). Stapedius reflex abnormalities in multiple sclerosis. *Audiology 14*, 63–71.

Cox, L.C. Infant assessment: developmental and age-related considerations; in Jacobson, The auditory brainstem response (College-Hill Press, San Diego 1985).

Daugherty, W.T., Lederman, R.J., Nodar, R.H., & Conomy, J.P. (1983). Hearing loss in multiple sclerosis. *Arch Neurol. 40*, 33–35.

Dayal, V.S., & Swisher, L.P. (1967). Pure tone thresholds in multiple sclerosis. *Laryngoscope 77*, 2169–2177.

Fifer, R.C., Jerger, J.F., Berlin, C.I., Tobey, E.A., & Campbell, J.C. (1983). Development of a dichotic sentence identification test for hearing-impaired adults. *Ear Hear. 4*, 300–305.

Gollegly, K.M., Kibbe-Michal, K., Reeves, A.G., & Musiek, F.E. Auditory behavioral and electrophysiological results in multiple sclerosis. Paper presented at the ASHA Convention, Washington DC, 1985.

Grenman, R., Lang, H., Panelius, M., Salmivally, A., Laine, H., & Rintamaki, J. (1984). Stapedius reflex and brainstem auditory evoked responses in multiple sclerosis patients. *Scand. Audiol. 13*, 109–113.

Hannley, M., Jerger, J.F., & Rivera, V.M. (1983). Relationships among auditory brain stem responses, masking level differences and the acoustic reflex in multiple sclerosis. *Audiology* 22, 20–33.

Häusler, R., & Levine, R.A. (1980). Brain stem auditory potentials are related to interaural time discrimination in patients with multiple sclerosis. *Brain Res. 191*, 589–594.

Hayes, D., & Jerger, J. (1979). Low-frequency hearing loss in presbyacusis. A central interpretation. *Archs Otolar. 105*, 9–12.

Hayes, D., & Jerger, J. (1982). Signal averaging of the acoustic reflex: diagnostic application of amplitude characteristics. *Scand. Audiol.*, suppl. 17, pp 31–36.

Hess, K. (1979). Stapedius reflex in multiple sclerosis. *J. Neurol. Neurosurg. Psychiat. 42*, 331–337.

Jacobson, J., Deppe, U., & Murray, R.J. (1983). Dichotic paradigms in multiple sclerosis. *Ear Hear. 4*, 311–317.

Jerger, J., & Jerger, S. (1975). Clinical validity of central auditory tests. *Scand. Audiol. 4*, 147–163.

Jerger, J., & Mauldin, L. (1978). Prediction of sensorineural hearing level from the brainstem evoked response. *Archs Otolar. 104*, 456–461.

Jerger, J., Brown, D., & Smith, S. (1984). Effect of peripheral hearing loss on the masking level difference. *Archs Otolar. 110*, 290–295.

Jerger, J., Oliver, T.A., Rivera, V., & Stach, B.A. (1986). Abnormalities of the acoustic reflex in multiple sclerosis. *Am. J. Otolar. 7*, 163–176.

Kjaer, M. (1980). Variations of brain stem auditory evoked potentials correlated to duration and severity of multiple sclerosis. *Acta Neur. Scand. 61*, 157–166.

Kjaer, M. (1983). Evoked potentials. With special reference to the diagnostic value in multiple sclerosis. *Acta Neur. Scand. 67*, 67–89.

Kofler, B. (1985). Visuell und akustisch evozierte Potentiale bei der multiplen Sklerose. *Wien. Med. Wschr. 135*, 35–38.

Kofler, F., Oberascher, G., & Pommer, B. (1984). Brain-stem involvement in multiple sclerosis: a comparison between brain-stem auditory evoked potentials and the acoustic stapedius reflex. *J. Neurol. 231*, 145–147.

Lacquaniti, F., Benna, P., Gilli, M., Troni, W., & Bergamasco, B. (1979). Brain stem auditory evoked potentials and blink reflex in quiescent multiple sclerosis. *Electroenceph. Clin. Neurophysiol. 47*, 607–610.

Luxon, L.M. (1980). Hearing loss in brainstem disorders. *J. Neurol. Neurosurg. Psychiat. 43*, 510–515.

McDonald, W.I. The role of evoked potentials in the diagnosis of multiple sclerosis; in Bauer, Poser, Ritter, Progress in multiple sclerosis research (Springer, New York 1980).

Maurer, K., Schafer, E., Hopf, H.C., & Leitner, H. (1980). The location by early auditory evoked potentials (EAEP) of acoustic nerve and brainstem demyelination in multiple sclerosis (MS). *J. Neurol. 223*, 43–58.

Noffsinger, D., Olsen, W.O., Carhart, R., Hart, C.W., & Sahgal, V. (1972). Auditory and vestibular aberrations in multiple sclerosis. *Acta oto-lar. 303*, suppl., pp. 1–63.

Oberascher, G. (1985). Otoneurologische Untersuchungsmöglichkeiten bei der multiplen Sklerose. *Wien. med. Wschr. 135*, 31–33.

Olsen, W., Noffsinger, D., & Kurdziel, S. (1975). Speech discrimination in quiet and in white noise by patients with peripheral and central lesions. *Acta Otolar. 80*, 375–382.

Olsen, W.O., Noffsinger, D., & Carhart, R. (1976). Masking level differences encountered in clinical populations. *Audiology 15*, 287–301.

Parving, A., Elberling, C., & Smith, T. (1981). Auditory electrophysiology: findings in multiple sclerosis. *Audiology 20*, 123–142.

Purves, S.J., Low, M.D., Galloway, J., & Reeves, B. (1981). A comparison of visual, brainstem auditory, and somatosensory evoked potentials in multiple sclerosis. *Can. J. Neurol. Sci. 8*, 15–19.

Robinson, K., & Rudge, P. (1977). The early components of the auditory evoked potential in multiple sclerosis. *Prog. Clin. Neurophysiol., 2*, 58–67.

Russolo, M., & Poli, P. (1983). Lateralization, impedance, auditory brainstem response, and synthetic sentence audiometry in brainstem disorders. *Audiology 22*, 50–62.

Sears, E.S., McCammon, A., Bigelow, R., & Hayman, L.A. (1970). Maximizing the harvest of contrast enhancing lesions in multiple sclerosis. *Neurology 20*, 1–59.

Stach, B., & Jerger, J. (1984). Acoustic reflex averaging. *Ear Hear. 5*, 289–296.

Stockard, J.J., Stockard, J.E., & Sharbrough, F.W. (1977). Detection and localization of occult lesions with brainstem auditory lesions. *Mayo Clin. Proc. 52*, 761–769.

Tackmann, W., Strenge, H., Barth, R., & Sojka-Raytscheff, A. (1980). Auditory brain stem evoked potentials in patients with multiple sclerosis. *Eur. Neurol. 19*, 396–401.

Waksman, F.H., & Reynolds, W.E. Research on multiple sclerosis (National Multiple Sclerosis Society, New York 1982).

ARTICLE SIX

SELF-ASSESSMENT QUESTIONS

1. Which combination of tests provided the greatest identification rate of patients with multiple sclerosis:
   (a) acoustic reflex measures or speech audiometry
   (b) masking level difference or auditory brainstem response testing
   (c) speech audiometry or masking level difference
   (d) acoustic reflex, speech audiometry, or auditory brainstem response testing
   (e) b and c

2. The most commonly observed abnormality in auditory brainstem response testing was:
   (a) selective loss of late waves
   (b) absence of wave I
   (c) poor morphology
   (d) reduced amplitude of all waves
   (e) prolonged latency of all waves

3. The most prevalent abnormality found on speech audiometry was:
   (a) rollover of the PI-PB function
   (b) reduced PB max score
   (c) reduced SSI-ICM score
   (d) reduced DSI score

4. The present study argues that one test may be overrated in its ability to identify multiple sclerosis. This test is:
   (a) speech audiometry
   (b) auditory brainstem response testing
   (c) suprathreshold acoustic reflex testing
   (d) masking level difference

5. This study indicates that there is a:
   (a) high prevalence of auditory abnormality in multiple sclerosis
   (b) great value in using a battery of tests, rather than a single test, for diagnostic procedures
   (c) all of the above
   (d) none of the above

Case Studies in Binaural Interference: Converging Evidence from Behavioral and Electrophysiologic Measures

James Jerger*
Shlomo Silman†
Henry L. Lew*
Rose Chmiel*

Abstract

We present four case reports of elderly hearing-impaired persons demonstrating a binaural interference effect. Performance measures were poorer when stimulation was binaural than when it was monaural. In the first case the effect is shown for aided speech recognition scores. In the second case it is shown in topographic brain maps of the middle-latency auditory evoked potential. In the third and fourth cases it is shown for both aided speech recognition and the middle-latency response. The effect may be analogous to the phenomenon of binocular rivalry in the visual domain.

Key Words: Binaural, binaural interference, binocular rivalry, cued-listening task, MLR, middle-latency response, monaural, speech recognition, topographic brain mapping

Evidence for binaural advantage in the normal auditory system is well documented. In general, when both ears are stimulated the result is better than for stimulation of either ear alone. When, for example, listeners are asked to compare the loudness of monaural and binaural pure tones, the monaural stimulus must be 6 to 10 dB more intense than the binaural stimulus to be judged equally loud (Haggard and Hall, 1982). Many investigators have also reported better speech understanding in the binaural as compared to the monaural mode (Harris 1965; Dirks and Wilson, 1969; Kaplan and Pickett, 1981). Using the Word Intelligibility by Picture Identification (WIPI) test (Yonovitz et al, 1979), the Modified Rhyme Test (MRT) (Nabelek and Robinson, 1982), the Sentence Identification in Noise (SIiN) test (Davis et al, 1990), and the Synthetic Sentence Identification (SSI) test (Kaplan and Pickett, 1981), investigators have reported binaural advantages ranging from 5 to 21 percent.

A number of studies have demonstrated binaural advantage in the amplitudes of auditory evoked potentials (Dobie and Berlin, 1979; Debruyne, 1984; Kelly-Ballweber and Dobie, 1984; Ito et al, 1988; McPherson et al, 1989). In general, subjects show larger auditory evoked response amplitudes to binaural than to monaural stimulation. Many researchers have reported that the earlier waves of the auditory brainstem response to binaural stimulation are reasonably identical to the algebraic summation of the two monaural responses (Ainslie and Boston, 1980; Debruyne, 1984; Dobie and Wilson, 1985). Specifically, for waves I and III, there is a 100 percent increase in amplitude with binaural as compared to monaural stimulation. At higher levels in the central auditory system, however, the binaural effect is apparently more complex than the simple summation of the two monaural responses (Dobie and Norton, 1980; Hosford-Dunn et al, 1981; Wrege and Starr, 1981; Prasher et al, 1982). Prasher and associates, for example, reported only a 68.7 percent increase in wave V amplitude from monaural to binaural stimulation in normal subjects.

Fewer binaural effects have been reported using longer latency auditory evoked potentials. Studies investigating the middle latency re-

---

*Division of Audiology, Baylor College of Medicine, Houston, Texas; † Department of Speech, Brooklyn College of the City University of New York, New York, New York

Reprint requests: James Jerger, NSC, NA 200, 6565 Fannin St., Houston, TX 77030

sponse (MLR) have shown that the binaural amplitude of the positive peak P_a is greater than the monaural amplitude, but smaller than the algebraic sum of the two monaural responses (Dobie and Norton, 1980; Debruyne, 1984; Kelly-Ballweber and Dobie, 1984; Woods and Clayworth, 1985). In the late response (LR), binaural and monaural amplitudes of the N_1 and P_2 are almost identical (Debruyne, 1984).

In the normal visual system, an analogous binocular advantage is also well documented. The effect has been demonstrated behaviorally by Snellen acuity (Barany, 1946), brightness threshold (Levelt, 1965), and contrast sensitivity (Legge, 1984). There is also evidence for binocular advantage in visually evoked potentials (VEPs). Typically, the amplitudes of the VEPs are compared under monocular and binocular conditions. When identical visual stimuli are delivered to each eye, the binocular VEP shows a larger amplitude than the monocular VEP, resulting in binocular advantage (Pardhan et al, 1990).

However, while binocular stimulation provides improvement in persons with normal vision, it introduces binocular rivalry in patients with strabismus, congenital cataract, or astigmatism (Von Noorden, 1974; Pickwell, 1989). As a result of binocular rivalry, amblyopia may develop. In humans with amblyopia (Wanger and Nilsson, 1978) or other defective binocular functions (Katsumi et al, 1986, 1988), responses to binocular stimulation may be poorer than responses to monocular stimulation. This phenomenon has been described as binocular inhibition, binocular rivalry, or binocular interference.

In the present paper we ask whether a similar effect might be observed in the auditory domain. In spite of the theoretical advantages of binaural amplification for individuals with bilateral hearing loss, for example, clinicians have long recognized that some persons, especially elderly persons, prefer to use one rather than two hearing aids. There are several possible explanations for this observation. In many such cases it is entirely possible that the individual views hearing aid use as a sign of aging and feels that the use of two hearing aids connotes twice the age-related handicap as the use of one. Other possible factors are cost, poor manual dexterity, cognitive deficits, or other general health problems. Finally, there may be genuine peripheral and/or central disorders that could lead to a binaural interference effect, perhaps not unlike the phenomenon of binocular rivalry leading to amblyopia in the visual system. Such

a binaural interference effect, in which the response from the poorer ear actually interferes with the response from the better ear, might lead to poorer performance with binaural than with monaural aids.

The concept of binaural interference in the auditory domain is not new. As early as 1971, for example, Arkebauer, Mencher, and McCall theorized that speech understanding might be reduced when differently distorted signals are received by the two ears. They hypothesized that, in patients with asymmetric hearing loss, there may be an inability to integrate or separate two speech signals. They also presented preliminary evidence suggesting that, when the poorer ear was excluded from testing, speech understanding improved. More recently, Hood and Prasher (1990) studied the effect of simulated bilateral cochlear impairment on speech understanding. They showed that, when speech was asymmetrically distorted at the two ears of normal subjects, the speech understanding score in response to binaural stimulation was poorer than the best monaural score.

These considerations suggest that at least some hearing-impaired individuals may, indeed, function better with one than with two hearing aids; that a binaural interference effect may nullify the theoretical advantage of binaural amplification. Our purpose, in presenting the following series of case reports, is to offer converging evidence for such a binaural interference effect from both behavioral and electrophysiologic measures of monaural and binaural function. We present detailed findings in four cases. The first case illustrates the binaural interference phenomenon in the behavioral evaluation of hearing aid performance. The second case illustrates the phenomenon in an electrophysiologic measure of auditory function, the middle latency response (MLR). The third and fourth cases illustrate both kinds of binaural interference in elderly hearing aid users.

CASE REPORTS

Case 1: Behavioral Example of Binaural Interference

Mrs. AW, a 71-year-old woman, reported that her hearing problems are age related. She first noticed a hearing problem about 15 years previously and it became gradually worse with time. She was fitted with a hearing aid in her left ear 10 years previously and has used it

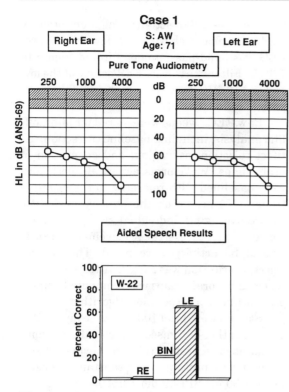

Figure 1 Audiograms and aided W-22 scores of case 1. Aided binaural score is significantly poorer than aided left-ear score.

almost continuously since that time. She recently returned to the audiology clinic for re-evaluation and a check on the performance of her hearing aid.

Figure 1 shows the results of this evaluation. The pure-tone audiogram, at the top, showed a relatively severe bilateral sensitivity loss. In spite of this symmetry in pure-tone sensitivity, there was a substantial difference in unaided suprathreshold word recognition. When W-22 lists were presented at a sensation level of 30 dB, scores were 50 percent for the left ear but 0 percent for the right ear. This difference in interaural word recognition cannot be attributed to greater sensitivity loss in the right ear. Indeed, hearing sensitivity was actually slightly better in the right ear than in the left ear.

In order to compare monaural and binaural conditions, we fitted patient AW with binaural behind-the-ear aids. These aids were initially selected on the basis of real-ear measures of frequency response according to the Berger rule. That is, aids were selected for evaluation based on the frequency response yielding, at each audiometric test frequency, a real-ear gain equivalent to the gain recommended by the Berger rule at that frequency. Further selection

was based on informal reports of sound quality until a single aid, representing the patient's overall preference in terms of perceived sound quality, was chosen. These aids were used in all subsequent tests of speech understanding in the monaural and binaural modes. The gain control of each aid was set, by the patient, to comfort level for continuous discourse presented at a level of 60 dB SPL. This adjustment was made separately for each condition of stimulation (i.e., right ear, left ear, and binaural).

The bottom panel of Figure 1 shows aided performance in the sound field. Target stimuli were 50-word W-22 lists delivered from a loudspeaker mounted at eye level directly in front of the patient (0-degree azimuth) at a distance of about 1 meter. The presentation level was 50 dB HL. When the left ear was aided, the behavioral performance score was 64 percent. When the right ear was aided, the analogous performance score was 0 percent. This difference was, of course, not unexpected in view of the 50 percent interaural difference in unaided W-22 scores. Of particular note, however, is the performance score obtained when both ears were aided (binaural condition). This score was only 22 percent, or 42 percent poorer than the score in the aided-left condition. If in the binaural condition the input to the right ear were having no effect on overall performance, then the binaural score would be expected to be a repeat of the left-ear aided score (i.e., 64%). The observed binaural score of 22 percent suggests that the right-sided input not only was having no effect on aided performance, but was also actually detrimental to aided performance. When the left ear alone was aided, performance was 64 percent. But when both ears were aided performance dropped to only 22 percent. We interpret this difference as evidence of binaural interference in aided speech recognition.

In order to determine whether this 42 percent performance difference was statistically significant we analyzed 95 percent critical difference scores for percentages according to the binomial model proposed by Thornton and Raffin (1978). According to this model, the observed difference of 42 percent was significant (p < .05).

Finally, in order to assure ourselves that W-22 scores were reliable in this patient, we repeated the binaural condition after a rest interval of 1 hour. This second binaural score was also 22 percent, identical to the original binaural score.

We suggest that this case illustrates a behavioral binaural interference phenomenon for aided speech recognition.

Case 2: Electrophysiologic Example of Binaural Interference

Mr. RC is a 66-year-old-man with a history of viral encephalitis. Since recovery he has complained of a hearing problem in his left ear.

Figure 2 shows RC's pure-tone audiogram. The right ear showed a mild loss below 2000 Hz. Both ears showed a steeply sloping loss above 6000 Hz. Word recognition for PB-50 word lists was within normal limits (90%) in both ears, but synthetic sentence identification (Jerger et al, 1968) was relatively poor. Maximum SSI scores were 20 percent in the right ear and 40 percent in the left ear.

We studied the auditory middle latency response (MLR) in patient RC by means of topographic brain mapping (Neuroscan System). Gold cup electrodes were affixed to the scalp according to the 10–20 International System (Jasper, 1958). No interelectrode impedance exceeded 5000 ohms. Eighteen channels of electroencephalogram (EEG) activity were referred to linked earlobes as reference. In addition, electro-ocular activity was monitored by electrodes placed above and below the left eye. EEG was band-pass, analog filtered from 5 to 120 Hz. Filter skirts were 6 dB/octave at the low end and 12 dB/octave at the high end of the band pass. The duration of each epoch was 100 msec.

Raw EEG sweeps were stored for later, off-line analysis, including baseline correction, artifact rejection, averaging, and generation of brain maps. Waveforms across all electrodes were baselined with reference to the negative trough (N_a) preceding the positive peak (P_a). Before averaging, individual sweeps were rejected if either excessive eye movement or excessive alpha activity were noted. The artifact rejection criterion was $\pm 5\,\mu V$. After averaging, topographic brain maps were computed using a 4-point linear interpolation algorithm.

Stimuli were brief 1000-Hz tone pips with a total duration of 5 msec (2-1-2 configuration). Stimulus presentation rate was always 4.1/sec. Stimuli were presented at a constant intensity level of 80 dB SPL under three conditions: (1) sound to right ear, (2) sound to left ear, and (3) sound to both ears (binaural). A total of 1000 stimuli were presented in each of the three conditions. Finally, to maintain an alert state, and to minimize eye-movement artifact, the patient was permitted to view the video portion of a videotaped cartoon during the testing period.

Figure 3 compares topographic brain maps of the MLR of patient RC with analogous maps obtained from a young adult with normal hearing and no history of brain disease. All maps represent the topographic distribution of electrical activity at the P_a latency, defined at electrode F_z. In the case of the normal control, the expected symmetric distribution of positivity across the anterior portion of the skull was observed. The area of maximum positivity was slightly larger for left-ear stimulation than for right, and larger still for binaural stimulation. In the case of patient RC, right-ear stimulation produced a relatively normal distribution of anterior positivity, but left-ear stimulation produced a distinctly abnormal distribution over the left temporoparietal region. Finally, binaural stimulation produced less activity than right-ear stimulation alone. In the binaural mode, the presence of the left-ear input apparently interfered with the right-ear input in such a way that the binaural response was substantially poorer than the response to right-ear stimulation alone.

We suggest that case 2 provides electrophysiologic evidence of binaural interference.

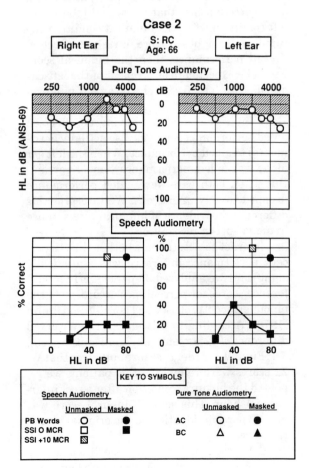

Figure 2 Audiograms and unaided speech audiometric results in case 2.

Case 3: Example of Both Behavioral and Electrophysiologic Evidence of Binaural Interference

Mr. BV is an 80-year-old man with a history of left-sided cerebrovascular insult. Figure 4 shows his pure-tone audiogram. The left ear shows a mild loss in the low-frequency region below 1000 Hz and a steeply sloping loss above 1000 Hz. The right ear shows a similar high-frequency loss and a slightly greater low-frequency loss. Under earphones, the W-22 score at a sensation level of 30 dB was 80 percent in the left ear and 36 percent in the right ear. A hearing-aid evaluation was carried out in the same fashion as case 1. The bottom panel of Figure 4 shows the results. When the left ear was aided monaurally, the W-22 score was 76 percent. When the right ear was aided monaurally, the word recognition score was 8 percent. During this test BV reported that in the right ear he heard only noise. When both ears were aided (binaural condition) the W-22 score fell to only 54 percent, a statistically significant decline (p < .05). In order to assess the reliability of these findings, we retested BV in all three aided conditions 3 weeks later. On this occasion the left ear score was 72 percent, the right ear score was 0 percent, and the binaural score was 42 percent. A further retest of the binaural condition 1 hour later yielded a score of 38 percent. It is noteworthy that even though the right ear seemed to be contributing nothing to word recognition, the presence of the right-ear input appeared to have an interfering effect on word recognition from left-ear stimulation.

In order to determine whether there might be concomitant electrophysiologic evidence of binaural interference, we measured the middle-latency auditory evoked potential under the three conditions of stimulation: signal to right ear, signal to left ear, and signal to both ears (binaural). The eliciting signal was a 1000-Hz tone pip with a total duration of 6 msec (2-2-2 configuration) presented at the rate of 9.7/sec. The presentation level was 115 dB peSPL. The active electrode was at C_z, the reference electrode at the ipsilateral earlobe, and the common electrode at the contralateral earlobe. EEG was filtered from 10 to 250 Hz, epoch length was 60 msec, and 2000 sweeps were averaged.

Figure 5 shows two replications of each waveform. Stimulation of the left ear produced a robust response. The latency at P_a was 36 msec, and the amplitude at that peak was 1.83 µV. When the right ear was stimulated, the amplitude at P_a was substantially reduced to only 0.90 µV. It could be argued that this reduction was to be expected in view of the 15 dB difference in sensitivity at 1000 Hz shown in the pure-tone audiogram. Not to be expected, however, was the reduction in amplitude of the response to binaural stimulation. Here the amplitude of 0.97 µV is substantially less than the response from the left ear alone. If the right ear were simply contributing nothing to the response, then the binaural MLR should be a repeat of the left ear MLR. The fact that the binaural response was so much smaller suggests an interference effect when the right and left ears were stimulated simultaneously.

In case 3, then, we have evidence of binaural interference from both behavioral and electrophysiologic measures. The W-22 score declined from 76 percent, when only the left ear was aided, to 54 percent when both ears were aided, and the amplitude of the MLR declined from 1.83 µV, when only the left ear was stimulated, to 0.97 µV, when both ears were stimulated.

Case 4: Example of Both Behavioral and Electrophysiologic Evidence of Binaural Interference

Mr. JB is an 81-year-old man who reported a gradual onset of mild hearing difficulty over the past decade. There is no history of stroke or other cardiac problem. He reports difficulties only in certain social situations. Figure 6 shows the pure-tone and speech audiometric results. We see the bilateral high-frequency loss pattern typical of presbyacusis. The sensitivity loss is slightly greater in the left ear. Unaided speech audiometry under earphones yielded a maximum PB score for PAL-50 words of 100 percent in the right ear and 60 percent in the left ear. The maximum score for SSI sentences was 80 percent in the right ear and 10 percent in the left ear.

Topographic brain maps of the middle latency response were derived using the signals, recording techniques, and algorithms summarized earlier for case 2. Figure 7 shows the waveform of the MLR at the electrode F_z under each of the three conditions of stimulation. When the right ear was stimulated, there was a robust response with a positive peak at 35 msec. The amplitude at this latency was 1.6 µV. When the left ear was stimulated there was no observable MLR. Nor was there a repeatable response when both ears were stimulated (binaural con-

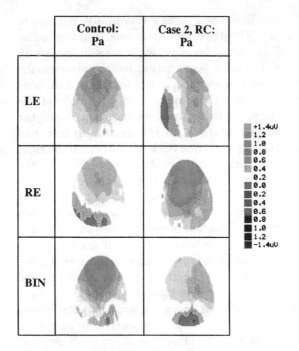

Figure 3 Topographic brain maps of the middle-latency averaged evoked potential at positive peak P_a. Right panels, case 2; left panels, normal young adult.

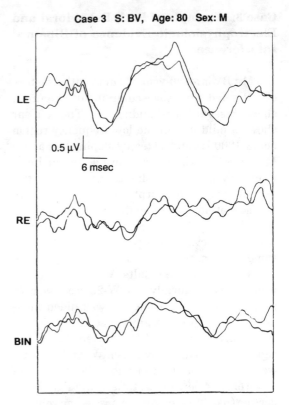

Figure 5 Waveforms of the middle-latency averaged evoked potential in case 3. Amplitude is less for binaural stimulation than for left-ear stimulation.

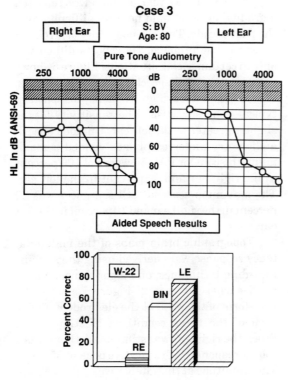

Figure 4 Audiograms and aided W-22 scores of case 3. Aided binaural score is significantly poorer than aided left-ear score.

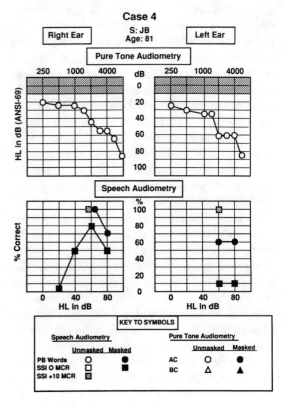

Figure 6 Audiograms and unaided speech audiometric results in case 4.

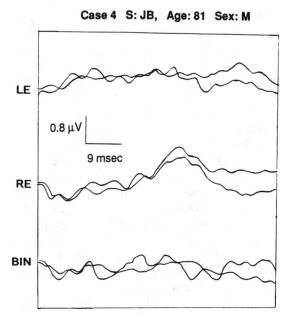

Case 4 S: JB, Age: 81 Sex: M

Figure 7 Waveforms of the middle-latency averaged evoked potential in case 4. Amplitude is less for binaural stimulation than for the right-ear stimulation.

dition). Figure 8 shows topographic brain maps of the MLR at P_a. For right-ear stimulation, positivity was distributed symmetrically across the anterior region in normal fashion. For left-ear stimulation, there was a much smaller response over the right frontal area. When both ears were stimulated, the map showed positivity only over the left frontotemporal area. Stimulation of the left ear appeared to interfere with the normal response from stimulation of the right ear.

Interestingly there was no evidence of binaural interference in the auditory brainstem response. Figure 9 shows that, when click stimuli (100 μsec pulses of alternating polarity) were delivered binaurally, wave V amplitude (0.31 μV) was larger than the amplitude for either the right ear alone (0.23 μV) or the left ear alone (0.15 μV).

We evaluated JB's aided performance using the Cued-Listening Task (Jerger and Jordan, 1992). The patient was seated in the center of a sound-treated room and equidistant between two loudspeakers, one directly to his right (azimuth = 90 degrees) and the other directly to his left (azimuth = 270 degrees). A third loudspeaker was mounted on the ceiling directly above his head. Continuous discourse of a male talker reading an adventure story, written in the first person, was presented to both the left and right loudspeakers. The story from one loudspeaker was offset by about 60 seconds

relative to the story from the other loudspeaker. Thus, different parts of the same story were presented simultaneously from the left and right sides. The patient responded by pressing a response button each time he heard the personal pronoun "I" from the direction cued by a signal light. Multitalker babble was played through the loudspeaker mounted above the patient's head. Before testing began, the presentation level of the story was adjusted to a comfortable listening level by playing the same recording, but without time offset, through both loudspeakers. The intensity level of the multi-talker babble was then adjusted to a message-to-competition ratio (MCR) of –5 dB.

For each aided condition (right ear aided, left ear aided, both ears aided), we presented 100 target "I"s, 50 from the patient's right and 50 from his left. The 50 targets from a particular side were presented in 5 blocks of 10 targets each. The order in which the 10 blocks (5 from the right, 5 from the left) were presented was quasi-randomized with the constraint that no condition (listen right or listen left) was presented more than twice in succession. The direc-

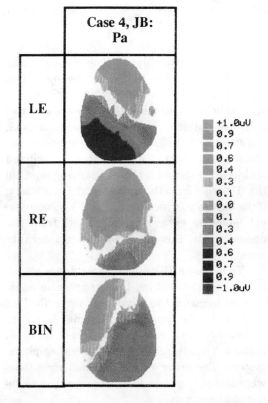

Figure 8 Topographic brain maps of the middle-latency average evoked potential at positive peak P_a in case 4. When stimulation is to right ear only, topographic distribution is normal. When stimulation is binaural, topographic distribution is abnormal.

Case 4 S: JB, Age: 81 Sex: M

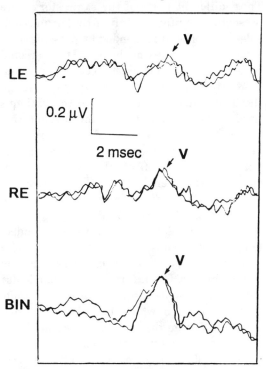

Figure 9 Waveforms of the auditory brainstem response in case 4. When stimulation is binaural, amplitude at wave V is larger than when stimulation is either to the right ear alone or to the left ear alone.

tion from which the targets came in a particular block was precued to the patient by one of two signal lights, one labelled "listen right" and the other labelled "listen left." There were also two response buttons, one for right-sided targets, the other for left-sided targets. A response was accepted and scored as correct if it occurred within a 1.5 second interval following onset of the "I" target from the correct side. Conversely, if the button push occurred with a 1.5 sec interval following onset of a target "I" from the noncued side, this was scored as a laterality error.

To evaluate JB's aided performance we fitted him with two behind-the-ear programmable aids set to match the target gain prescribed for each ear by the Australian National Acoustics Laboratory (NAL) rule, (Byrne and Dillon, 1986) using a Virtual, model 340 probe-microphone system. The order in which aided conditions were tested (right vs left vs binaural) was selected at random.

Figure 10 summarizes aided performance in terms of both correct identifications (A) and incorrect laterality errors (B). In the unaided condition, JB's correct identifications, averaged

across both target directions, totalled 61 percent. In the aided right condition he scored 37 percent, in the aided left condition 18 percent, and in the aided binaural condition 34 percent. In terms of laterality errors he scored 17 percent in the unaided condition, 17 percent in the aided right condition, 15 percent in the aided left condition, and 28 percent in the aided binaural condition. In order to derive a performance index combining both correct identifications and laterality errors, we treated the correct identifications as "hits," the laterality errors as "false alarms," and computed the detectability index d' (Clarke and Bilger, 1973). These results are summarized in Figure 11. For the right-ear aided condition the d' was 0.62, for the left-ear aided condition 0.11, and for the binaural-aided condition 0.17. Thus, overall performance in the binaural condition was only slightly better than left-ear aided alone, and substantially worse than right-ear aided alone. Detailed analysis of laterality errors revealed that the high error score in the binaural condition was due to unu-

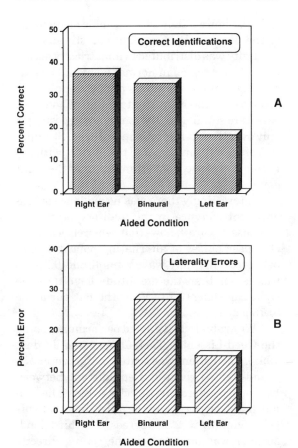

Figure 10 Performance of case 4 on a cued-listening task. A...Correct identifications, B...laterality errors. When both ears are aided correct identifications are smaller, and laterality errors are larger, than when only the right ear is aided.

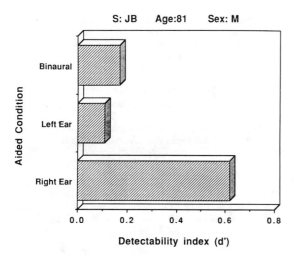

Figure 11 Performance of case 4 on the cued-listening task, expressed as the detectability index, d'.

sual difficulty when targets came from the left side. In this condition, the laterality error score was 21 percent in the aided-right condition, 29 percent in the aided-left condition, and 56 percent in the aided-binaural condition. In other words, when the target came from JB's left side he showed least laterality errors when only the right ear was aided, slightly more errors when only the left ear was aided, and almost twice as many errors when both ears were aided. It was as if the binaural aids hampered his ability to make successful left-right localizations.

In summary, we have seen in this case both electrophysiologic and behavioral evidence of binaural interference.

DISCUSSION

The present results suggest that a binaural interference phenomenon, perhaps analogous to binocular rivalry in the visual system, can be observed in the auditory domain. In the present paper we have demonstrated such a phenomenon both behaviorally, in the context of the evaluation of hearing aid performance, and electrophysiologically, in the context of the middle-latency auditory evoked potential.

It is appropriate to ask whether the binaural interference effect can be explained by audiometric asymmetries. In cases 3 and 4, for example, can the interference effect be explained by the fact that there was apparently more peripheral hearing sensitivity loss on the poorer functioning ear? The answer would appear to be negative. No degree of audiometric asymmetry can explain the observation of poorer response when both ears are stimulated than when only

one is stimulated. If there were no hearing at all in one of the two ears, we should still expect that the response to binaural stimulation would be at least as good as stimulation of the other ear alone. If stimulation of the better ear produces a given response, and stimulation of both ears produces a poorer response, then it must be concluded that stimulation of the poorer ear has, in some way, interfered with the response from the better ear. And this would be true no matter what the degree of interaural audiometric asymmetry.

In the absence of definitive data, it is difficult to estimate the prevalence of binaural interference in the population of potential hearing aid users. In our own audiology service we compared monaural and binaural aided performance in a small sample of 37 elderly persons who had been evaluated for hearing aid use. Hearing aid performance was measured in the sound field using the SSI paradigm described by Jerger and Hayes (1976). If we defined a significant difference in performance as an SSI difference in excess of 30 percent, then 3 of the 37 candidates performed less well in the binaural mode than in the best monaural mode. On this basis, we can estimate the prevalence of the problem, very roughly, to be about 8 to 10 percent among elderly hearing aid users, but better data are needed before a definitive answer to the question of prevalence can be given.

The exact mechanism of the binaural interference effect is not clear. It would appear, however, that by virtue of asymmetric distortion, either on a peripheral or central basis, the input to one auditory pathway suppresses or inhibits the input to the other pathway. The effect is, perhaps, analogous to binocular rivalry, leading to amblyopia in the visual system.

REFERENCES

Ainslie P, Boston J. (1980). Comparison of brain stem auditory evoked potentials for monaural and binaural stimuli. *EEG Clin Neurophysiol* 49:291–302.

Arkebauer HJ, Mencher GT, McCall C. (1971). Modification of speech discrimination in patients with binaural asymmetrical hearing loss. *J Speech Hear Disord* 36: 208–212.

Barany E. (1946). A theory of binocular visual acuity and an analysis of the variability of visual acuity. *Acta Ophthalmol* 24:63–92.

Byrne D, Dillon H. (1986). The National Acoustic Laboratories' (NAL) new procedure for selecting the gain and frequency response of a hearing aid. *Ear Hear* 7:257–265.

Clarke FR, Bilger RC. (1973). The theory of signal detectability and the measurement of hearing. In: Jerger J, ed. *Modern Developments in Audiology*. 2nd ed. New York: Academic Press.

Davis A, Haggard M, Bell I. (1990). Magnitude of diotic summation in speech-in-noise tasks: performance region and appropriate baseline. *Br J Audiol* 24:11–16.

Debruyne F. (1984). Binaural interaction in early, middle and late auditory evoked responses. *Scand Audiol* 13: 293–296.

Dirks D, Wilson R. (1969). Binaural hearing for aided and unaided conditions. *J Speech Hear Res* 12:650–664.

Dobie R, Berlin C. (1979). Binaural interaction in brainstem-evoked responses. *Arch Otolaryngol* 105: 391–398.

Dobie R, Norton S. (1980). Binaural interaction in human auditory evoked potentials. *EEG Clin Neurophysiol* 49:303–13.

Dobie R, Wilson M. (1985). Binaural interaction in auditory brain-stem responses: effects of masking. *EEG Clin Neurophysiol* 62:56–64.

Haggard M, Hall J. (1982). Forms of binaural summation and the implications of individual variability for binaural hearing aids. *Scand Audiol* 15 (Suppl): 47–63.

Harris J. (1965). Monaural and binaural speech intelligibility and stereophonic effects based upon temporal cues. *Laryngoscope* 75:428–446.

Hood J, Prasher D. (1990). Effect of simulated bilateral cochlear distortion on speech discrimination in normal subjects. *Scand Audiol* 19:37–41.

Hosford-Dunn H, Mendelson T, Salamy A. (1981). Binaural interactions in the short-latency evoked potentials of neonates. *Audiology* 20:394–408.

Ito S, Hoke M, Pantev C, Lutkenhoner B. (1988). Binaural interaction in brainstem auditory evoked potentials elicited by frequency-specific stimuli. *Hear Res* 35:9–20.

Jasper H. (1958). The ten-twenty electrode system of the International Federation. *EEG Clin Neurophysiol* 10:371–375.

Jerger J, Speaks C, Trammel J. (1968). A new approach to speech audiometry. *J Speech Hear Disord* 33:318–327.

Jerger J, Hayes D. (1976). Hearing aid evaluation. *Arch Otolaryngol* 102:214–225.

Jerger J, Jordan C. (1992). Age increases asymmetry on a cued-listening task. *Ear Hear* 13:272–277.

Kaplan H, Pickett J. (1981). Effects of dichotic/diotic versus monotic presentation on speech understanding in noise in elderly hearing-impaired listeners. *Ear Hear* 2:202–207.

Katsumi O, Tanino T, Hirose T. (1986). Effect of aniseikonia on binocular function. *Invest Ophthalmol Vis Sci* 27:601–604.

Katsumi O, Hirose T, Tanino T, Uemura Y. (1988). Pattern reversal VER as a tool for evaluating unbalanced visual inputs between two eyes. *Jpn J Ophthalmol* 32: 86–97.

Kelly-Ballweber D, Dobie R. (1984). Binaural interaction measured behaviorally and electrophysiologically in young and old adults. *Audiology* 23:181–264.

Legge G. (1984). Binocular contrast summation — I. Detection and discrimination. *Vision Res* 24:373–383.

Levelt W. (1965). Binocular brightness averaging and contour information. *Br J Psychol* 56:1–13.

McPherson D, Tures C, Starr A. (1989). Binaural interaction of the auditory brain-stem potentials and middle latency auditory evoked potentials in infants and adults. *EEG Clin Neurophysiol* 74:124–130.

Nabelek A, Robinson P. (1982). Monaural and binaural speech perception in reverberation for listeners of various ages. *J Acoust Soc Am* 71:1242–1248.

Pardhan S, Gilchrist J, Douthwaite W. (1990). Binocular inhibition: psychophysical and electrophysiological evidence. *Optom Vis Sci* 67:688–691.

Pickwell D. (1989). *Binocular Vision Anomalies: Investigation and Treatment.* 2nd ed. London:Butterworths, 101–111.

Prasher D, Sainz M, Gibson W. (1982). Binaural voltage summation of brainstem auditory evoked potentials: an adjunct to the diagnostic criteria for multiple sclerosis. *Ann Neurol* 11:86–91.

Thornton A, Raffin M. (1978). Speech-discrimination scores modeled as a binomial variable. *J Speech Hear Res* 21:507–518.

Von Noorden GV. (1974). Factors involved in the production of amblyopia. *Br J Ophthalmol* 58:158–164.

Wanger P, Nilsson B. (1978). Visual evoked responses to pattern-reversal stimulation in patients with amblyopia and/or defective binocular functions. *Acta Ophthalmol* 56:617–627.

Woods D, Clayworth C. (1985). Click spatial position influences middle latency auditory evoked potentials (MAEPs) in humans. *EEG Clin Neurophysiol* 60: 122–129.

Wrege K, Starr A. (1981). Binaural interaction in human auditory brainstem evoked potentials. *Arch Neurol* 38:572–580.

Yonovitz A, Dickenson P, Miller D, Spydell J. (1979). Speech discrimination in children: auditory and auditory/visual processing with binaural and monaural presentation. *J Am Audiol Soc* 5:60–64.

Clinical Forum

Otoacoustic Emissions, Audiometric Sensitivity Loss, and Speech Understanding: A Case Study

James Jerger*
Ali Ali*
Karen Fong*
Ewen Tseng*

Abstract

The clinical measurement of otoacoustic emissions can assist in differentiating between peripheral and central explanations for deficits in speech understanding. We present audiometric and distortion-product emission data in a case with sensorineural hearing loss and a deficit in speech understanding. The presence of evoked emissions argues against attributing the speech audiometric loss to cochlear defect.

Key Words: Otoacoustic emissions, sensorineural hearing loss, speech understanding, peripheral hearing loss, central hearing loss, central auditory processing disorders

The interpretation of speech audiometric deficits is often limited by inability to separate the effects of peripheral sensitivity loss from the effects of central processing disorder (Helfer and Wilber, 1990; Humes and Roberts, 1990; Humes and Christopherson, 1991). If a patient has both a speech audiometric deficit and depressed audiometric sensitivity, especially in the frequency range above 1000 Hz, it may be difficult to determine how much of the speech understanding deficit should be attributed to central processing disorder versus how much should be attributed to peripheral (i.e., cochlear) hearing loss. Even in the case of patients with normal audiograms one cannot rule out the possibility of a subtle cochlear defect, sufficient to impact measures of speech understanding, but not sufficient to cause audiometric sensitivity loss for pure-tone signals (Bredberg, 1968). As long as the pure-tone audiogram served as the sole index of cochlear normality there was no easy solution to this problem.

With the advent of clinically viable methods for measuring otoacoustic emissions, especially distortion-product emissions, however, the distortion-product audiogram provides invaluable complimentary information about cochlear status. It is now widely accepted that, with only rare exceptions (e.g., Prieve et al, 1991), the presence of otoacoustic emissions at normal levels indicates normal outer-hair-cell function (Lonsbury-Martin and Martin, 1990; Norton and Widen, 1990). This places a powerful interpretive tool at our disposal. If it can be shown that a patient with a speech audiometric deficit has normal otoacoustic emissions, then it cannot be easily argued that the speech understanding deficit is attributable to cochlear deficit. This will be true irrespective of the level of the pure-tone audiogram.

In the present paper we report findings in such a case. The patient had speech audiometric deficits, depressed behavioral audiograms, but normal distortion-product emissions. We argue that the presence of emissions supports a central rather than a peripheral interpretation of the deficit in speech understanding.

METHOD

Distortion-product emissions were measured by means of commercially available system consisting of a microcomputer (Dynova 286), an Ariel board, an Etymotic ER10B probe

---

*Department of Otolaryngology & Communicative Sciences, Baylor College of Medicine, Houston, Texas

Reprint requests: James Jerger, 11922 Taylorcrest Rd., Houston, TX 77024

microphone system, two Etymotic ER2 tube-phones, and software developed by Jont Allen. For pairs of probe tones, f_1 and f_2, the amplitude, in dB SPL, of the cubic distortion product, $2f_1 - f_2$, was measured at the frequency f_2. Over the range from 1000 to 8000 Hz, 14 pairs of probe tones at approximately equally spaced logarithmic units of frequency were presented. The intensity levels, L_1 and L_2, corresponding to the probe-tone frequencies f_1 and f_2, were always 65 dB SPL. Thus the L_1/L_2 ratio was always 1.0. The f_2/f_1 frequency ratio was always 1.2. Normal values for the noise floor in this report are based on the distribution of test results in ten ears of five young adults with normal hearing and no hearing complaints. In subsequent figures the dashed lines denoting the normal limits for the noise floor encompass 90 percent of the expected normal range (± 1.65 standard deviations).

Conventional audiometric data were obtained during the course of routine clinical audiometric assessment. For pure-tone audiograms we used the Virtual 320 system, controlled by a MacIntosh II microcomputer. For speech audiometric measures tape-recorded phonetically balanced (PB) word lists and synthetic sentence identification (SSI) materials were delivered through the Virtual system. Immittance measures were obtained with an Amplaid 720 system.

CASE REPORT

Patient LS, a 29-year-old woman, had shown symptoms of multiple sclerosis (MS) for approximately 10 years. A diagnosis of definite MS was made 3 years prior to the present audiologic evaluation. Magnetic resonance imaging (MRI) of the brain, with and without contrast, revealed white matter lesions near the lateral ventricles, an extensive region of abnormality in the midline involving the entire superior margin of the corpus callosum, and a lesion in the deep left temporal white matter. She was referred to us with the complaint of progressive hearing loss in the right ear. Figure 1 summarizes the results of the conventional audiometric assessment. The left ear showed a mild low-frequency sensitivity loss, but was well within normal limits over the frequency range from 2000 to 8000 Hz. At no frequency on the left ear did the pure-tone threshold level exceed 20 dB HL. The score for PB words, presented at 80 dB HL, was 100 percent, and the maximum score for SSI at 0 dB MCR was 90 percent.

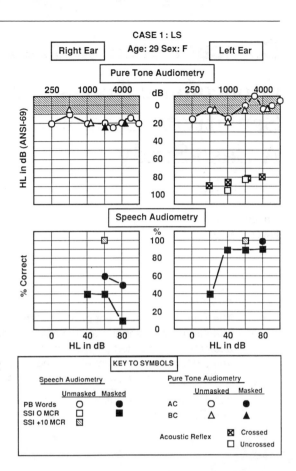

Figure 1 Audiometric results for a 29-year-old woman with multiple sclerosis. Note pure-tone and speech-audiometric deficits on the right side.

Results from the right ear, however, showed significant deficits. The pure-tone audiogram showed only a mild, relatively flat, sensitivity loss. The poorest threshold, at 3000 Hz, was 25 dB HL. In spite of this relatively mild sensitivity loss, however, speech understanding showed a marked deficit. The maximum PB score was only 60 percent, and the maximum SSI score was only 40 percent. In addition, there was significant rollover of the performance versus intensity (PI) function for SSI. The score decreased from 40 percent at 60 dB HL to 10 percent at 80 dB HL. Scores on the Dichotic Sentence Identification Test (DSI) in the focused attention mode were 100 percent on the left ear and 20 percent on the right ear.

Middle-ear function, as assessed by tympanometry, was normal bilaterally. With signals to the left ear, acoustic reflex thresholds, in both the crossed and uncrossed modes, varied from 80 to 95 dB HL over the frequency range from 500 to 4000 Hz. With signal to the right ear, however, neither crossed nor uncrossed acoustic reflexes could be elicited at any test frequency at intensity levels up to 110 dB HL.

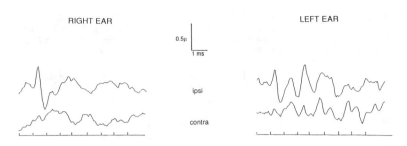

Figure 2 Auditory brainstem responses for the 29-year-old woman with multiple sclerosis.

The auditory brainstem response (ABR) was recorded from a convential four-electrode montage. The active electrode was at the vertex (c_z), reference electrodes at the earlobes, and the ground electrode on the forehead. The ABR was elicited by 100-microsecond pulses presented at the rate of 21.1 per second. The EEG was filtered from 150 to 3000 Hz. A total of 2,048 individual sweeps were averaged to define each ABR waveform.

Figure 2 shows that the ABR was within normal limits for clicks delivered to the left ear, but for right ear stimulation there were no repeatable waves beyond wave I.

The poor speech audiometric scores for the right ear are, of course, well outside the limits to be expected from patients with cochlear deficits at the 20 to 25 dB level (Yellin et al, 1989). Although extremely unlikely, one cannot rule out the possibility that the right ear's sensitivity loss might reflect a subclinical cochlear defect sufficient to account for the reduction in PB and SSI scores. If this were the case, however, we would expect that otoacoustic emissions would be reduced or absent from the right ear. Figure 3 shows that this was not the case. Across the f_2 range from 1000 to 8000 Hz the $2f_1 - f_2$ distortion product emissions were robust from both ears. We cannot, therefore, account for the poor speech audiometric scores from this patient's right ear on the basis of a right cochlear defect in spite of the slight apparent reduction in pure-tone sensitivity on the right side. Clearly,

a processing deficit at a more central site in the auditory system must be invoked.

COMMENT

This case (LS) illustrates how otoacoustic emissions can be useful in ruling out subtle cochlear defect as an explanation for deficits in speech understanding. There was a marked asymmetry in speech audiometric scores along with a slight asymmetry in pure-tone sensitivity levels. The presence of distortion-product otoacoustic emissions from both ears argues for a more central locus of the speech processing disorder.

Of course, this argument rests on the assumption that, in persons with sensorineural hearing loss, outer hair cell loss, evoked otoacoustic emissions, and audiometric threshold levels are highly correlated measures. It is possible, however, that the combination of substantial sensitivity loss and good otoacoustic emissions is the result of selective loss of inner hair cell function, with preservation of outer hair cells and the otoacoustic emissions generated by them. This was, indeed, the mechanism suggested by Prieve et al (1991) to explain their unusual results in a subject with severe sensorineural loss and an apparently normal tone-burst evoked emission. This is not, however, an attractive hypothesis to explain results in the present case. Although late waves of the right-ear ABR were abnormal, there was a robust wave I at levels of 60 and 80 dB nHL.

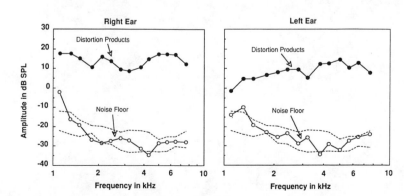

Figure 3 Distortion-product emissions are robust from both ears, in spite of pure-tone and speech-audiometric deficits on the right side.

We conclude, therefore, that the asymmetric speech audiometric deficit reflects central rather than peripheral asymmetry in auditory processing.

Acknowledgment.   We are grateful to the Dunn Foundation for partial support of this study, and to Charles Berlin and Linda Hood for helpful suggestions.

REFERENCES

Bredberg G. (1968) Cellular pattern and nerve supply of the human organ of Corti. *Acta Otolaryngol* (Stockh) Suppl 236.

Helfer K, Wilber L. (1990) Hearing loss, aging, and speech perception in reverberation and noise. *J Speech Hear Res* 33:149–155.

Humes L, Christopherson L. (1991) Speech identification difficulties of hearing-impaired elderly persons: the contributions of auditory processing deficits. *J Speech Hear Res* 34:686–693.

Humes L, Roberts L. (1990) Speech recognition difficulties of the hearing-impaired elderly: the contributions of audibility. *J Speech Hear Res* 33:726–735.

Lonsbury-Martin B, Martin G. (1990) The clinical utility of distortion-product otoacoustic emissions. *Ear Hear* 11:144–154.

Norton S, Widen J. (1990) Evoked otoacoustic emissions in normal-hearing infants and children: emerging data and issues. *Ear Hear* 11:121–127.

Prieve B, Gorga M, Neely S. (1991) Otoacoustic emissions in an adult with severe hearing loss. *J Speech Hear Res* 34:379–385.

Yellin MW, Jerger J, Fifer RC. (1989) Norms for disproportionate loss in speech intelligibility. *Ear Hear* 10:231–234.

Central Auditory Processing Disorder

Paula Tallal of Rutgers University, has a t-shirt decorated with the familiar anatomical drawing of the outer, middle, and inner ears. At conferences concerned with auditory processing she likes to hold up the t-shirt, turn it from side to side, and ask:

"What's wrong with this picture?"

Answering her own question she notes that there is no brain connected to the ear.

Regrettably, too many of us, in our zeal to understand how the ear works, neglect the fact that it is connected to a very complicated brain. We accept the concept that, if there is trouble in the ear, there can be a hearing problem, but many of us seem reluctant to accept the equally reasonable notion that, if there is trouble in the auditory pathways in the brain, there can also be a hearing problem. One of my early teachers at Northwestern, Helmer Myklebust, pioneered the idea that at least some of the language development problems of children might be the result of central auditory processing disorders. Another early influence on my thinking in this area was the unpublished doctoral dissertation of another early teacher, John Gaeth. This may very well be the most-cited unpublished dissertation in the history of scholarship. It has been a major

motivator of countless later studies and still appears in bibliographies on aging, although the research was carried out more than 45 years ago. Gaeth showed that, in many elderly persons with presbyacusic audiometric losses, speech recognition scores were unusually poor, poorer than could be reasonably accounted for by the degree of pure-tone loss. I always supposed that this reflected the influences of changes in the central auditory pathways, and subsequent experience has certainly verified this early supposition.

Today, the notion of central auditory processing disorder (CAPD) is fairly widespread. There is a perception that the academic problems of many children may be related to specifically auditory, as opposed to more general attentional, deficits. And indeed, intervention with assistive-listening devices to focus sound input and optimize signal-to-noise ratio has been remarkably successful. Similarly, we have come to understand that at least some of the communicative difficulties encountered by elderly persons are the result of age-related central auditory changes rather than the concomitant peripheral hearing loss, and that such problems are complex and may not necessarily be helped by conventional amplification.

But acceptance of the reality of CAPD has been slow and painful. In the early days, before acoustic reflexes, evoked potentials, and other electroacoustic and electrophysiologic tests, the only evidence we could marshal was based on behavioral tests, especially tests involving speech understanding under various conditions of degradation. But such evidence was never very convincing to our medical colleagues, especially in neurology. "Where," they were fond of asking, "is the *hard* evidence?" Where is the evidence that there really is something abnormal in the brain mechanisms of these children and elderly persons? In those days, hard evidence was abnormality in the EEG. Today, it is abnormalities revealed by imaging studies like computed tomography (CT), magnetic resonance imaging (MRI), or positron emission tomography (PET), the acoustic reflex, and auditory evoked potentials.

The first step in developing our own lines of "hard evidence" was to show that our tests did, indeed, reveal abnormalities in the central auditory system when such abnormalities were known to exist. And this was the direction that many investigators took in the 1960s and 1970s. Our own work along these lines is illustrated by the first four papers in this section: "Auditory Disorders Following Bilateral Temporal Lobe Insult" (*Journal of Speech and Hearing Disorders*, 1972), "Auditory Findings in Brain Stem Disorders" (*Archives of Otolaryngology*, 1974), "Clinical Validity of Central Auditory Tests" (*Scandinavian Audiology*, 1975), and "Neuroaudiologic Findings in Patients with Central Auditory Disorder" (*Seminars in Hearing*, 1983).

In each of these four papers, the main thrust is the effect that localized, confirmed brain lesions have on speech recognition. The object is to show how sensitive speech audiometric paradigms can be in revealing the effects of known lesions to the central auditory system and to show that such paradigms are specifically auditory, that is, not affected by CNS lesions that do not affect the auditory system.

The next paper, "Development of a Dichotic Sentence Identification Test for Hearing Impaired Adults" (*Ear & Hearing*, 1983) was the culmination of collaborative work between our laboratory at Baylor and the Kresge Hearing Research Laboratory at Louisiana State University in New Orleans. As a result of the pioneering work by Charles Berlin and his colleagues at the Kresge laboratory during the 1970s on Vietnam war veterans with closed head injuries, it became clear that the dichotic paradigm was going to be a powerful technique for the study of CAPD. The only problem was that the speech materials being used, digits, CVs, and spondees, were notoriously affected by high-frequency hearing loss. If there was substantial asymmetry in high-frequency sensitivity, therefore, it was often difficult to separate the central dichotic effect from the peripheral hearing loss effect.

Berlin was impressed by the fact that our SSI sentences were quite resistant to the effects of high-frequency loss, and suggested that our two laboratories might collaborate in the construction of a dichotic test, based on such sentences, to minimize the high-frequency loss problem. The result was the Dichotic Sentence Identification (DSI) test, in which the speech targets are two different third-order SSI sentences. We have been using the DSI test routinely at the Methodist Hospital audiology service for the past several years and find that it is becoming a valuable adjunct to the routine test battery for audiometric assessment. Because of its resistance to the effects of high-frequency loss, it is particularly valuable in the evaluation of elderly persons with presbyacusic audiometric contours.

The next two papers, "Specific Auditory Perceptual Dysfunction in a Learning Disabled Child" (*Ear & Hearing*, 1987), and "Central Auditory Processing Disorder: A Case Study" (*Journal of the American Academy of Audiology*, 1991), illustrate how a research approach to clinical evaluation can be used to gain a better understanding of the nature of CAPD.

In the first case, an 11-year-old boy with severe learning disability, Susan Jerger, Randi Martin, and I show how analysis of relative performance measures, both within and across tasks, can be used to differentiate an auditory-specific disorder from either an attention deficit disorder or a linguistic-cognitive disorder. In the second case, we illustrate the sensitivity of dichotic listening tests as a screen for CAPD and how valuable they can be in differentiating auditory from cognitive deficits. Interestingly, in both cases the acoustic reflex provided "hard" evidence of central auditory disorder in a manner less equivocal than evoked potentials.

Finally, in the last paper, "Phase Coherence of the Middle Latency Response in the Elderly" (*Scandinavian Audiology*, 1992), my Egyptian colleague, Alia A. Ali, and I showed a clear difference between elderly persons with and without disproportionately poor speech recognition scores. By analyzing sequential samples of the middle latency response (MLR), we were able to show that the phase coherence (essentially a measure of latency) of selected Fourier components of the MLR waveform, was less stable from sample to sample in the group with speech audiometric deficits than in the group with normal speech audiometric findings. In so doing we were, perhaps, providing "hard evidence" of a central auditory basis for the phenomenon John Gaeth described so many years ago.

In summary, the concept of central auditory processing disorder, both in children and in the elderly, has been with us for many years. The papers reprinted in this section are representative of our efforts to develop and refine better tests of CAPD, to understand its nature, and to provide "hard evidence" of central auditory dysfunction.

AUDITORY DISORDER FOLLOWING BILATERAL TEMPORAL LOBE INSULT: REPORT OF A CASE

James Jerger

Baylor College of Medicine, Houston, Texas

Larry Lovering and Max Wertz

Good Samaritan Hospital, Phoenix, Arizona

Audiologic data are presented for a patient with bilateral temporal lobe damage. Neuropathologic examination of the brain at autopsy confirmed site of lesion. Audiologic results on this patient are contrasted to results obtained in 1969 by Jerger et al. on another patient with presumed bilateral lesions of the temporal lobe. The two patients showed striking similarities. Both experienced transient aphasia but no hearing problems after the first (left-sided) episode. Both reported severe hearing loss after the second (right-sided) episode. In both cases, the presumed sensitivity loss had essentially recovered within three months of the second episode. Both showed marked inability to recognize either single words or sentences. This profound deficit did not improve significantly, even under ideal listening conditions, in either patient during the period of study. In contrast to the striking similarities between the two patients, there was one significant difference. Whereas the 1969 patient could not localize sounds in space, the present patient's sound localization ability was unimpaired. This finding seemed related to an interaural imbalance in the relation between loudness and signal duration. The 1969 patient had such an imbalance and could not localize effectively. The present patient did not have an imbalance and localized accurately. This finding indicates that impairment in sound localization is not an invariable concomitant of temporal lobe disease.

In 1969, Jerger et al. presented extensive audiologic data obtained from a single patient with presumed bilateral lesions of the temporal lobe consequent to bilateral partial cerebral hemisphere infarction. Since the patient survived the ordeal, neuropathologic confirmation of the site of the lesion was not possible.

This paper presents similar audiologic data on a second patient who sustained similar cerebral damage. This patient, however, subsequently expired, permitting neuropathologic examination of the brain. In addition to this unique feature, the second patient's findings demonstrate both points of similarity and interesting contrasts with the first patient's results.

Reprinted from the *Journal of Speech and Hearing Disorders*
November 1972, Vol. 37, No. 4

CLINICAL HISTORY[1]

First Admission. The patient, a 62-year-old, right-handed male, was first admitted to Barrow Neurological Institute, St. Joseph's Hospital and Medical Center, in Phoenix, Arizona, in June 1969. He had a three-week history of intermittent aphasia. Just before the patient's admission his verbal expression had changed markedly, although his verbal comprehension seemed intact. Additionally, his right arm had become numb.

The results of physical and neurologic examinations at admission were essentially within normal limits except for the mild aphasia. The results of routine laboratory studies were within normal limits. The VDRL test was nonreactive. The electrocardiogram was normal. The brain scan was negative. A percutaneous *left* carotid arteriogram showed occlusive disease involving the horizontal portion of the middle cerebral artery as it approached the sylvian fissure, with anastomotic circulation filling the sylvian branches.

The aphasia cleared rapidly and the patient was dismissed with only mild left-sided headache. There had been no subjective complaint or objective evidence of hearing loss throughout this period of observation. Audiometric studies, however, were not carried out.

Second Admission. In October 1970, the patient developed right periorbital headache and nausea lasting approximately two days. He subsequently lost consciousness momentarily and became rigid in all four extremities. He was treated at the emergency room at St. Joseph's Hospital. At admission, he could hear quite well and denied any visual difficulties, weakness or numbness of extremities, or other neurological abnormalities.

During this examination the patient experienced a relatively sudden "hearing loss" characterized primarily by a loss in the ability to understand speech. He described his difficulty as "I can hear you talking, but I can't translate it."

The patient returned in two days for reevaluation. On this date his expressive speech was normal and he was able to read and interpret written instructions well. The neurological findings were normal. However, there was continued loss in speech understanding. Spoken language was largely incomprehensible. The patient was hospitalized and treated with intravenous histamine and nicotinic acid.

Results of laboratory studies at this admission were within normal limits. The electrocardiogram was normal. The electroencephalogram was moderately abnormal with focal theta and sharp wave activity in the right temporal region. A percutaneous carotid cerebral angiogram showed occlusion of the major middle cerebral trunk with anastomotic filling in a retrograde manner from the parieto-occipital branch of the *right* posterior cerebral artery. There was no evidence of aneurysm, arteriovenous malformation, tumor stain, or significant arteriosclerotic disease.

---

[1]For a more detailed description of this patient's physical findings, see Kanshepolsky, Kelley, and Waggener (in press).

The patient was discharged from the hospital to be followed monthly on an outpatient basis. Approximately two months later (December 1970), comprehensive audiologic tests were administered at the Audiology Service, Good Samaritan Hospital. The results are presented in detail below.

Third Admission. In April 1971, the patient suffered an acute cerebral infarction with right hemiplegia and aphasia. He was readmitted to the hospital for appropriate therapy. One week following admission, he suddenly became unresponsive and had a short period of cyanosis. The electrocardiogram showed acute myocardial infarction. Supportive therapy was instituted. The patient progressed to flaccid quadriplegia with Cheyne-Stokes respirations, however, and died. At autopsy, death was attributed to acute myocardial infarction secondary to left coronary artery thrombosis.

NEUROPATHOLOGY EXAMINATION[2]

Examination of the surface of the brain revealed bilateral and symmetrical areas of softening in the posterior segments of the superior temporal gyri. At the pial surface these measured 2 cm in maximum width. A smaller lesion occupied the right middle temporal gyrus, posteriorly. Except for minimal atrophy, the remaining gyri were unremarkable. The major arteries displayed moderate atherosclerosis. There was no evidence of embolism.

Coronal sectioning of the cerebrum revealed the bilateral areas of temporal softening to represent cystic infarcts. The adjacent tranverse gyri were also involved. A more recent hemorrhagic infarct involved the basal ganglia and internal capsule on the left. Other areas of the cerebrum were intact. A 1-mm, old infarct was found in the superior lateral medulla.

AUDIOLOGIC PROCEDURES

Auditory tests were administered during two days of intensive examination, December 17, 1970, and January 15, 1971. All testing was conducted in a sound-treated suite of the Audiology Service, Good Samaritan Hospital, in Phoenix. Basic test instruments included a two-channel clinical audiometer (Allison, model 22), a Bekesy audiometer (Grason-Stadler, model E800), and an electronic switch (Grason-Stadler, model 829S).

The patient was alert, cooperative, and well-motivated throughout both testing days. At no time did the examiners feel that poor performance resulted from malaise, lack of cooperation, lack of motivation, or other extra-auditory factors. Because of the patient's consistently high level of cooperation, we are confident that failure to perform normally on any of the tests administered can, with reasonable certainty, be attributed to specific central auditory disorder.

---

[2] For a more detailed description of this patient's neuropathologic findings, see Kanshepolsky, Kelley, and Waggener (in press).

Results are summarized below under two general categories: tests involving pure-tone signals, and tests involving speech signals.

Pure-Tone Signals

Pure-tone signals were used to measure threshold sensitivity, loudness discrimination, threshold-duration functions, sound localization, temporal ordering, and binaural loudness balance.

Threshold Sensitivity. Threshold audiograms were obtained for each ear by means of a standard Bekesy-type audiometer (Grason-Stadler, type E800). Frequency changed at the rate of 1 octave/min, intensity changed at the rate of 2.5 dB/sec, and the signal was periodically interrupted at the rate of 2.5 ips. The tracing width was relatively large (15-25 dB) on both ears, but the threshold tracings were otherwise unremarkable. Figure 1 shows the air-

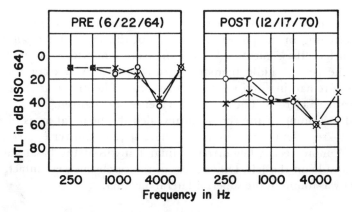

Figure 1. Pure-tone audiograms obtained six years before and three months after second (right-sided) CVA.

conduction audiogram obtained from the midpoints of the threshold tracings on December 17, 1970 (right-hand panel). By good fortune the patient had been tested at the Good Samaritan Hospital approximately five years before the cerebrovascular episodes that occurred late in 1969. This audiogram (June 22, 1964) is shown on the left panel of Figure 1. We see that, in 1964, the threshold audiogram was within normal limits except for a mild notch or dip at 4000 Hz.

Comparison of the two audiograms, pre- and post-CVA, shows that sensitivity has definitely decreased, especially at low frequencies on the left ear. Yet the change is not great. After allowing for the expected sensitivity loss from normal aging over the six-year period from 1964 to 1970 (ages 56 to 62), we are left with little more than a 10-30-dB sensitivity loss, somewhat larger on the left ear than on the right. It is quite possible that the sensitivity was profoundly depressed immediately after the second episode (October 3, 1970) and that it slowly recovered to the relatively good levels shown in Figure 1.

This seemed to be the case in the patient with bilateral temporal lobe lesions previously reported by Jerger et al. (1969). On the other hand, sensitivity levels for pure tones may have changed very little. The patient's report of marked bilateral "hearing loss" may have simply reflected his sudden, rather profound loss in the ability to understand speech signals, a phenomenon well-documented below.

Loudness Discrimination. Loudness discrimination was tested by the quantal psychophysical method (Stevens, Morgan, and Volkmann, 1941). Short-intensity increments (200 msec) were added to a steady-state, pure-tone signal at 5-sec intervals. Increments were presented in blocks of 20. Increment size was constant within each block, but varied over successive blocks in order to construct psychometric functions over the response range from 0-100% correction detection. The hearing level (HTL) of the steady-state signal was 60 dB at 500, 1000, and 2000 Hz and 80 dB at 4000 Hz. Figure 2 shows psychometric functions for both right and left ears at each of the four test frequencies. Performance is reasonably good on the right ear, but relatively poor on the left ear. At 500 Hz, for example, 100% correct detection is not achieved until the increment size is 5 dB. At 2000 Hz even 5 dB is not sufficient. Performance on the left ear never exceeds 70%. Interestingly, at 4000 Hz both ears show amazingly good loudness discrimination. An increment of only 1 dB produces 100% correct detection in both right and left ears. This is, of course, a "positive SISI" score and undoubtedly derives from the isolated cochlear defect in the 4000-Hz region demonstrated on the pre-insult audiogram. In any event, frequencies below 4000 Hz show a pronounced deficit in loudness discrimination in the left ear. A similar effect was noted in the right ear of the patient previously described by Jerger et al. (1969).

Sound Localization. To assess gross spatial sound localization, the patient was seated, blindfolded, in the center of a sound-treated room (IAC, Series 1200) about 11 ft square. By means of a Rudmose Warblet, a frequency-modulated, 3000-Hz tone burst could be presented at various azimuths. The sound signal was 3 meters from the patient's head, at an SPL of 80 dB. Informal observation revealed no obvious difficulty in sound localization in either hemisphere of acoustic space. A fairly difficult localization task was then presented. Over a series of 10 listening trials the sound source was positioned either 5° to the left or 5° to the right of midline. On all 10 trials, 5° to the right and 5° to the left, the patient correctly named the direction of the 5° deviation. We conclude, therefore, that his ability to localize sounds in space was not demonstrably impaired.

Threshold-Duration Functions. In the patient with bilateral temporal lobe disorder previously reported by Jerger et al. (1969), pure-tone threshold changed dramatically as a function of signal on-time. The effect was substantially greater in one ear than the other. Jerger et al. suggested that this ear difference in the apparent rate of loudness increase with duration might underlie the patient's extraordinary difficulty with the localization of point sources in space.

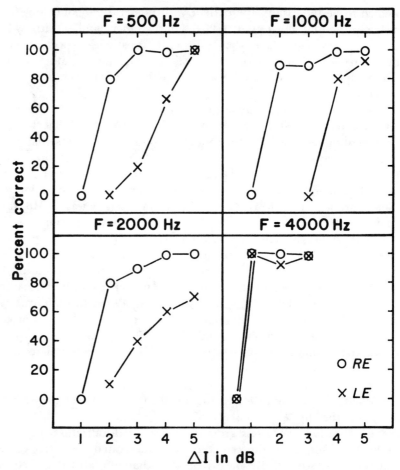

Figure 2. Psychometric functions for loudness discrimination at four test frequencies. Note consistently poorer performance on left ear, except at 4000 Hz, where previous cochlear defects produced heightened loudness discrimination (positive SISI score) in both ears.

In the present patient, threshold for 1000 Hz was explored as a function of signal on-time with off-time held constant. Figure 3 shows the threshold-duration functions for both right and left ears as the on-time was varied over the range from 25 to 2000 msec. Two important findings are evident. First, threshold-duration functions show the same abnormality evidenced by the patient reported in 1969. As on-duration becomes very short, sound intensity must be raised appreciably (20-25 dB) to maintain the threshold-response. In normal patients the effect would be less than 10 dB.

Temporal Order. Temporal ordering refers to the patient's ability to identify the order in which different auditory events occur in time. The phenomenon is of interest in central auditory disorders because of mounting evidence (Efron, 1963; Edwards and Auger, 1965) that the ability to identify

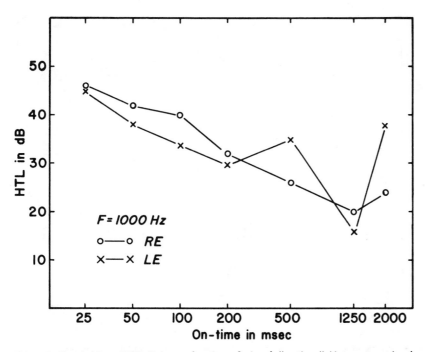

Figure 3. Threshold at 1000 Hz as a function of signal "on-time." Note symmetric abnormality of threshold-duration functions in both ears.

temporal order may be severely compromised in patients with aphasia. In the present patient, temporal ordering was tested by presenting a pair of pure tones, widely separated in frequency, and with the onset of one delayed relative to the onset of the other. Frequencies were 300 Hz and 3000 Hz, signal duration was 1000 msec, and intersignal delay was varied from 750 to 20 msec. Trials were presented in blocks of 20 in a two-alternative, forced-choice (2AFC) paradigm. Within each block of 20 trials the lower pitched tone (300 Hz) was delayed relative to the higher pitched tone (3000 Hz) on 10 randomly chosen trials. The higher pitched tone was delayed relative to the lower pitched tone on the other 10 trials. Temporal delay was constant within a given block of 20 trials, but varied over successive blocks. The signal level was always 80 dB HTL.

Figure 4 shows the resulting psychometric function for both right and left ears. Results are well within normal limits for both ears. The value of Δt yielding 75% correct performance is close to 150 msec. In a normal standardization group the analagous average delay was 139 msec, with a range from 20-200 msec. Although just detectable temporal delays in this range are considerably larger than the 20-40-msec values obtained on trained subjects, they are in the expected range for relatively untrained listeners taking the test for the first time. It is especially significant that, on temporal order, we do not see the ear difference so evident for intensity discrimination.

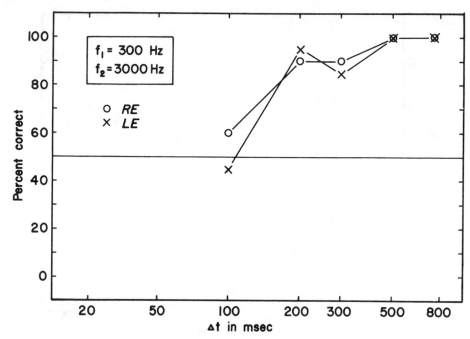

Figure 4. Psychometric functions for temporal order discrimination. Fifty percent performance is chance level.

Binaural Loudness Balance and Median-Plane Localization. The alternate binaural loudness balance test procedure was attempted, but results were unsatisfactory. Like the 1969 patient of Jerger et al. the present patient was unable to make reliable judgments of interaural loudness. Binaural signals were then presented simultaneously rather than alternately, and the patient was asked to adjust the interaural intensity until the sound image was localized in the median plane. For a pure-tone signal of 1000 Hz this task was executed with considerably greater reliability than the loudness judgments. At high levels (90-100 dB HTL), results were quite normal. Equal physical intensities produced median-plane localization. At lower levels, however, (60-80 dB) median-plane localization required somewhat greater intensity (10-15 dB) in the left ear.

Speech Signals

Spondees and Phonetically Balanced (PB) Monosyllables. The patient was unable to repeat correctly any PB word at any presentation level. His PB scores were 0% on both ears. This extreme deficit in speech intelligibility effectively limited the extent to which spondee words could be used to obtain conventional spondee thresholds. However, by the use of the single word *cowboy,* speech detection thresholds could be established at the 20-dB level (HTL) on both ears, a level in good agreement with the pure-tone audiogram.

Synthetic Sentence Identification (SSI). To explore speech understanding deficits, it was necessary to employ a speech audiometric technique characterized by greater redundancy than conventional PB materials. Accordingly, the synthetic sentence identification (SSI) procedure (Jerger, Speaks, and Trammell, 1968) was used. The patient hears a sequence of 10 artificially or synthetically constructed sentences. After each sentence has been presented he must search a visually presented, closed set of the 10 sentences, select or identify the sentence heard, and press an appropriate response button.

When the sentences are presented in quiet, the listening task is relatively easy and performance is normally excellent. The difficulty of the task may be manipulated, however, either by distorting the speech signal or by adding a competing speech signal to the sentences. The latter competition can be added either to the same ear as the sentence or to the opposite ear.

Figure 5 shows SSI results on each ear when sentences were presented in

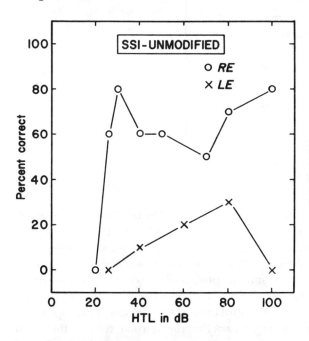

Figure 5. Performance-intensity (PI). functions for synthetic sentence identification (SSI). Test sentences are presented in quiet without modification or competition of any kind.

quiet without distortion or competition of any kind. Here we see dramatic evidence of the profound effects that central auditory lesions can exert on speech intelligibility. In spite of the extreme redundancy of the speech signals, and the essentially low level of difficulty posed by this test procedure, the patient's performance never exceeds 30% on the left ear. On the right ear, performance is erratic but plateaus at 70-80 % over a considerable range of speech levels.

Figure 6 shows the result when sentences are presented to one ear and a competing speech message (CM) is added to the ipsilateral ear (ICM) or to the contralateral ear (CCM). For these tests the sentences were presented at a constant level of 60 dB HTL, and the level of the competing message was

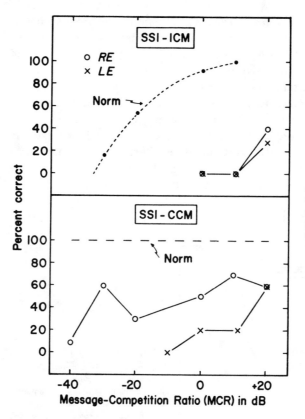

Figure 6. Synthetic sentence identification (SSI) performance in the presence of both ipsilateral competition (ICM) and contralateral competition (CCM).

varied such that the ratio between sentence and competition, the message-competition ratio (MCR), covered the range from +20 dB to −40 dB. The upper panel of Figure 6 shows that ipsilateral competition, even when it is relatively weak (MCR = +20 dB), virtually destroyed sentence identification. Contralateral competition had a similar profound effect. Poor performance on this test configuration (CCM) is, in our experience, specific to temporal lobe disorder. Here both ears show significant abnormalities, but, again, the left ear is much worse than the right ear. For the normal subject the CCM test configuration is a relatively easy listening task, even at an MCR of −40 dB. It is simply a matter of attending to the sentence in one ear while ignoring or suppressing the competing signal in the other ear. As the present results demonstrate, this ability to "selectively attend" may be profoundly affected by temporal lobe lesions.

Other forms of signal distortion had equally profound effects on sentence identification. Low-pass filtering of the sentences at 2000 Hz had little effect, but filtering at 1000 Hz reduced performance to 0%. Both temporal interruption, at virtually any rate, and 50% temporal compression also reduced performance to 0%.

In general, speech intelligibility, even under the most favorable conditions, was severely impaired in this patient. Almost any form of signal distortion further reduced performance to 0%. Even contralateral competition (CCM), a relatively easy listening task, had a profound effect on SSI in both ears.

DISCUSSION

Virtually all of our knowledge concerning the auditory manifestations of temporal lobe disorders comes from the study of patients with unilateral lesions. We know that, in these patients, there is ordinarily no loss of audiometric sensitivity in either ear, that the intelligibility of undistorted speech signals is usually quite good, but that sufficient distortion of the speech signal may reveal a relative deficit in the ear contralateral to the affected side of the brain. In general, the effects are quite subtle and not readily demonstrable by conventional audiometric evaluation.

It is of considerable interest to ask, therefore, how bilateral temporal lobe disorder modifies this overall picture. The present patient is, to our knowledge, only the second well-documented case report of bilateral temporal lobe lesion where auditory function has been systematically studied. Jerger et al. presented the first in 1969. The two patients show striking similarities. Both experienced transient aphasia but no apparent hearing problem after the first (left-sided) episode. Both reported severe hearing loss following the second (right-sided) episode. In both cases, however, the presumed sensitivity loss had largely disappeared within two to three months of the second episode. In the 1969 patient the gradual return of pure-tone sensitivity was documented audiometrically. In the present patient, however, we do not know whether a true loss of sensitivity did occur, or whether his report of a sudden bilateral deafness merely reflected his sudden inability to understand speech.

In any event, it is clear that, although bilateral temporal lobe lesions may produce an initial loss in auditory sensitivity, the effect is apparently only temporary. We are in basic agreement with DiCarlo, Kendall, and Goldstein (1962), therefore, that substantial loss in sensitivity is not a permanent characteristic of either unilateral or bilateral temporal lobe lesion.

On the other hand, the ability to understand speech is apparently profoundly impaired by bilateral temporal lobe disorder. Both patients showed a marked inability to recognize either single words or sentences, even under ideal listening conditions. The addition of virtually any form of signal distortion quickly eliminated even this residual intelligibility.

Here we see a fundamental point of sharp contrast between unilateral and bilateral disorder. Whereas the unilateral deficit in speech understanding is subtle and can be elicited only by creating a rather difficult listening task, the bilateral deficit is profound and may be demonstrated even under the easiest of listening conditions.

Another point of striking similarity between these two patients is that both showed systematic ear differences on a variety of psychoacoustic tasks, but no ear difference for temporal order. In the 1969 patient, the right ear was consistently poorer than the left ear on tasks involving speech intelligibility and loudness discrimination. This ear difference undoubtedly reflected the fact that the left temporal lobe had sustained somewhat greater damage than the right. In the present patient, the left ear was consistently poorer than the right on all speech-intelligibility and loudness-discrimination tasks. This ear difference undoubtedly reflects greater damage to the right hemisphere. In both patients, however, no ear difference was observed on temporal ordering. These findings further substantiate Efron's (1963) view that temporal ordering does not have bilateral representation but is, instead, localized in the hemisphere dominant for speech. In this connection, it is interesting that in the 1969 patient, with greatest damage to the left hemisphere, temporal ordering showed a pronounced bilateral deficit. In the present patient, on the other hand, damage was greatest in the right hemisphere and no significant deficit in temporal order occurred on either ear.

In contrast to the striking similarities between these two patients there is one significant difference. Whereas the 1969 patient could not localize sounds in space, the present patient's sound localization ability seemed unimpaired. This finding lends further support to our earlier hypothesis that impairment in sound localization in the patient with temporal lobe disorder is not due to the fact that the temporal lobes, per se, play a vital role in sound localization, but to the presence of an interaural imbalance in the relation between loudness and signal duration. The 1969 patient had such an imbalance and could not effectively localize. The present patient did not have an imbalance and localized accurately and without difficulty.

This finding shows that impairment in sound localization is not an invariable concomitant of temporal lobe disease. We should expect, however, in view of the high incidence of unilateral lesions with consequent interaural imbalance in threshold-duration functions, that the incidence of impaired sound localization ability will be quite high.

ACKNOWLEDGMENT

This study was supported, in part, by Public Health Research Grant NS08542 from the National Institute of Neurological Diseases and Stroke. We are indebted to Jose Kanshepolsky and John J. Kelley, Division of Neurological Surgery, and John D. Waggener, Division of Neuropathology, Barrow Neurological Institute of St. Joseph's Hospital and Medical Center, Phoenix, Arizona, for assistance in the preparation of this manuscript, especially details of the patient's clinical history and neuropathologic findings. It is a pleasure also to acknowledge our continuing debt to Charles Berlin, Louisiana State University School of Medicine, whose innovative studies of temporal lobe disease are a constant inspiration to students of central auditory disorder. Requests for reprints of this article should be addressed to James Jerger, 11922 Taylorcrest Road, Houston, Texas 77024.

REFERENCES

DiCarlo, L. M., Kendall, D. C., and Goldstein, R., Diagnostic procedures for auditory disorders in children. *Folia phoniat.,* 14, 206-264 (1962).

EDWARDS, A., and AUGER, R., The effect of aphasia on the perception of precedence. *Proceedings of the Seventy-Third Convention of the American Psychological Association,* pp. 207-208 (1965).

EFRON, R., Temporal perception, aphasia, and deja vu. *Brain,* **86,** 403-424 (1963).

JERGER, J., SPEAKS, C., and TRAMMELL, J., A new approach to speech audiometry. *J. Speech Hearing Dis.,* **33,** 318-328 (1968).

JERGER, J., WEIKERS, N., SHARBROUGH, F., and JERGER, S., Bilateral lesions of the temporal lobe: A case study. *Acta otolaryng.,* Suppl. 258 (1969).

KANSHEPOLSKY, J., KELLEY, J., and WAGGENER, J., A cortical auditory disorder: Report of a case. *Neurol.* (in press).

STEVENS, S., MORGAN, C., and VOLKMANN, J., Theory of the neural quantum in the discrimination of loudness and pitch. *Amer. J. Psychol.,* **54,** 315-335 (1941).

Auditory Findings
in Brain Stem Disorders

James Jerger, PhD, Susan Jerger, MS, Houston

Audiometric tests were administered to 16 patients with intra-axial brain stem lesions. Eight patients showed some audiometric loss in one or both ears. Maximum speech intelligibility (PB) scores were at least 80% in 10 patients. In the remaining, depressed PB maximum performance was found either on both ears or on the ear contralateral to the site of lesion. Performance-intensity (PI) functions for PB words yielded a consistent difference between ears across all intensity levels in nine patients.

Performance on synthetic sentence identification (SSI) materials was disporportionately poor for sentences in the presence of ipsilateral competing speech messages (ICM). In the presence of contralateral competing speech messages (CCM), SSI performance generally remained within the normal range. A relatively greater performance deficit for the ICM task than for the CCM task was an important characteristic of brain stem disorder.

Previous studies of patients with brain stem lesions fail to describe a consistent pattern of auditory findings. Results to date are both inconsistent and contradictory. For example, pure-tone sensitivity in these patients has been categorized as essentially normal,[1-5] as mildly impaired, particularly in the high-frequency region;[6-9] and as severely impaired on one or both ears.[10-12] Reports on speech intelligibility also reflect this unusual inconsistency. Some studies[4,5] have reported normal speech intelligibility scores; others[1,2,7,8,13] have reported mild to severe speech intelligibility problems, particularly on the contralateral ear. The studies on Bekesy audiometry also produced conflicting results. Some studies[1,13,14] found normal Bekesy tracing in these patients whereas others[3,4,7,8,12,15,16] found abnormal results. These observations have led some previous investigators[7,8,17] to conclude that the audiometric pattern characterizing brain stem lesions is essentially indistinguishable from the pattern in eighth nerve disorders.

Our review of the existing literature suggests that some of the inconsistencies surrounding previous studies may have been due, in part at least, to a lack of distinction between extra-axial and intra-axial brain stem lesions. Unless one carefully excludes extra-axial brain stem disorders, the possibility exists that auditory symptoms can be produced by direct involvement of the eighth nerve trunk rather than the brain stem pathway. The purpose of the present study is to describe auditory brain stem symptoms in a series of

Accepted for publication May 23, 1973.

From the Department of Otorhinolaryngology and Communicative Sciences, Baylor College of Medicine, Texas Medical Center, Houston.

Reprint requests to Department of Otolaryngology, Baylor College of Medicine, Houston, TX 77025 (Dr. J. Jerger).

that the levator palatini plays a major role in the mesial movement of the lateral pharyngeal walls; yet, this muscle is largely responsible for palatal elevation and apparently has no effect on active opening of the eustachian tube. Though the tensor palatini is known to be capable of opening the eustachian orifice, it has no known bearing on the narrowing of the pharynx.

If the levator palatini does, in fact, account in large measure for mesial movements of the lateral pharyngeal walls as well as posterosuperior movements of the velum, what accounts for the lack of strong relationship among palatal and pharyngeal muscle activity and eustachian tube function in the present study? It may be that, in some patients, the presence of substantial amounts of scar tissue in the oropharyngeal tissues, particularly the palatopharyngeal fold, would tend to inhibit palate elevation while allowing a relatively uninhibited mesial excursion of the pharyngeal walls.

It is likely that two or more muscles are accountable for the finding that

normal eustachian tube activity and good pharyngeal wall movement occur simultaneously in the great majority of subjects. Recent research[25,26] confirms the long-standing subjective impression that the prevalence of middle ear disease is reduced following surgical closure of the cleft palate. Although an extensive muscle complex is affected by palatal closure, the tensor and levator palatini and the palatopharyngeus muscles are most directly affected. Of these, the tensor and levator palatini would seem to be implicated most directly in the present findings. Curiously though, two recent reports dealing with unilateral hamulotomy or hamulus fracture performed during surgical closure of the cleft palate, revealed no difference in eustachian tube function and no increase in the incidence of middle ear disease.[26,27]

In spite of the lack of any obvious anatomic explanation, the data are compelling. Of the 56 subjects tested, only four (two experimental and two control) yielded data inconsistent with the apparent relationship between eustachian tube activity and

pharyngeal wall activity.

From the results of this investigation, it would appear that poorer than normal eustachian tube function is not characteristic of the cleft palate condition, per se, at least not in the young-adult age group. Eustachian tube function does appear, however, to be related to observed pharyngeal wall activity. Granting this relationship, the fact that a greater number of experimental group subjects had poor pharyngeal wall activity than in the control group may be related to the consistently smaller means for the cleft palate group during the eustachian tube test.

The sound-conduction method continues to hold promise as a rapid and accurate method of assessing eustachian tube function under normal and pathologic conditions. Modifications of the test procedure in the direction of less bulky and less expensive equipment, introduced by Satoh and his group,[23] add the advantages of simplicity and practicality.

This study was supported by Public Health Service Grant DE 02172.

References

1. Graham MD: A longitudinal study of ear disease and hearing loss in patients with cleft lips and palates. *Ann Otol Rhinol Laryngol* 73:34-47, 1964.
2. Pannbacker M: Hearing loss and cleft palate. *Cleft Palate J* 6:50-56, 1969.
3. Heller JC, Hochberg I, Milano G: Audiologic and otologic evaluation of cleft palate children. *Cleft Palate J* 7:774-783, 1970.
4. Drettner B: The nasal airway and hearing in patients with cleft palate. *Acta Otolaryngol* 52:131-142, 1960.
5. Holborow CA: Conductive deafness associated with the cleft palate deformity. *Proc R Soc Med* 55:305-309, 1962.
6. Schultz RC: Surgically produced cleft palates in rabbits: A study of resulting middle ear infections. *Plast Reconstr Surg* 33:120-127, 1964.
7. Stool S: Diagnosis and treatment of ear disease in cleft palate children, in Grabb WC et al (eds): *Cleft Lip and Palate: Surgical, Dental, and Speech Aspects*. Boston, Little Brown & Co, 1971, pp 868-877.
8. Bluestone CD: Eustachian tube obstruction in the infant with cleft palate. *Ann Otol*, suppl 2, 1971, pp 1-30.
9. Bluestone CD, Wittel RA, Paradise JL: Roentgenographic evaluation of eustachian tube function in infants with cleft and normal pal-

ates. *Cleft Palate J* 9:93-100, 1972.
10. Yule CT: On the mechanism of opening and closing the eustachian tube. *J Anat Physiol* 8:127-132, 1873.
11. Rich AR: A physiologic study of the eustachian tube and its related muscles. *Johns Hopkins Hosp Bull* 352:206-214, 1920.
12. Simkins CS: Functional anatomy of the eustachian tube. *Arch Otolaryngol* 38:476-484, 1943.
13. Perlman HB: Mouth of the eustachian tube: Action during swallowing and phonation. *Arch Otolaryngol* 53:353-369, 1951.
14. Kriens OB: Fundamental anatomic findings for an intravelar veloplasty. *Cleft Palate J* 7:27-36, 1970.
15. Ross MA: Functional anatomy of the tensor palati. *Arch Otolaryngol* 93:1-8, 1971.
16. Politzer A: Über subjective gehörsempfindungen. *Wien Med Wochenschr* 15:1710-1717, 1865.
17. Gyergyay A: Neue wege zur erkennung der physologie und pathologie der ohrtrompete. *Monatsschr Ohrenheilkd* 66:769-773, 1932.
18. Perlman HB: The eustachian tube: Abnormal patency and normal physiologic state. *Arch Otolaryngol* 30:212-238, 1939.
19. Perlman HB: Observations on the eustachian tube. *Arch Otolaryngol* 53:370-385, 1951.
20. Tsukamoto A: On the measurement of pa-

tency of the auditory tube by sound waves. *Jap J Otol* 60:901-919, 1957.
21. Elpern BS, Naunton RF, Perlman HB: Objective measurement of middle ear function: The eustachian tube. *Laryngoscope* 74:359-371, 1964.
22. Naunton RF, Galluser J: Measurements of eustachian tube function. *Ann Otol Rhinol Laryngol* 76:455-471, 1967.
23. Satoh I, Watanabe I, Sainoo T: Measurement of eustachian tube function. *Arch Otolaryngol* 92:329-334, 1970.
24. Dickson DR, Dickson WM: Velopharyngeal anatomy. *J Speech Hear Res* 15:372-381, 1972.
25. Paradise JL, Bluestone CE: More on the universal occurrence of otitis media in infants with cleft palate and a preliminary evaluation of its treatment. Read before the 29th Annual Meeting of the American Cleft Palate Association, Pittsburgh, April 23, 1971.
26. Bluestone CD, et al: Certain effects of cleft palate repair on eustachian tube function. *Cleft Palate J* 9:183-193, 1972.
27. Noone RB, et al: The effect of hamulus fracture on middle ear disease in children with cleft palate. Read before the 30th Annual Meeting of the American Cleft Palate Association, Phoenix, Ariz, April 14, 1972.

carefully selected patients with well-defined mass lesions involving the intra-axial brain stem pathways. In particular, no patient with inflammatory, viral, or suspected lesions of the brain stem pathways participated in this study. We sought to delineate the pattern and variability characterizing auditory test results in patients with intra-axial brain stem lesions when all possible extra-axial brain stem disorders had been eliminated.

Methods

Subjects.—Subjects were 16 patients with intra-axial brain stem lesions referred to the Audiology Service, The Methodist Hospital, Houston, between 1967 and 1972. Of these patients, 12 were male and 4 were female. The average age was 24.4 years and ranged from 6 to 48 years. Brain stem lesions were confirmed surgically in eight patients. Final diagnosis from histopathologic report was pontine glioma in four patients and melanoma, astrocytoma, ependymoma, or arteriovenous malformation in the remaining four patients. Brain stem lesions in the eight patients without surgical intervention were defined radiographically, usually by pneumoencephalographic technique. All eight patients had pontine gliomas.

In these 16 patients, the lesion was primarily on the left side of the brain in seven patients, primarily on the right side in eight patients, and bilaterally symmetrical in one patient.

Test Battery.—The following series of tests was attempted on all patients:

Pure-Tone Sensitivity.—Threshold hearing levels (International Standards Organization [ISO-1964]) at octave frequencies between 250 and 8,000 Hz were obtained by either manual or Bekesy technique. For manual audiometry, threshold sensitivity was determined by the Hughson-Westlake method.[18] For Bekesy audiometry, threshold levels were obtained by a line visually fitted to the midpoints of the tracing.

Bekesy Audiometry.—Sweep-frequency tracings for interrupted and continuous signals were obtained over the frequency range from 200 to 8,000 Hz. Frequency changed at a rate of one octave per minute, and intensity changed at a rate of 2.5 dB per second.

Acoustic Reflex.—Acoustic reflex thresholds were obtained as one of the three basic components of impedance audiometry. Reflex contractions were elicited at frequencies of 500, 1,000, 2,000, and 4,000 Hz. Threshold levels were recorded as the lowest hearing level in decibels (ISO-1964)

that produced reliable, observable deflections of the balance meter when sound was presented to the ear opposite the ear containing the impedance bridge probe-tip.

Performance-Intensity Phonetically Balanced Functions.—Performance-intensity (PI) functions for monosyllabic phonetically balanced (PB) word lists (PI-PB) were constructed by presenting half-lists of 25 words each at several intensities until the shape of the function was well defined. Generally PI-PB functions ranged from that speech level yielding 0 to 20% correct up to a maximum speech intensity of 110 dB sound pressure level (SPL). Performance was measured by having the patient repeat each word to a tester who scored it as correct or incorrect. Whenever the speech level was sufficiently intense to cross over and be heard in the nontest ear, white-noise masking was presented to the nontest ear at a level 20 dB less than the speech level in the test ear.

Synthetic Sentence Identification.—Synthetic sentence identification (SSI) materials consisted of a single list of ten synthetic sentences, seven words each, representing a third-order approximation to actual English sentences. Sentence construction and test procedures are described in detail elsewhere.[19,20] In brief, the patient was seated before a console containing a list of the ten synthetic sentences, a column of ten push buttons, and two lights labelled "listen" and "rest." After each sentence had been presented, the patient had approximately five seconds to select or identify the sentence he heard from the list in front of him and to push the appropriate response button. The same ten sentences were used throughout the entire test session, but were presented in different random orders. The sentence message set was presented at an intensity level yielding 100% correct performance in both ears. For most patients, this level was 50 dB SPL. However, a few patients required louder presentation levels in order to meet our criterion of 100% correct in both ears. The sentence identification task was made difficult by the presence of a competing speech message. The competing message was a passage concerning events in the life of a Texas pioneer and was recorded on tape by the same talker who recorded the sentences. Results were gathered by measuring performance at various message-to-competition ratios (MCRs) for both a contralateral competing message (CCM) and an ipsilateral competing message (ICM). For the CCM condition (sentences to the test ear and competition to the opposite ear), MCRs were varied in 20-dB steps over the range from 0 dB to −40 dB. Normal listeners' performance on this task re-

mains at 100% correct, even at the most unfavorable MCR condition. For the ICM condition (sentences and competition to the same ear), MCRs were varied in 10-dB steps over the range from +10 dB to −30 dB. These MCRs define performance in normal listeners from 100% to about 20% correct.

Instrumentation.—Pure-tone audiograms were obtained with either a standard audiometer (Beltone, model 10D) or a Bekesy audiometer (Grason-Stadler, model E800). Impedance audiometry was carried out with an electroacoustic impedance bridge (Madsen, type ZO-70) and an associated pure-tone audiometer (Beltone, model 10D). Speech audiometry was performed with six PB-50 word lists[21] and a single list of ten synthetic sentences.[19] All speech materials were prerecorded on magnetic tape by the same male talker. The tape playback system was a dual channel instrument (Ampex, AG440) played through a speech audiometer (Grason-Stadler, type 162) to earphones (Telephonic, type TDH-39) housed in circumaural cushions (CZW-6). Speech level was defined as the SPL of a 1,000-Hz signal recorded at the average level of frequent peaks of the speech as monitored on a meter (VU).

Procedure.—Patients were tested in a sound-treated booth at the Audiology Service, The Methodist Hospital, Houston, in a single test session of two to three hours duration. Pure-tone sensitivity measures and PI-PB functions were obtained on both ears of all 16 patients. However, due to a variety of factors, it was not always possible to obtain successful results for all patients on the other tests in our battery. Eleven of the sixteen patients successfully completed Bekesy audiometry and SSI testing on both ears, and 12 patients had complete acoustic reflex results at all frequencies on both ears.

Results

Findings on pure-tone audiometry, speech audiometry, and impedance audiometry are presented below in terms of the ear "ipsilateral" or "contralateral" to the affected side of the brain. For example, in a patient with a pontine glioma eccentric to the right, the right ear is referred to as the ipsilateral (I) ear and the left ear is termed the contralateral (C) ear.

Pure-Tone Sensitivity.—Pure-tone sensitivity measures in this series of patients were analyzed in two ways: first, in terms of group averages and, second, in terms of individual audiometric configurations. For the first analysis, Fig 1 shows average hearing threshold levels (HLs) and their ranges at octave intervals between 500 and 4,000 Hz for all 16 patients. Results for the I and C ears are plotted separately. Average threshold levels were approximately 10 to 15 dB from 500 to 2,000 Hz and 20 to 25 dB at 4,000 Hz. The average hearing levels shown in Fig 1 agree with the observations of several previous investigators.[1-5] However, large variability among individual patient's audiograms is reflected in Fig 1 by a range of at least 40 dB at each of the four frequencies. Note that, in spite of this variability, there is no evidence of substantial ear difference in the average results for the two ears.

Pure-tone sensitivity measures for individual patients could be divided into two distinct patterns. One group showed relatively normal pure-tone sensitivity; the other group showed some hearing impairment. Specifically, hearing threshold levels for frequencies between 500 and 4,000 Hz were within the normal range (≤ 25 dB, ISO-1964) for eight of the 16 patients. The remaining eight patients had mild to moderate hearing impairment (≤ 70 dB, ISO-1964) on at least one ear for at least one frequency between 500 and 4,000 Hz. In general, the pattern of loss in these eight patients revealed bilaterally sloping configurations with greater loss for high than for low frequencies. Five patients had sensitivity loss on both ears, and three patients had a loss on one ear only. Pure-tone average (PTA) results for 500, 1,000, and 2,000 Hz in these eight patients ranged from 1 to 38 dB on the I ear and from 7 to 35 dB on the C ear.

In contrast to patients with extra-axial brain stem lesions and eighth nerve involvement, the eight patients in this series with abnormal audiograms generally did not show a sensitivity difference between ears. The average difference between ears (PTA) was 7 dB with a range from 0 to 20 dB. Only three patients had an average ear difference greater than 5 dB. Results on these eight patients affirm the observations of Calearo and Antonelli[22] and Nakamura[23] that ear differences are not predictably re-

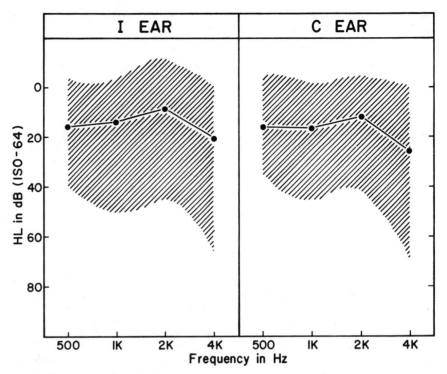

Fig 1.—Average threshold hearing levels and range at octave frequencies between 500 and 4,000 Hz for 16 patients with intra-axial brain stem lesions.

lated to the site of the brain stem lesion. In the present three patients with substantial ear difference, two showed greater sensitivity loss on the C ear and one showed greater loss on the I ear.

All eight patients had sloping audiometric contours on at least one ear. Seven patients had sloping configurations on both ears and one patient had a sloping loss on the I ear only. The presence of bilaterally sloping audiometric configurations in most patients is consistent with the observations of several previous investigators.[3,6,9,24] In the present eight patients, audiometric contours were sometimes symmetrical on both ears, sometimes more severe on the C ear, and other times more severe on the I ear.

In summary, pure-tone sensitivity was essentially within the normal range for 8 of the 16 patients in this series with intra-axial brain stem disorder. The remaining eight patients showed some hearing impairment for at least one frequency on at least one ear. Audiometric contours in these latter eight patients were generally

characterized by sloping losses in both ears with slightly greater impairment in the high frequency region than in the low frequency region. However, the maximum hearing loss (PTA) observed in any patient was relatively mild, 38 dB.

Bekesy Audiometry.—Eleven of the sixteen patients completed Bekesy audiometry. The results are shown below.

Type I on both ears	8
Type II on both ears	1
Type IV on the ear	
Type I on other ear	2

In general, Bekesy tracings were normal on both ears. This finding agrees with the previous results of Jerger[1] and Owens.[14] Eight of the eleven patients in this group had type I tracings on both ears. One other patient, a 41-year-old man, had type II tracings on both ears. The possibility of hearing loss due to noise exposure in an industrial setting existed for this patient. In fact, hearing loss had been noted on an industrial medical examination at least one year prior to the onset of brain stem symptoms.

The two remaining patients had

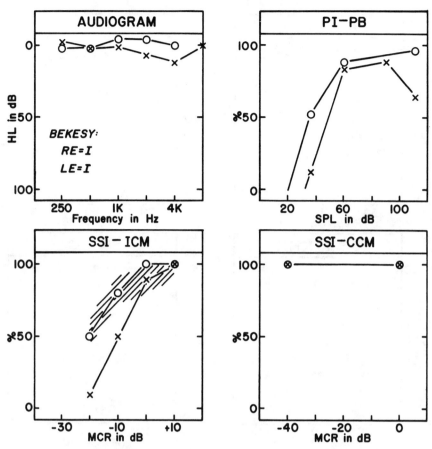

Fig 2.—Summary of diagnostic test results for 8-year-old boy with intra-axial brain stem lesion eccentric to the right. Hatched area represents normal range for SSI-ICM.

sistently higher HLs on the C ear. The difference between ears was as large as 25 dB even though audiometric contours on the two ears were essentially symmetrical.

Three of the twelve patients showed unexpected reflex abnormalities. Even though sensitivity was at best only mildly impaired on either ear at any frequency for all three patients, no reflex response to an auditory signal at 110 dB HL could be detected at some frequencies. In all three patients, tympanograms were normal, and there was no other evidence of middle ear disorder.

Absent stapedial muscle reflex contractions have been previously described by Greisen and Rasmussen[25] in two patients with brain stem disorder. The pattern of reflex abnormality in the present three patients was not consistent, however. Two patients had absent reflexes on both ears, and one patient had missing reflexes on the I ear only. Reflex abnormalities in the latter patient could be attributed to facial nerve paresis on the side of the head containing the impedance bridge probe-tip. And, indeed, reflex responses in this patient's other ear were present and brisk at all frequencies. Reflex contractions were inexplicably absent in the other two patients, however. One patient had absent reflexes at all frequencies on both ears. The other patient had absent reflexes at all frequencies on the I ear and at 2,000 and 4,000 Hz on the C ear. Reflex contractions were observed at 500 and 1,000 Hz on the C ear in this patient. Threshold HLs were 110 and 100 dB, respectively; however, levels were at the high end of the normal range.

In summary, acoustic reflex responses were present in most of these patients with intra-axial brain stem disorders. Only 3 of the 12 patients tested had missing reflexes on one or both ears. The pattern of reflex abnormality was not consistent among these three patients, however. Sometimes abnormal results were seen on both ears, sometimes on one ear only.

PI-PB Functions.—Performance-intensity functions for monosyllabic PB word lists were obtained for each ear of the 16 patients. In evaluating PI-

type I Bekesy tracings on one ear, but type IV Bekesy tracings on the other ear. Abnormal Bekesy tracings have been previously reported by many studies[3,4,8,12,15,16] that usually presented audiometric findings for only one or two patients with brain stem disorder. In our two patients, the type IV tracing was observed on the I ear in one patient and on the C ear in the other patient. Neither patient had an unusual sensitivity loss in the ear with the abnormal Bekesy tracing. One patient had a PTA of 23 dB and a mildly sloping audiometric contour revealing slightly greater loss in the high-frequency region. The other patient had a PTA of 14 dB and a moderately sloping audiometric contour with greater loss in the high-frequency region.

In summary, Bekesy audiometry generally produced type I tracings for both ears of patients with brain stem disorder. When an abnormal Bekesy pattern did emerge, the ear yielding the unusual finding was not consistent. Type IV tracings were observed on the I ear for one patient and on the C ear for one patient.

Acoustic Reflex.—Acoustic reflex thresholds for 500, 1,000, 2,000, and 4,000 Hz were obtained by impedance audiometric technique in 12 patients. Nine of these patients had normal reflex contractions on both ears at all frequencies. On closer examination, however, three of these nine patients showed an unusual ear difference in reflex threshold HLs. Two patients showed consistently higher HLs on the I ear, and one patient had con-

PB functions in these patients, it was necessary to consider two factors: first, absolute performance scores and, second, performance differences between ears. In terms of absolute performance, the following summary shows the maximum percent correct (PBmax) scores for all patients in this series.

80% to 100% on both ears	10
24% to 52% on both ears	2
90% to 100% on I ear and 60% to 75% on C ear	3
90% to 100% on I ear and 36% on C ear	1

In 10 of the 16 patients, PBmax scores were relatively good, at least 80%, on both ears. The remaining six patients had unusually poor maximum performance scores on PI-PB testing, however. Two patients had unusually poor PBmax scores on both ears. Four patients had difficulty on the C ear only. This variability in maximum PI-PB performance scores from relatively good to unusually poor on both ears is reflected in previous reports that document essentially normal PBmax performance,[4,5] disproportionately reduced PBmax scores,[1,2,8,13] or inconsistent findings[3,6,9,16,22,26] in patients with brain stem disorders.

The relation between PBmax scores and PTAs in the 16 patients yielded diverse findings. Eight of the eleven patients with PTAs of less than 20 dB had PBmax scores of at least 80% correct on both ears. The remaining three patients with PTAs between 0 and 19 dB had unusually poor PI-PB performance, however. Performance deficits in this group were observed on the C ear only. This finding agrees with previous investigators,[2,6,9] who noted that performance deficits in brain stem patients are usually observed on the ear contralateral to the affected side of the brain. Even though sensitivity was essentially the same on both ears in these patients, a large difference between ears emerged on PI-PB testing.

The four patients with PTAs of 20 to 35 dB on both ears did not yield consistent findings on PI-PB testing. Two patients had relatively good PBmax scores on both ears. Two pa-

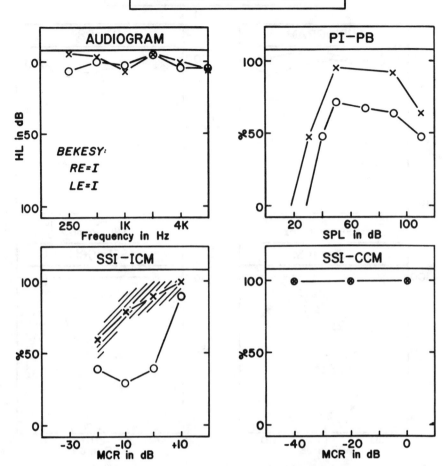

Fig 3.—Summary of diagnostic test results for 17-year-old girl with intra-axial brain stem lesion on the left. Hatched area represents normal range for SSI-ICM.

tients had relatively poor PBmax scores on both ears. The remaining patient, with a mild loss in one ear only, also showed a unilateral problem on PI-PB testing. Both the PI-PB loss and the hearing loss were observed on the ear contralateral to the affected side of the brain stem.

In short, when PBmax deficits were observed in these patients, they were generally found on both ears or on the C ear only. Average PBmax scores for the I and C ears seem to reflect the presence of more PBmax deficits on the C ear. The average PBmax scores were 85.5% for the I ear and 78.0% for the C ear. The range of performance scores for each ear was essentially the same, however, approximately 28% to 100% correct.

In our opinion, absolute perform-

ance scores in these patients failed to reflect the most important aspect of PI-PB testing, namely the consistency of the performance difference between ears across all PI-PB intensity levels, rather than the absolute PBmax scores. For example, some patients in this series showed only a slight PBmax difference (4% to 8%) between ears. However, the direction of the ear difference in these patients was consistent at all intensity levels and, furthermore, was frequently accentuated at very low and very high speech levels. To us, in view of the symmetrical pure-tone audiograms, these patients with consistently poorer performance on one ear than the other for PI-PB testing had substantial ear differences even though the PBmax ear difference had to be

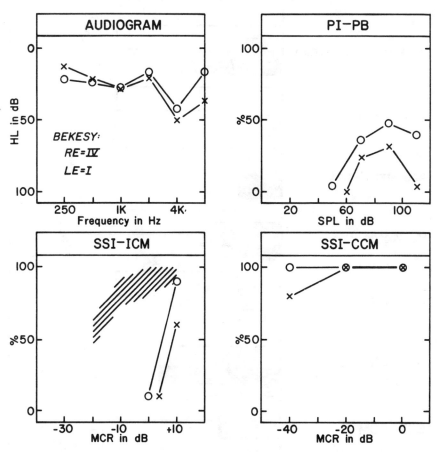

Fig 4.—Summary of diagnostic test results for 35-year-old man with intra-axial brain stem lesion on the right. Hatched area represents normal range for SSI-ICM.

considered within the range of normal variability.

In order to examine ear differences in greater detail than PBmax scores would permit, we divided patients into two groups according to whether the direction of ear differences was consistent or inconsistent across all intensity levels. Group A consisted of seven patients with interweaving PI-PB functions and no consistent ear differences. Group B was composed of nine patients with a consistent PI-PB ear difference. In these patients, the direction of the difference was the same at all intensity levels tested.

Poorer performance scores in group B were generally observed on the ear contralateral to the site of disorder. Only one of the nine patients had consistently poorer performance scores on the I ear. Although the direction of

the difference was generally the same in these patients, poorer performance on the C ear than on the I ear, the absolute difference between ears varied considerably. When ear differences were averaged across all intensity levels tested, we obtained an average difference of approximately 8% in two patients, 20% in three patients, 36% in three patients, and 50% in one patient. Interestingly enough, if we had considered only PBmax scores instead of the entire PI-PB function, three of these nine patients with consistent ear differences would have been unnoticed since PBmax measures were above 90% correct on both ears of all three patients.

In summary, only 6 of the 16 patients in this series had PBmax scores of less than 80% in either ear. Poor PBmax scores in these six patients

were generally found on the C ear only, but sometimes on both ears. Consistent performance differences between ears on the entire PI-PB function were found in nine of the 16 patients. Ear differences averaged approximately 25% and ranged from about 10% to 50%.

PI-PB Roll Over.—In some patients the PI-PB function reached a maximum, then declined substantially with further increase in speech level. This performance drop-off or "roll over"[27] at high speech intensities was quantified for patients in this series by analyzing each PI-PB function for PBmax and PB minimum (min). Phonetically balanced maximum was defined as the maximum discrimination score at any speech level; PBmin was defined as the lowest discrimination scores at any speech level above PBmax. The difference between these two scores (PBmax and PBmin) defined degree of roll over.

Patients with relatively good PBmax scores on both ears generally did not show a substantial roll over effect. In seven of the ten patients with PBmax scores on both ears of at least 80% correct, the amount of roll over was approximately 4%, a difference that is well within the range of normal variability. The remaining three patients showed a roll over effect of approximately 28%. The pattern of results was inconsistent in these three patients, however. Two patients had roll over on the C ear only, and one patient showed a roll over effect on both ears.

The two patients with relatively poor PBmax scores (24% to 52%) on each ear both showed the roll over phenomenon. Again, however, the pattern was not consistent. One patient showed a roll over effect of about 24% on both ears. One had roll over of 28% on the C ear only.

The four patients with a PBmax deficit only on the C ear showed varying patterns of roll over. Two patients showed roll over effect of 28% and 64% respectively on the C ear only; one showed roll over of about 28% on both ears; and one had essentially no roll over, less than 20%, on either ear.

In summary, a roll over effect was

more frequently observed in patients with a PBmax deficit on at least one ear than in patients with good PBmax scores (≥ 80%) on both ears. When abnormal roll over occurred, the ear yielding the unusual drop-off was not predictable. Roll over was observed on the C ear only for some patients, on the I ear only for others, and on both ears for still others.

SSI.—Performance for SSI materials in the presence of an ICM and a CCM was obtained on 11 patients. Results for SSI-ICM tasks in this series of patients were unusually consistent, in marked contrast to the pattern of results characterizing other audiometric tests. In short, ICM tasks produced unusually poor performance scores in all 11 brain stem patients. Six patients. had difficulty on both ears, and five patients had abnormal scores on the C ear only. No patient had poor performance on the I ear only, however.

In the six patients with ICM performance deficits for both ears, scores for the C ear were generally poorer than scores for the I ear. However, the difference between ears was usually not great. Performance scores averaged across MCRs of 0, −10, and −20 dB were approximately 37% on both the I and C ears. Performance averaged across these MCRs in normal listeners is 76%. Ear differences were dramatic in the remaining five patients with abnormal scores on the C ear only. Average scores for MCRs of 0, −10, and −20 dB were 82% on the I ear and 44% on the C ear.

Results for SSI-CCM tasks in this series of patients were strikingly different from results on SSI-ICM tasks. In 8 of the 11 patients, performance on the CCM task remained at 90% to 100% correct, even at the most unfavorable MCR condition (−40 dB). Relatively normal performance for CCM tasks in these eight patients was in dramatic contrast to the substantial ICM deficits observed.

The remaining three patients in this series had an average performance score for MCRs of 0, −20, and −40 dB of approximately 70% correct on the CCM task. Performance deficits were confined to the C ear only. The most striking finding in

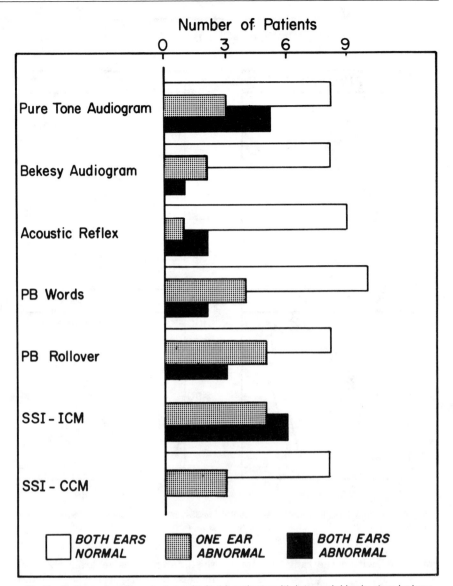

Fig 5.—Pattern of auditory test results in 16 patients with intra-axial brain stem lesions. For each test, number of patients with normal findings on both ears, abnormal results on one ear only, and abnormal scores on both ears is presented.

these patients was that the performance deficit for ICM was considerably more dramatic than the relatively slight CCM deficit. Interestingly, auditory function in two of the three patients with abnormal CCM scores was monitored at frequent intervals during a course of radiologic treatment. The rate of recovery in auditory symptoms was drastically different for CCM and ICM tasks. Both patients quickly climbed to 100% on CCM tasks although ICM performance deficits continued to be pronounced.

In summary, ICM performance

scores were consistently poor in all patients in this series. The C ear generally showed the more severe deficit, although both ears were severely affected in some patients. CCM performance scores generally remained at 90% to 100% in these patients. Only three patients had difficulty with CCM tasks. In all three of these patients, moreover, the ICM deficit was much greater than the CCM deficit on the involved ear. Performance deficits for CCM were confined to the C ear only. The most important finding was that CCM deficits were consistently less severe than ICM deficits.

Illustrative Cases.—Figures 2, 3, and 4 present diagnostic test results in three patients with pontine gliomas. These cases were selected to illustrate the unusual variability characterizing speech audiometric results in this series of patients. However, in each patient, the overall pattern of diagnostic results was valuable in distinguishing a brain stem site. Figure 2 presents results for an 8-year-old boy with a lesion eccentric to the right. The audiogram shows normal sensitivity on both ears. Sweep-frequency Bekesy audiograms were type I on both ears. The PI function for PB words (PI-PB) showed consistently poorer performance on the left (C) ear than the right (I) ear at all intensity levels. The slight roll over on the left (C) ear is unusual but not sufficiently severe to be diagnostic; PBmax scores were 88% on the left (C) ear and 96% on the right (I) ear. On SSI-ICM, there is a performance deficit when signals are presented to the left (C) ear. Relatively normal SSI-ICM results were obtained on the right (I) ear. No difficulty was observed on either ear for SSI-CCM. The presence of a performance deficit for ICM tasks and normal performance for CCM tasks was a typical finding in this series of patients.

Figure 3 shows results for a 17-year-old girl with a pontine glioma primarily on the left. Sensitivity is within the normal range on both ears. Bekesy audiograms are type I. Performance for PI-PB shows unusually poor performance on the right (C) ear and some roll over on both ears. The SSI-ICM task shows impaired performance on the right (C) ear and normal performance on the left (I) ear. Performance for SSI-CCM is unimpaired on either ear. Speech intelligibility deficits in this patient are observed only on the ear contralateral to the affected side of the brain stem.

Figure 4 shows results for a 35-year-old man with a pontine glioma eccentric to the right. The audiogram shows a mild bilateral loss, slightly greater at high frequencies. Bekesy audiograms were type I on the left (C) ear and type IV on the right (I) ear; PI-PB functions show severely reduced performance on both ears,

slightly greater on the left (C) ear. Performance on SSI tasks shows severely reduced scores on both ears for SSI-ICM. On SSI-CCM, a slight deficit was observed on the left (C) ear only. In this patient, the distinction between a brain stem disorder and an eighth nerve disorder is complicated by the type IV Bekesy tracing on the right (I) ear. The differentiation between these two sites of disorder is only possible in this patient on the basis of speech audiometric results. In a patient with right eighth nerve disorder, performance deficits for PI-PB functions and SSI-ICM tasks would be observed on the right ear only. In contrast, both ears of this patient show severe performance deficits on both PI-PB and SSI-ICM tests.

Comment

Auditory findings in this series of patients with intra-axial brain stem disorder varied considerably on any one absolute index of auditory function. Listening tasks that were very easy for some patients seemed unusually difficult for other patients. Results for the three representative patients illustrate well the variability characterizing any one auditory test. For example, in these three patients, performance on PI-PB functions ranged from relatively normal on both ears to abnormal on the C ear only to severely impaired on both ears. Performance on SSI-ICM tasks at any one level of difficulty also reflected this wide variability. In these three patients, performance at 0 MCR varied over the range from 10% to 90%.

Figure 5 summarizes the pattern of auditory test results in the entire series of patients. For each test, the number of patients with normal findings on both ears, abnormal results on one ear only, or abnormal scores on both ears is presented. This figure dramatically illustrates the diversity of test results characterizing any one test. The roll over phenomenon for PB words is a good example of this inconsistency. Results were within normal limits for eight patients, abnormal on one ear only for five patients, and abnormal on both ears for three patients. The only test that

yielded uniformly impaired performance in all patients tested was the SSI-ICM procedure. About one half of the patients showed abnormal scores on both ears, and the other half had impaired performance on the C ear only.

In spite of this inevitable variability, there is a thread of consistency that seems to suggest a constellation of auditory findings unique to an intra-axial brain stem disorder. The patients in this series presented an "over all" picture of brain stem symptoms that was generally characterized by (1) slight, if any, loss of pure-tone sensitivity below 1,000 Hz on either ear; (2) little or no evidence of abnormal adaptation on Bekesy audiometry; (3) mild, if any, impairment in PBmax scores; (4) consistent impairment for SSI materials in the presence of ipsilateral competition (SSI-ICM); and (5) either contralateral or bilateral symptoms. The diagnostic value of this brain stem syndrome is, of course, necessarily limited by the variability characterizing each auditory test. However, it does seem possible to differentiate an eighth nerve or extra-axial brain stem site from an intra-axial brain stem site on the following basis. Eighth nerve and extra-axial patients generally show (1) some unilateral sensitivity loss, (2) abnormal adaptation on Bekesey audiometry, (3) moderate to severe reduction in PBmax scores, and (4) ipsilateral symptoms.

This study was supported by Public Health Service research grant NB-08542 from the National Institute of Neurological Diseases and Stroke.

Dr. Robert A. Evans, Radiology Service, and Dr. James M. Killian, Neurology Service, The Methodist Hospital, cooperated in this investigation.

References

1. Jerger J: Audiological manifestations of lesions in the auditory nervous system. *Laryngoscope* 70:417-425, 1960.
2. Jerger J: Auditory tests for disorders of the central auditory mechanism, in Fields WS, Alford BR (eds): *Neurological Aspects of Auditory and Vestibular Disorders.* Springfield, Ill, Charles C Thomas, 1964, pp 77-93.
3. Parker W, Decker R, Richards N: Auditory function and lesions of the pons. *Arch Otolaryngol* 87:228-240, 1968.
4. Liden G: The scope and application of cur-

rent audiometric tests. *J Laryngol Otol* 83:507-520, 1969.

5. Korsen-Bengtsen M: Auditory patterns in diseases of the acoustic nerve, brain stem, and cortex, in Rojskaer C (ed): *Speech Audiometry*. Odense, Denmark, Second Danavox Symposium, 1970, pp 184-190.

6. Antonelli A, Calearo C, DeMetri T: On the auditory function in brain stem diseases. *Int Aud* 2:55-61, 1963.

7. Miller M, Daly J: Cerebellar atrophy simulating acoustic neurinoma. *Arch Otolaryngol* 85:383-386, 1967.

8. Shapiro I: Progression of auditory signs in pontine glioma. *Laryngoscope* 79:201-212, 1969.

9. Antonelli A: Sensitized speech tests: Results in brain stem lesions and diffusive CNS diseases, in Rojskaer C (ed): *Speech Audiometry*. Odense, Denmark, Second Danavox Symposium, 1970, pp 130-139.

10. Horrax G: Differential diagnosis of tumors: Primarily pineal, primarily pontile. *Arch Neurol Psychiatr* 17:179-192, 1927.

11. Sloan P, Persky A, Saltzman M: Midbrain deafness: Tumor of the midbrain producing sudden and complete deafness. *Arch Neurol Psychiatr* 49:237-243, 1943.

12. Eichel B, Hedgecock L, Williams H: A review of the literature on the audiologic aspect of neuro-otologic diagnosis. *Laryngoscope* 76:1-29, 1966.

13. Jerger J: Diagnostic significance of SSI test procedures: Retrocochlear site, in Rojskaer C (ed): *Speech Audiometry*. Odense, Denmark, Second Danavox Symposium, 1970, pp 163-175.

14. Owens E: Bekesy tracings and site of lesion. *J Speech Hear Dis* 29:456-468, 1964.

15. Katz J: Audiologic diagnosis: Cochlea to cortex. *Menorah Med J* 1:25-38, 1970.

16. Owens E: Audiologic evaluation in cochlear versus retrocochlear lesions. *Acta Otolaryngol* suppl 283, 1971, p 45.

17. Courville C: Intracranial tumors. *Bull Los Angeles Neurol Soc* 32:43-46, 1967.

18. Carhart R, Jerger J: Preferred method for clinical determination of puretone thresholds. *J Speech Hear Dis* 24:330-345, 1959.

19. Jerger J, Speaks C, Trammell J: A new approach to speech audiometry. *J Speech Hear Dis* 33:318-328, 1968.

20. Jerger J: Diagnostic audiometry, in Jerger J (ed): *Modern Developments in Audiology*, ed 2. New York, Academic Press, 1973, pp 75-115.

21. Egan J: Articulation testing methods. *Laryngoscope* 58:955-991, 1948.

22. Calearo C, Antonelli A: Audiometric findings in brain stem lesions. *Acta Otolaryngol* 66:305-319, 1968.

23. Nakamura T: A supplement to auditory findings in cases of brain tumor. *Otorhinolaryngol Clin* 57:347-365, 1964.

24. Chladek V: Audiometric diagnosis of brain stem lesions. *Excerpta Med* 11:22, 1969.

25. Greisen O, Rasmussen P: Stapedius muscle reflexes and otoneurological examinations in brain stem tumors. *Acta Otolaryngol* 70:366-370, 1970.

26. Parker W, Decker R, Gardner W: Auditory function and intracranial lesions. *Arch Otolaryngol* 76:425-435, 1962.

27. Jerger J, Jerger S: Diagnostic significance of PB word functions. *Arch Otolaryngol* 93:573-580, 1971.

Scand Audiol 4: 147–163, 1975

CLINICAL VALIDITY OF CENTRAL AUDITORY TESTS

J. Jerger and S. Jerger

From the Department of Otorhinolaryngology and Communicative Sciences, Baylor College of Medicine and the Methodist Hospital, Houston, Texas

ABSTRACT

Clinical validity of central auditory tests. Jerger, J. and Jerger, S. (Baylor College of Medicine and The Methodist Hospital, Houston, Texas, USA).
Scand Audiol 1975, 4 (147–163).

Six audiometric procedures were administered to seventy patients divided into seven groups: normal, eighth nerve, brain stem, temporal lobe, non-auditory CNS, aphasic, and amyotrophic lateral sclerosis (ALS). Pure-tone sensitivity was equated among groups. For the eighth nerve group, performance was consistently poor for all measures. For the brain stem group, performance was consistently depressed for difficult monotic speech tasks. For the temporal lobe group, performance was most severely affected for difficult dichotic speech messages. For the aphasic group, performance was generally poor for both monotic and dichotic speech procedures. For the non-auditory CNS and ALS groups, results were normal. Inter- and intra-group variability were substantial.

INTRODUCTION

In order to establish the validity of any proposed test procedure for the evaluation of auditory disorders, it is necessary to demonstrate (1) that the test yields the expected result in patients with auditory disorders and (2) that false-positive results usually do not appear in patients without auditory disorders.

In the case of central auditory disorder, we can identify at least four potential sources of error. First is the possibility that ill patients may perform poorly on difficult auditory tests due entirely to physical malaise rather than a central auditory problem. Second is the possibility that patients with *any* disorder of the central nervous system (CNS) may perform poorly on central auditory tests even though there is no direct involvement of the central auditory pathways per se. Third is the possibility that the presence of a language disorder in some patients with temporal lobe site may compromise the diagnostic value of degraded speech audiometry. Fourth, and finally, is the possibility that auditory test results may not be "site-specific" in some patients with either eighth nerve or brain stem auditory disorder because of secondary symptoms that masquerade as independent lesions. For example, is it possible for a patient with a brain stem disorder to show the same configuration of results as a patient with an eighth nerve site?

The present paper attempts to evaluate these potential sources of error by comparing the performance of groups of patients with central auditory disorders to the performance of patients in various control groups.

METHOD

Subjects

Seventy patients, tested by the Audiology Service, The Methodist Hospital, between 1968 and 1973, were divided into seven groups of ten patients each on the basis of the final medical diagnosis. Two were experimental groups composed of patients with either brain stem or temporal lobe disorders. Five were control groups divided into one normal group, one eighth nerve group, and three CNS groups.

Experimental groups

Brain stem. Site of lesion was confirmed surgically and/or radiographically in all 10 intra-axial brain stem patients. Final diagnosis from histopathologic report or pneumoencephalographic report was pontine glioma in 9 patients and arteriovenous malformation in 1 patient. Subjects were 2 females and 8 males. The average age was 26.0 years and ranged from 8 to 48 years. The brain stem lesion was primarily on the right side in 6 patients, primarily on the left side in 3 patients, and bilaterally symmetrical in 1 patient.

Temporal lobe. Site of lesion was confirmed surgically and/or radiographically in 6 patients. Final diagnosis in these patients was astrocytoma in 2 patients, and either ependymoma, glioblastoma multiforme, glioma, or ischemia in the other four patients. The final medical diagnosis in the remaining patients was temporal lobe encephalopathy in 2 patients, temporal lobe embolyst in 1 patient, and skull trauma in 1 patient. Diagnosis was based on neurological findings, electrograms, clinical course, and history of onset. Subjects were 7 males and 3 females. The average age was 47.8 years and ranged from 24 to 63 years. The temporal lobe lesion was on the right side in 7 patients and on the left side in 3 patients. Patients in this group did not show any obvious language dysfunction accompanying the temporal lobe disorder.

Control groups

Normal. Subjects were classified as normal on the basis of (1) hearing threshold levels less than or equal to 25 dB (ISO-64) between 250 and 4 000 Hz, (2) normal findings on impedance audiometry, and (3) no evidence of intracranial disorder. Medical examination usually revealed a clinical history of dizziness and no other significant findings. Patients in this group did not have specific hearing complaints. Subjects were 6 females and 4 males. The average age was 41.1 years and ranged from 29 to 63 years. The purpose of the normal control group was to provide "baseline" information against which to compare the performance of the other control groups and the experimental groups. We referred all other test results to the data obtained in this normal group.

Eighth nerve. Site of lesion was confirmed surgically in all patients. Final diagnosis from histopathologic report was acoustic neuroma in 5 patients, glomus jugularae tumor in 1 patient, cerebellopontine angle meningioma in 1 patient, cerebellopontine angle glioblastoma in 1 patient, jugular foramen neurofibroma in 1 patient, and clivus meningioma in 1 patient. Seven subjects were female and 3 were male. The average age was 40.7 years and ranged from 10 to 64 years. The lesion was on the right side in 5 patients and on the left side in 5 patients. The purpose of the eighth nerve control group was to determine whether eighth nerve auditory symptomatology may be confused with brain stem auditory symptomatology due to possible overriding secondary symptoms produced by either primary mass.

Aphasic. All patients had a final medical diagnosis of aphasia. Histories revealed either a cerebrovascular accident or skull trauma. Eight patients were concurrently receiving aphasia therapy by the Speech Pathology Service of The Methodist Hospital. All of the 10 patients in this group could understand the verbal instructions for the audiometric tests. However, five patients were expressively impaired to the extent that speech tests involving oral repetition could not be carried out. The remaining five patients performed all speech tasks easily. The length of time between the onset of the aphasia and the audiologic evaluation varied from 1 month to 28 years. Three patients were 1 to 3 months post-insult, three were 4 to 5 months post-insult, three were 10 to 12 months, and one was 28 years. Subjects were 5 females and 5 males. The average age was 46.5 years and ranged from 12 to 72 years. The purpose of the aphasic control group was to evaluate performance on speech intelligibility tests in patients with a language disorder in addition to possible temporal lobe disorder. We sought to determine whether auditory test results based on the perception of speech materials might be uniquely compromised by the presence of aphasia.

Non-auditory CNS. Patients in this group had intracranial lesions that did not affect the central auditory pathways. Site of lesion was confirmed surgically and/or radiographically in all patients. Final diagnosis from histopathology, pneumoencephalography, or angiography was parietal glioblastoma in 1 patient, Arnold-Chiari malformation in 1 patient, pituitary tumor in 2 patients, midbrain glioma in 2 patients, vertebral artery aneurysm in 2 patients, parietal astrocytoma in 1 patient, and frontal falx meningioma in 1 patient. Subjects were 5 females and 5 males. The average age was 39.3 years and ranged from 22 to 53 years. The lesion was on the right side of the brain in 3 patients and on the left side in 3 patients. The remaining 4 patients had midline brain lesions. The purpose of the non-auditory CNS control group was to insure that abnormal test results were specific only to patients with direct involvement of the central auditory pathways.

ALS. Patients in this group had amyotrophic lateral sclerosis (ALS), a degenerative motor neuron disease. Degeneration generally involves the Betz cells of the motor cortex, the motor nuclei of the brain stem, or the anterior horn cells of the spinal cord (Wolfgram & Myers, 1973). Subjects were 6 females and 4 males. The average age was 52.4 years and ranged from 31 to 66 years. The purpose of the ALS control group was to evaluate the effects on performance due to extreme physical malaise, (a characteristic of patients in this group), and to insure that "false-positive" results did not occur in patients with non-auditory brain stem disorders.

Test battery

Six audiometric test procedures were attempted on all patients. These procedures have been described in detail previously (Jerger & Jerger, 1974*a*) and are briefly summarized below.

Pure tone sensitivity. Threshold hearing levels (ISO-64) at octave frequencies between 250 and 4 000 Hz were obtained by either conventional manual or Békésy techniques.

Békésy audiometry. Sweep frequency tracings for interrupted and continuous signals were obtained over the frequency range from 200 to 8 000 Hz. Frequency changed at a rate of one octave per minute. Intensity changed at a rate of 2.5 dB per second.

Acoustic reflex. Acoustic reflex thresholds were measured at octave frequencies between 500 and 4 000 Hz. Threshold levels were defined as the lowest hearing level (HL) in dB that produced reliable deflections of the balance meter when sound was presented to the ear opposite the ear containing the impedance bridge probe. The maximum intensity used to elicit reflex contractions was 110 dB HL.

PI–PB functions. Performance-intensity functions for monosyllabic (PB) word lists (PI–PB) were constructed by presenting blocks of 25 words at each of several suprathreshold levels. Generally, performance was defined from that intensity level yielding 0 to 20% correct up to a maximum speech intensity of 110 dB sound pressure level (SPL). The patient repeated each word to a tester who scored it as correct or incorrect. White noise masking was presented to the nontest ear whenever the speech level was sufficiently intense to cross over and be heard in the nontest ear.

Synthetic sentence identification (SSI). SSI materials (Jerger et al., 1968) consisted of a single list of ten synthetic sentences, seven words each, representing a third-order approximation to actual English sentences. The patient was seated before a console containing a list of the ten sentences and a corresponding column of push buttons. After each sentence had been presented, the patient identified the sentence he heard from the list in front of him and pushed the appropriate button. Different random presentations of the same ten sentences were used throughout the test session. Sentences were presented at an intensity level yielding 100% correct performance in both ears. For most patients, this level was 50 dB SPL. However, a few patients required louder presentation levels to achieve a criterion of 100% in both ears. The SSI task was made difficult by a competing speech message concerning the life of a Texas pioneer (Davy Crockett). Performance was measured at several message-to-competition ratios (MCR's) for both a contralateral competing message (CCM) and an ipsilateral competing message (ICM). For the CCM condition (sentences to the test ear and competition to the opposite ear) MCR's were varied in 20 dB steps over the range from 0 dB to −40 dB. For the ICM condition (sentences and competition to the same ear) MCR's were varied in 10 dB steps over the range from +10 dB to −20 dB.

Staggered Spondaic Word (SSW) test. The SSW test (Katz, 1962) was composed of 40 pairs of partially overlapping spondaic words. The time sequence for an illustrative word pair (*upstairs* and *downtown*) consisted of the patient hearing *up* in one ear, then *stairs* and *down* simultaneously in both ears, then *town* in the opposite ear. We called the first monosyllable the *leading* condition, the simultaneous monosyllables the *competing* condition, and the last monosyllable the *lagging* condition. The 40 spondaic pairs were alternated between ears so that each ear received the leading monosyllable one-half of the time. The patient was instructed to repeat all the words he heard in either ear. The presentation level was the intensity yielding maximum performance on PI–PB testing. The percent correct scores for the leading, competing and lagging conditions were obtained for each ear. The leading and lagging conditions were averaged in some groups to obtain one *non-competing* score. Results for each group were also scored according to the method recommended by Katz (1968).

Table I. *Number of patients in each group with successful results on both ears for each of the seven test procedures*

Test procedure	Groups							Total (N = 70)
	Normal	VIIIth nerve	Brain stem	Temporal lobe	Aphasic	Non-auditory CNS	ALS	
Pure-tone sensitivity	10	10	10	10	10	10	10	70
Békésy audiogram	10	10	8	4	7	8	3	50
Acoustic reflex	10	6	9	5	5	6	10	51
PI–PB	10	10	10	10	5	10	7	62
SSI–ICM	10	10	10	10	7	10	8	65
SSI–CCM	10	10	10	10	8	10	8	66
SSW	10	1	3	6	3	4	5	32

Instrumentation and test materials

Pure-tone audiograms were obtained with either a manual audiometer (Beltone, model 10D) or a Békésy audiometer (Grason-Stadler, model E800). Impedance audiometry was carried out with an electroacoustic impedance bridge (Madsen, type ZO-70) and an associated pure-tone audiometer (Beltone, model 10D). Speech materials consisted of six PB-50 word lists (Egan, 1948), one list of ten synthetic sentences (Jerger et al., 1968), and one SSW list of 40 spondaic pairs (Katz, 1962). All materials were prerecorded on magnetic tape by the same male talker. The tape playback system (Ampex, AG440) was routed through a speech audiometer (Grason-Stadler, type 162) to earphones (Telephonic, type TDH-39) housed in CZW-6 cush-

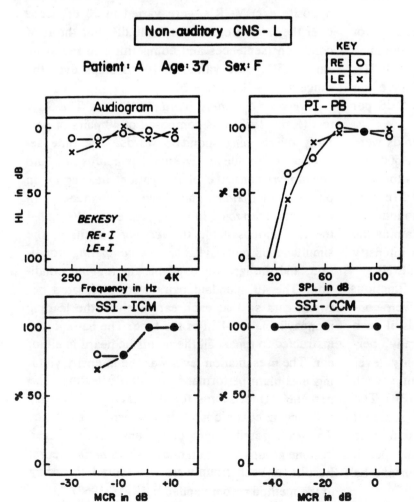

Fig. 1. Summary of diagnostic test results for a 37-year-old female with a non-auditory CNS lesion on the left. Stippled area represents the normal range for SSI–ICM.

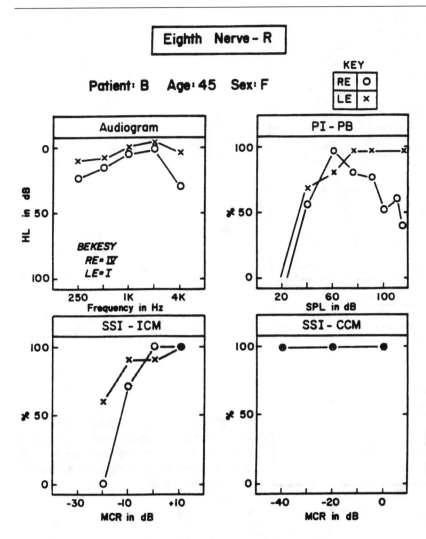

Fig. 2. Summary of diagnostic test results for a 45-year-old female with an eighth nerve disorder on the right. The stippled area represents the normal range for SSI–ICM.

ions. Speech level was defined as the SPL of a 1 000 Hz signal recorded at the average level of frequent peaks of the speech as monitored on a VU meter.

Procedure

Patients were tested in a single session of two to three hours duration. The entire test battery was attempted on all patients, but it was not possible to obtain all procedures on both ears of every subject. Patients that did not complete the entire test battery either were unusually ill, were young children, or had other tests (i.e. radiograms) scheduled and could not stay for the entire session. Table I presents the number of patients in each group with successful results on both ears for each of the seven tests. All 70 patients completed pure tone sensitivity testing on both ears. At least 62 of the 70 patients had complete results for PI–PB functions, SSI–ICM, and SSI–CCM. Békésy audiometry and acoustic reflex measures were obtained in both ears in approximately 50 patients. The SSW test was successfully completed in 32 of the 70 patients.

RESULTS

Illustrative cases

Patient A. Fig. 1 summarizes auditory findings for a 37-year-old female with a non-auditory CNS lesion on the left. Surgical exploration revealed a well circumscribed glioblastoma in the left temporoparietal region underlying the gyrus posterior to the junction of the occipital and temporal lobes and lower parietal region. The audiogram showed essentially normal sensitivity on both ears. Békésy audiograms were type I on both ears. The PI–PB functions were normal on both ears. The maximum PB (PB_{max}) scores were 100% on the right ear and 96% on the left ear. SSI–ICM scores were within the normal range, as indicated by the stippled area, on both ears. SSI–CCM scores remained at 100% on both ears at all MCR's. All diagnostic test results were negative. There was no evidence of eighth nerve or central auditory pathway involvement on either ear.

Patient B. Fig. 2 shows results for a 45-year-old female with an eighth nerve disorder on the right.

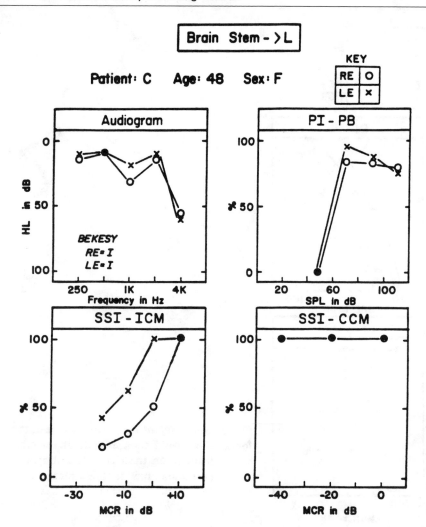

Fig. 3. Summary of diagnostic test results for a 48-year-old female with an intra-axial brain stem disorder primarily on the left side. Stippled area represents the normal range for SSI–ICM.

An acoustic neurilemoma was removed at surgery. The audiogram showed normal sensitivity on the left ear and a mild sensori-neural loss on the right ear. Impedance audiometry showed normal, type A, tympanograms and normal static compliance in both ears. However, acoustic reflexes were absent at all frequencies with sound in the right ear. With sound in the left ear, reflexes were present at normal HL's at 500, 1000, and 2000 Hz, but absent at 4000 Hz. The absence of acoustic reflexes at 4000 Hz only in the left ear probably has no diagnostic significance. Békésy audiograms were type IV in the right ear and type I in the left ear. The PI–PB function was normal on the left ear but showed substantial rollover on the right ear. PB$_{max}$ scores were 96% correct on both ears. SSI–ICM scores showed unusually poor performance on the right ear only. SSI–CCM performance was unimpaired on either ear. Note that auditory deficits—sensitivity loss, abnormal adaptation on Békésy audiometry, substantial PI–PB rollover, and SSI–ICM loss—were observed on the right ear only, the ear showing the radiographic abnormality.

Patient C. Fig. 3 presents results for a 48-year-old female with an intra-axial brain stem disorder primarily on the left side. Left vertebral angiography revealed a large intra-axial neoplasm extending from the caudal pons to the upper cervical cord and centered at the medulla oblongata with infiltration into the left cerebellar hemisphere. A shunt was performed to relieve increased ventricular pressure. Surgery confirmed the presence of a brain stem glioma. The audiogram showed a moderate high frequency loss in both ears. Acoustic reflexes were present at normal HL's for all test frequencies on both ears. Békésy audiograms were type I on both ears. PI–PB functions showed slightly reduced maximum performance on the right ear and a mild rollover effect on the left ear. PB$_{max}$ scores were 96% on the left ear and 84% on the right ear. SSI–ICM performance showed a deficit on the right ear only. SSI–CCM scores remained at 100% on both ears. Substantial SSI–ICM losses in the presence of normal or near normal SSI–CCM performance is a distinguishing characteristic of brain stem disorder. Note that speech intelligibility

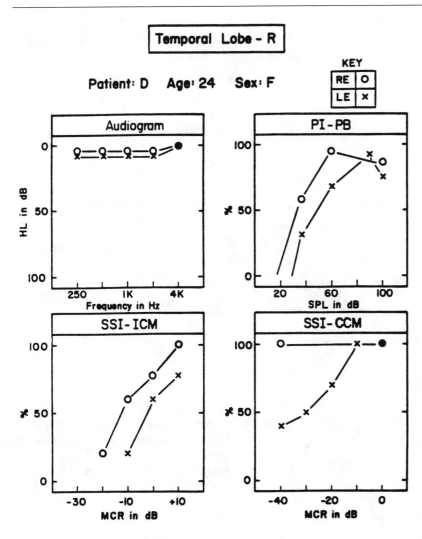

Fig. 4. Summary of diagnostic test results for a 24-year-old female with a temporal lobe disorder on the right. Stippled area represents the normal range for SSI–ICM.

deficits are observed on the right ear, the ear opposite the affected side of the brain stem.

Patient D. Fig. 4 shows results for a 24-year-old female with a temporal lobe disorder on the right. Angiography showed an ischemic area in the right temporal area with extensions into the frontal and parietal areas accompanied by cerebral edema and hydrocephalus. The audiogram showed normal sensitivity in both ears. Acoustic reflexes were observed at normal HL's for all test frequencies on both ears. The PI–PB functions showed normal maximum scores and insignificant rollover, but the left ear showed an unusually slow rise to maximum performance. PB_{max} scores were 96% on the right ear and 88% on the left ear. SSI–ICM scores showed performance deficits on both ears with poorer performance on the left ear. SSI–CCM scores were normal on the right ear but showed a substantial deficit on the left ear. Marked difficulty on SSI–CCM tasks is a distinguishing feature of temporal lobe disorder.

Patient E. Fig. 5 presents test results for a 54-year-old male with aphasia. The patient sustained a cerebrovascular accident approximately one year prior to audiometric evaluation. The audiogram showed normal sensitivity in both ears. Acoustic reflexes were present at HL's within the normal range for all test frequencies on both ears. Békésy audiograms were type I in both ears. PI–PB functions could not be obtained (CNE) due to the patient's limited expressive ability. SSI–ICM and SSI–CCM (which require only a manual response) were within the normal range on the left ear and showed moderate impairment on the right ear. The aphasic patient usually shows a general deficit in speech intelligibility that is apparent for both monotic and dichotic listening tasks.

Distribution of auditory findings

Audiometric group data are presented in terms of the ear ipsilateral (I) and contralateral (C) to the site of disorder. For example, in a patient with a lesion on the right side, the right ear would be the I ear and left ear would be the C ear. In the ALS group with non-unilateral lesions, the right ear and the left ear

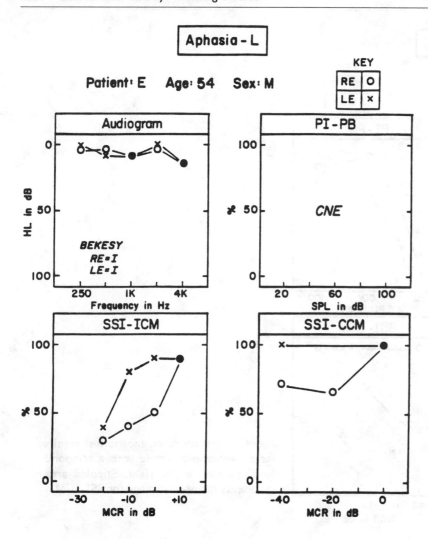

Fig. 5. Summary of diagnostic test results for a 54-year-old male with aphasia. PI–PB performance could not be established (CNE) due to the patient's limited expressive ability. Stippled area represents the normal range for SSI–ICM.

were randomly selected to represent the I or the C ear one-half of the time. Results for each test procedure are referred to results obtained in the normal group.

Pure-tone sensitivity. Patients in this study were purposefully selected on the basis of normal hearing or, at most, a very mild hearing impairment in either ear. We attempted to equate sensitivity among groups in order to minimize any effects on performance due to differences in threshold HL's rather than differences in site of disorder. As a result of this selection procedure, a substantial sensitivity loss was unlikely in any group. Fig. 6 shows the average threshold HL's at octave intervals between 500 and 4000 Hz for the six groups. All HL's are plotted relative to average sensitivity levels in the normal group. With the exception of the eighth nerve group, average sensitivity levels for all groups were within the normal range on both ears at all frequencies. The eighth nerve group showed an average mild loss, approximately 10 to 20 dB, on the I ear and normal sensitivity on the C ear.

Békésy audiometry. Fig. 7 summarizes Békésy tracings on the I and C ears of patients in the six groups. Tracings for the normal group were type I on both ears of all patients and are not shown. Type I and II patterns are consistent with normal hearing or a cochlear site; type III and IV tracings are consistent with a retrocochlear disorder (Jerger, 1960b). Type I or II Békésy audiograms characterized both ears of all patients in the temporal lobe, aphasic, non-auditory CNS, and ALS groups. None of these patients showed a retrocochlear pattern on either ear.

Seven of eight brain stem patients showed normal, type I, tracings on both ears. This finding is consistent with the observations of Jerger (1960a) and Owens (1964, 1971). However, one patient, a 35-year-old male, had a type I tracing on the C ear and a type IV pattern on the I ear. Pure-tone sensitivity in this patient showed a bilaterally symmetrical loss with a pure-tone average (PTA) at 500, 1000, and 2000 Hz of 17 dB on each ear. Surgical findings revealed a pontomesencephalic glioma with an exophytic extension to the right (I) side

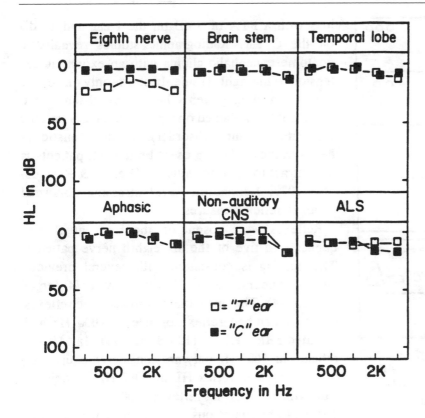

Fig. 6. Average threshold hearing levels at octave frequencies between 500 and 4 000 Hz for six patient groups. Results are plotted relative to sensitivity levels in normal group.

which may have indirectly involved the eighth nerve fibers.

Six of the 10 eighth nerve patients showed a type III or IV pattern on the I ear. This finding is consistent with the results of Johnson (1968), Owens (1971), and Jerger (1973). Conversely, four eighth

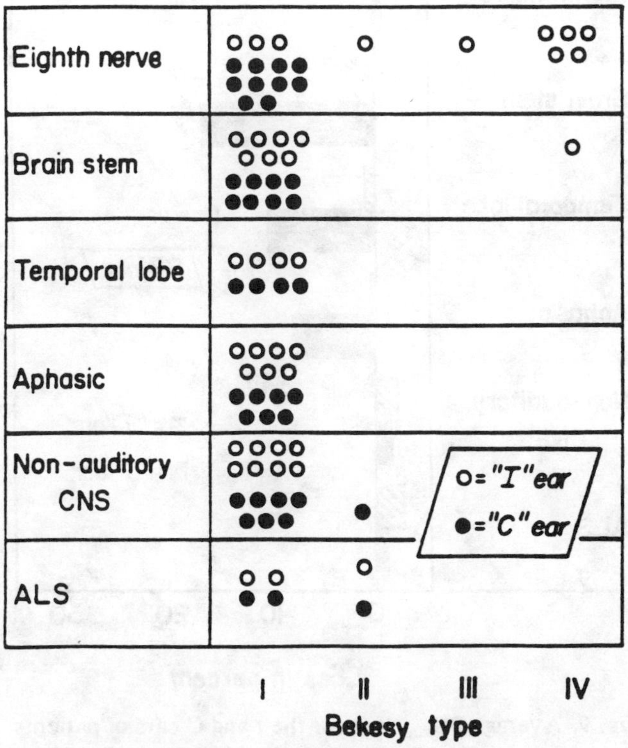

Fig. 7. Type of Békésy audiogram found on I and C ears of patients in each group.

nerve patients had a type I or II tracing on the I ear. However, two of these four patients with normal Békésy tracings showed positive, retrocochlear, results for modified Békésy audiometry. One patient had a significant discrepancy between continuous-forward versus continuous-backward sweep frequency tracings (Palva et al., 1970; Jerger et al., 1972b). The other patient had a positive (retrocochlear) pattern on Békésy comfortable loudness (BCL) audiometry (Jerger & Jerger, 1974b). In short, Békésy audiometry was consistent with a retrocochlear site in eight of the 10 eighth nerve patients when the conventional procedure was supplemented by either continuous-forward versus continuous-backward tracings or BCL tracings. All eighth nerve patients had normal, type I, tracings on the C ear.

Acoustic reflex. Fig. 8 shows acoustic reflex results for the I and C ears of all patients in the six groups. Reflexes for the normal group were present at all frequencies on both ears and are not presented. Reflexes were usually absent (at 110 dB HL) in the eighth nerve group, sometimes absent in the brain stem group, and generally present in the four remaining groups.

Acoustic reflexes were present at all frequencies on both ears of patients in the temporal lobe and aphasic groups. In the non-auditory CNS and ALS groups, reflexes were present at all frequencies on

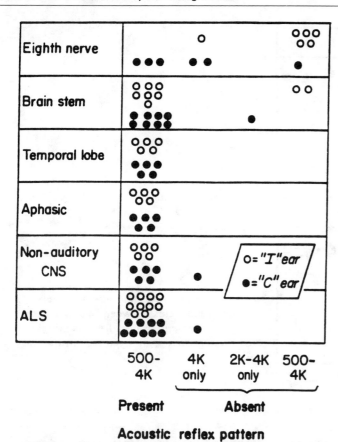

Fig. 8. Pattern of acoustic reflexes for the I and C ears of patients in each group.

loss with a PTA of 9 dB on the I ear and 11 dB on the C ear. Radiographic studies revealed a pontomesencephalic glioma with an exophytic extension to the right (I) side. In short, only one of the nine brain stem patients had reflex absence that could not be explained on a peripheral basis (middle ear or motor-neuron disorder). Normal acoustic reflexes in most of the present brain stem patients is in contrast to previous studies (Greisen & Rasmussen, 1970; Lehnhardt, 1973) stressing abnormal acoustic reflex measures.

Reflexes were absent on the I ear at all frequencies in five of the six eighth nerve patients. This finding is consistent with several previous studies (Anderson et al., 1969; Sheehy, 1974; Jerger et al., 1974). The one patient with acoustic reflexes on the I ear had reflex absence at 4 000 Hz and elevated reflex HL's (110 dB) at 2 000 Hz. Absent reflexes at 4 000 Hz only are considered equivocal, but the elevated reflex HL at 2 000 Hz in conjunction with the missing reflex at 4 000 Hz is unusual enough to be suspicious in our experience. According to this criterion, all six eighth nerve patients had reflex patterns on the I ear suggesting the possibility of retrocochlear disorder.

the I ear, but absent at 4 000 Hz only for two patients on the C ear. Generally, we disregard reflex absence at 4 000 Hz only on a single ear. About 4% of patients with otherwise normal ears have missing reflexes at this frequency on one ear for no apparent reason (Jerger et al., 1972a). Results for the I ear of one patient in the non-auditory CNS group are not presented since reflex measures were equivocal due to a slight middle ear disorder in the ear containing the probe.

Acoustic reflexes were present at all frequencies on both ears for seven of the nine brain stem patients. Only two patients had abnormal reflexes. One patient had reflex absence on the I ear only. Reflex abnormality in this patient could be attributed to facial nerve paresis on the side of the head containing the impedance bridge probe. Reflexes in this patient's other ear were present at all frequencies. The other patient had absent reflexes at all frequencies on the I ear and at 2 000 and 4 000 Hz on the C ear. Reflexes were observed at 500 and 1 000 Hz on the C ear, but threshold HL's were 110 dB and 100 dB respectively, levels at the high end of the normal range. Pure-tone sensitivity showed a moderate, bilaterally symmetrical, high frequency

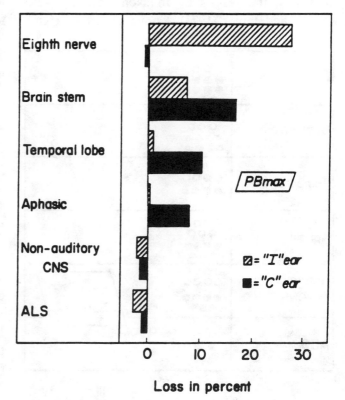

Fig. 9. Average PB$_{max}$ loss for the I and C ears of patients in each group. Results are plotted relative to performance in the normal group.

On the C ear, reflexes were present at all frequencies or absent at 4 000 Hz only in five of the six eighth nerve patients. The remaining patient had reflex absence at all frequencies on the C ear as well as the I ear. Pure-tone sensitivity showed a mild loss on both ears, with a PTA of 34 dB on the I ear and 26 dB on the C ear. Surgical findings revealed a 35-mm angular neurilemoma that had produced displacement, deformity, and rotation of the brain stem. At least two possible explanations for reflex absence on the C ear exist in this patient. One is that reflex absence may be due to the considerable displacement of the brain stem noted at surgery. The other is that reflex absence may be due to seventh nerve involvement on the I ear. Medical examination at the time of hospitalization did not record any specific seventh nerve abnormality on either side. However, clinical records noted that the patient's mouth "drooped" on the I side, the side of the head containing the impedance bridge probe when sound was introduced to the C ear.

PI–PB functions. Fig. 9 shows the average PB_{max} losses for each ear of patients in the six groups. All results are plotted relative to performance in the normal group. The eighth nerve group showed a loss on the I ear only; the brain stem group showed a loss on both ears, but greater on the C ear; the temporal lobe and aphasic groups showed a loss on the C ear only; and the non-auditory CNS and ALS groups showed normal scores on both ears.

The largest PB_{max} deficit was observed for patients with eighth nerve disorder. Even though the average hearing loss on the impaired ear was only 18 dB, the PB_{max} score for this group was approximately 30% poorer than normal performance. Unusually poor performance for PB word tests has long been recognized as a distinguishing characteristic of eighth nerve site (Goodman, 1957; Flower & Viehweg, 1961; Johnson, 1970; Katz, 1970).

The brain stem group had a PB_{max} deficit of 17% on the C ear and 7% on the I ear even though sensitivity measures were within the normal range on both ears. Bilateral speech intelligibility deficits, with greatest impairment on the C ear, have been reported previously in patients with intra-axial brain stem lesions (Parker et al., 1962, 1968; Calearo & Antonelli, 1968; Antonelli, 1970). However, PB_{max} deficits in the present group reflect, at most, only a mild impairment on either ear for this repetition task.

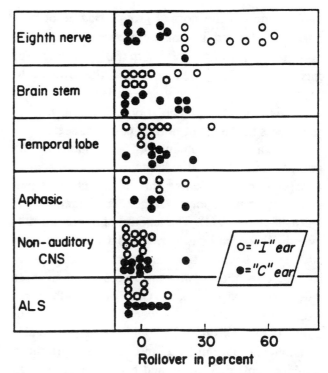

Fig. 10. Distribution of PI–PB rollover indices for I and C ears of patients in each group. Results are plotted relative to performance in normal group. The stippled area represents the normal range.

Performance scores on the C ear of the temporal lobe group and the aphasic patients who could perform the task were approximately 10% poorer than normal performance. PB_{max} scores on the I ear were unimpaired in both groups. The observation of slight PB_{max} deficits, on the C ear only, agrees with the findings of some previous investigators (Jerger, 1964, 1973; Berlin et al., 1965; Korsan-Bengtsen, 1970, 1973). However, in the past, PB_{max} performance in temporal lobe patients has generally been considered normal (Antonelli et al., 1963; Lynn & Gilroy, 1972; Liden & Korsan-Bengtsen, 1973). Maximum scores on both ears have been within the "normal" range and slight ear differences, if present, have been presumed to be within the range of normal variability. However, our experience suggests that a very real, although slight, deficit is present on the C ear. In this project, we carefully constructed PI–PB functions across many intensity levels and found consistently poorer performance on the C ear although pure-tone sensitivity was the same on both ears. Furthermore, the performance deficit was frequently more pronounced at very low and very high intensities.

PI–PB rollover. Fig. 10 shows the distribution of rollover indices for both ears of all patients in the six groups. Rollover indices are plotted relative to performance in the normal group. Degree of roll-over was defined by the difference between the maximum (PB$_{max}$) and minimum (PB$_{min}$) scores. For this purpose, PB$_{min}$ was defined as the lowest percent correct score at any speech level above that level yielding PB$_{max}$. The stippled area in Fig. 10 represents the range of normal performance.

The rollover phenomenon differed among the six groups. Abnormal rollover occurred on the I ear of all eighth nerve patients. This finding is consistent with previous reports (Jerger & Jerger, 1971; Igarashi et al., 1974). The amount of abnormal roll-over in these patients varied from approximately 20% to 60% more than the normal group. And, indeed, only the eighth nerve group had rollover effects of more than 35%. Only one eighth nerve patient had abnormal rollover on the C ear also. Surgical reports on this patient noted an angular meningioma, 35 mm by 25 mm, that had produced displacement, deformity, and rotation of the brain stem. Bilateral rollover in this patient may have reflected the extensive amount of brain stem involvement noted at surgery.

Abnormal rollover occurred in four of the 10

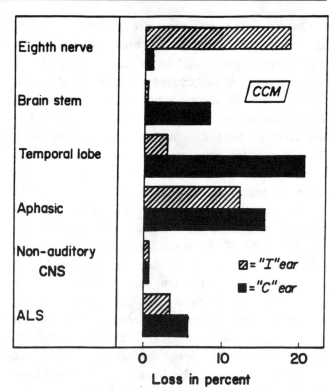

Fig. 12. Average SSI–CCM loss on the I and C ears of patients in each group. Performance was averaged across message-to-competition ratios of 0, −20, and −40 dB. Results are plotted relative to performance in the normal group. The stippled area represents the range of normal findings.

brain stem patients. Two patients had abnormal rollover on both ears and two patients had abnormal rollover on the C ear only. The amount of rollover was approximately 20% on both the I and C ears of all four patients.

Rollover effects were generally within normal limits for the temporal lobe, aphasic, non-auditory CNS and ALS groups. Abnormal rollover effects occurred in only two temporal lobe patients, on the I ear only and on the C ear only; in one aphasic patient on both ears; and in one non-auditory CNS patient on the C ear only.

SSI functions (SSI–ICM and SSI–CCM). Fig. 11 shows the average loss on each ear for the six groups on the ICM task. Performance was averaged across MCR's of 0, −10, and −20 dB. All results are plotted relative to performance in the normal group. The stippled area represents the range of normal findings. ICM results were within normal limits on both ears of the non-auditory CNS and ALS groups.

The eighth nerve and brain stem groups had performance deficits on one ear only. However, the ear reflecting the ICM loss differed in the two

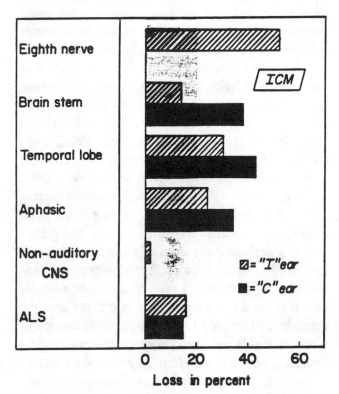

Fig. 11. Average SSI–ICM loss on the I and C ears of patients in each group. Performance was averaged across message-to-competition ratios of 0, −10, and −20 dB. Results are plotted relative to performance in the normal group. The stippled area represents the range of normal findings.

groups. The eighth nerve group had a loss of approximately 50% on the I ear only; the brain stem group had a loss of about 40% on the C ear only.

The temporal lobe and aphasic groups had a loss on both ears, but greater on the C ear. Average performance deficits in the temporal lobe group were approximately 30% on the I ear and 40% on the C ear. Average losses in the aphasic group were abot 25% on the I ear and 35% on the C ear.

Fig. 12 summarizes the average loss for each ear on the CCM task. Performance was averaged across MCR's of 0, −20, and −40 dB. All scores are plotted relative to results in the normal group. The stippled area presents the range of normal findings. CCM results were within normal limits for both ears of the brain stem, non-auditory CNS, and ALS groups. The eighth nerve group had a loss, on the I ear only, of approximately 18%. The temporal lobe group had a performance deficit on the C ear only of approximately 20%. The aphasic group showed poor performance on both ears, with a loss of 12% on the I ear and 16% on the C ear.

For SSI performance, diagnostic information is provided by two indices: (1) the relative configuration of results for ICM and CCM tasks and (2) the ear reflecting the performance deficits. For eighth nerve patients, the SSI procedure is characterized by poor performance on both ICM and CCM tasks. All deficits are confined to the I ear only. For brain stem patients, the SSI procedure shows poor performance for ICM and relatively good performance for CCM. The ICM deficits are observed on the C ear only and CCM performance is within normal limits on both ears. Although this "brain stem" pattern is observed in most brain stem patients, a few patients may present slightly different results. In these later patients there may be ICM deficits on both ears, instead of the C ear only, and/or a relatively mild CCM deficit on the C ear only, instead of normal performance on both ears. However, the observation of relatively more difficulty on ICM tasks than on CCM tasks holds for all brain stem patients in our experience.

For temporal lobe patients, the SSI procedure yields poor performance on both ICM and CCM. The ICM deficits are observed on both ears and the CCM deficit is observed on the C ear only. The exceptions to the expected "temporal lobe" pattern are that some temporal lobe patients may have an ICM deficit on the C ear only or normal ICM performance on both ears. The overriding principle

Table II. *Loss in percent relative to normal group for SSW test and PB word test in both ears of three control groups*

Group	Ear	SSW			PB
		Lead	Compete	Lag	
ALS	C	−1	3	−2	1
	I	2	7	0	−1
Ear difference			4		2
Non-auditory CNS	C	−1	7	5	−3
	I	2	5	−4	−2
Ear difference			2		1
Aphasic	C	8	6	−2	0
	I	3	15	8	0
Ear difference			9		0

in these patients is relatively more difficulty for CCM tasks than for ICM tasks.

For aphasic patients, SSI performance deficits did not seem to be more obvious on CCM tasks than on ICM tasks. The overriding principle for the present patients seemed to be a general speech intelligibility deficit that characterized both monotic and dichotic listening paradigms. Abnormally poor SSI scores occurred on both ears, usually with slightly greater deficits observed on the C ear than on the I ear.

SSW test. Tables II and III show the average loss for the leading, competing, and lagging SSW conditions in the ALS, non-auditory CNS, aphasic, brain stem, and temporal lobe groups. The average PB word loss for the patients completing the SSW test is also shown. All results are presented relative to performance in the normal group. Results for the eighth nerve group are not included since only one patient completed the test.

As shown in Table II, the ALS and non-auditory CNS groups had ear deficits of less than 10% on all three SSW conditions. The difference between ears for the competing monosyllables was small, approximately 3%, in both groups. The aphasic group had performance deficits of less than 10% on the leading and lagging conditions. On the competing condition, the C ear was essentially normal but the I ear showed a 15% loss. An ear difference of 10% was observed for competing and lagging conditions although no ear difference was observed for PB words.

In our experience, results for these three groups

Table III. *Loss in percent relative to normal group for SSW test and PB word test on both ears of experimental groups*

Group	Ear	SSW Lead	SSW Compete	SSW Lag	PB
Brain	C	22	44	26	44
Stem	I	7	16	3	21
Ear difference			28		23
Temporal	C	36	65	30	14
Lobe	I	6	10	8	5
Ear difference			55		9

are essentially negative and do not suggest the presence of central auditory disorder. SSW results for the three groups scored according to Katz's method (1968) were in the range between normal (upper limit of 5) and mildly abnormal (upper limit of 15). Katz's total corrected SSW scores were 7 for the ALS group, 11 for the non-auditory CNS patients, and 14 for the aphasics. This finding of "mildly abnormal" SSW results agrees with Katz's observations (1968) on "central non-auditory" patients, but disagrees with Balas' (1971) comments. The latter investigator reported completely normal scores in all of his patients with non-auditory lesions involving either the frontal, parietal, or occipital lobes.

Table III shows the SSW results and the PB_{max} deficits for the brain stem and temporal lobe groups. The brain stem group showed a performance deficit for the leading, competing, and lagging conditions on the C ear. On the I ear, depressed performance was observed for the competing condition only. A difference between ears of approximately 15% to 25% was observed for competing and non-competing words. However, this ear difference was observed on traditional PB word tests as well as the SSW test. PB_{max} deficits were 44% on the C ear and 21% on the I ear. If we correct for PB_{max} deficits as suggested by Katz (1968), the corrected SSW scores for "condition", "ear", and "total" measures are well within Katz's normal range. For example, the "total" corrected SSW score was −5 for the brain stem group. The negative value reflects a slightly greater loss for PB words than for SSW monosyllables. Poorer performance for PB words than for SSW conditions also characterized some of the patients studied by

Lynn and his colleagues (1972). This performance difference suggests that PB monosyllables presented in isolation may be a more difficult listening task for some patients than SSW monosyllables presented in spondaic units. To us, the present difference is not unreasonable in view of the constraints on syllabic sequence imposed on monosyllables presented in the SSW paradigm.

SSW results for the temporal lobe group were essentially normal on the I ear, but showed large deficits for the non-competing and competing conditions on the C ear. The loss on the C ear was approximately 33% for the non-competing conditions and 65% for the competing condition. PB_{max} deficits were within normal limits, 5%, on the I ear and showed only a very slight loss, 14%, on the C ear. Katz's corrected "ear" scores were 11 (normal) on the I ear and 39 (moderately abnormal) on the C ear. Abnormal performance on the C ear only for temporal lobe patients has been previously reported by Katz (1968), Balas (1971), Berlin & Lowe (1972), Lynn and his colleagues (1972) and Gilroy & Lynn (1974).

In short, only the temporal lobe group showed significant SSW performance deficits according to Katz's criterion. The other four groups had essentially negative results when PB_{max} losses were subtracted from the SSW deficits.

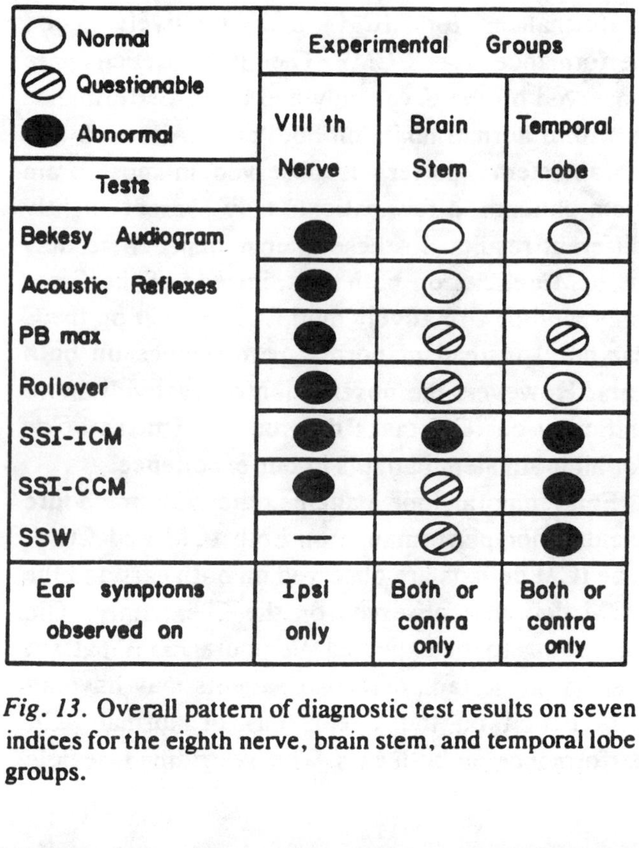

Fig. 13. Overall pattern of diagnostic test results on seven indices for the eighth nerve, brain stem, and temporal lobe groups.

COMMENT

Auditory findings in these six patient groups varied considerably on any one individual test of auditory function. For example, one of the present intra-axial brain stem patients had an abnormal, type IV, Békésy audiogram. This pattern would be expected in a patient with peripheral eighth nerve disorder, but is not expected in a patient with a brain stem site. On the other hand, two of the present eighth nerve patients had type I or II conventional Békésy audiograms and no abnormalities on either of the modified Békésy procedures. This result is expected in patients with brain stem disorder, but is a false-negative result for eighth nerve site. Acoustic reflex results also produced confusing findings in a few isolated patients. For example, one eighth nerve patient in this series had abnormal reflexes on both ears, instead of the I ear only. This pattern is more typical of an intra-axial brain stem site than of a peripheral eighth nerve disorder.

In spite of these inconsistencies on individual test procedures, the overall battery of test results seemed to produce a pattern unique to each of the six groups. Fig. 13 summarizes the overall pattern characterizing the three groups with specific auditory disorders: either eighth nerve, brain stem, or temporal lobe. The overall pattern of results differed significantly among these groups. The eighth nerve group was usually characterized by abnormal Békésy audiograms, absent or decaying acoustic reflexes, relatively poor PB_{max} scores, substantial PI–PB rollover, SSI–ICM loss, SSI–CCM loss, and auditory symptoms on the ipsilateral ear only. The eighth nerve control group contrasted sharply with the intra-axial brain stem group. The latter group was generally characterized by normal Békésy audiograms; normal acoustic reflexes; mild, if any, PB_{max} deficits; mild, if any, PI–PB rollover; substantial SSI–ICM deficits; relatively normal SSI–CCM performance; relatively normal SSW results; and auditory symptoms on both ears or the contralateral ear only. In distinction to the above two groups, the temporal lobe group was usually characterized by normal Békésy audiograms, normal acoustic reflexes; mild, if any, PB_{max} loss; no PI–PB rollover; SSI–ICM deficits; SSI–CCM deficits; abnormal SSW results; and auditory symptoms on both ears or on the contralateral ear only. The unique difference between the brain stem and temporal lobe groups was that the brain stem group had more difficulty with degraded monotic signals and the temporal lobe group had more difficulty with dichotic signals.

At the present time, we are not suggesting that the test procedures shown in Fig. 13 comprise the perfect test battery. However, the combination of the SSI procedure and the SSW test did seem to offer an unusually effective diagnostic tool for differentiating brain stem and temporal lobe sites. In the present study, the SSW test offered unique assistance in differentiating temporal lobe disorders, but did not consistently identify patients with brain stem disorders. Conversely, the SSI procedure provided unique assistance in differentiating brain stem site, but did not consistently identify temporal lobe site. For example, the temporal lobe patients usually showed substantial SSW deficits, but the SSI–CCM deficits varied considerably. Some temporal lobe patients had clearcut SSI–CCM losses; other patients performed better than we expected. On the other hand, the brain stem patients consistently showed striking SSI–ICM deficits, but SSW results varied considerably. Some brain stem patients had no SSW deficits; others had unusually poor SSW performance. Also, the relation between PB_{max} scores and SSW scores varied in the brain stem patients. Sometimes SSW scores could be corrected by PB_{max} deficits to within the normal range; at other times, however, SSW deficits remained, even when corrected; and still other times the PB_{max} deficits were so much more severe than SSW deficits that a negative corrected SSW score appeared. The overriding principle that characterized the combination of the two procedures was that the brain stem patients consistently showed SSI–ICM deficits whereas temporal lobe patients consistently showed SSW deficits.

CONCLUSIONS

1. Does the physical discomfort characterizing patients with central nervous system disease produce abnormal test results on a central auditory test battery? *Probably not.* For example, findings in the present ALS control group were consistently within normal limits, although these patients were typically extremely ill and uncomfortable.

2. Does *any* central nervous system disorder produce abnormal auditory test results even though there is no direct involvement of the auditory pathways, per se? *Probably not.* For example, findings in the present non-auditory CNS control group were consistently within the normal range.

3. Does the presence of aphasia in patients with temporal lobe disorder compromise the diagnostic value of degraded speech audiometry? *To some extent.* The present aphasic patients usually showed a performance deficit on both ears for difficult speech tasks, rather than the expected deficit only on the ear contralateral to the affected side of the brain. Further, performance deficits seemed just as pronounced for monotic listening conditions as for dichotic conditions.

4. Can auditory test results differentiate brain stem disorders from eighth nerve disorders? *Yes, fairly well.* In the present eighth nerve and brain stem groups, there were no patients in whom secondary symptoms masked the primary site of disorder when results for the entire test battery were considered. However, isolated test procedures showed some overlap between the two groups. Whenever individual patients showed both eighth nerve and brain stem auditory symptomatology, surgical and/or radiographic findings usually noted either (1) eighth nerve neoplasms rotating, distorting, and/or compressing the brain stem, or (2) brain stem neoplasms critically invading the cerebellopontine angle.

ACKNOWLEDGEMENTS

This project was supported by Public Health Service research grants NB-08542 and NS-10940 from the National Institute of Neurological Diseases and Stroke.

REFERENCES

Anderson, H., Barr, B. & Wedenberg, E. 1969. Intra-aural reflexes in retrocochlear lesions. In *Nobel symposium 10: Disorders of the skull base region* (ed. C. Hamberger & J. Wersäll), p. 49. Almqvist & Wiksell, Stockholm.

Antonelli, A. 1970. Sensitized speech tests: Results in lesions of the brain. In *Speech audiometry* (ed. C. Røjskjær), p. 176. Second Danavox Symposium, Odense, Denmark.

Antonelli, A., Calearo, C. & DeMitri, T. 1963. On the auditory function in brain stem diseases. *Int Audiol 2*, 55.

Balas, R. 1971. Staggered spondaic word test: Support. *Ann Otol 80*, 1.

Berlin, C. & Lowe, S. 1972. Temporal and dichotic factors in central auditory testing. In *Handbook of clinical audiology* (ed. J. Katz), p. 280. The Williams & Wilkins Co., Baltimore.

Berlin, C., Chase, R., Dill, A. & Hagepanos, T. 1965. Auditory findings in patients with temporal lobectomies. *Amer Speech Hearing Assoc 7*, 386.

Calearo, C. & Antonelli, A. 1968. Audiometric findings in brain stem lesions. *Acta Otolaryngol* (Stockholm) *66*, 305.

Egan, J. 1948. Articulation testing methods. *Laryngoscope 58*, 955.

Flower, R. & Viehweg, R. 1961. A review of audiologic findings among patients with cerebellopontine angle tumors. *Laryngoscope 71*, 1105.

Gilroy, J. & Lynn, G. 1974. Reversibility of abnormal auditory findings in cerebral hemisphere lesions. *J Neurol Sci 21*, 117.

Goodman, A. 1957. Some relations between auditory function and intracranial lesions with particular reference to lesions of the cerebellopontine angle. *Laryngoscope 67*, 987.

Greisen, O. & Rasmussen, P. 1970. Stapedius muscle reflexes and otoneurological examinations in brain stem tumors. *Acta Otolaryngol* (Stockholm) *70*, 366.

Igarashi, M., Jerger, J., Alford, B. & Stasney, R. 1974. Functional and histological findings of bilateral acoustic tumor. *Arch Otolaryngol* (Chicago) *99*, 379.

Jerger, J. 1960a. Audiological manifestations of lesions in the auditory nervous system. *Laryngoscope 70*, 417.

— 1960b. Békésy audiometry in the analysis of auditory disorders. *J Speech Hearing Res 3*, 275.

— 1964. Auditory tests for disorders of the central auditory mechanism. In *Neurological aspects of auditory and vestibular disorders* (ed. W. Fields & B. Alford), p. 77. Charles C. Thomas, Springfield, Ill.

— 1973. Diagnostic audiometry. In *Modern developments in audiology*, 2nd ed. (ed. J. Jerger), p. 75. Academic Press, New York.

Jerger, J. & Jerger, S. 1971. Diagnostic significance of PB word functions. *Arch Otolaryngol* (Chicago) *93*, 573.

— 1974a. Auditory findings in brain stem disorders. *Arch Otolaryngol* (Chicago) *99*, 342.

— 1974b. Diagnostic value of Békésy comfortable loudness tracings. *Arch Otolaryngol* (Chicago) *99*, 351.

Jerger, J., Jerger, S. & Mauldin, L. 1972a. Studies in impedance audiometry. I. Normal and sensori-neural ears. *Arch Otolaryngol* (Chicago) *96*, 513.

— 1972b. The forward–backward discrepancy in Békésy audiometry. *Arch Otolaryngol* (Chicago) *96*, 400.

Jerger, J., Speaks, C. & Trammell, J. 1968. A new approach to speech audiometry. *J Speech Hearing Dis 33*, 318.

Jerger, J., Harford, E., Clemis, J. & Alford, B. 1974. The acoustic reflex in eighth nerve disorders. *Arch Otolaryngol* (Chicago) *99*, 409.

Johnson, E. 1968. Auditory findings in 200 cases of acoustic neuromas. *Arch Otolaryngol* (Chicago) *88*, 598.

— 1970. Auditory test results in 268 cases of confirmed retrocochlear lesions. *Audiology 9*, 15.

Katz, J. 1962. The use of staggered spondaic words for assessing the integrity of the central auditory nervous system. *J Aud Res 2*, 327.

— 1968. The SSW test: An interim report. *J Speech Hearing Dis 33*, 318.

— 1970. Audiologic diagnosis: Cochlea to cortex. *Menorah Med Jour 1*, 25.

Korsan-Bengtsen, M. 1970. Some comparisons between ordinary and sensitized speech tests in patients with central hearing loss. In *Speech audiometry* (ed. C. Røjskjær), p. 123. Second Danavox Symposium, Odense, Denmark.

— 1973. Distorted speech audiometry. *Acta Otolaryngol* (Stockholm) Suppl. *310*, 34.

Lehnhardt, E. 1973. Audiometric localization of brain stem lesions. *Z Laryng Rhinol Otol 52*, 11.

Liden, G. & Korsan-Bengtsen, M. 1973. Audiometric manifestations of retrocochlear lesions. *Scand Audiol 2*, 29.

Lynn, G. & Gilroy, J. 1972. Neuro-audiological abnormalities in patients with temporal lobe tumors. *J Neurol Sci 17*, 167.

Lynn, G., Benitez, J., Eisenbrey, A., Gilroy, J. & Welner, H. 1972. Neuroaudiological correlates in cerebral hemisphere lesions. Temporal and parietal lobe tumors. *Audiology 2*, 115.

Owens, E. 1964. Békésy tracings and site of lesion. *J Speech Hearing Dis 29*, 456.

— 1971. Audiologic evaluation in cochlear versus retrocochlear lesions. *Acta Otolaryngol* (Stockholm) Suppl. *283*, 1.

Palva, T., Karja, J. & Palva, A. 1970. Forward vs. reversed Békésy tracings. *Arch Otolaryngol* (Chicago) *91*, 449.

Parker, W., Decker, R. & Garner, W. 1962. Auditory function and intracranial lesions. *Arch Otolaryngol* (Chicago) *76*, 425.

Parker, W., Decker, R. & Richards, N. 1968. Auditory function and lesions of the pons. *Arch Otolaryngol* (Chicago) *87*, 228.

Sheehy, J. 1974. Impedance audiometry in otologic practice. Cited in Jerger, J.: 2nd International Symposium on Impedance Measurement, Houston, Texas. *Audiology 13*, 271.

Wolfgram, F. & Myers, L. 1973. Amyotrophic lateral sclerosis: Effect of serum on anterior horn cells in tissue culture. *Science 179*, 579.

Received February 2, 1975

Address for reprints:

11922 Taylorcrest
Houston, Texas 77024
USA

NEUROAUDIOLOGIC FINDINGS IN PATIENTS WITH CENTRAL AUDITORY DISORDER

*Susan Jerger, M.S. and
James Jerger, Ph.D.*

In this article, we present results of four audiometric procedures—pure tone, immittance, speech, and auditory evoked response audiometry— on seven patients with surgically or radiographically confirmed central auditory disorder. Results are grouped into five different categories of disease that may affect the central auditory pathways: tumors, vascular and hypoxic, trauma, infections, and demyelinative disease (see Neely, elsewhere in this issue of *Seminars*). Whenever possible, we detail audiometric findings for both adults and children. Patient data are organized into history, results, and impression, with the latter containing the diagnostic impression formed by the overall pattern of audiometric results. Specific abnormalities supporting the interpreted site of auditory disorder are detailed.

In adults, speech audiometry was carried out with monosyllabic phonetically balanced [PB] word materials and synthetic sentence identification [SSI] materials (Jerger and Jerger, 1981). In children younger than 7 years of age, speech audiometry was carried out with the newly developed pediatric speech intelligibility (PSI) test materials (Jerger et al., 1983). For PSI results, the degree of performance deficit required to classify results as "abnormal," rather than within the normal range of variability, had been determined previously in a group of normal young children. We based our interpretation of the probable site of auditory disorder associated with abnormal PSI results on our clinical experience with the same speech audiometric paradigms in adults. For example, if the PSI performance intensity (PSI-PI) function showed the rollover phenomenon (an abnormal decrease in speech intelligibility performance as the intensity of the speech signal was increased above the level yielding maximum performance), then PSI-PI test results were interpreted as consistent with retrocochlear disorder.

Department of Otorhinolaryngology, Baylor College of Medicine, Texas Medical Center, Houston, Texas

Publisher: Thieme-Stratton Inc., 381 Park Avenue South, New York, NY 10016

Likewise, if the PSI ipsilateral competing message (PSI-ICM) function showed abnormal performance, results were interpreted as consistent with a central auditory disorder, especially at the brainstem level. Interpreting PSI results according to the principles that underlie the interpretation of diagnostic speech audiometry in adults seemed a reasonable first step in the clinical application of these new pediatric speech materials, especially in view of the fact that the PSI test was modeled on extant adult procedures.

NEOPLASTIC AND NON-NEOPLASTIC TUMORS

Case 1

A 6-year 4-month old girl with an extra- and intra-axial brainstem disorder primarily on the right side, had a final medical diagnosis of a congenital extra-axial porencephalic cyst with associated hydrocephalus.

History

At birth, skull x-rays and needle ventriculography indicated a large porencephalic cyst occupying most of the right hemicranium. Marked hydrocephalus was apparent. Air could not be detected within the third and fourth ventricles or the aqueduct. The child was not expected to survive and no shunting procedure was carried out. However, at 9 months of age, the hydrocephalus arrested. Neurological status improved, although developmental delay continued to be apparent. At 2½ years of age, a ventriculoperitoneal shunting procedure was performed. Between 2½ and 6 years of age, the child underwent multiple shunt revisions.

About 5 months before the audiologic evaluation, the child was admitted to the hospital for deterioration of neurological function, lethargy, abdominal pain, incontinence, and headache, pre-

Key to Symbols

SPEECH AUDIOMETRY

	Isolation	Competition
Adult Materials		
PB Words	○	—
SSI Sentences	□	■
Pediatric Materials		
PSI Words	○	●
PSI Sentences	□	■

PURE TONE AUDIOMETRY

	Unmasked	Masked
Air Conduction	○	●
Bone Conduction	△	▲
	Crossed	Uncrossed
Acoustic Reflex	⊠	□

sumably due to shunt malfunction. Neurological examination revealed extensor plantar responses, ataxic gait, and dysmetria on coordination testing. Clonic responses were noted in the ankles. The child underwent six shunt revisions. At the last revision, an additional shunt was placed in the porencephalic cyst.

At the time of the audiologic evaluation, neurological and physical examinations were essentially normal except for an ataxic gait, extensor plantar responses, and diplopia. The child was wearing an eyepatch for the diplopia. The mother

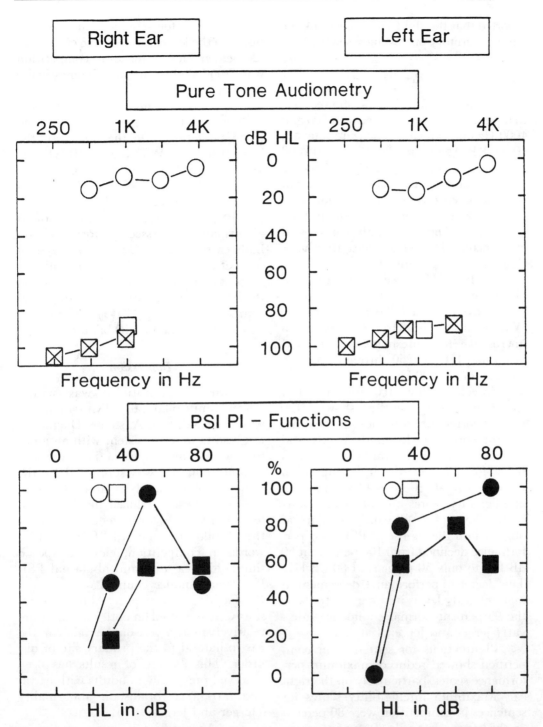

Figure 1. A 6-year 4-month-old girl with an extra- and intra-axial brainstem disorder primarily on the right side had a final medical diagnosis of congenital extra-axial porencephalic cyst with associated hydrocephalus. a: Audiogram, acoustic reflex thresholds, and PSI-PI functions for words and sentences. The MCR was held constant across intensity levels at +4 dB (words) or 0 dB (sentences). The competing message was presented to the same earphone or the same loudspeaker that received the test sentences. When appropriate, masking noise was presented to the nontest ear. The SnT score on the right ear was determined by the 25 percent intelligibility level, instead of the 50 percent intelligibility level, due to depressed maximum performance.

reported that the child's teachers think she has an "auditory processing disorder."

Results

The audiogram (Fig. 1a) showed normal pure-tone sensitivity between 500 and 4000 Hz on both ears. The pure-tone average (PTA) scores at 500, 1000, and 2000 Hz were 14 dB hearing level (HL) on the right ear and 13 dB HL on the left ear. Tympanometry (not shown) showed a normal, type A, configuration on both ears. With sound to the right ear, crossed and uncrossed acoustic reflex thresholds (Fig. 1a) were present at normal HLs at 500 and 1000 Hz. However, reflex thresholds were elevated at 250 Hz and absent (>110 dB HL) at 2000 and 4000 Hz. With sound to the left ear, crossed and uncrossed reflex thresholds were present at normal HLs at 250 through 2000 Hz and absent at 4000 Hz.

Speech audiometry for the PSI speech materials (Fig. 1a) showed 100 percent correct performance for the quiet control condition for both words and sentences bilaterally. Similarly, PI functions for PSI words in competition showed normal (100 percent) maximum intelligibility scores on both ears. However, rollover of the PI word function was observed on the right ear. PSI word performance declined from 100 percent at 50 dB HL to only 50 percent at 80 dB HL. This degree of performance decrement at high intensity levels is abnormal (outside the 95 percent normal confidence interval) (Jerger and Jerger, 1982).

PI functions for sentences in competition showed reduced maximum performance scores, particularly on the right ear. Maximum intelligibility scores for sentences in competition were 80 percent on the left ear, but only 60 percent on the right ear. The difference between performance in quiet versus competition was within normal limits on the left ear, but was abnormal (outside the 95 percent normal confidence interval) on the right ear. No significant rollover was observed on either ear for sentences in competition. On the left ear, the degree of rollover (20 percent) for sentences in competition was too slight to be diagnostically significant.

Speech thresholds were elevated with respect to average pure-tone sensitivity bilaterally. On the right ear, the word threshold (WT) was 31 dB HL; the sentence threshold (SnT) was 35 dB HL. On the left ear, the WT was 24 dB HL and the SnT was 27 dB HL.

PSI-ICM functions (Fig. 1b) showed abnormally depressed performance on both ears. Results at 0 dB message-to-competition ratio (MCR) were only 20 percent on the right ear and 60 percent on the left ear. In contrast, PSI contralateral competing message (CCM) performance was within normal limits bilaterally.

Impression

Pure-tone sensitivity was within normal limits bilaterally. Tympanometry was a normal, type A, shape. Diagnostic test results were consistent with an auditory disorder at the level of the brainstem. A brainstem site was supported by the presence of elevated or absent crossed acoustic reflexes, reduced maximum intelligibility scores for sentences in competition, rollover of the PSI-PI function for words in competition, elevated speech threshold measures, and abnormal PSI-ICM performance coupled with normal PSI-CCM performance. Abnormal results were observed on both ears, but were relatively more severe on the right ear, the ear ipsilateral to the primary site of disorder. This pattern of results has been observed previously in adults with extra- and intra-axial brainstem abnormality (Jerger and Jerger, 1975).

CASE 2

An 11-year-old girl had an intra-axial brainstem disorder, eccentric to the right side. Surgery and histopathological

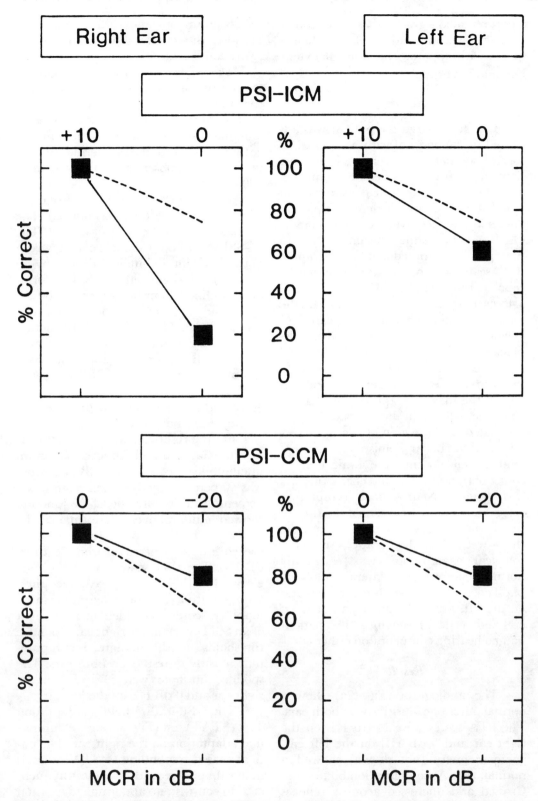

Figure 1b: ICM and CCM functions for PSI sentence materials (P = 30 dB HL). The dashed lines represent the limits of the 95 percent normal confidence interval.

report revealed a grade IV astrocytoma of the right vermis and cerebellar hemisphere with apparent peduncular extension into the brainstem.

History

One month ago the patient was admitted to the hospital with a 6-week history of somnolence, lethargy, headache, nausea, recurrent projectile vomiting, and ataxia. A neurological examination noted bilateral papilledema, diplopia, and bilateral positive Babinski reflexes. On Romberg testing, the patient *fell* to the right. A computed axial tomographic (CT) scan, arteriogram, and pneumoencephalogram revealed hydrocephalus and a large mass lesion in the region of the mesencephalon. The mass appeared to extend into the thalamus with displacement of the third ventricle.

The patient underwent a surgical shunt procedure. At surgery, the true extent of the mass was appreciated for the first time. A large infiltrating mass lesion originated in the region of the right vermis and cerebellar hemisphere and extended well up into the brainstem. A course of radiotherapy and chemotherapy was begun. Neurological symptomatology improved markedly. At the time of the audiologic evaluation (during the third week of radiotherapy), the neurological examination was essentially normal except for bilateral resolving papilledema, a mild sixth nerve weakness on the left, a slightly ataxic gait, and lateral and vertical nystagmus. The patient had no hearing complaint on either ear.

Results

The audiogram (Fig. 2a) showed normal pure-tone sensitivity on both ears. The PTA scores were 13 dB HL on the right ear and 5 dB HL on the left ear. Tympanometry (not shown) showed a normal, type A, configuration bilaterally. Crossed and uncrossed acoustic reflexes (Fig. 2a) were present at normal HLs at 500 to 4000 Hz on both ears. However, the contour of reflex thresholds with sound to the left ear showed an unusual rising configuration.

The reflex decay test on the right ear was normal at 500 Hz, but showed positive reflex decay at 1000 Hz (Fig. 2b). Reflex amplitude at 1000 Hz declined to less than one-half the initial magnitude within a 10-second test period. Reflex decay was not observed on the left ear at 500 or 1000 Hz.

The shape of the PI-PB function (Fig. 2a) on the left ear was normal. The PBmax score was 96 percent correct. The PI-SSI function on the left ear showed a normal maximum intelligibility score (90 percent), but slight rollover. SSI performance declined from 90 percent at 60 dB HL to only 60 percent at 80 dB HL. The speech threshold for the PI-PB function (the PBT score) on the left ear, 10 dB HL, agreed with average pure-tone sensitivity levels. In contrast, the PI-SSI speech threshold (the SSIT score) on the left ear, 46 dB HL, was elevated with respect to average sensitivity levels.

On the right ear, the PI-PB and PI-SSI functions showed reduced maximum intelligibility scores. The PBmax score was 40 percent; the SSI max score was 0 percent. Additionally, the PI-PB function showed mild rollover. Performance declined from 40 to only 16 percent as speech intensity increased from 50 to 80 dB HL. The PBT score, 45 dB HL, was elevated with respect to average pure-tone sensitivity. Poor maximum intelligibility scores precluded measurement of an SSIT score on the right ear. Spondee thresholds (not shown) agreed with pure-tone sensitivity results on both ears. The spondee thresholds were 14 dB HL on the right ear and 0 dB HL on the left ear.

The Suprathreshold Adaptation Test (STAT) test (Fig. 2c) showed abnormal adaptation on the right ear. The patient ceased responding to STAT signals in less than 30 seconds at all test frequencies. In contrast, no abnormal adaptation was observed on the left ear at any frequency.

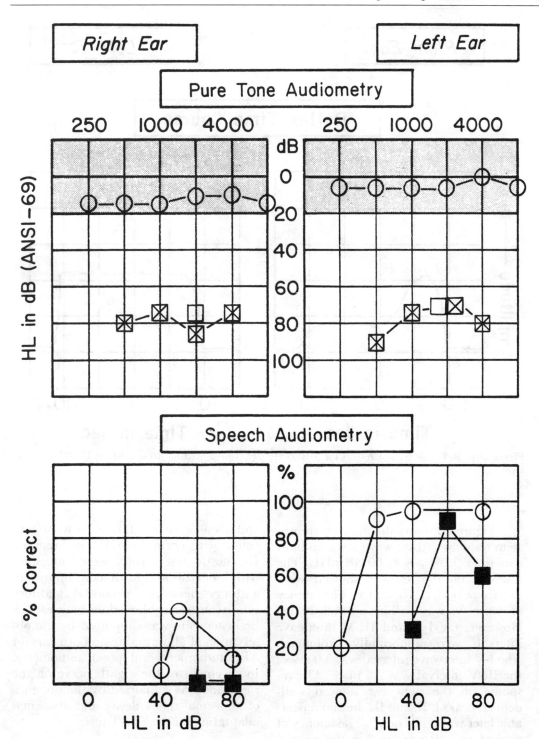

Figure 2. An 11-year-old girl with an intra-axial brainstem disorder, eccentric to the right side had a final medical diagnosis of astrocytoma of the right vermis and cerebellar hemisphere with peduncular extension into the brainstem. a: Audiogram, acoustic reflex thresholds, and PI functions for PB words and SSI sentences. For the PI-SSI function, the MCR was held constant across intensity levels at 0 dB. The competing message was presented to the same earphone that received the test sentences. When appropriate, masking noise was presented to the nontest ear. The PBT score on the right ear was determined by the 25 percent intelligibility level, rather than the 50 percent level, due to depressed maximum performance.

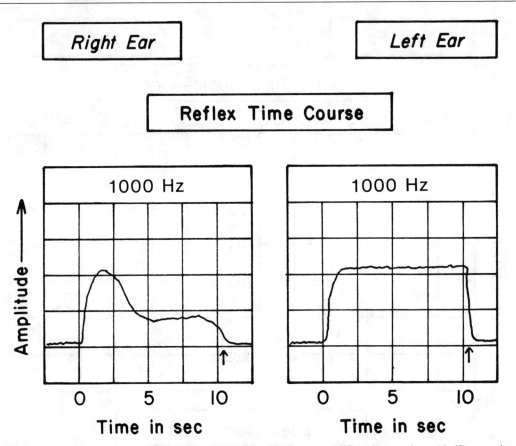

Figure 2b: Reflex decay test results for a 1000 Hz signal presented for 10 seconds at 10 dB sensation level.

Figure 2d shows the auditory brainstem response (ABR) wave form on both ears to click signals at 80 dB nHL. The response on the left ear showed well-formed peaks I, II, III, and V. The latency of wave V was within normal limits. However, the I-V and III-V interwave intervals were abnormally prolonged. The I-V interwave interval was 5.0 msec; the III-V interval was 2.8 msec. The response on the right ear showed well-defined peaks I, II, and III, but no repeatable later waves (IV or V). The latency of peaks I and III were within the normal range.

Impression

Pure-tone sensitivity was within normal limits bilaterally. Tympanometry and acoustic reflex thresholds were consistent with normal middle ear function. Diagnostic test results were consistent with an extra- and intra-axial brainstem auditory disorder. Abnormal auditory symptoms were observed on both ears. A brainstem site was supported by the observation of abnormality on both ears for ABR audiometry and speech audiometry. Involvement of the eighth nerve on the right side was supported by the presence of abnormal reflex decay and abnormal adaptation on the STAT test.

VASCULAR DISORDERS

CASE 3

A 3-year 8-month-old boy had a left temporal lobe disorder due to a cere-

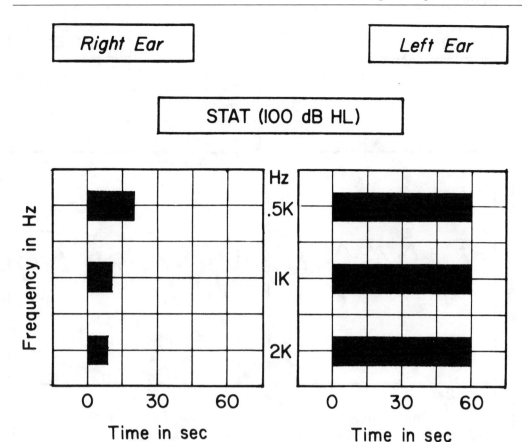

Figure 2c: STAT test.

brovascular accident in the left hemisphere, probably secondary to congestive cardiomyopathy.

History

The child's growth and development appeared normal until 17 months of age. At that time, during lunch, he suddenly cried out and became limp. He was taken immediately to a hospital. At admission, neurological examination noted right hemiparesis, increased deep tendon reflexes, increased muscle tone in the right extremities, mild right facial asymmetry, a positive Babinski reflex on the right, and a persistent deviation of the eyes to the left.

A chest x-ray revealed cardiomegaly. Left cardiac angiography indicated dif-

fuse cardiomyopathy of the congestive type. A CT scan revealed an area of decreased density in the expected distribution of the middle cerebral artery on the left. Convolutional markings were more prominent over the left hemisphere Electroencephalographic (EEG) findings showed a focus of low voltage slow wave activity in the left temporal region. The child was placed on appropriate medications. Intensive physical and occupational therapy was begun.

At the time of the audiologic examination (approximately 2 years post-insult), the child's neurological symptomatology had improved markedly. However, physical examination and neurological evaluation noted weakness, but no paralysis, of the right side and general delay in growth and development, in-

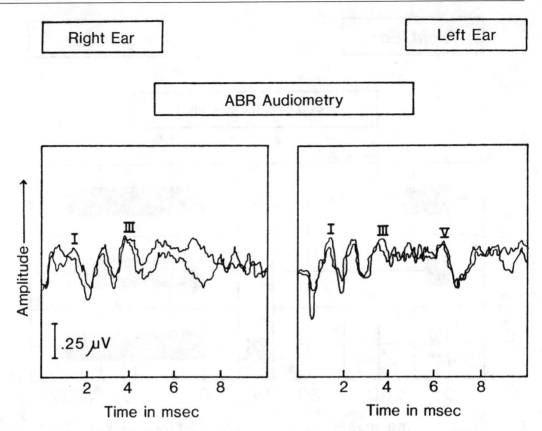

Figure 2d: ABR wave form to click signals at 80 dB nHL. Signal presentation rate was 20 clicks/second.

Results

The audiogram (Fig. 3a) showed pure-tone sensitivity within normal limits at 500, 1000, and 4000 Hz on the right ear and at 500 and 4000 Hz on the left ear. Pure-tone testing was not carried out at other frequencies due to the child's apprehensiveness. Tympanometry and static compliance measures (not shown) were normal bilaterally. Crossed and uncrossed acoustic reflexes (Fig. 3a) were present at normal HLs from 500 to 4000 Hz on both ears.

Sound–field speech audiometric results for the PSI speech materials (Fig. 3a) showed maximum intelligibility scores of 80 to 100 percent correct for both words and sentences. The SnT threshold, 8 dB HL, crosschecked the presence of normal pure-tone sensitivity.

PSI-ICM functions (Fig. 3b) (obtained via earphones) were within normal limits at the most difficult test MCR (0 dB) on both ears. In contrast, PSI-CCM functions (obtained via earphones) showed substantial performance deficits bilaterally. The PSI-CCM deficit was relatively greater on the right ear, the ear contralateral to the affected side of the brain.

Impression

Pure-tone sensitivity was within normal limits. Immittance audiometry was consistent with normal middle ear function. Diagnostic test results were consistent with a central auditory disorder at the level of the temporal lobe. A temporal lobe site was supported by sub-

cluding speech and language abilities. The child was enrolled in a special preschool program for speech and language development.

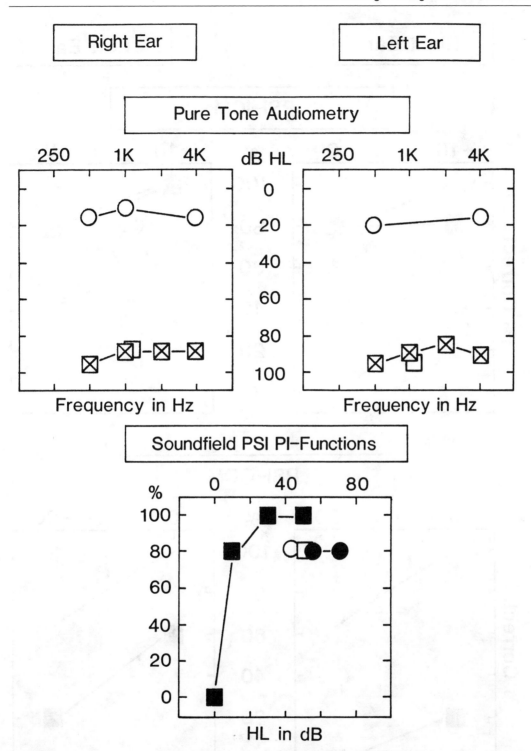

Figure 3.   A 3-year 8-month-old boy had a left temporal lobe disorder. The final medical diagnosis was a cerebrovascular accident in the left hemisphere. EEG findings showed abnormal activity in the left temporal region. a: Audiogram, acoustic reflex thresholds, and sound field PSI-PI functions for words and sentences.

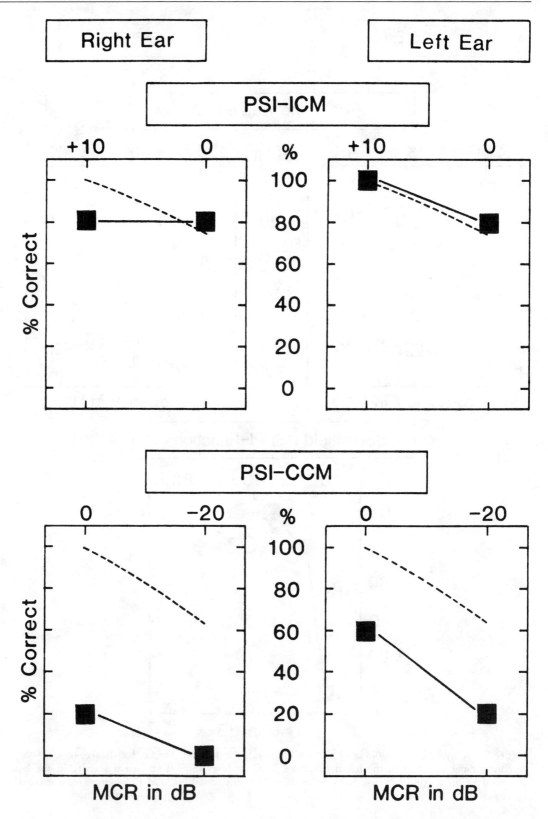

Figure 3b: ICM and CCM functions (obtained via earphones) for PSI sentences (P = 30 dB HL).

stantial PSI-CCM deficits in the presence of relatively normal PSI-ICM performance.

Case 4

A 57-year-old woman had arteriosclerotic cerebrovascular disease.

History

The patient has received medical treatment for 20 years for hypertensive cardiovascular disease and vascular headaches. She reported that her mother and several brothers have heart disease, artherosclerotic disease, and/or stroke. At the present hospitalization, the patient's chief complaints were dizziness, recent onset of left-side numbness, and headaches with olfactory and gustatory auras. Carotid and vertebral arteriography showed occlusive disease in the right vertebral artery and the posterior inferior cerebellar artery.

Results

The audiogram (Fig. 4a) showed mild, bilateral, sensorineural hearing loss. The PTA scores were 17 dB HL on both ears. Tympanometry and static compliance measures (not shown) were within normal limits bilaterally. Crossed and uncrossed acoustic reflexes (Fig. 4a) on both ears were present at normal HLs between 250 and 4000 Hz. Reflex decay (not shown) was not observed on either ear at 500 or 1000 Hz.

PI-PB functions (Fig. 4a) showed normal maximum intelligibility scores bilaterally: 100 percent on the right ear and 96 percent on the left ear. PI-SSI functions showed maximum intelligibility scores of 100 percent on the left ear, but only 70 percent on the right ear. The shape of the PI-PB and PI-SSI functions was normal on both ears.

Speech thresholds on each ear agreed with average pure-tone sensitivity. The PBT scores were 18 dB HL on the right ear and 16 dB HL on the left ear. The SSIT scores were 20 dB HL bilaterally.

SSI-ICM functions (Fig. 4b) showed reduced performance on both ears. Average SSI-ICM scores (0, -10, and -20 dB MCR) were 27 percent on the right ear and 53 percent on the left ear. SSI-CCM performance was unimpaired on either ear. SSI-CCM scores were 100 percent at all test conditions.

Staggered spondaic word (SSW) results (not shown) were within normal limits for all test conditions on both ears. Average performance scores for the competing condition were 85 percent bilaterally.

ABR audiometry (Fig. 4c) showed normal wave V and interwave latency measures on both ears. A well-formed response (waves I through V) was observed bilaterally. Late vertex (V) potentials (Fig. 4d) were also normally formed and symmetric on the two ears. In contrast to these results, middle latency wave forms (Fig. 4e) showed a well-formed response on the left ear, but a degraded wave form on the right ear.

Impression

There was a mild, bilateral, sensorineural hearing loss. Immittance audiometry was consistent with normal middle ear function on both ears. Diagnostic test results were consistent with a central auditory disorder at a rostral brainstem level. A brainstem site was supported by a discrepancy between PB max and SSI max scores, reduced performance on SSI-ICM, and abnormal middle latency responses. Involvement of caudal brainstem auditory pathways was rendered unlikely by normal acoustic reflexes and normal ABR audiometry. Involvement of temporal lobe structures was rendered unlikely due to normal SSI-CCM results, normal SSW results, and normal late vertex (V) responses.

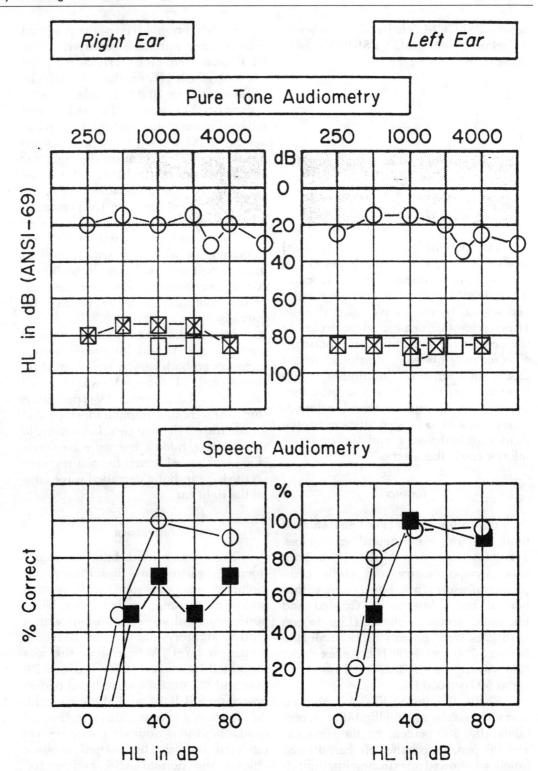

Figure 4. A 57-year-old woman had arteriosclerotic cerebrovascular disease characterized by occlusive disease in the right vertebral artery and the posterior inferior cerebellar artery. a: Audiogram, acoustic reflex thresholds, and PI-PB and PI-SSI functions.

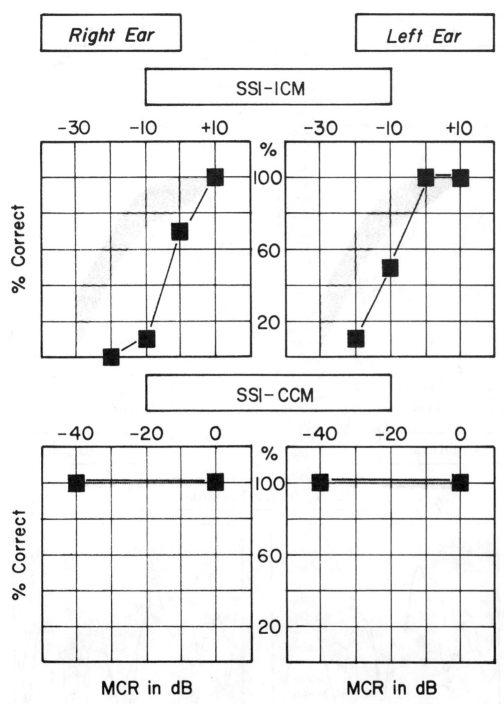

Figure 4b: ICM and CCM functions for SSI sentences (P = 30 dB HL).

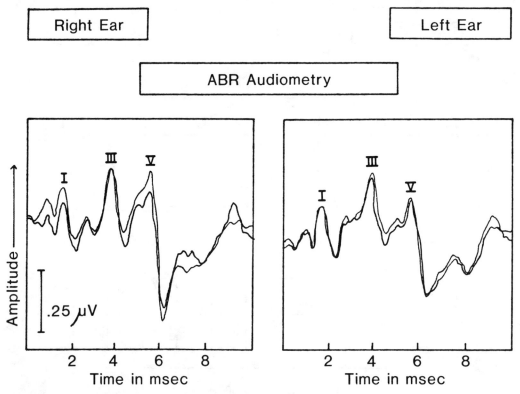

Figure 4c: ABR wave form to click signals at 80 dB nHL. Signal presentation rate was 20 clicks/second.

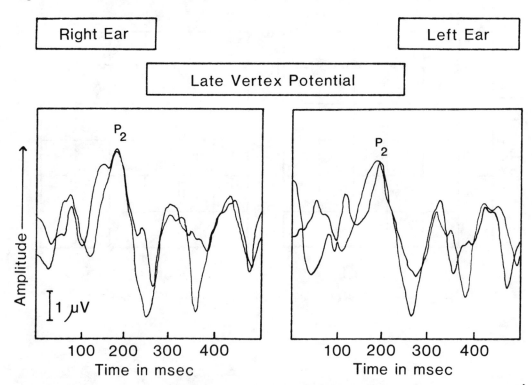

Figure 4d: Late vertex (V) potentials to click signals at 80 dB nHL. Signal presentation rate was 1 click per 2-second interval.

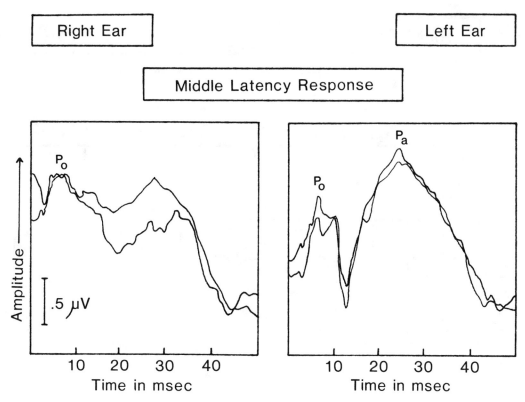

Figure 4e: Middle latency responses to click signals at 80 dB nHL. Signal presentation rate was 8 clicks/seconds.

TRAUMA

CASE 5

A 28-year-old woman had brainstem and cerebral contusion.

History

Approximately 9 months ago, the patient was admitted to the hospital with severe neurological deficits due to head trauma received in an automobile accident. She was intermittently decerebrate. Angiograms and skull X-rays were within normal limits. EEG findings showed a diffuse disturbance in cerebral function apparently related to multiple regions of cerebral contusion involving cortical and subcortical structures. During the next 30 days, serial EEG testing showed marked improvement, although diffuse slow activity continued to be noted. The patient's neurological symptomatology improved substantially.

At the present hospitalization, the patient was being reevaluated for labored speech problems, dizziness, and numbness of the right side of the body. She had not noticed any unusual hearing difficulties on either ear.

Results

The audiogram (Fig. 5a) showed normal pure-tone sensitivity on both ears. The PTA scores were 3 dB HL on the right ear and 7 dB HL on the left ear. Immittance audiometry showed normal, type A, tympanograms (not shown) and normal static compliance measures bilaterally. Crossed and uncrossed acoustic reflexes (Fig. 5a) were present at normal

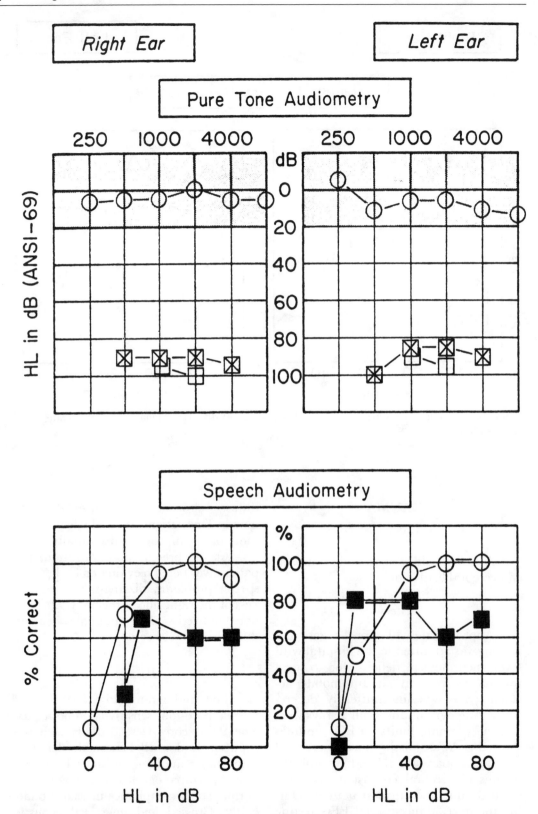

Figure 5. A 28-year-old woman had brainstem and cerebral contusion due to head trauma. a: Audiogram, acoustic reflex thresholds, and PI-PB and PI-SSI functions.

HLs on both ears. Reflex decay (not shown) was not observed at 500 or 1000 Hz on either ear.

PI-PB functions (Fig. 5a) on both ears showed normal (100 percent) maximum intelligibility scores. In contrast to PI-PB functions, PI-SSI functions showed reduced maximum intelligibility scores bilaterally. The SSI max scores were 70 percent on the right ear and 80 percent on the left ear. The shape of the PI-PB and PI-SSI functions was within normal limits on both ears.

PBT thresholds, 12 dB HL on the right ear and 10 dB HL on the left ear, agreed with average pure-tone sensitivity bilaterally. The SSIT speech threshold agreed with pure-tone sensitivity results on the left ear, but was abnormally elevated with respect to pure-tone sensitivity on the right ear. The SSIT scores were 5 dB HL on the left ear, but 24 dB HL on the right ear.

SSI-ICM performance (Fig. 5b) was slightly below the normal range on both ears. Average performance scores were 53 percent on the right ear and 47 percent on the left ear. SSI-CCM performance was normal (100 percent) at all MCRs on both ears. SSW results (not shown) for the competing condition showed a performance difference of 25 percent between ears. Average performance for the competing monosyllables was 83 percent on the right ear, but only 58 percent on the left ear.

ABR audiometry (Fig. 5c) yielded normal wave V latencies on both ears. Absolute and interwave latencies of all component waves were within normal limits. Repeatable wave V responses were elicited at intensity levels down to 40 dB nHL on both ears.

Impression

Pure-tone sensitivity was within normal limits bilaterally. Immittance audiometry was consistent with normal middle ear function on both ears. Diagnostic test results were consistent with a central auditory disorder at the level of the upper midbrain or temporal lobe. A central auditory disorder was supported by a bilateral discrepancy between PBmax and SSI max scores, bilateral SSI-ICM deficits, and a performance deficit for the competing condition on the SSW test. The performance deficit on the SSW task was observed on the left ear only. The involvement of caudal brainstem structures was rendered unlikely due to normal acoustic reflex thresholds and a normal reflex time course.

INFECTION

Case 6

A 3-year 3-month old boy had meningitis.

History

The patient was admitted to the hospital with chief complaints of fever, ataxia, intermittent headaches, stiff neck, vomiting, and difficulty with standing. Neurological evaluation was essentially normal except for the ataxia. A CT scan and skull x-rays were within normal limits. The child's growth and development prior to the present illness were normal. However, at approximately 1 year of age, he had undergone heart surgery to correct pulmonary stenosis. The final medical diagnosis was meningitis. The 'child received antibiotic therapy with a meningitic regimen. The audiologic evaluation was obtained just prior to the child's release from the hospital.

Results

The audiogram (Fig. 6) showed pure-tone sensitivity within normal limits (15 dB HL) at 500, 1000, and 2000 Hz. Pure-tone testing was not conducted at other frequencies. Immittance audiometry was not carried out due to the child's apprehensiveness.

Sound field PSI-PI functions (Fig.

6a) showed normal (100 percent) maximum intelligibility scores for the quiet control condition for both words and sentences. In contrast, PSI-PI functions in competition showed unusually reduced performance for both types of speech materials. Maximum intelligibility scores in competition were only 60 percent for sen-

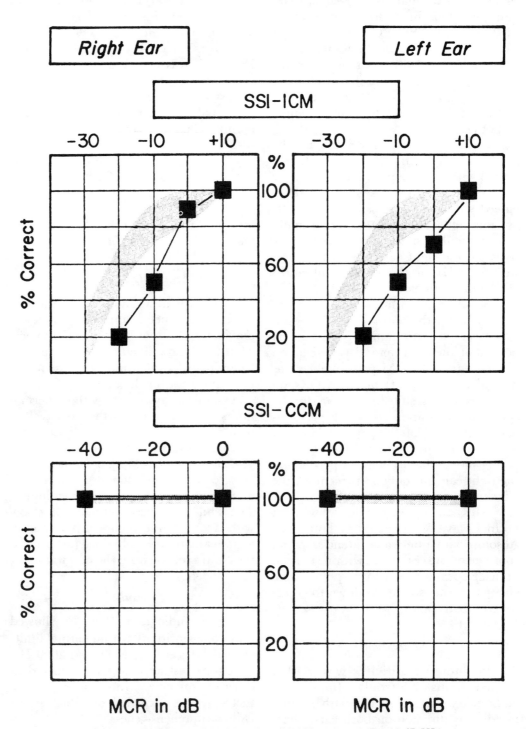

Figure 5b: ICM and CCM functions for SSI sentences (P = 30 dB HL).

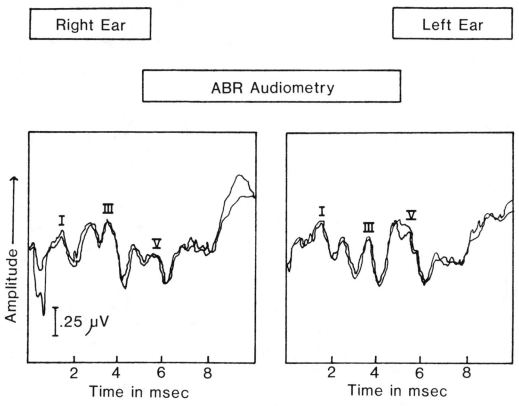

Figure 5c: ABR wave form to click signals at 80 dB nHL. Signal presentation rate was 20 clicks/second.

tences and 40 percent for words. The difference between performance in quiet versus competition was abnormal (outside the 95 percent normal confidence interval). The shape of the PSI-PI function in competition was normal for words, but showed the rollover phenomenon for sentences. Sentence performance declined from 60 to 20 percent as speech intensity increased from 30 to 70 dB HL.

Sound field speech thresholds for the quiet condition, 5 dB HL for words and 12 dB HL for sentences, cross checked the presence of normal sensitivity for the frequencies important for speech understanding. The SnT score in competition, 18 dB HL, also agreed with pure-tone sensitivity. However, the WT in competition, 38 dB HL, was elevated with respect to average pure-tone results.

PSI-ICM performance (obtained via earphone) (Fig. 6b) showed reduced scores on both ears. Performance at 0 dB MCR was 60 percent on the right ear and 40 percent on the left ear. PSI-CCM performance (obtained via earphone) showed a substantial performance deficit bilaterally. At the easiest test condition (0 dB MCR), performance was only 20 to 30 percent on either ear.

Impression

Pure-tone sensitivity was within normal limits at 500 to 2000 Hz. Diagnostic speech audiometric results were consistent with a central auditory disorder. Central auditory dysfunction was supported by abnormality of performance in competition for PI, ICM, and CCM functions.

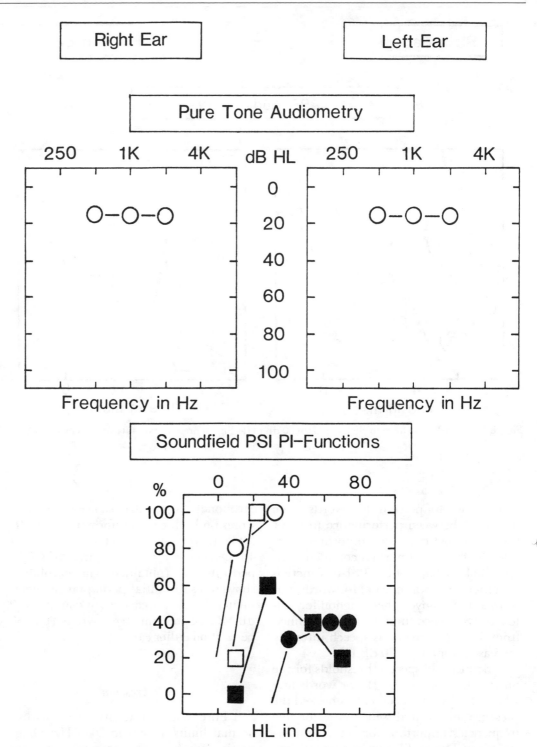

Figure 6. A 3-year 3-month-old boy had meningitis. a: Audiogram and sound field PSI-PI functions for words and sentences. Speech threshold in competition were determined by the 25 percent intelligibility levels.

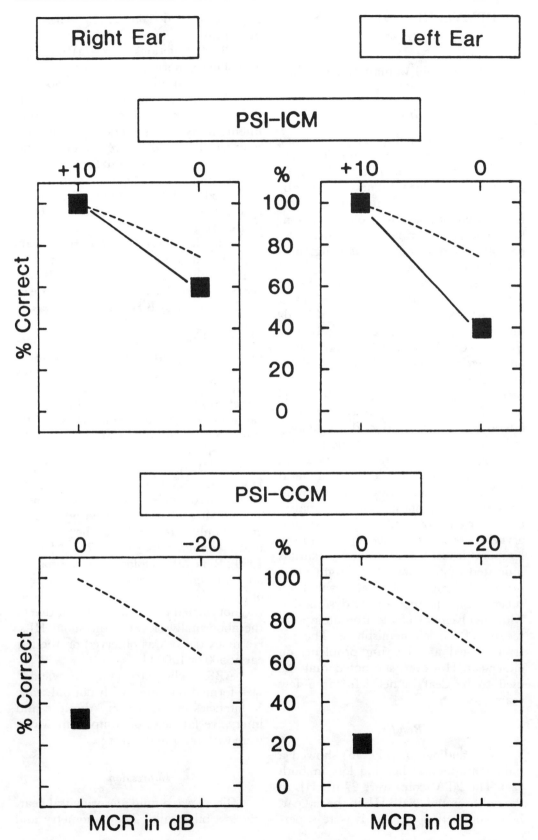

Figure 6b: ICM and CCM functions (obtained via earphones) for PSI sentences (P = 40 dB HL).

DEMYELINATIVE DISEASE

CASE 7

A 26-year-old woman had multiple sclerosis.

History

This patient had an 11-year history of multiple sclerosis. During previous hospitalizations, the patient complained of seizures, right-sided weakness and numbness, incoordination, intention tremor, intermittent double vision, blurred vision, headaches, and urinary problems. The patient had received various drug therapies for many years.

Presently, the patient was being reevaluated because she had a seizure 5 days earlier. Chief complaints at this admission were headaches, abnormally slow speech, weakness of the legs and hands, and the seizure episode. Neurological examination revealed right homonymous hemianopia, papilledema, ataxia, intermittent slurred speech, restricted right lateral gaze, hyperactive deep tendon reflexes on the right side, clonic patellar jerks bilaterally, abnormal gait, bilateral extensor plantar responses, and bilateral Hoffmann's signs. EEG findings were consistent with a nonspecific abnormality characterized by moderately slow and asynchronous low voltage activity in the temporal leads. Visual evoked potentials indicated dysfunction of the right optic nerve. Neuropsychological evaluation suggested moderate cerebral dysfunction with involvement of the frontotemporal regions of the left hemisphere. The patient denied any hearing problems on either ear. However, she noted that she used to be deaf in her left ear a few years ago.

Results

The audiogram (Fig. 7a) showed a mild sensorineural hearing loss in both ears. The PTA scores were 27 dB HL in the right ear and 28 dB HL in the left ear. Bone conduction thresholds were superimposed on air conduction sensitivity bilaterally.

PI-PB functions (Fig. 7a) on both ears showed normal (100 percent) maximum intelligibility scores and no rollover. In contrast to PI-PB functions, PI-SSI functions showed reduced maximum intelligibility scores bilaterally. The SSI max scores were 80 percent on each ear. The shape of the PI-SSI functions was abnormal on both ears. Performance decreased 40 percent bilaterally as the speech intensity was increased from 60 to 80 dB HL.

Speech thresholds on both ears agreed with average pure-tone sensitivity. On the right ear, the PBT was 22 dB HL; the SSIT was 28 dB HL. On the left ear, the PBT was 22 dB HL; the SSIT was 26 dB HL.

Immittance audiometry showed normal type A tympanograms (not shown) and normal static compliance measures bilaterally. Crossed and uncrossed acoustic reflexes (Fig. 7a) with sound to the left ear were present at normal HLs at 500 through 4000 Hz. With sound to the right ear, uncrossed reflexes were present at normal HLs between 500 and 4000 Hz. However, crossed reflexes were elevated at all four frequencies. This rare pattern of abnormality, elevated crossed reflexes on one ear only, is referred to as the "unibox" reflex configuration (Fig. 7b) (Jerger, 1980). Reflex thresholds are abnormal for only the crossed condition on one ear only. Reflex decay testing (not shown) was not carried out on the right ear due to the abnormally elevated threshold HLs. No reflex decay was observed on the left ear at 500 or 1000 Hz.

ABR audiometry (Fig. 7c) yielded well-formed responses with normal wave V latencies on both ears. Absolute and interwave latencies of component waves were within normal limits.

Impression

There was a mild sensorineural hearing loss bilaterally. Tympanometry and

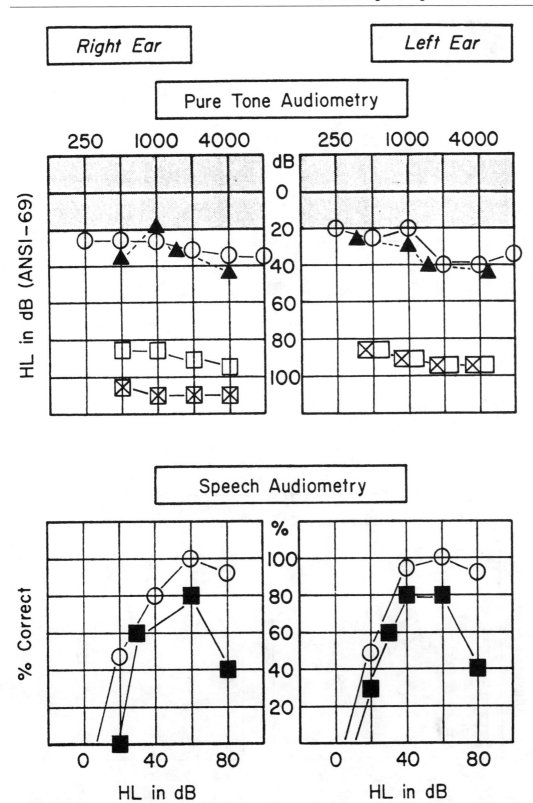

Figure 7. A 26-year-old woman had multiple sclerosis. a: Audiogram, acoustic reflex thresholds, and PI-PB and PI-SSI functions.

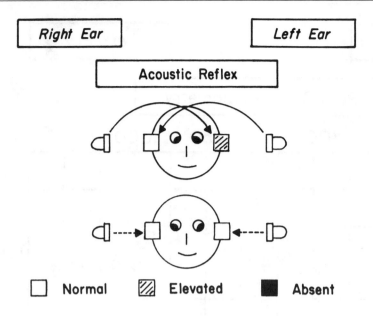

Figure 7b: "Unibox" reflex pattern of abnormality. For an explanation of the four reflex array summarizing relations among crossed and uncrossed thresholds, see Jerger (1975).

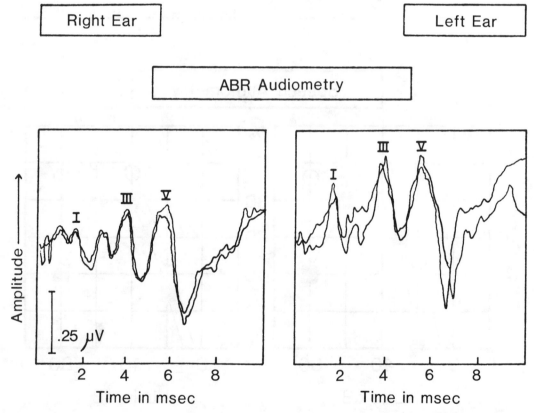

Figure 7c: ABR wave form to click signals at 80 dB nHL. Signal presentation rate was 20 clicks/seconds.

static compliance measures were consistent with normal middle ear function on both ears. Results of ABR audiometry were normal on each ear. However, a discrepancy between PB max and SSI max performance, rollover of the PI-SSI functions, and abnormal elevation of crossed reflexes with sound to the right ear suggested the presence of central auditory disorder.

ACKNOWLEDGMENTS

Preparation of this chapter was supported, in part, by Public Health Service Research Grant NS-10940 from the National Institute of Neurological and Communicative Disorders and Stroke. We thank Mrs. Sue Abrams and Dr. Deborah Hayes for their assistance. Patient results were obtained in the Audiology Service or the Children's Hearing Center, Baylor College of Medicine and the Neurosensory Center.

REFERENCES

Jerger, J.: Diagnostic use of impedance measures. In Jerger, J. (Ed.): *Handbook of Clinical Impedance Audiometry*. New York: American Electromedics Corp. 1975, pp. 149–174.

Jerger, S.: Diagnostic application of impedance audiometry in central auditory disorders. In Jerger, J., and Northern, J. (Eds.): *Clinical Impedance Audiometry*, Acton, Mass.: American Electromedics Corp. 1980, pp. 128–140.

Jerger, S., and Jerger, J.: *Auditory Disorders. A Manual for Clinical Evaluation.* Boston: Little, Brown, & Co., 1981.

Jerger, S., and Jerger, J.: Pediatric speech intelligibility test: performance—intensity characteristics. *Ear and Hearing* 1982, *3:* 325–334.

Jerger, S., and Jerger, J.: Extra- and intra-axial brain stem auditory disorders. *Audiology* 1975, *14:* 93–98.

Jerger, S., Jerger, J., and Abrams, S.: Speech audiometry in the young child. *Ear and Hearing* 1983, *4:* 56–66.

ARTICLE FIVE

SELF-ASSESSMENT QUESTIONS

1. Patient 1: In this patient with an extra- and intra-axial brainstem disorder, abnormality of performance was:
   (a) symmetric on the two ears
   (b) relatively more severe on the ear ipsilateral to the primary site of disorder
   (c) relatively more severe on the ear contralateral to the primary site of disorder

2. Patient 2: In this patient with an intra-axial brain stem disorder, concommitant involvement of the eighth nerve on the primary side of the disorder was indicated by:
   (a) abnormal reflex decay
   (b) abnormal adaptation on STAT
   (c) depressed maximum speech intelligibility scores
   (d) a and b
   (e) a, b, and c

3. Patient 4: In this patient with a non-localized disorder (arteriosclerotic cerebrovascular disease), involvement of caudal brain stem auditory pathways was considered unlikely due to:
   (a) normal ABR audiometry
   (b) normal acoustic reflexes
   (c) normal PI-PB functions
   (d) a and b
   (e) a, b, and c

4. Patient 6: In this young 3-year-old child with meningitis, PSI performance in isolation was helpful in:
   (a) obtaining a speech threshold to crosscheck pure tone sensitivity results
   (b) providing a control condition to assure that the child was capable of the motor-cognitive-linguistics demands of the task
   (c) both of the above

5. Patient 7: In this patient with multiple sclerosis, the results presented in this chapter will probably:
   (a) be stable over time
   (b) vary over time
   (c) be consistently worse over time

Development of a Dichotic Sentence Identification Test for Hearing-Impaired Adults

Robert C. Fifer, James F. Jerger, Charles I. Berlin, Emily A. Tobey, and John C. Campbell

Department of Otorhinolaryngology and Communicative Sciences, Baylor College of Medicine, Houston, Texas [R. C. F., J. F. J.], Kresge Hearing Research Laboratory of the South, New Orleans, Louisiana [C. I. B., E. A. T.], and Wilford Hall United States Air Force Medical Center, SGHSOS, Lackland AFB, Texas [J. C. C.]

ABSTRACT

Third-order synthetic sentences were aligned to make them suitable for dichotic presentation. These dichotic sentence materials were then administered to 14 normal listeners and 48 hearing-impaired subjects to determine the influence of peripheral hearing loss on test performance. Results suggest that the Dichotic Sentence Identification test is resistant to the influence of peripheral hearing loss until the pure-tone average of 500, 1000, and 2000 Hz exceeds approximately 50 dB. Beyond this level, degree of peripheral hearing loss limits its value for detecting central auditory disorder. Data are also provided on six persons with either confirmed or suspected lesions involving retrocochlear structures.

Virtually all speech audiometric procedures designed to evaluate auditory function share a common problem. They are influenced, to a greater or lesser extent, by peripheral hearing loss.[8, 10, 12] The Dichotic Sentence Identification (DSI) test was developed in an attempt to devise a dichotic listening test only minimally affected by peripheral hearing loss. The basic test paradigm is illustrated in Figure 1. Two different sentences are presented simultaneously to the two ears. Onsets and offsets of the two sentences are aligned with an accuracy of 100 μsec. Each sentence pair is randomly chosen from among the 10 seven-word, third-order approximations that constitute the closed message set for the conventional Synthetic Sentence Identification (SSI) test. Ninety randomly chosen pairs are presented successively. The subject's task is to scan the list of 10 sentences and report the two numbers corresponding to the two sentences that he heard. The purpose of this paper is to present preliminary findings on the DSI test in both normal and hearing-impaired listeners.

METHOD

Subjects

A total of 68 subjects participated in this study. Fourteen listeners had normal hearing bilaterally. Pure-tone thresholds were equal to or better than 20 dB HL (ANSI, 1969). Forty-eight subjects had varying degrees of sensorineural (presumably cochlear) hearing loss. They were subdivided into two subgroups: (1) subjects with a poorer ear pure-tone average of 500, 1000, and 2000 Hz (PEPTA1) less than 50 dB ($n = 28$); and (2) subjects with a PEPTA1 greater than 50 dB ($n = 20$).

We also tested six persons with either confirmed or suspected lesions involving retrocochlear structures. Two individuals had advanced diabetes mellitus: a 60-yr-old male with vascular and circulatory complications, and a 64-yr-old male with ophthalmic complications and stocking glove neuropathy. One patient, a 54-yr-old male, reported a long history of alcohol abuse and was undergoing detoxification at the time of testing. The fourth individual was a 45-yr-old male with a history of right middle cerebral artery occlusion and subsequent bypass surgery. Also in this group was a 60-yr-old male who had a foreign object penetration of his left temporal bone resulting in severe brain injury in the left temporal/parietal regions. The last person included in this group was a 19-yr-old male who presented initially with viral encephalitis. Shortly after his hospital admission for treatment, his condition was complicated by an intracranial hemorrhage in the region of the left temporal lobe. Five of these individuals had bilateral high-frequency sensorineural hearing loss with PEPTA1 less than 50 dB. The sixth person had normal hearing sensitivity bilaterally.

The normal listeners ranged in age from 23 to 55 yrs with a mean of 35.6 yrs. In the hearing-impaired group, age ranged from 24 to 67 yrs with a mean of 52.0 yrs. Criteria for acceptance as a participant in either group included a negative history of neurologic and otologic problems other than sensorineural hearing loss. Each person was required to speak English as his/her primary language and to have reading skills adequate to recognize the test sentences.

Materials

The basic materials for this test were the third-order synthetic sentences described by Speaks and Jerger[13] (Table 1). Sentences from the standard SSI tape were entered from an Ampex 440G two-channel tape recorder into a Perkin-Elmer 8/32 computer via a 12-bit analog-to-digital (A/D) converter at a 10 kHz rate. Before processing, the sentences were passed through a low-pass, 5 kHz Ithaca filter (model 4251). Subsequent to filtering, the test items were edited and equaled for overall intensity. Overall duration of each sentence was adjusted to 2 sec by editing out or expanding the vowel segments in the sentences. Edited sentences were then paired, randomized, and recorded on a two-channel

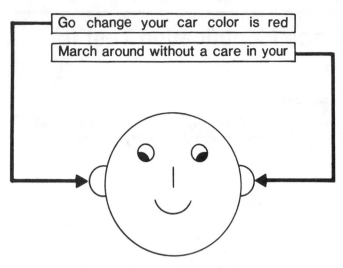

Go change your car color is red

March around without a care in your

Figure 1. Schematic representation of the test paradigm.

Table 1. The 10 third-order synthetic sentences used in the DSI test

DSI Synthetic Sentences
1. Small boat with a picture has become
2. Built the government with the force almost
3. Go change your car color is red
4. Forward march said the boy had a
5. March around without a care in your
6. That neighbor who said business is better
7. Battle cry and be better than ever
8. Down by the time is real enough
9. Agree with him only to find out
10. Women view men with green paper should

Ampex 440G tape recorder. The intensity level of the calibration tone was set to the average intensity of the vowel segments and recorded before the stimuli.

The tape was played on a dual-channel tape recorder connected to a dual-channel clinical diagnostic audiometer and routed to matched TDH-49 earphones. For the normal listeners, items were presented at an intensity level of 50 dB HL. In the hearing loss group, however, if PEPTA1 was less than 50 dB, then the intensity level on each ear was set in two different ways: (1) at a constant hearing level of 50 dB; and (2) at a constant sensation level of 50 dB referred to the pure-tone average of 500, 1000, and 2000 Hz (PTA1) for the respective ear. The order of presentation (50 dB HL versus 50 dB SL) was counterbalanced. Subjects with PEPTA1 greater than 50 dB listened to the test items at a level 1½ times the PTA1 value for each ear since this intensity best approximates normal use gain of personal amplification units.[1] If a loudness tolerance problem was encountered for any hearing-impaired subject, the sentences were presented at the most comfortable loudness level.

Procedure

Subjects were seated in a sound-treated audiometric booth with an adequate acoustic environment and sufficient illumination to see the printed list of synthetic sentences. Each participant was instructed to listen for two sentences presented dichotically, find the sentences from among a printed list numbered 1 through 10, and write the corresponding numbers of the sentences onto an answer form. The last 30 sentence pairs of the test were presented as practice items to ensure understanding of the task.

Each listener heard the first 10 practice items monaurally, five in each ear. The remaining 20 practice items were presented dichotically. Following the practice, the 90-item test was administered. The stimulus duration was 2 sec, followed by an 8-sec response period. The test required approximately 25 min to administer for the persons with normal sensitivity or with PEPTA1 greater than 50 dB. Those with PEPTA1 less than 50 dB required approximately 40 min to complete both test conditions. Test results were scored as percent correct identification for each ear separately. The resulting DSI score was the basic datum of subsequent analysis.

RESULTS

Table 2 shows the means and standard deviations of the DSI scores for each ear of the normal subjects. The means for the right and left ears are 94.2 and 93.5%, respectively. Despite the appearance of a slight right ear advantage, a statistical test on the difference between the means was not significant at the 0.05 level ($t = -0.484$; $p = 0.64$).

Figure 2 compares the means and standard deviations of DSI ear scores in the subgroup of hearing-impaired listeners with PEPTA1 less than 50 dB. In this subgroup we were particularly interested in comparing results ob-

Table 2. Mean DSI ear scores for the right and left ears of 14 normal subjects

	Mean DSI Ear Score	S.D.	t	p
Right ear	94.2%	9.6		
			−0.48	0.64
Left ear	93.5%	7.5		

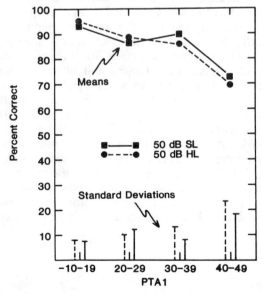

Figure 2. Means and standard deviations of the DSI scores for the 50 dB HL and the 50 dB SL presentation levels for subjects with PEPTA1 < 50 dB (n = 28). The *squares connected by the solid line* represent the 50 dB HL means; the *circles connected by the dashed line* represent the 50 dB SL means. The magnitude of the standard deviations shown by the *solid* and *dashed lines* correspond to the 50 dB HL and the 50 dB SL scores, respectively.

tained for constant HL and constant SL test conditions. We found no statistically significant differences between the mean scores for the two presentation levels at any PTA1 interval. Note that as PTA1 increased, there was a slight concomitant increase in variability. In the −10 to 19 dB interval, the standard deviations were essentially equal. In the 20 to 29 dB interval, the constant SL results showed a slightly greater standard deviation. At 30 to 39 dB and 40 to 49 dB, however, the constant HL standard deviations were consistently larger than the corresponding constant SL values. Despite this trend in variances as PTA1 increased, the F-ratios for evaluation of differences between the variances at each of the four levels were not significant at the 0.05 level. Therefore, we chose to consider only the 50 dB SL results in all further analyses.

Figure 3 is a scatter plot of 124 individual ear scores for both the right and left ears of the 14 normal listeners and 48 cochlear hearing loss subjects. The abscissa is the PTA1 value of the test ear; the ordinate is the DSI ear score. The hatched area delineates the region of chance performance, and the dashed line represents an empirically fitted lower boundary of normal performance based on a false-positive rate of 5%. For PTA1 in the range from −4 to 20 dB, normal values range from 100% to 75%. As the hearing loss increases beyond a PTA1 of 20 dB, the variability of the ear scores also increases, resulting in a negatively sloping lower boundary. At a PTA1 of 50 dB, the percentage point corresponding to the lower boundary value is approximately 32%. Above PTA1 = 50 dB, the distance between the lowest acceptable normal score and the chance performance level is less than 25%. Hence, the normal boundary beyond 50 dB leaves little area beneath it with which to distinguish abnormal from chance performance. Seven of the 124 noncentral ears scored below

this empirically defined normal range for a false-positive rate of 5.6%.

Figure 4 shows the individual ear scores of the six suspected retrocochlear subjects. In the subject with viral encephalitis, both ear scores fell into the abnormal range. In the other five individuals, the better ear scored within the normal area whereas the poorer ear scored outside the normal area. None of the retrocochlear subjects scored within the normal range on both ears.

Another aspect of performance on the DSI test is the interaural difference score. The ear difference scores of the 54 subjects with PEPTA1 between −10 and 59 dB are plotted in relation to bilateral pure-tone asymmetry in Figure 5. The dashed line encompasses the difference scores of a subgroup with PEPTA1 between −10 and 39 dB. These subjects had a maximum PTA1 asymmetry of 20 dB and a binaural performance difference of 16% or less. As PTA1 asymmetry increased, the variability of the ear difference scores also increased. As a result, 38% was established as the maximum normal difference in interaural DSI scores for persons with PEPTA1 between 40 and 59 dB. One subject had a difference score of 68%, thus yielding a false-positive rate of 1.9%.

The interaural differences in DSI performance for the retrocochlear subjects, shown in Figure 6, reflect the abnormal performance of the poorer ear. The abscissa of this graph is the absolute value of the PTA1 difference between ears. The ordinate is the percent difference in DSI scores between the right and left ears of each subject. The shaded area in the left portion of the figure is the normal response area for PEPTA1 values from −10 to 39 dB and in the right portion for PEPTA1 values between 40 and 59 dB. The subject with viral encephalitis had an interaural performance difference of 8%, thus falling in

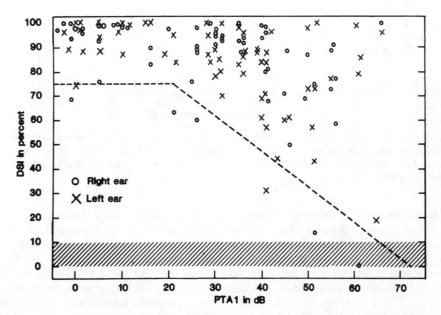

Figure 3. Scatter plot of 124 DSI scores for the right and left ears of 14 normal hearers and 48 hearing-impaired subjects. The data are plotted with the PTA1 value of each ear along the *abscissa* and the corresponding DSI score along the *ordinate*. The *dashed line* represents an empirically fitted lower boundary of "normal performance." The *hatched area* corresponds to the chance performance level of the test.

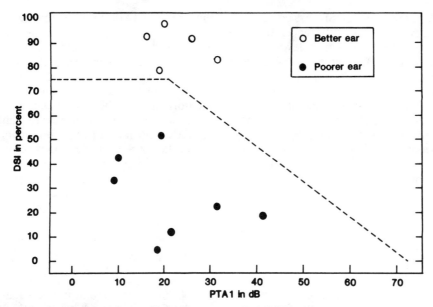

Figure 4. Scatter plot of the DSI ear scores for six suspected retrocochlear subjects. The *dashed line* is taken from Figure 3 and corresponds to the lower boundary of normal performance. The *open circles* represent the better performing ear for five subjects; the *filled circles* represent the abnormal contralateral ear scores. In one subject both ears scored in the abnormal range.

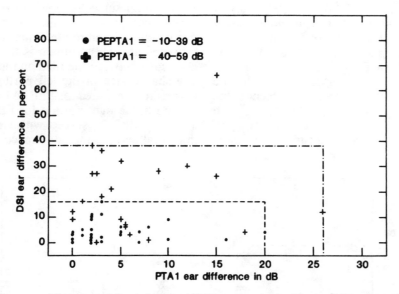

Figure 5. DSI interaural performance differences relative to interaural PTA1 asymmetry for 14 normal listeners and 40 hearing-impaired subjects. The *ordinate* is the DSI difference score (right ear minus left ear). The *abscissa* is the PTA1 difference score (right ear minus left ear). The *dashed line* encloses values obtained from subjects with PEPTA1 between −10 and 39 dB. The *dot-dashed line* is an empirically drawn normal boundary for subjects with PEPTA1 ranging from 40 to 59 dB.

the normal region. Both ears of this subject performed poorly with individual ear scores of 30 and 38%. Consequently he was abnormal with regard to absolute performance and would not be counted as a false negative. The remaining ear difference scores for PEPTA1 less than 40 dB were well beyond the normal response area. On the right side of Figure 6, the PEPTA1 range of 40 to 59 dB includes one person with a PEPTA1 of 43 dB and an interaural performance difference of 64%. When the performance asymmetry criteria were combined with the

absolute performance levels, there were no ambiguous test results for these six retrocochlear subjects.

In Figure 7 the effect of hearing loss on the DSI is compared to analogous results for the Staggered Spondaic Word (SSW),[2] Dichotic Digits, and Dichotic Consonant-Vowels (CVs).[10] Comparison of the present results with these previous studies shows that, with the exception of SSW, a surprising variety of test materials are all about equally affected by increasing sensorineural loss. The studies of Roeser et al.[10] using digits and CVs show that, although absolute performance is poorer, the effect of sensorineural hearing loss is about the same as for the DSI. In the case of SSW, however, the study of Arnst[2] shows a somewhat greater effect on test performance as PTA1 exceeds 50 dB.

DISCUSSION

The results of this study indicate that the DSI is applicable for use in ears having a PTA1 value up to 49 dB.

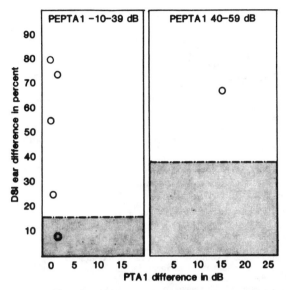

Figure 6. DSI interaural performance differences relative to interaural PTA1 asymmetry for six suspected retrocochlear subjects. The *hatched area beneath the dot-dashed line* represents the range of normal difference scores. *Left*, results for the five subjects with PEPTA1 between −10 and 39 dB. *Right*, result for the single subject with PEPTA1 between 40 and 59 dB.

Furthermore, binaural PTA1 asymmetries with a PEPTA1 less than 40 dB should have an interaural performance difference on the DSI of 16% or less. Binaural asymmetries with the poorer ear worse than 40 dB should result in a DSI difference score of 38% or less.

Relatively few studies exist which examine the influence of peripheral hearing loss on the speech materials used for central auditory evaluation. Kurdziel et al.[7] report reduced intelligibility in their hearing-impaired subjects for all conditions of time compressed consonant-nucleus-consonant monosyllables. Miltenberger et al.[9] found a strong interaction between the configuration of the hearing loss and the test results from the Dichotic Sentence test described by Willeford, low-pass filtered speech, a binaural fusion task, and rapidly alternating speech. Of their 70 neurologically normal, hearing-impaired subjects, 77% failed one or more of the tests. Roeser et al.[10] investigated the effect of hearing loss on Dichotic CVs and Dichotic Digits. Their hearing-impaired subjects consistently performed more poorly than the normal control subjects and demonstrated worse performance as the degree of hearing loss increased. Moreover, large individual ear differences were found in their hearing-impaired group, particularly for Dichotic Digits. Roeser and his co-workers concluded that their sensorineural subjects showed poorer recall due to peripheral distortion and reduced discrimination ability. Lynn and Gilroy[8] summarized their experience with dichotic tests by stating that abnormal test results in the presence of hearing impairment may reflect multiple sites of involvement, including peripheral hearing loss.

The SSW test[6] attempts to compensate for peripheral impairment. The test is administered on the assumption that a high correlation exists between the speech discrimination score for monosyllabic words and the raw SSW score. Lynn and Gilroy[8] criticized this assumption because an unrelated peripheral impairment may coexist with a

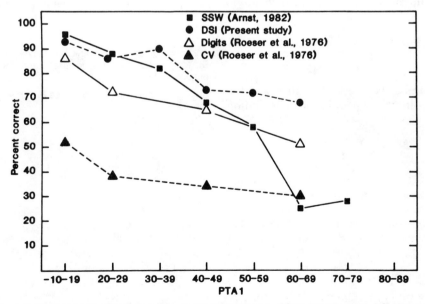

Figure 7. Comparison of the influence of peripheral hearing loss on the mean scores of four dichotic tests. DSI (*filled circle*), SSW (*filled square*), dichotic digits (*open triangle*), and dichotic CVs (*filled triangle*).

central auditory deficit.[12] It may be difficult, therefore, to separate the "peripheral components" in a person with central auditory disorder. Consequently, both peripheral and central factors may contribute to a reduced monosyllabic discrimination score.[8] Furthermore, use of a correction factor introduces another source of measurement error. Arnst[2] examined the raw and the corrected SSW percent error as a function of PTA1. Seventy-six percent of his hearing-impaired subjects scored in the normal, overcorrected, or mild categories, whereas 24% scored in the moderate to severe categories due to the degree of hearing loss. He concluded that caution must be exercised for interpretation of corrected SSW scores with PTA1 values greater than 40 dB.

Caferelli et al.[3] evaluated the SSW in patients with Meniére's disease. They found great intersubject and intrasubject variability in their hearing-impaired listeners. Similar to Arnst,[2] they recommended conservative interpretation of the SSW test results in the presence of hearing loss.

It has been well established that monosyllables and single words rely heavily on acoustic information above 1000 Hz.[4] In contrast, the synthetic sentences have a pivotal frequency of approximately 725 Hz.[11] Jerger and Hayes[5] demonstrated the importance of the pivotal frequencies for words and sentences in subjects with cochlear impairment. They found that with flat audiograms, the shape and the maxima of the performance-intensity functions for words and sentences were very similar. A rising audiometric configuration resulted in a poorer SSI score. Conversely, persons with sloping high-frequency hearing loss had poorer discrimination scores for words than for sentences. The magnitude of performance difference for the two materials was directly proportional to the steepness of the audiometric slope and inversely proportional to the frequency at which the slope began. Consequently, the dependence on low-frequency energy for the sentences gives them a distinct intelligibility advantage over monosyllabic words for persons with high-frequency sloping hearing losses.

SUMMARY

The DSI holds promise as a test of central auditory function in the hearing-impaired population. The findings of the present study suggest that the DSI is applicable for use in auditory assessment of impaired ears through PTA1 values up to 49 dB. The test results may be evaluated with regard to the absolute performance of each ear or, in the case of pure-tone asymmetries, the relative performance of the right and left ears. For subjects with PEPTA1 less than 40 dB, the ear difference score should not exceed 16%. Persons with PEPTA1 between 40 and 59 dB should show interaural performance differences of 38% or less. Finally, these data indicate that it does not matter whether the materials are presented to the two ears on a constant HL or a constant SL basis.

References

1. Alpiner, J. 1975. Hearing aid selection in adults. pp. 145–205. *in* M. Pollack, ed. *Amplification for the Hearing Impaired.* Grune & Stratton, New York.
2. Arnst, D. 1982. SSW test results with peripheral hearing loss. pp. 287–293. *in* D. Arnst, and J. Katz, eds. *Central Auditory Assessment: the SSW Test. Development and Clinical Use.* College Hill Press, San Diego.
3. Cafarelli, D., R. Nodar, M. Collard, and D. Larkins. 1982. SSW test results on patients with Meniere's disease. pp. 282–286. *in* D. Arnst, and J. Katz, eds. *Central Auditory Assessment: the SSW Test. Development and Clinical Use.* College Hill Press, San Diego.
4. French, N., and J. Steinberg. 1947. Factors governing the intelligibility of speech sounds. J. Acoust. Soc. Am. **19**, 90–119.
5. Jerger, J., and D. Hayes. 1977. Diagnostic speech audiometry. Arch. Otolaryngol. **103**, 216–222.
6. Katz, J. 1962. The use of spondaic staggered words for assessing the integrity of the central auditory nervous system. J. Aud. Res. **2**, 327–337.
7. Kurdziel, S., W. Rintelmann, and D. Beasley. 1975. Performance of noise-induced hearing-impaired listeners on time-compressed consonent-nucleus-consonent monosyllables. J. Am. Aud. Soc. **1**, 54–60.
8. Lynn, G., and J. Gilroy. 1977. Evaluation of central auditory dysfunction in patients with neurological disorders. pp. 177–222. *in* R. W. Keith, ed. *Central Auditory Dysfunction.* Grune & Stratton, New York.
9. Miltenberger, G., G. Dawson, and A. Raica. 1978. Central auditory testing with peripheral hearing loss. Arch. Otolaryngol. **104**, 11–15.
10. Roeser, R., D. Johns, and L. Price. 1976. Dichotic listening with sensorineural hearing loss. J. Am. Aud. Soc. **2**, 19–25.
11. Speaks, C. 1967. Intelligibility of filtered synthetic sentences. J. Speech Hear. Res. **10**, 289–298.
12. Speaks, C. 1975. Dichotic listening: a clinical research tool? pp. 1–25. *in* M. Sullivan, ed. *Central Auditory Processing Disorders.* Proceedings of a conference held at the University of Nebraska Medical Center, Omaha, NE.
13. Speaks, C., and J. Jerger. 1965. Method for measurement of speech identification. J. Speech Hear. Res. **8**, 185–194.

Acknowledgments: We thank Dr. James Olsson, Dr. Mel Shadowens, Dr. Martha Wofford, and Dr. Lois Sutton for their assistance with this project.

Address reprint requests to James F. Jerger, 11922 Taylorcrest, Houston, TX 77024.

Specific Auditory Perceptual Dysfunction in a Learning Disabled Child*

Susan Jerger, Randi C. Martin, and James Jerger

Baylor College of Medicine (Audiology) [S. J., J. J.], and Rice University (Psycholinguistics) [R. C. M.], Houston, Texas

ABSTRACT

An 11½ year old child with learning disability was evaluated with a battery of auditory and linguistic test procedures: electrophysiologic (auditory brain stem, middle latency response, and late potentials), electroacoustic (stapedial reflexes), and behavioral (measures of phonetic-phonologic, syntactic, and semantic processing). The overall pattern of results suggested the presence of an isolated auditory-phonologic processing disorder. Results supported an auditory-perceptual, as opposed to a linguistic-cognitive, model of learning disability.

Increasing numbers of children with language-learning disabilities are being referred to audiologists for evaluation of possible "central auditory processing disorders." Audiologic assessment is frequently included in the initial diagnostic evaluation because, in some circumstances, these children act as if they are hearing impaired. To date, however, the nature of the relation between auditory-perceptual and language-learning abilities has not been clearly established (1). With few exceptions (e.g., 2, 3), previous studies have not related auditory-perceptual and linguistic functions in the same child. Such data are crucial, however, in establishing the nature of the link, if any, between auditory-perceptual and language-learning skills.

Recently, we systematically investigated auditory-perceptual and linguistic abilities in a child diagnosed as learning-disabled. A single case experimental approach to the study of interrelationships between auditory-perceptual and linguistic-symbolic functions was considered desirable due to the heterogeneity of deficits and symptoms characterizing learning-disabled subjects (4–6). In this circumstance, forming homogeneous subject groups is difficult and averaging results across heterogeneous subject types may, of course, yield misleading findings (7, 8). The single case study was conducted within an information-processing theoretical framework (9).

Contemporary information processing theories (e.g., 10–12) view speech comprehension as a complex, rather than a unitary, phenomenon. Information processing models organize speech comprehension into a hierarchy of levels, including auditory, phonetic-phonologic, syntactic, and semantic. Interrelations among the different levels of processing are studied with componential performance measures. Global measures, such as traditional speech audiometric procedures, are considered undesirable because they do not reveal the nature of the complex interactive processes underlying performance (9). In view of these considerations, the test protocol of the present study did not emphasize traditional speech audiometric procedures. Instead, a wide range of specific test materials that attempted to isolate a particular auditory-perceptual or linguistic processing component were used.

The goal of the present report is to highlight findings in the learning-disabled child on auditory perceptual measures. Results are discussed in terms of both auditory and phonetic-phonologic levels of processing. Linguistic abilities in terms of syntactic and semantic levels of processing, however, are only briefly summarized. Detailed information on the child's language function is presented elsewhere (13).

METHOD

Subjects

Experimental Subject The child was a 11 yr 5 mo old male Caucasian. Antenatal and neonatal history were unremarkable. Growth and development proceeded normally until 6 yr of age. At age 6, the child began to experience episodes preceded by an auditory aura, described as a high-pitched tone. During the episodes, speech perception was apparently altered (reported as muffled and unintelligible) and automatisms involving swallowing and pinching movements of right forefinger and thumb were observed. The episodes were usually brief although one continued for approximately 15 minutes. Results of a comprehensive physical evaluation and neurologic examination at a Clinic for Pediatric Neurology were normal. Routine audiologic assessment (performed elsewhere) was reported as "completely normal." Electroencephalographic testing, however, showed spike and slow wave activity in the left temporal region. Medical diagnosis was mild seizure disorder. The child received medication to control seizure activity.

At age 9 yr, the child was reevaluated. No seizures had been observed within the past 2 yr. The child's chief complaint at reevaluation was difficulty in understanding verbal instructions in the classroom. Neurologic, physical, and audiologic (performed elsewhere) evaluations were within normal limits. No social or emotional problems were evident. Speech-language

* This research was supported in part by National Institutes of Health (NINCDS) grants NS-19652 (R. C. M.) and NS-10940 (J. J.).

evaluation indicated normal speech articulation and grammatical usage. Psychoeducational evaluation indicated intelligence (I.Q.) within the normal range. The Peabody Picture Vocabulary Test (14) yielded an I.Q. score of 95. The WISC-R (15) yielded a full-scale I.Q. score of 94 (verbal score = 98; performance score = 91). In spite of normal intelligence, however, the child had considerable academic difficulties in reading, mathematics, and written language. The final diagnosis, made by a team consisting of a pediatric neurologist, clinical psychologist, educational psychologist, and social worker, was attentional deficit disorder and learning disability without hyperactivity.

At age 11 yr 5 mo, the child was referred to the Children's Hearing Center because he continued to complain of hearing problems. He reported difficulty in understanding his teachers and sometimes the other children. He spends one-half of each school day in a support program for children with learning disability.

Normal Subjects For contrast and comparison, the experimental test battery was administered to three boys with a normal educational history. One child, termed N1, completed the entire protocol (48 hr of testing). The remaining children, termed N2 and N3, completed only a restricted set of procedures. Physical, neurologic, and routine audiologic assessment were within normal limits in all children. Growth and developmental milestones were also consistently normal. The educational performance level in each child was termed "average." The primary normal subject, N1, was 11 yr 3 mo of age. I.Q. scores were 91 on the Peabody Picture Vocabulary Test and 106 (full-scale) on the WISC-R (verbal score = 103; performance score = 109). The two secondary normal subjects, N2 and N3, were 11 yr 1 mo and 12 yr 1 mo of age, respectively. I.Q. scores on the Peabody Picture Vocabulary Test were 104 (N2) and 105 (N3). The WISC-R was not administered to the two secondary normal subjects. To approximate the probable degree of normal variability characterizing experimental procedures, the three normal children were carefully selected to represent personalities ranging from easy-to-test and attentive (N2) to hard-to-test and restless (N1).

Materials and Procedure

Electrophysiologic Measures Three auditory evoked potentials were obtained: auditory brain stem response (ABR), middle latency response (MLR), and late vertex potential. All potentials were evoked by click stimuli at 80 dB nHL. Recording parameters for each potential are summarized in Table 1. Instrumentation and procedural details have been elaborated elsewhere (16). Children were tested while awake and actively attending to the auditory signals.

Electroacoustic Measures Crossed and uncrossed acoustic reflex waveforms were obtained by signal averaging technique. Details of the experimental procedure and apparatus have been described previously (17). In brief, a dual-probe assembly presented signals alternately between ears such that the crossed reflex from one ear and the uncrossed reflex from the other ear

were measured simultaneously. Responses to eight successive signals on each ear were signal-averaged. Three reflex-eliciting signals were used: broadband noise, 500 Hz, and 2000 Hz. Routine immittance measures were also obtained with an electroacoustic bridge (Madsen, Z0–72).

Behavioral Measures Hearing sensitivity was defined by conventional manual technique at octave intervals between 250 and 8000 Hz with a standard pure-tone audiometer (Beltone, model 10D).

General Procedure and Instrumentation The tests detailed below were administered at a conversational loudness level, 60 dB sound pressure level (SPL). The tape playback system consisted of a multichannel tape recorder (Sony TC-788-4) fed through amplifying, attenuating, and mixing circuits (Broadcast Electronics, series Audio Console 8S150) to a loudspeaker (Phillips, type 22RH544/64R) or to earphones (Telephonic, TDH-39) mounted in circumaural cushions (CZW-6). For procedures with a competing signal in the background, the competition was always white noise at a signal-to-noise (S/N) ratio of 0 dB. The S/N ratio was selected on the basis of pilot data in adults, indicating that performance at 0 dB S/N ratio remained near ceiling (80 to 100%) on all test procedures. Below 0 dB S/N ratio, performance systematically declined; above this ratio, performance was consistently 100%.

Phoneme Discrimination was measured with a specially constructed Nonsense Syllable Detection Test (NSDT). The NSDT consisted of 33 different pairs of consonants differing in only one distinctive feature ("minimal" pairs) (18). The set of minimal pairs assessed discrimination of phonemes contrasting in seven different binary distinctive features: voicing, labiality, continuancy, back/front, sibilancy, sonorancy, and nasality. Consonant minimal pairs (e.g., b-p) were recorded onto magnetic tape (male talker) as consonant-vowel (CV) pairs by adding the vowel /a/ (e.g., ba-pa). All possible combinations of each CV pair (e.g., ba-pa, ba-ba, pa-pa, and pa-ba) were randomized, yielding a recorded series of 132 trials. The inter-item interval (ITI) was 6 sec. The carrier phrase was "Number . . .". The listener's task was to indicate whether the CV pairs were the same or different in a two alternative forced choice paradigm (50% a priori probability). An examiner monitored the subject's verbal responses and scored them as correct or incorrect. Previous investigators (19, 20) have demonstrated that children as young as 3 to 5 yr of age can successfully perform this type of phoneme feature-opposition task.

Phoneme Identification was measured with a set of CV stimuli that were generated on a speech synthesizer at the University of Oregon. The CVs were three formant patterns that differed in the acoustic parameter of voice onset time (VOT). The VOT continuum ranged from 0 to 70 msec in 10 msec increments. Normal listeners perceive the series of stimuli in terms of two discrete categories (ba-pa). Tape recorded stimuli (random series of 30 examples of each VOT variant) were presented monaurally. The ITI was 5 sec. The subject labeled each target that he heard (two alternative forced choice paradigm) as "ba" or "pa." An examiner monitored the subject's verbal responses and scored them as correct or incorrect.

Phoneme Analysis was studied with the sound analysis test of the Goldman-Fristoe-Woodcock (GFW) Sound-Symbol Subtest (21). Test items were nonsense words consisting of 2 to 3 phonemes (e.g., chid). The subject was instructed a priori to indicate either the first, middle, or last sound of the string.

Phoneme Blending skills were studied with the GFW Sound Blending subtest. Component sounds of words were presented in isolation in the correct order (k—a—t). The subject responded with the word that was formed by combining the ordered sounds. Test items ranged from 2 to 7 components.

Table 1. Recording parameters for ABR, MLR, and late auditory evoked potentials

Parameter	ABR	MLR	Late
Signal	Click	Click	Click
Intensity in dB nHL	80	80	80
Rate per sec	21.1	8.8	0.5
Epoch in msec	10	50	500
EEG passband in Hz			
Low cutoff	30	10	1
High cutoff	3000	1000	100

Phoneme Repetition skills were measured with the GFW Sound Mimicry subtest. Test items were nonsense words consisting of 1 to 3 syllables. Items varied from English word-like ("tash") to less word-like ("abfim") in the combinations of phonemes.

Word Discrimination was measured with a specially constructed picture word test. The subject's task was to decide whether an orally presented word matched a picture in a two alternative (yes-no) forced choice paradigm. One hundred (100) trials—50 matching and 50 nonmatching—were presented. Nonmatching items were constructed to represent three different confusion categories: phonemic (clown versus crown), semantic (fork versus spoon), and unrelated (roof versus shoe). All test items were common concrete nouns. An examiner monitored the subject's verbal responses and scored them as correct or incorrect.

Word Identification was measured with two sets of monosyllabic (PB) word materials: PAL PB-50 word lists (22) and the Northwestern University Children's Perception of Speech (Nu-chips) lists (23). Tape recorded stimuli were presented monaurally. For adult materials, an examiner monitored the subject's verbal responses and scored them as correct or incorrect.

RESULTS

Routine Audiologic Findings

Audiometric findings in both experimental (E) (Fig. 1, *top*) and normal (N1-3) (Fig. 1, *bottom*) subjects showed normal hearing sensitivity on both ears. Pure-tone average (PTA) scores at 500, 1000, and 2000 Hz ranged from 2 to 8 dB hearing level (HL). Maximum intelligibility scores for Nu-chips words were 96 to 100% correct in all subjects. Immittance audiometry showed normal, type A, tympanograms and normal static compliance measures on each ear of each subject. In E, unmasked bone conduction thresholds were superimposed on air conduction thresholds.

Acoustic Reflexes

Crossed and uncrossed acoustic reflex thresholds in the normal subjects (Fig. 1) were present at normal HLs between 500 to 2000 Hz on both ears. At 4000 Hz, crossed acoustic reflexes were within normal limits in N1 and N3, but were absent (greater than 110 dB HL) bilaterally in N2. Reflex absence at 4000 Hz only was considered a normal variant (24). In E, crossed acoustic reflex thresholds were elevated or absent on both ears. Uncrossed reflex thresholds at 1000 Hz were elevated on the left ear and within normal limits on the right ear. Abnormal crossed and uncrossed acoustic reflex thresholds in children with learning disability have been observed previously (25, 26).

Figure 2 shows averaged acoustic reflex waveforms to a 1000 Hz signal at 10 dB sensation level in E and N1. In N1, crossed and uncrossed reflex amplitudes and latencies (both onset and offset) were within normal limits. Reflex indices (afferent, efferent, and central pathway) were normal (27). In E, averaged reflex waveforms were degraded on both ears. As seen in Figure 2, *top*, crossed reflex activity was barely discernible on either ear. Uncrossed

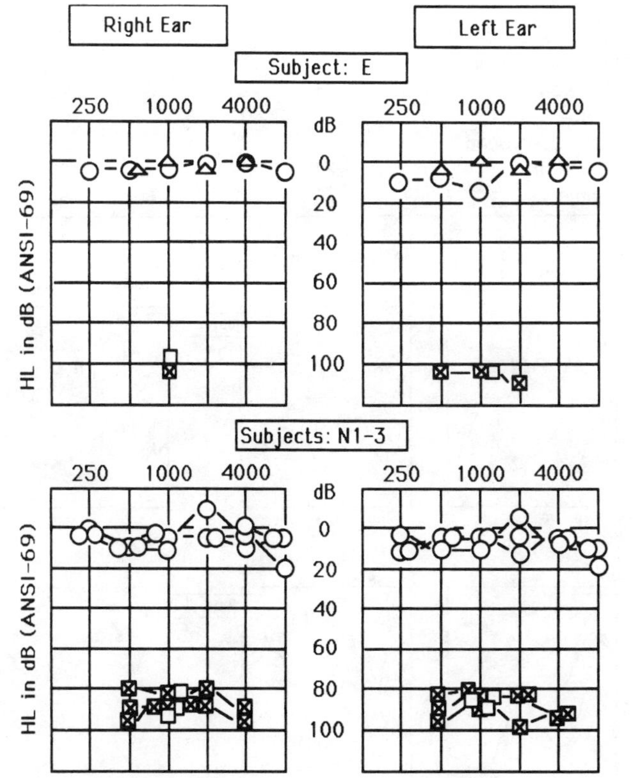

Figure 1. Pure-tone sensitivity results and crossed (⊠) and uncrossed (□) acoustic reflex thresholds in experimental (E) and three normal (N1-3) subjects. Air conduction: unmasked (O), masked (●); bone conduction: unmasked (△), masked (▲).

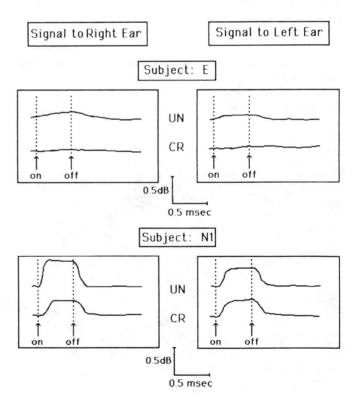

Figure 2. Averaged acoustic reflex waveforms for uncrossed (UN) and crossed (CR) conditions in the experimental (E) and one of the normal (N1) subjects. The reflex eliciting signal was a 1000 Hz tone at 10 dB sensation level.

reflex waveforms showed slight deflections from baseline at signal onset and offset. Uncrossed reflex amplitude, however, was severely reduced on both ears. Latency severity of reflex waveform degradation. The possibility that reflex abnormalities in E could be due to middle ear disorder was rendered unlikely by the observation of normal tympanograms on both ears and overlapping threshold measures for air conduction and unmasked bone conduction bilaterally. Reflex abnormalities in E supported the presence of central auditory dysfunction.

Auditory Evoked Potentials

Figure 3 shows auditory evoked potentials in E and N1. Responses were recorded between the vertex and each earlobe. Tracings represent simultaneous evoked activity in the hemisphere ipsilateral (I) and contralateral (C) to the ear stimulated. ABR results (Fig. 3A) in both subjects showed well-defined wave IV–V peaks at normal latencies bilaterally. Interwave latency measures were within normal limits on both ears of each subject. In E, however, waveform morphology on the right ear appeared degraded for peak waves I, II, and III. Waveform morphology on the left ear was normal. Contralateral hemisphere tracings are not available in E through technical error. Previous investigators (25, 28–32) have reported both normal and abnormal ABR waveforms in children described as having either learning disability, dyslexia, or minimal brain dysfunction.

In N1, MLR results (Fig. 3B) showed a normal configuration bilaterally. A prominent Pa component occurred at approximately 30 to 35 msec in both ipsilateral and contralateral recordings. In contrast to these results, MLR tracings in E were degraded bilaterally. Waveform morphology (both ipsilateral and contralateral recordings) exhibited both poor definition and replicability for peaks Na-Pa and Pa-Nb on both ears. Late vertex potentials (Fig. 3C) in both N1 and E were normal and well-formed on

both ears. In short, abnormality of auditory evoked potentials in E was characterized by bilaterally degraded MLR potentials and unilaterally atypical ABR waveforms. Abnormal ABR and MLR recordings in children with language-learning disabilities have been observed previously (25).

Phoneme Discrimination and Identification

Table 2 summarizes performance on the phoneme discrimination task in E and N1-3. The task was administered in the sound field both in quiet and in noise. Results for the quiet condition were characterized by a ceiling effect in all subjects (95 to 100%). In the noise condition, overall performance remained near ceiling (average performance: 83%) in N1-3 but dropped to 74% in E. The necessity of increasing task difficulty in order to explore auditory perceptual skills has been stressed previously (33–35). In E and N1-2, similar performance for both "same" and "different" trials indicated that response bias was not influencing results. In N3, however, a bias in favor of "different" responses was noted.

To dissect the performance difference between E and the normal subjects in the noise condition, discrimination

Table 2. Phoneme discrimination ability (percent correct) for same and different trials in experimental (E) and normal (N1–3) subjects. Test items were presented both in quiet and against a noise background.

Response Category	Subjects			
	E	N1	N2	N3
Quiet background				
Different	95	96	100	99
Same	98	97	98	99
Noise background				
Different	74	82	88	85
Same	73	89	86	68

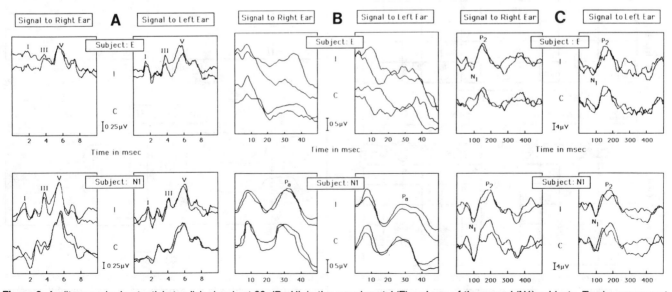

Figure 3. Auditory evoked potentials to click signals at 80 dB nHL in the experimental (E) and one of the normal (N1) subjects. Tracings represent simultaneous evoked activity in the hemisphere both ipsilateral (I) and contralateral (C) to the ear stimulated. A, Auditory brain stem response (ABR)—contralateral hemisphere tracings are not available in E; B, middle latency response (MLR); C, late (V) potential.

ability for each of the distinctive feature categories was analyzed (Table 3). Results are based on performance scores for different trials only. Same trials were not considered since the basis for responding same is not analyzable in terms of specific distinctive features.

Average performance in the normal subjects remained between 80 to 100% for all distinctive feature categories. Performance in E also remained near or at ceiling for four of the categories: sonorant, nasal, sibilant, and voice. Results across studies in the literature are not easily related due to the observation (36–38) that phoneme recognition may vary as a function of the characteristics of the noise spectrum, vowel context, and the S/N ratio. As a general comment, however, the present results agree with previous data (36, 39) from phoneme recognition tasks in noise, emphasizing the perceptual robustness of the voicing and nasality features.

Consistent with Miller and Nicely's (39) emphasis on the perceptual independence of distinctive features, results in E and the normal subjects were similar on the above categories, but divergent on the remaining categories. In particular, a striking performance difference between E and N1-3 occurred on the features of labiality (e.g., ba-da) and continuancy/obstruency (e.g., ha-ka). Performance for these two features was, on average, 81 to 83% in N1-3, but only 33 to 57% in E. Abnormal phoneme discrimination ability for synthesized tokens differing in place of articulation has been reported previously in dyslexic children (40) and learning disabled adults (41). The pattern of errors in E was consistent with the developmental pattern of consonant accuracy characterizing children (nasals > stops > continuants), both normal and language delayed (42). In the present subjects, interpretation of performance differences is difficult due to the lack of an isomorphic relation between specific acoustic cues and specific phonetic features in natural speech tokens (37, 43). Normal performance in E for some categories does stress, however, that performance deficits were due to specific perceptual deficits, rather than nonspecific task-related variables.

Phoneme identification ability was explored in subjects with a series of stimuli representing a ba-pa continuum. Identification functions were gathered both in quiet and in noise. Table 4 tabulates category boundary values of the obtained functions. Data represent the crossover point

Table 3. Phoneme discrimination ability (percent correct for "different" trials only) for seven binary distinctive feature categories in experimental (E) and normal (N1–3) subjects. Data represent performance for test items presented in a noise background.

Distinctive Feature	Subjects			
	E	N1	N2	N3
Sonorant	100	100	100	100
Nasal	100	100	100	100
Voice	100	100	86	93
Sibilant	90	70	100	70
Back	75	83	83	91
Labial	57	79	93	71
Continuant	33	67	92	91

Table 4. Phoneme identification ability as defined by the category boundary (voice onset time in msec yielding 50% correct) for a ba-pa continuum in experimental (E) and normal (N1–3) subjects. Data represent performance for test items presented both in quiet and against a noise background.

Background	Subjects			
	E	N1	N2	N3
Quiet	33	27	31	25
Noise	20	23	31	24
Difference	13	4	0	1

of the functions; in other words, the voice onset time at which 50% of stimuli were identified as "ba" (or conversely, 50% as "pa"). Absolute category boundary values in all subjects were generally consistent with results observed in adults (20 to 30 msec) (44, 45). Normal phoneme boundaries for synthesized speech tokens differing in either voicing or place of articulation have been observed previously in both children with dyslexia and young adults with learning disability (40, 41, 46).

Although absolute category boundary values were similar across subjects, the relation between crossover points in quiet versus noise noticeably differed between E and the normal subjects. Performance in E showed an unusual shift in the category boundary between conditions. Whereas category boundaries in N1-3 remained unchanged (0 to 4 msec) in quiet versus noise backgrounds, the category boundary for E shifted more than one step on the continuum, from 33 msec in quiet to only 20 msec in noise.

In summary, phoneme discrimination and identification abilities in E were characterized by an unusual performance difference between quiet and noise conditions. This observation is consistent with the findings of several previous investigators. Abnormal results in degraded listening conditions only has been a prevalent finding in studies of children with learning and/or reading disabilities (e.g., 35, 47, 48) and in patients with confirmed central auditory dysfunction (e.g., 49).

Without further data, the above pattern of abnormality is not unequivocally interpretable, however. The difference in performance between quiet and noise conditions is consistent with either of two hypotheses. One possible hypothesis is that E has a phonologic processing disorder. The disorder is manifest, however, only on tasks that place some degree of stress, such as competing noise, on the speech perception mechanism. Another, equally tenable, hypothesis is that E has a selective attention disorder. In this hypothesis, E is considered to have normal phonologic processing abilities but simply cannot attend selectively to test stimuli in a competing-inputs task.

To address the issue of whether E had abnormal phonologic processing abilities or abnormal selective attention abilities, three tasks that presented speech stimuli in quiet but required some phonologic operation on the stimuli were administered. If E's difficulties on the previous phoneme tasks were related to a selective attention disorder, he should have no difficulty with these new tasks. If, on the other hand, E's difficulties were related to a phonologic processing disorder, performance on these more difficult tasks presented in quiet should also reveal deficits.

Phoneme Processing Skills in Quiet

Table 5 presents results for E and N1 on the GFW subtests of sound analysis, blending, and mimicry. Performance in E was consistently impaired. Percentile scores ranged from only the 1st to the 28th percentiles. Results indicate that E's perceptual difficulties with phoneme discrimination and identification cannot be attributed solely to difficulty with selectively attending to test items in the presence of a competing input. These results argue for a phonologic processing disorder and against a selective attention deficit as the explanation of E's difficulties. Both Pelham (50) and Elliott and her colleagues (41, 51) have also theorized that attentional difficulties were not an adequate explanation of the deficits observed in their subjects—poor readers and learning disabled young adults and children. The next series of test procedures investigated whether E's phonologic processing difficulties extended to the perception of words.

Word Discrimination and Identification

Table 6 shows word discrimination ability on the specially constructed picture-word task in E and N1-3. Performance was measured both in quiet and in noise. Results for the quiet condition and for matching trials (both quiet and noise conditions) are not enumerated in Table 6 because performance was characterized by a ceiling effect (at least 95% correct) in all subjects. In noise, performance for nonmatching trials remained near ceiling (85 to 100%) for all categories in N1-3. In E, performance remained at ceiling for the semantic and unrelated conditions, but dropped to only 20% for the phonemically similar trials.

Table 7 summarizes word identification ability in E and N1-3. Word identification ability was evaluated with a set

Table 5. Phonologic ability on subtests of the Goldman-Fristoe-Woodcock Test of auditory discrimination in the experimental (E) subject and one of the normal (N1) subjects

Subtest	Subjects	
	E	N1
	Percentile score	
Sound analysis	28th	56th
Sound blending	7th	68th
Sound mimicry	1st	43rd

Table 6. Word discrimination ability (percent correct for nonmatching trials) in experimental (E) and normal (N1–3) subjects. Data represent performance for test items presented in a noise background.

Confusion Category	Subjects			
	E	N1	N2	N3
Unrelated	90	100	100	100
Semantic confusion	90	100	100	100
Phonemic confusion	20	95	95	85

Table 7. Word identification ability (percent correct) in experimental (E) and normal (N1–3) subjects for low-frequency (estimated frequency per million occurrence of less than 100) words. Data represent performance for test items presented in a quiet background.

Estimated Frequency per Million	Subjects			
	E	N1	N2	N3
Less than 10[a]	77	92	100	100
10–99[b]	86	100	100	100

Example words:
  [a] *vamp, corpse, mange.*
  [b] *cloud, cane, folk.*

of uncommon, termed low-frequency, words. Selected test items had an estimated frequency per million occurrence in children's literature of less than or equal to 100 (52). The value of a corpus of low-frequency words to the present study was to place some degree of stress, other than a competing signal, on the speech perception mechanism. According to Morton's (53, 54) Logogen Theory of word recognition, low-frequency words require more extensive auditory and phonologic processing in order to be identified than high frequency words. The necessity for more extensive perceptual processing of low-frequency words is attributed to (1) experiential factors and/or (2) differences in the structural, phonotactic, characteristics of the words per se (55, 56).

As seen in Table 7, word identification ability for low-frequency words presented in quiet was at ceiling (92 to 100%) in N1-3 but only 77 to 86% in E. Consistent with theoretical expectations (57), however, performance in E improved as word frequency increased. Poor identification of low-frequency words in E was consistent with his poor performance on the GFW sound mimicry subtest (Table 5).

In summary, word discrimination and identification abilities in E were characterized by normal performance for easy listening conditions and abnormal performance for difficult listening conditions. The lack of a performance decrement for semantic and unrelated trials on the picture-word test in noise (Table 6) again votes against a selective attention deficit hypothesis as the basis for E's perceptual disorder. Inability to attend selectively should have impaired performance for all items presented in noise relative to the quiet condition. Instead, performance declined for phonemically similar trials only. In short, E's difficulty in the identification of speech was not limited to nonsense syllables but extended to the perception of words as well. We should note, however, that some low-frequency word targets of the present study may have represented "nonsense" words to E. The unfamiliarity of the words apparently stressed the speech perception mechanism to the extent that pronounced auditory-phonologic processing difficulties were revealed.

Linguistic Abilities

Semantic abilities, defined by both standardized and experimental measures, were normal in E. In the present paper, examples of normal semantic abilities were (1) vocabulary skills consistently at or above age level on the Peabody Picture Vocabulary Test and the WISC-R and (2) normal performance on the picture-word test (Table 6) for semantic confusion trials, requiring correct discrimination between semantically related concepts. Syntactic abilities and short-term memory (STM) skills have been thoroughly detailed elsewhere (13). In brief, E's ability to process the syntactic information conveyed by word order and grammatical markers was assessed with sentence materials ranging in difficulty from simple one-clause active sentences to complex embedded relative-clause sentences containing a passive form. Results for syntactic measures varied as a function of the presentation mode. With visual presentation, E's performance for all sentence types was normal. With auditory presentation, however, results were depressed, particularly for the more syntactically complex sentences. Normal performance on the visual control condition indicated that E's knowledge of syntactic structures per se was normal. Abnormal results on the auditory condition therefore have to be attributed to some processing factor specific to the auditory modality.

A possible source of the auditory sentence-comprehension difficulty was disrupted auditory STM. E exhibited a restricted STM span for tests requiring memory for order. In contrast, memory skills for tasks that drew on semantic information were consistently normal. Other aspects of E's STM performance indicated a specific disruption of the ability to retain phonological information, It was hypothesized (13) that the observed phonological retention deficit was the source of E's auditory sentence processing difficulties. An association between impaired phonological processing and impaired memory for order has been observed repeatedly by previous investigators (e.g., 58).

DISCUSSION

Implication of Results in Terms of Information Processing Model of Speech Comprehension

Figure 4 lists (1) the hypothetical levels of processing involved in speech comprehension in an information processing theoretical model (10, 11) and (2) the measures we used to study each processing component. First is an auditory stage that transforms the speech waveform into a neurally encoded signal. Next are the phonetic and phonologic stages that analyze the transformed acoustic pattern into phonetic features and bundle the features into a particular phoneme. The final two stages involve linguistic functions that organize the phonologic segments into a grammatical structure (syntactic level) and specify the semantic content in order to form a conceptual representation.

The functional adequacy of each of the levels of processing was predicted from the present data as shown in Figure 4. In terms of the auditory stage of processing, results suggested that the acoustic waveform was not being transformed into an appropriate neurally encoded signal. Evidence for abnormal auditory transformation was provided by abnormal electrophysiologic and electroacoustic measures of auditory function. Although late vertex (P2 component) potentials and wave IV–V peaks of the ABR

Level of Processing	Test	Outcome
AUDITORY	Acoustic Reflex	■
	ABR	◨
	Middle Latency	■
	Late V Potential	□
PHONETIC-PHONOLOGIC	Phoneme Discrimination	■
	Identification	■
	Word Discrimination	■
	Identification	■
	Phonologic Processing	■
SYNTACTIC	Sentence Identification (auditory)	■
	(visual)	□
SEMANTIC	Word Identification	□
	Vocabulary	□
	Naming to Definition	□

■ Abnormal   □ Normal

Figure 4. Hypothetical levels of processing involved in speech comprehension in an information processing theoretical model and the functional adequacy of each level as predicted from the componential measures of the present study.

were normal, middle latency responses, ABR waveform morphology, and acoustic reflex thresholds and morphology were abnormal. The overall pattern of results emphasizes the diagnostic value of electrophysiologic evaluation at multiple levels within the auditory system, a point that is beginning to recur in the literature (59–62, although see 63 for a precaution).

In terms of the phonetic-phonologic stages, results suggested that the transformed acoustic patterns were not being mapped onto appropriate phonologic representations. Alternatively, the transformed acoustic patterns may have been degraded to the extent that appropriate phonologic representations could not be consistently determined. Evidence for abnormal phonetic-phonologic processing was provided by abnormal discrimination and identification abilities for both phoneme and word measures. Further evidence was the abnormality for phoneme processing skills (sound analysis, blending, and mimicry) and performance for uncommon words. These latter two performance measures were obtained in a quiet background, thus arguing against any hypothesis that involves a selective attention disorder as the basis for perceptual difficulties. Finally, results suggested that the syntactic and semantic levels were functioning normally. In contrast to the abnormalities observed on measures of auditory-phonetic abilities, syntactic and semantic abilities were normal, except when syntactic measures were presented via the auditory modality.

Data from the present experiment may be interpreted

Table 8. Profiles of two different theoretical models of learning disability

	Models	
Topics	Linguistic	Auditory
Problem	Conceptual	Perceptual
Deficit	Symbolic	Precursor
	Behaviors	Behaviors
Linguistic factors	Primary	Secondary

not only within an information processing framework but also in terms of theoretical orientations to learning disability. The following section addresses the issue of whether learning disability reflects symbolic or perceptual dysfunction.

Implication of Results in Terms of Perceptual versus Linguistic Models of Learning Disability

Table 8 summarizes basic aspects of two different theoretical approaches to learning disability, termed the linguistic and auditory models (for in-depth discussion of these issues in children with learning disability and/or developmental language disability, see 1, 41, 64–68). Distinctions between strong versions of the two viewpoints may be briefly highlighted as follows: The orientation of the linguistic model is that conceptual factors are the basis for learning disability. Learning-disabled children are viewed as having a problem in representational or symbolic behaviors, rather than perceptual processes. The linguistic model hypothesizes that linguistic-cognitive deficits are the primary problem.

In contrast to this viewpoint, the auditory model hypothesizes that auditory-perceptual factors are the basis for learning disability. The auditory model does not view linguistic-cognitive deficits as primary problems but as secondary concomitants of a more basic auditory perceptual impairment. Learning-disabled children are viewed as having a problem in the precursor behaviors necessary for developing normal higher level functioning. In other words, learning disability in this model involves a deficit in the processes that are presumed to be prerequisites for normal linguistic cognitive development. The auditory model assumes that certain auditory skills are fundamental to normal language acquisition and learning.

Data in E are not consistent with the linguistic model's assumption that the basis for learning disability is linguistic-symbolic factors. The present data argue instead for the existence of isolated auditory perceptual deficits as a potential factor in the problem of the learning disabled. Further evidence in this regard is that E seemed to have intact internal phonologic representations based on (1) his ability to identify and discriminate phonemes presented in quiet, and (2) his normal speech production abilities (see subject description section). To us, E's difficulty was not a central phonologic disorder but a disorder in transforming auditory input into the correct phonologic representation in difficult listening tasks. In terms of the speech perception model discussed by Blumstein (69), E had a deficit in acoustic phonetics.

This interpretation has important implications for an appropriate remediation strategy. If our hypothesis is correct—that the basis of E's learning disability was auditory perceptual dysfunction—then a remediation program based on the linguistic-cognitive model would, of course, be inappropriate. Relative to a broader viewpoint, however, we should reiterate that learning-disabled children present a heterogeneity of deficits that probably require varying remediation strategies.

Implication of Results in Terms of Audiologic Evaluation of Children

These data stress the need for more subtle auditory tasks than pure-tone and PB word tests in order to demonstrate the presence of central auditory abnormality in children with learning disability. This child had voiced auditory complaints since he was 6 yr old. On three different occasions, at ages 6, 9, and 11 yr, he was referred for audiologic evaluations. Results of the first two evaluations were consistently reported as "normal."

The auditory disorder in this child was not recognized for 5 yr due to the inadequacy of routine audiologic test procedures in detecting subtle auditory perceptual dysfunction. This fact places a unique responsibility on clinical audiologists. A critical aspect of the clinical audiologic evaluation of children is to be alert to the possibility of central auditory processing disorders. Pediatric audiologic evaluations must be expanded beyond the narrow confines of pure-tone thresholds and simple PB word scores for adequate assessment of auditory function. Helpful discussion of the general problem of evaluating central auditory processing skills in children is presented in a commendable chapter by Keith (68).

SUMMARY

A child with learning disability demonstrated a selective deficit in auditory perceptual function. Analysis of relative performance measures (both within and across tasks) consistently argued for a specific auditory-phonologic processing disorder and against either a primary linguistic-cognitive deficit, a selective attention disorder, or some other nonspecific task-related dysfunction.

References

1. Supple M de Montfort. Auditory perceptual function in relation to phonological development. Br J Audiol 1983;17:59–68.
2. Tallal P. Auditory processing disorders in children. In: Levinson P, Sloan C, eds. Auditory processing and language. Clinical and research perspectives. New York: Grune & Stratton, 1980:81–100.
3. Tallal P. Language disabilities in children: perceptual correlates. Int J Pediatr Otorhinolaryngol 1981;3:1–13.
4. Keogh B. Research in learning disabilities: a view of status and need. In: Das J, Mulcahy R, Wall A, eds. Theory and research in learning disabilities. New York: Plenum Press, 1982.
5. Willeford J. Assessment of central auditory disorders in children. In: Musiek F, Pinheiro M, eds. Assessment of central auditory dysfunction. Foundations and clinical correlates. Baltimore: Williams & Wilkins, 1985:239–55.
6. Johnson D, Blalock J. Young adults with learning disabilities. Orlando: Grune & Stratton, 1986.
7. Hersen M, Barlow D. Single case experimental designs. Strategies for studying behavior change. New York: Pergamon Press, 1978.
8. Caramazza A, Martin R. Theoretical and methodological issues in the study of aphasia. In: Hellige J, ed. Cerebral hemisphere asymmetry: method, theory, and application. New York: Praeger Scientific Publishers, 1983.
9. Siegler R. Information processing approaches to development. In: Mussen P,

ed. Handbook of child psychology. 4th ed, Kessen W, ed. Vol 1: History, theory, and methods. New York: John Wiley & Sons, 1983:129–202.

10. Pisoni D. Speech perception. In: Estes W, ed. Handbook of learning: linguistic functions in cognitive theory. Baltimore: Lawrence Erlbaum, 1978:166–233.

11. Pisoni D. Speech perception: some new directions in research and theory. J Acoust Soc Am 1985;78:381–8.

12. Kuhl P. Speech perception: an overview of current issues. In: Lass N, McReynolds L, Northern J, Yoder D, eds. Speech, language and hearing. vol 1: normal processes. Philadelphia: WB Saunders, 1982:286–321.

13. Martin R, Jerger S, Breedin S. Syntactic processing of auditory and visual sentences in a learning disabled child: relation to short-term memory. Develop Neuropsychol (in press).

14. Dunn L, Dunn L. Manual for forms L and M of the Peabody Picture Vocabulary Test—revised. Circle Pines, MN: American Guidance Service, 1981.

15. Wechsler D. Manual for the Wechsler Intelligence Scale for Children—revised. New York: The Psychological Corporation, 1974.

16. Jerger J, Mauldin L. Prediction of sensorineural hearing level from the brainstem evoked response. Arch Otolaryngol 1978;104:456–61.

17. Stach B, Jerger J. Acoustic reflex averaging. Ear Hear 1984;5:289–96.

18. Singh S. Distinctive features. Theory and validation. Baltimore: University Park Press, 1976.

19. Graham L, House A. Phonological oppositions in children: a perceptual study. J Acoust Soc Am 1971;49:559–66.

20. Stewart J, Singh S, Hayden M. Distinctive feature use in speech perception of children. Lang Speech 1979;22:69–79.

21. Goldman R, Fristoe M, Woodcock R. The Goldman-Fristoe-Woodcock test of auditory discrimination. Circle Pines, MN: American Guidance Service, 1970.

22. Egan J. Articulation testing methods. Laryngoscope 1948;58:955–91.

23. Elliott L, Katz D. Development of a new children's test of speech discrimination. St Louis: Auditec, 1980.

24. Jerger J, Jerger S, Mauldin L. Studies in impedance audiometry. I. Normal and sensorineural ears. Arch Otolaryngol 1972;96:513–23.

25. Kraus N, Ozdamar O, Stein L, Reed N. Absent auditory brain stem response: peripheral hearing loss or brain stem dysfunction? Laryngoscope 1984;94:400–6.

26. Thomas W, McMurry G, Pillsbury H. Acoustic reflex abnormalities in behaviorally disturbed and language delayed children. Laryngoscope 1985;95:811–7.

27. Hayes D, Jerger J. Signal averaging of the acoustic reflex: diagnostic applications of amplitude characteristics. Scand Audiol 1982;(suppl 17):31–36.

28. Sohmer H, Student M. Auditory nerve and brainstem evoked responses in normal, autistic, minimal brain dysfunction and psychomotor retarded children. Electroencephalogr Clin Neurophysiol 1978;45:577–84.

29. Welsh L, Welsh J, Healy M, Cooper B. Cortical, subcortical, and brainstem dysfunction: a correlation in dyslexic children. Ann Otol Rhinol Laryngol 1982;91:310–5.

30. Greenblatt E, Bar A, Zappulla R, Hughes D. Learning disability assessed through audiologic and physiologic measures: a case study. J Commun Dis 1983;16:309–13.

31. Tait C, Roush J. Normal ABR's in children classified as learning disabled. J Aud Res 1983;23:56–62.

32. Roush J, Tait C. Binaural fusion, masking level differences, and auditory brain stem responses in children with language-learning disabilities. Ear Hear 1984;5:37–41.

33. Goetzinger C, Dirks D, Baer C. Auditory discrimination and visual perception in good and poor readers. Ann Otol Rhinol Laryngol 1960;69:121–36.

34. Dillon H. The effect of test difficulty on the sensitivity of speech discrimination tests. J Acoust Soc Am 1983;73:336–44.

35. Brady S, Shankweiler D, Mann V. Speech perception and memory coding in relation to reading ability. J Exp Child Psychol 1983;35:345–67.

36. Wang M, Bilger R. Consonant confusions in noise: a study of perceptual features. J Acoust Soc Am 1973;54:1248–66.

37. Dubno J, Levitt H. Predicting consonant confusions from acoustic analysis. J Acoust Soc Am 1981;69:249–61.

38. Gordon-Salant S. Phoneme feature perception in noise by normal-hearing and hearing-impaired subjects. J Speech Hear Res 1985;28:87–95.

39. Miller G, Nicely P. An analysis of perceptual confusions among some English consonants. J Acoust Soc Am 1955;27:338–52.

40. Godfrey J, Syrdal-Lasky A, Millay K, Knox C. Performance of dyslexic children on speech perception tests. J Exp Child Psychol 1981;32:401–24.

41. Elliott L, Clifton L. Auditory processing by learning-disabled young adults. In: Johnson D, Blalock J, eds. Young adults with learning disabilities. Orlando: Grune & Stratton, 1986.

42. Leonard L. Phonological deficits in children with developmental language impairment. Brain Lang 1982;16:73–86.

43. Soli S, Arabie P. Auditory versus phonetic accounts of observed confusions between consonant phonemes. J Acoust Soc Am 1979;66:46–59.

44. Pisoni D, Lazarus J. Categorical and noncategorical modes of speech perception along the voicing continuum. J Acoust Soc Am 1974;55:328–33.

45. Friedrich F, Glenn C, Marin O. Interruption of phonological coding in conduction aphasia. Brain Lang 1984;22:266–91.

46. Brandt J, Rosen J. Auditory phonemic perception in dyslexia: categorical identification and discrimination of stop consonants. Brain Lang 1980;9:324–37.

47. Farrer S, Keith R. Filtered word testing in the assessment of children's central auditory abilities. Ear Hear 1981;2:267–9.

48. Musiek F, Gollegly K, Baran J. Myelination of the corpus callosum and auditory processing problems in children: theoretical and clinical correlates. Semin Hear 1984;5:231–41.

49. Jerger S, Jerger J. Auditory disorders. A manual for clinical evaluation. Boston: Little, Brown, 1981.

50. Pelham W. Selective attention deficits in poor readers? Dichotic listening, speeded classification, and auditory and visual central and incidental learning tasks. Child Dev 1979;50:1050–61.

51. Elliott L, Connors S, Kille E, Levin S, Ball K, Katz D. Children's understanding of monosyllabic nouns in quiet and in noise. J Acoust Soc Am 1979;66:12–21.

52. Carroll J, Davies P, Richman B. Word frequency book. Boston: Houghton Mifflin, 1971.

53. Morton J. A functional model for memory. In: Norman D, ed. Models of human memory. New York: Academic Press, 1970:203–54.

54. Morton J. Facilitation in word recognition: experiments causing change in the logogen model. In: Kolers P, Wrolstad M, Bouma H, eds. Processing of visible language. vol 1. New York: Plenum Press, 1978:259–68.

55. Landauer T, Streeter L. Structural differences between common and rare words: failure of equivalence assumptions for theories of word recognition. J Verb Learn Verb Behav 1973;12:119–31.

56. Pisoni D, Nusbaum H, Luce P, Slowiaczek L. Speech perception, word recognition and the structure of the lexicon. Speech Commun 1985;4:75–95.

57. Morton J. Word recognition. In: Morton J, Marshall J, eds. Psycholinguistics 2: structures and processes. Cambridge: MIT Press, 1979:109–56.

58. Campbell R, Butterworth B. Phonological dyslexia and dysgraphia in a highly literate subject: a developmental case with associated deficits of phonemic processing and awareness. Quart J Exp Psychol 1985;37A:435–75.

59. Kileny P. Middle latency (MLR) and late vertex auditory evoked responses (LVAER) in central auditory dysfunction. In: Pinheiro M, Musiek F, eds. Assessment of central auditory dysfunction, foundations and clinical correlates. Baltimore: Williams & Wilkins, 1985:87–102.

60. Kileny P, Berry D. Selective impairment of late vertex and middle latency auditory evoked responses. In: Mencher G, Gerber S, eds. The multiply handicapped hearing impaired child. New York: Grune & Stratton, 1983:233–58.

61. Jerger S, Jerger J. Audiologic applications of early, middle, and late auditory evoked potentials. Hear J 1985;38:31–6.

62. Mason S, Mellor D. Brain stem, middle latency and late cortical evoked potentials in children with speech and language disorders. Electroencephalogr Clin Neurophysiol 1984;59:297–309.

63. Kraus N, Smith D, Reed N, Stein L, Carter C. Auditory middle latency responses in children: effects of age and diagnostic category. Electroencephalogr Clin Neurophysiol 1985;62:343–56.

64. Rees N. Auditory processing factors in language disorders: the view from Procrustes' bed. J Speech Hear Disord 1973;38:304–15.

65. Rampp D. Hearing and learning disabilities. In: Bradford L, Hardy W, eds. Hearing and hearing impairment. New York: Grune & Stratton, 1979:381–9.

66. Levinson P, Sloan C. Auditory processing and language. Clinical and research perspectives. New York: Grune & Stratton, 1980.

67. Lubert N. Auditory perceptual impairments in children with specific language disorders: a review of the literature. J Speech Hear Disord 1981;46:3–9.

68. Keith R. Central auditory tests. In: Lass N, McReynolds L, Northern J, Yoder D, eds. Speech, language, and hearing. III. Hearing disorders. Philadelphia: WB Saunders, 1982:1015–38.

69. Blumstein S. Phonological aspects of aphasia. In: Sarno M, ed. Acquired aphasia. New York: Academic Press, 1981.

Acknowledgments: We thank Terrey Oliver, Rose Chmiel, Sarah Breedin, and Tammi Leong for assistance on this project. We gratefully acknowledge the friend-colleagues who critically reviewed the presubmitted version of this paper.

Address reprint requests to Susan Jerger, Ph.D., Division of Audiology and Speech Pathology, Baylor College of Medicine, Neurosensory Center NA200, Texas Medical Center, Houston, TX 77030.

Received October 10, 1986; accepted November 20, 1986.

Clinical Forum

Central Auditory Processing Disorder: A Case Study

James Jerger*
Karen Johnson*
Susan Jerger*
Newton Coker*
Francis Pirozzolo[†]
Lincoln Gray[‡]

Abstract

We carried out extensive audiologic, electrophysiologic, and neuropsychologic testing on a young woman who complained that she had difficulty hearing in her educational environment. Conventional audiometric results, including pure-tone, speech, and immittance audiometry, were all within normal limits. The subject performed normally on tests involving the processing of rapidly changing temporal information, interaural time and intensity difference detection, and both absolute and relative sound localization. Early, middle, late and task-related auditory evoked potentials were essentially normal, although some asymmetry was observed in the middle latency (MLR) and late (LVR) responses. There was, however, a consistent left-ear deficit on dichotic sentence identification, on threshold and suprathreshold speech measures in the left sound field when various types of competition were delivered in the right sound field, and on cued-target identification in the left sound field in the presence of multitalker babble. Results suggest a central auditory processing disorder characterized by an asymmetric problem in the processing of binaural, noncoherent signals in auditory space. When auditory space was structured such that the target was directed to the left ear, and the competition to the right ear, unwanted background was less successfully suppressed than when the physical arrangement was reversed.

Key Words: Central auditory processing disorder, auditory-perceptual disorders, auditory-diseases-central, auditory evoked potentials

The concept of central auditory processing disorder (CAPD) in children arose from observations by teachers and parents that some children appear to have difficulty in hearing even though their pure-tone audiograms indicate normal peripheral sensitivity. Observers have described problems in hearing the teacher in the presence of background noise, in executing a sequence of auditory instructions and commands, and in sustaining attention to auditory input (Cohen, 1980; Keith, 1981; Lasky, 1983; Willeford, 1985). The common thread in this "symptom complex" is the consistent description of a child who appears to have a "hearing loss," especially in the classroom situation, but whose pure-tone audiogram is invariably within normal limits (Cohen, 1980; Gerber and Mencher, 1980; Jerger et al, 1988; Musiek and Guerkink, 1980; Rampp, 1979; Willeford, 1985).

The construct that such problems may be related to dysfunction in the central auditory system follows from the rich literature on the

*Department of Otolaryngology and Communicative Sciences, Baylor College of Medicine, Houston, Texas

[†]Department of Neurology, Baylor College of Medicine, Houston, Texas

[‡]Department of Otolaryngology, University of Texas Health Science Center, Houston, Texas

Reprint requests: James Jerger, Baylor College of Medicine, 6501 Fannin, NA 200, Houston, TX 77030

behavioral manifestations of documented brain lesions affecting the central auditory pathways and centers (cf., Calearo and Antonelli, 1968; Berlin et al, 1972; Liden and Korsan-Bengsten, 1973; Jerger, 1960; Jerger and Jerger, 1974, 1975; Lynn et al, 1972; Speaks et al, 1975). Patients with demyelinating disease, intra-axial tumor, or cerebrovascular insult typically show a similar symptom complex if the brain lesion affects the central auditory system. Peripheral hearing sensitivity, as indicated by the pure-tone audiogram, is within normal limits, but the ability to process suprathreshold auditory signals may be mildly to severely compromised, especially in the presence of competing background sounds. This similarity in symptomatology invites speculation that at least some of the apparent auditory problems observed in children without known brain lesions may be manifestations of as-yet-undetected dysfunction of the central auditory system (Barr, 1972; Gerber and Mencher, 1980; Jerger et al, 1988; Musiek et al, 1984).

Complicating the issue, however, is the fact that the combination of apparent auditory processing disorder and academic difficulty has also invited speculation, among educators, that at least some of the problems subsumed under the rubric of "learning disorder" or "learning disability" may be due to such auditory deficits (cf., Beasley and Freeman, 1977; Katz and Illmer, 1972; Keith, 1981; Knox and Roeser, 1980; Rampp, 1979; Sloan, 1980). Similarly, the frequently observed association between receptive and expressive language function has invited speculation that at least some of the language disorders of children may be attributed to CAPD (cf., Lubert, 1981; Sloan, 1980; Tallal, 1980; Tallal et al, 1985a, b). In the absence of substantial experimentally-controlled data such speculation has invited counter speculation challenging the reality of the phenomenon of a specifically-auditory processing disorder (Bloom and Lahey, 1978; Lyon, 1977; Rees, 1973, 1981). The association, for example, between attentional deficits and performance on auditory tests (cf., Campbell and McNeil, 1985; Gascon et al, 1986) has suggested to some investigators that the presumed auditory problem may, in fact, be a manifestation of impaired attention (DeMarco et al, 1989; Robin et al, 1989).

In the present paper we present a considerable body of data from a single subject with what we believe to be an auditory-specific central processing disorder. This young woman complained of hearing and understanding difficulties in her educational environment. She felt that her problems were sufficient to consider use of a hearing aid. Basic audiologic measures, including pure tone audiometry, acoustic immittance measures, and routine speech audiometry were all within normal limits. We noted on routine examination, however, an abnormality in dichotic listening; specifically, a left ear deficit on the Dichotic Sentence Identification (DSI) test and set out to explore the nature of this apparent deficit in greater detail. We believe that our findings address many of the persistent issues surrounding the controversial area of CAPD.

DESCRIPTION OF SUBJECT

History

The subject was an 18-year-old woman who complained that, for the past 2 years, she had experienced difficulty in hearing and understanding her high-school teachers. She complained that she frequently missed the teacher's verbal assignments. The most difficulty was experienced when the classroom was noisy. She did not complain of hearing loss in the sense of reduced sensitivity to sound. Rather, she described her problem as a difficulty in understanding the teacher when there was interference from background noise. The subject also reported difficulties in group social situations, while watching TV, and in using the telephone. She had no problem with the telephone on the right ear but reported that the sound was "not as good" when listening on the left ear. She felt that her problems were sufficient to consider use of a hearing aid.

On the Self Assessment of Communication (SAC) scale she scored 38 percent, a value associated with mild auditory handicap (Schow and Tannahill, 1977). She reported particular difficulty on question 3 ("Do you experience communication difficulties while listening to someone speak to a large group?") and question 5 ("Do you experience communication difficulties when you are in an unfavorable listening environment?"). Nevertheless she had just graduated from high school without obvious academic difficulty and was college-bound as a music major.

Physical Findings

Physical examination revealed an alert, well-developed, young adult. Both external auditory canals and tympanic membranes were normal. There was no evidence of pathology in the middle ear clefts. Extraocular muscle movements were normal. Pupils were equally round and reactive to light and accommodation. Nasal cavity, oral cavity, pharynx, and larynx were normal. Neck findings were negative. Cranial nerves III to XII were intact.

Routine laboratory studies included a normal complete blood count with normal sedimentation rate. Serum T4 and T3 levels as well as T3 uptake level were normal. Urinalysis was negative. Five-hour glucose tolerance test was normal. A magnetic resonance image (MRI) of the brain and posterior fossa was performed with the adminstration of gadolinium. No abnormalities were observed in the brain or in the region of the VIII nerve complex.

Basic Audiometric Evaluation

Figure 1 shows routine pure-tone and speech audiometric data. With the exception of the threshold at 250 Hz in the right ear (25 dB HL), all pure-tone thresholds were within normal limits. The PTA (average of pure-tone threshold hearing levels at 500, 1000, and 2000 Hz) was 12 dB HL for the right ear and 10 dB HL for the left ear. Results of basic speech audiometry were also within normal limits. The threshold for spondee words was 20 dB HL in each ear, the PB score at 80 dB HL was 96 percent in the left ear, 90 percent in the right ear, and the maximum of the performance versus intensity (PI) function for SSI sentences at 0 dB MCR function was 90 percent in the right ear and 100 percent in the left ear. Immittance audiometry showed a normal, type A, tympanogram in each ear, and acoustic reflex thresholds, both crossed and uncrossed, varied from 90-95 dB HL across the frequency range from 500 to 4000 Hz.

The masking level difference (MLD) for a 500-Hz pure tone in the presence of broad-band noise was 16 dB, well within the normal range. On the routine DSI test, however, the subject scored 97 percent on the right ear but only 79 percent on the left ear. This 18 percent interaural difference exceeds the normal boundary of 16 percent established by Fifer et al (1983).

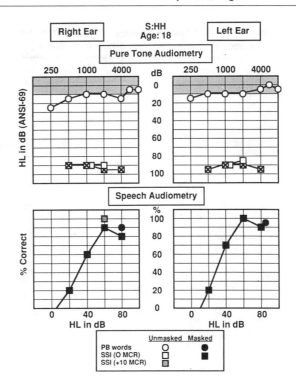

Figure 1 Pure-tone and speech audiometric findings in an 18-year-old woman who complained that she had difficulty hearing her high-school teachers.

NEUROPSYCHOLOGIC EXAMINATION

The subject underwent a neuropsychologic evaluation, including tests of cognitive, perceptual, perceptual-motor, simple and choice reaction times, and other neurobehavioral abilities. The evaluation, described in previous communications (Jerger et al, 1989), was administered and interpreted by a neuropsychologist. Findings are summarized in Tables 1 and 2. Table 1 shows scores on the various subtests of the Wechsler Adult Intelligence Scale (WAIS), the Wechsler Memory Scale, the Boston Naming Test, and the Spatial Orientation Memory Test. Table 2 lists simple auditory, simple visual, and 4-choice visual reaction times.

The profile of neuropsychologic abilities in this patient was remarkable for evidence of:

1. supranormal global intelligence
2. supranormal speed of mental processing
3. supranormal visual-spatial organizational abilities
4. supranormal higher cognitive abilities, including vocabulary and verbal similarities
5. discrepancy between global intelligence and fund of knowledge (information).

Table 1 Performance Scores of Experimental Subject on Selected Cognitive Measures

Cognitive Measure	Score
WAIS-R: Verbal Tests*	
Information	8
Vocabulary	13
Arithmetic	8
Comprehension	12
Similarities	17
Digit span	11
WAIS-R: Performance Tests*	
Picture completion	13
Picture arrangement	12
Block design	13
Object assembly	13
Digit symbol	13
WAIS-R: Summary	
Verbal IQ	105
Performance IQ	120
Full scale IQ	112
Wechsler Memory Scale†	
Passages	9.5
Visual reproduction	13
Associative learning	21
Boston Naming Test‡	57
Spatial Orientation Memory‡	14

*age-corrected scores
†scaled scores
‡raw scores

The subject reports "missing" auditory information in school tasks, a condition that may account for the relative weakness in fund of information in spite of high global intelligence. The arithmetic subtest of the WAIS-R is not only a test of mathematical abilities, but due to its format (auditory presentations of mathematical problems to be manipulated without benefit of pencil and paper) it should also be considered a test of auditory manipulation of arithmetic information. Parallel tests of attention span and memory for visual-spatial information and its manipulation (visual-motor tasks) did not reveal similar deficits. In fact, the subject performed in the supranormal range on these tests.

On the Hand Preference Questionnaire (Annett, 1970) the subject showed a profile associated with mixed handedness. She indicated preference for the right hand on eight items, the left hand on two items, and either hand on two items. In view of this finding it is interesting to note, in Table 2, that simple auditory and simple visual reaction times were shorter with the left hand than with the right hand.

EXPERIMENTAL AUDIOLOGIC EVALUATION

We administered a series of behavioral tests selected to evaluate monaural, binaural, and soundfield processing of auditory signals. Monaural and binaural tasks were administered via earphones, soundfield tasks via loudspeakers. In the following sections we present, for the sake of continuity, only enough information on methodology to permit an understanding of the figures and tables. Expanded descriptions of methodology are available to the interested reader as appended notes.

Monaural Tasks

Monaural tasks could be classified into two groups: (1) tasks involving the controlled study of rapid temporal analysis, and (2) a task involving the discrimination of differences in duration.

Rapid temporal analysis was studied in two ways; (1) variation in the onset of two pure tones, and (2) variation in the onset of voicing.

To measure variation in *pure-tone onset* we employed a technique modified from a paradigm originally described by Hirsh (1959) and Hirsh and Sherrick (1961),[1] in which two tones, differing in frequency and by an onset time difference, Δt, are presented simultaneously. In our modification the subject judged whether the two tones were "same" or "different." Figure 2 shows percent correct "different" judgments for each ear as a function of Δt. The false alarm rate, for trials with no onset difference ($\Delta t = 0$), was low in both ears (3 of 225 trials in the left ear; 0 of

---

[1] A pair of tone bursts was presented to the subject at a level of 70 dB SPL. The frequency of one tone burst was 800 Hz, the other 1200 Hz. The 800 Hz burst always had a duration of 500 msec. The onset of the 1200 Hz burst could be delayed, relative to the onset of the 800 Hz burst, by a variable amount. Both bursts, however, ended simultaneously. Thus the only clue to discrimination was the difference in onset times. Performance was measured over a single block of 300 successive pairs of tone bursts. The interpair interval was 2 seconds. The value of Δt was 25 msec in 25 pairs, 50 msec in 25 pairs, 100 msec in 25 pairs, and 0 msec (no onset difference) in the remaining 225 pairs. Thus the *a priori* probability of a difference was 0.33. We chose this value, rather than the more traditional 0.50, in order to force the subject to adopt a relatively more stringent response criterion. For this task the subject judged whether the two members of the pair were "same" or "different." Presumably a judgment of "different" was made on the basis of the perception of differing onset times.

Table 2   Norms and Performance Scores of Experimental Subject on Three Measures of Reaction Time

Reaction Time Measure	Norm*	Experimental Subject		
		Right	Left	Difference %
Simple auditory	221	220.8	190.1	– 13.9
Simple visual	253	223.0	199.2	– 10.7
Four-choice visual	454	441.9	459.2	3.9

*Reaction time in milliseconds, based on young adults with a mean age of 24.5 years. Mahurin R, Pirozzolo J. (1986). Chronometric analysis: clinical applications in aging and dementia. *Dev Neuropsych* 2: 345–362.

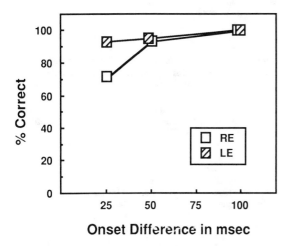

Figure 2   Perception of temporal order. Two tone bursts, differing in pitch, start at different times but end simultaneously. Percent correct discrimination as a function of difference in onset time.

225 trials in the right ear). In general, performance on this task was in good agreement with the 20 msec value reported by Hirsh (1959) for the 75 percent point of the psychometric function relating onset difference to judgment of temporal order. There was no evidence of a significant problem in the appreciation of small differences in onset times of tonal signals.

To measure variation in *voice-onset* we employed a set of consonant-vowel (CV) stimuli that had been generated on a speech synthesizer at the University of Oregon. The CVs were three formant patterns that differed in the acoustic parameter of voice onset time (VOT). The VOT continuum ranged from 0 to 70 msec in 10 msec increments. Normal listeners perceive the series of stimuli in terms of two discrete categories (ba-pa). Tape recorded stimuli (random series of 30 examples of each VOT var-

iant) were presented monaurally. The intertrial interval was 5 sec. The subject labeled each target that she heard as "ba" or "pa." The examiner recorded the subject's verbal responses. Signals were presented, without background competition, at 60 dB SPL.

Figure 3 plots percent correct "pa" judgments against voice-onset time in msec. Results are similar for the two ears and show the relatively sharp boundaries characteristic of categoric perception. The voice onset time corresponding to the 50 percent point of the identification function is about 30 msec, a value in close agreement with a range of 25 to 31 msec reported by Jerger et al, (1987) using the same taped tokens on three normal children in the 11 to 12 year age range.

Duration discrimination was measured using a three-tone sequence paradigm suggested by Musiek (1989).[2] Results showed no overall difficulty with duration discrimination. Scores were 97 percent correct on the right ear and 90 percent correct on the left ear. We did note, however, that performance was noticeably poorer for one of the six sequences (SLS) than for any of the other five. For the SLS sequence performance was 80 percent for the right ear, and only 50 percent for the left ear. Figure 4 shows the percentage of errors as a function of the sequence. Included also, in Figure 4, are normative data (mean percent errors and their standard errors), obtained from 10 young adults. The isolated abnormality for the SLS sequence in comparison with results or the other five sequences, in our subject, is readily apparent. The fact that our subject's errors are specific to a

---

[2] The subject heard a sequence of three tone bursts. The duration of each burst was either 250 msec (short or S) or 500 msec (long L). There were 6 possible permutations of these two durations over a three-burst sequence (i.e., SLS, SSL, SLL, LSS, LSL, and LLS). Each permutation was presented 10 times. The interval between successive tone bursts was 100 msec. The frequency of each tone burst was 1000 Hz. Tones were presented via earphone at 70 dB SPL. A white noise at the same level (0 dB signal-to-noise or S/N ratio) was mixed with the test signal. The subject was seated before a console containing two response buttons. Above each button was a vertical bar. One bar was twice the length of the other. The subject was instructed to listen to a three-burst sequence, then respond by pushing the buttons in the proper order. She was instructed that the button aligned beneath the shorter bar represented the "short" sound, and the button aligned beneath the longer bar represented "long" sound. She was to press the buttons in the same pattern as the sequence of durations heard. The 60 sequences were presented in a predetermined quasi-random order, with the constraint that each of the 6 permutations was presented exactly 10 times.

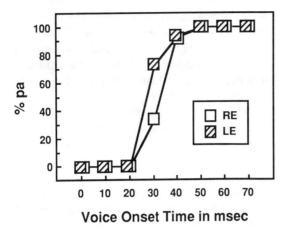

Figure 3 Identification functions for stimuli varying in voice-onset time. Percent "pa" judgments versus voice-onset time continuum.

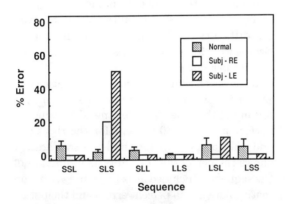

Figure 4 Duration discrimination. Stimulus is a three tone-burst sequence. Duration of each tone burst is either 250 msec ("short") or 500 msec ("long"). Percent errors for each possible sequence, compared with norms obtained on 12 young adults. Note apparently selective deficit for short-long-short (SLS) sequence.

particular sequence effectively rules out an attention deficit as an explanation for the finding.

Binaural Tasks

Binaural tasks could be classified into four groups: (1) a series of tasks involving detection of interaural time and intensity differences, (2) a binaural integration task, (3) a serial recall task, and (4) a series of dichotic listening tasks.

Interaural intensity difference detection was measured using two loudness balance procedures: (1) an alternating binaural loudness balance (ABLB) task and (2) a simultaneous binaural loudness balance (SBLB) task.[3] *Inter-*

aural temporal difference detection was studied through two paradigms; (1) a binaural temporal balance task (BTB) and (2) an adaptive interaural temporal discrimination task (ITD).[4]

Table 3 summarizes results on the four interaural difference detection tasks, along with the means and standard deviations for a refer-

---

[3] The stimuli for both procedures were gated clicks (100 μsec on and 100 msec off), presented in triplets at a rate of one triplet per second. In the ABLB task, click triplets were alternated between the ears. The subject was instructed to adjust the relative intensities of alternating clicks until she perceived them as equally loud in both ears. In the SBLB task, the clicks were presented simultaneously to both ears. The subject was instructed to adjust the relative intensities of clicks until she perceived them as located in the middle of her head. In both tasks, the subject controlled the intensity level of the clicks with a joy stick. When the stick was moved to the right, click intensity was simultaneously increased on the right and decreased on the left. When the stick was moved to the left, intensity changed in the reverse direction. Intensity changes were made in 2-dB increments. Three trials, each with a different starting point, were carried out for both the ABLB and SBLB tasks. The first trial was begun with equal intensities to both ears. In the second and third trials a 20 dB asymmetry was introduced between the ears; first in one direction, then in the opposite direction. The subject's interaural intensity difference, averaged over three trials, was 1.33 dB for each of the loudness balance tasks.

---

[4] The BTB task was analogous to the procedure described above for the SBLB. The subject was required to adjust the relative arrival times of simultaneous clicks until they were perceived at midline. The stimuli were click triplets presented at an overall intensity of 80 dB peak equivalent SPL. Adjustments in relative arrival time to the two ears were made in 20 μsec increments via joy stick. Again, three trials, with different starting points, were carried out. The temporal difference in arrival times between the two ears when perceived at midline, averaged over three trials, was 33.33 μsec.

The interaural temporal discrimination task was carried out using a four-interval, two-alternative, forced-choice, adaptive-test paradigm. Each trial consisted of clicks presented binaurally during each of four listening intervals, which were labeled sequentially on a computer terminal. In each trial, an interaural difference in arrival time was introduced during either the second or the third listening interval (0.50 *a priori* probability). The subject's task was to press a button during the interval in which a difference was detected. Differences in arrival times were initiated at 1000 μsec, with the right ear leading. Thereafter, interaural differences were adjusted according to a two-down, one-up rule (Levitt, 1971), wherein the interaural difference was decreased after two successive correct responses and increased after every incorrect response. Testing continued until fourteen response reversals had been obtained. Differences were changed by a factor of 2 through the fourth reversal and by a factor of the square root of 2 for the next 10 reversals. The mean of the last 10 reversals, 58.20 μsec, was taken as the subject's interaural temporal difference limen.

Table 3   Performance Scores of Experimental Subject on Measures of Interaural Difference Detection

Measure	Experimental Subject Score	Reference Group Mean (SD)
Alternate binaural loudness balance	1.33 dB	3.22 dB (1.75)
Simultaneous binaural loudness balance	1.33 dB	1.66 dB (1.89)
Binaural temporal balance	33.33 μsec	45.93 μsec (14.02)
Interaural temporal discrimination	58.20 μsec	56.37 μsec (25.77)

Also shown are means and standard deviations for a reference group of normal hearing subjects (N = 12).

ence group of 12 normal hearing subjects. On the ABLB, the subject's scores fell within 2 standard deviations of the mean. On the remaining three tasks, the subject's performance was within 1 standard deviation of the mean. Thus, there was no evidence of difficulty in detecting small time or intensity differences between the two ears.

The *Speech with Alternating Masking Index* (SWAMI; Jerger et al, 1960) was used to assess the subject's ability to integrate fragmentary speech information from the two ears.[5] Our subject achieved a maximum of 88 percent correct at both 80 and 100 dB SPL, falling within the range of expected performance for normal hearing listeners (Jerger et al, 1960).

The materials and procedures used in the *serial recall* task have been detailed previously (Jerger and Watkins, 1988).[6] Figure 5 compares the average percent correct score, across all serial positions, for the visual versus auditory conditions without a suffix, and for the three auditory conditions with and without suffixes. Comparison of the visual versus auditory conditions in the left-hand panel shows better recall

for the auditory presentation mode than for the visual mode, a normal modality effect. The auditory advantage was due to an increase in performance for the last one or two items of the auditory list—again, a normal finding, the auditory recency effect. Figure 6 illustrates the magnitude of the recency effect by detailing the serial-position curves for the two presentation modalities.

Results in the right hand panel of Figure 5 show that recall was reduced, as expected, when an irrelevant speech suffix was appended to the auditory list. As with normal subjects, the "suffix effect" did not occur with a noise suffix. Thus the normal distinction between speech and nonspeech suffixes in memory was observed.

In short, serial recall for lists of digits revealed what are widely regarded as cardinal characteristics of normal short-term memory; namely the modality effect, the auditory recency effect, and the speech suffix effect. As shown in Table 1, performance on the digit-span subtest of the WAIS was also within normal limits.

Dichotic listening was explored using three measures: (1) the Staggered Spondee Word (SSW) test (Katz, 1962), (2) the Competing Environmental Sounds (CES) tests (Katz, 1985),

---

[5] The test material consisted of a dual-channel tape-recording to monosyllabic word lists (PAL-PBs) on which were superimposed 500 msec noise bursts. The noise bursts, recorded at a level 20 dB more intense than the words, alternated between the two ears at a rate of one burst every 0.5 sec. When this tape is played through either earphone singly the words are virtually unintelligible; the periodic noise bursts effectively mask all or part of most of the words. When listening through both earphones, however, and provided that the two earphones are phase matched, the listener experiences an illusion in which the bursts of noise are localized to the ears, but the words are localized to the center of the head. The word fragments from each ear are "fused" into a single unitary image. As a result the words are easily understood and the performance score is in the 90 to 100 percent range. For the present subject a performance-intensity function was obtained by presenting 25 words at each of three intensity levels: 60, 80, and 100 dB SPL. The subject's task was to repeat each of the words. Performance was scored as percent correct at each of three intensity levels.

[6] In brief, the task required the subject to reproduce a list of 7 digits presented in one of two modes; auditory or visual. The lists were comprised of the digits 1 through 6 presented via microcomputer at a rate of one item per second. For the auditory mode, tests items were presented binaurally at 75 dB SPL. For the visual mode, items were flashed in numerical form on the computer screen. For the auditory mode, the subject was tested under three conditions: no suffix, speech suffix (the digit 9), and noise suffix (burst of white noise). For the visual mode, the subject was tested only under the no-suffix condition. Twenty practice items representing the conditions were administered. Then 10 test trials were gathered in each condition. For all trials, a light on a response panel signaled the subject when to begin recall. The subject's task was to reproduce the list. The subject responded by pushing buttons, labeled 1 through 6 on a response box, in the correct order.

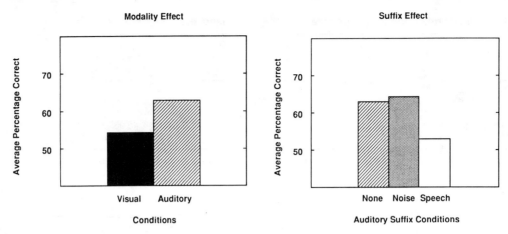

Figure 5 Summary of results of serial-recall paradigm. Average percent correct scores for modality effect (visual versus auditory) and suffix effect (no suffix versus noise suffix versus speech suffix).

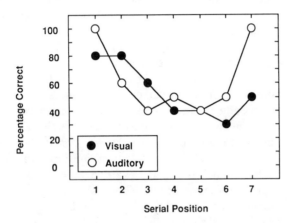

Figure 6 Serial position curves for auditory and visual modalities.

and the Dichotic Speech Intelligibility (DSI) test (Fifer et al, 1983).[7]

The *SSW* and *CES* were both administered at 60 dB SPL. For the SSW test, only raw scores were computed. The subject scored 100 percent correct for both ears in all noncompeting conditions. In the competing conditions, she scored 92.5 percent and 97.5 percent for the right and left ears, respectively. On the CES test, the subject scored 100 percent in both ears.

We expanded the Dichotic Sentence Identification (DSI) paradigm to include two monotic control conditions and three additional dichotic test conditions. In the first monotic condition (i.e., "single" sentence condition), the 20 sentences were presented sequentially via a single channel. The subject's task was simply to report the sentence heard. The purpose of this

condition was to ensure that the subject was able to perform the task, in each ear separately, when there was no competing sentence in the other ear. For the second monotic condition (i.e., "double-sequential" condition), pairs of sentences were recorded, one immediately following the other, onto a single channel of cassette tape. The subject's task in this condition was to report both sentences of the pair after the second sentence had been presented. This condition was incorporated to control for memory. If the subject can correctly report both of the sequential sentences presented monaurally, then memory, *per se*, cannot be invoked as a basis for poor dichotic performance.

The three dichotic conditions added to the battery differed from the conventional DSI paradigm (i.e., "free recall" condition) only in terms of the instructions to the subject. In the

---

[7] The *Dichotic Sentence Identification Test (DSI)* consists of 90 pairs of sentences randomly selected from the 10 seven-word, third-order sentence approximations comprising the Synthetic Sentence Identification (SSI) Test (Jerger et al, 1968). Each member of the sentence pair has been temporally aligned in the onset and offset to within 100 μsec of the other. In the conventional DSI, sentences are presented at the rate of one pair every ten seconds, via dual-channel cassette tape, simultaneously to the two ears. The 10 sentence targets are listed on a response panel situated in front of the subject. Beside each of the sentences is a response button. The subject is instructed to identify each member of the sentence pair by pushing the corresponding response buttons on the panel. Performance is scored as percent correct identification for each ear according to a free recall format, in which subjects can report either ear first and need not designate the ear in which a specific target was heard.

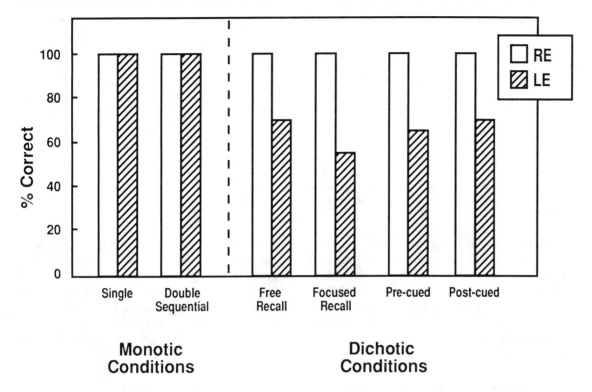

Figure 7 Dichotic sentence identification (DSI) scores in two monotic and four dichotic conditions.

second dichotic condition the subject was instructed to identify the sentences heard in one ear only (i.e., "focused recall"). By comparing performance in the "free-recall" versus "focused-recall" conditions, the effect of divided versus focused attention could be evaluated. The right ear was designated the ear-of-report for the first 20 items; the left ear for the second 20. In the third and fourth dichotic conditions, the subject was again instructed to report one ear only. In both of these conditions, however, the to-be-reported ear was designated by one of two lights, labeled "right" and "left," located on top of the response panel in front of the subject. In the "pre-cued" condition, the to-be-reported ear was signaled immediately prior to sentence delivery. This condition allowed us to evaluate the subject's ability to shift attention rapidly from one channel to the other. In the "post-cued" condition, the ear-to-be-reported was signaled immediately following sentence delivery. Thus, the subject was required to attend to, and remember, both sentences until the designated ear-to-be-reported was cued. The ear-of-report was randomized between the two ears in both conditions. In all conditions, sentences were presented at 60 dB SPL.

Figure 7 summarizes results for all DSI test conditions. In both of the monotic conditions,

the subject scored 100 percent correct identification in both ears. She also scored 100 percent for the right ear in all four dichotic conditions. However, performance was consistently depressed in the left ear across all dichotic conditions. Thus, while scoring 100 percent in both ears in each of the monotic conditions, the subject showed a relatively consistent ear asymmetry, of 30 to 40 percent, over all dichotic conditions, regardless of attention or memory demands. If such cognitive factors were playing a significant role in the ear asymmetry, we might expect, for example, performance on the left ear to improve, in the focused recall and pre-cued conditions. These conditions are more similar to the monotic conditions where one attends to, and reports, only one ear. Such performance shifts did not, however, occur. The relatively constant ear asymmetry, in spite of variation in cognitive demand, suggests an auditory-specific basis for the performance deficit on the left ear.

Soundfield Tasks

Soundfield studies could be classified into two groups: (1) localization tasks, and (2) tasks requiring the suppression of background noise.

Table 4   Performance Scores of Experimental Subject on Measures of Absolute Sound Localization

Measure	Experimental Subject's Score	Reference Group Mean (SD)
Horizontal localization		
Facing forward	1.90°	0.80° (0.74)
Left ear forward	11.20°	10.93° (4.32)
Right ear forward	8.50°	7.69° (2.96)
Vertical localization		
Facing forward	4.40°	5.85° (2.41)
Left ear forward	4.80°	6.22° (1.61)
Right ear forward	4.50°	6.06° (1.84)

Data are the mean absolute differences (degrees) between the selected and activated speakers. Also shown are mean absolute differences (± 1 standard deviation) for reference group of twelve normal hearing subjects on the same tasks.

Localization tasks included both the absolute localization of sound sources in space and the relative localization of a signal in one field with a different signal in the opposite field. Both studies were carried out in reverberant rooms.

For *absolute localization*[8] the subject was seated facing 12 loudspeakers mounted on the opposite wall at a distance of 2.7 m. The loudspeakers were arranged in the form of a cross, with the center loudspeaker located directly in front of the subject. Three loudspeakers were located at 9.8 degrees, 19.1 degrees, and 26.5 degrees to the right, left, and above the center loudspeaker. Two loudspeakers were located at 9.8 degrees and 19.1 degrees below center. The loudspeakers were labeled "1" to "7" from left to right, and "A" to "F" from top to bottom.

In the horizontal condition, the subject's mean absolute error was 1.9 degrees when facing the loudspeakers, 11.2 degrees with the left ear toward the loudspeakers, and 8.5 degrees with the right ear toward the loudspeakers. In the vertical condition, mean absolute errors were 4.4 degrees when facing the loudspeakers, 4.8 degrees with the left ear toward the loudspeakers, and 4.5 degrees with the right ear toward

the loudspeakers. These results, along with the means and standard deviations for a reference groups of young adults, are listed in Table 4. Results show that the subject performed normally in the absolute localization of clicks in either the horizontal or vertical plane.

For *relative localization*[9] the subject was seated facing a semicircular table containing two loudspeakers, one to the left of the subject's midline, the other to the right of midline. One of the two loudspeakers was arbitrarily defined as the "reference" or fixed loudspeaker, the other as the variable loudspeaker. Before each trial the reference loudspeaker was set to an azimuth position of 45 degrees. The variable loudspeaker was then positioned at one of nine azimuths in the opposite field. These positions varied in five-degree steps from 25 degrees to 65 degrees. Our subject consistently localized correctly (three

---

[8] Absolute localization was tested separately in the horizontal and vertical planes. Stimuli for both of the conditions were clicks presented at 84 dB peak equivalent SPL. For each trial, the subject's task was to identify the origin of the clicks. She responded by calling out the corresponding loudspeaker number, in the case of horizontal localization, and loudspeaker letter, in the case of vertical localization. For both conditions, the subject was oriented in each of three directions: facing loudspeakers, left ear toward the loudspeakers, and right ear toward the loudspeakers. Twenty-five trials were carried out for each of the three directions. For each trial, the difference in degrees between the selected and the activated loudspeaker was calculated. Accuracy of localization was quantified as the mean of the absolute differences between selected and activated loudspeakers.

[9] The reference loudspeaker was positioned in the right field on 50 percent of trials, in the left field on the remaining 50 percent of trials. The subject's head was a constant 2.8 m from each loudspeaker position. The test stimuli were pairs of tone bursts presented alternately to the two loudspeakers at 60 dB SPL. The frequency of the tone burst from the reference loudspeaker was always 800 Hz, from the variable loudspeaker always 1200 Hz. The interval between the two test tones was 500 msec. The subject's task was to indicate, after the presentation of each pair of tones, whether the angle of azimuth of the variable loudspeaker agreed with the angle of azimuth of the reference loudspeaker (i.e., was the tone from the variable loudspeaker as far to the right of midline as the tone from the reference loudspeaker was to the left of midline, or vice versa). The subject responded "same" when the variable tone was localized at the same azimuth, in its field, as the perceived azimuth of the reference tone in the opposite field. The subject responded "right" when the variable tone was localized to the right of the target azimuth in the variable field, and "left" when the variable tone was localized to the left of the target azimuth. Each condition was tested three times. Conditions were sequentially randomized in such a way that the same condition never occurred twice in succession.

out of three trials) when the difference between azimuths was 15 degrees. Nor were there significant field asymmetries. A normal control, a 23-year-old woman tested on the same apparatus, did not do as well, requiring a difference of 20 degrees to achieve the same level of performance. Thus we observed no apparent deficit in the relative localization of sounds.

Background suppression was studied in a sound-treated room. Figure 8 shows the experimental arrangement. The subject was seated equidistant between, and 1.6 meters from, two loudspeakers. A third loudspeaker was mounted on a stand and positioned 0.5 meters above, and slightly behind, the subject's head. A pair of signal lights, labeled "right" and "left", were mounted directly in front of the subject at eye level. The subject's ability to suppress auditory background while attending to auditory foreground was studied in three ways: (1) threshold effects; (2) suprathreshold effects; and (3) a cued target task.

Threshold effects were studied by presenting a target signal (auditory foreground) from either the left or right loudspeakers, while simultaneously presenting a competing signal (auditory background) from either the same or the opposite loudspeaker.[10] Figure 9 summarizes the experimental results. The difference between

thresholds in the ipsilateral competition (IC) and contralateral competition (CC) modes is represented by solid bars, for the right ear, and striped bars for the left ear. The height of each bar represents the effect of moving the competition from the same side to the opposite side of the head, that is, the extent to which threshold is improved by having the target and competition coming from opposite sides of the head rather than from the same side.

Figure 9 shows that, when the target was presented in the right auditory field, this advantage was typically about 20 dB. When the target was presented in the left auditory field,

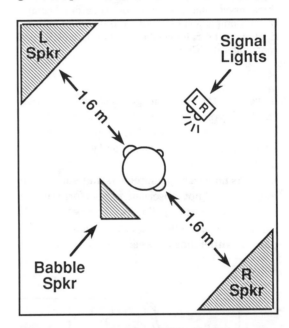

Figure 8   Arrangement of experimental apparatus for studies of background suppression.

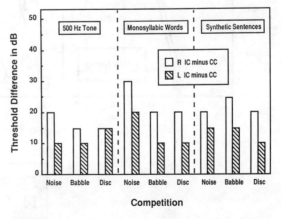

Figure 9   Combinations of three targets and three types of background competition. Comparison of threshold differences between conditions of ipsilateral competition (IC) and contralateral (CC) for each ear.

---

[10] With the intensity of the competition at a fixed level the intensity of the target was varied until threshold for the target had been defined. We employed three different targets; (1) 500 Hz tone bursts, (2) monosyllabic (PB) words, and (3) synthetic sentences (SSI). Each target was paired with one of three different types of competition; (1) white noise, (2) multitalker babble, and (3) the continuous discourse of a single talker.

The competing signal was always presented at an SPL of 50 dB. When the target and the competition were delivered by the same loudspeaker the condition is referred to as ipsilateral competition (IC). When the competition was presented from the loudspeaker in the opposite auditory field the condition is referred to as contralateral competition (CC). For purposes of analysis, data are displayed in the form of the difference between thresholds in the IC and CC modes. The difference is a measure of the extent to which the subject is able to suppress the competition when it comes from the auditory field opposite the target, as compared with her ability to suppress the competition when it comes from the same side as the target. All thresholds were measured in 5-dB steps according to a modified method of limits (Carhart and Jerger, 1959). Tone bursts had a 10 msec rise-decay time and a total duration of 500 msec. Monosyllabic words were taken from the PAL PB lists (Egan, 1948). Synthetic sentences were taken from the SSI lists (Jerger et al, 1968). The multitalker babble was taken from the SPIN test (Kalikow et al, 1977), the single-talker continuous discourse was taken from the SSI test.

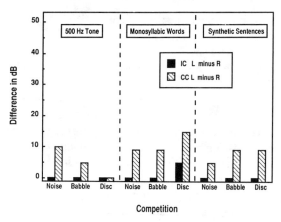

Figure 10   Same data as Figure 9. Combinations of three targets and three types of background competition. Comparison of threshold differences between right and left ears for conditions of ipsilateral (IC) and contralateral (CC) competition.

however, the advantage was consistently smaller, typically about 10 dB. The magnitude of this ear asymmetry did not appear to be related to either type of target or type of competition.

It is noteworthy, moreover, that such asymmetries were not observed for performance in any condition of ipsilateral competition. In Figure 10 the same data are replotted to compare the difference between the two sides when the competition was ipsilateral versus the difference between the two sides when the competition was contralateral. When target and competition were presented from the same side (IC mode), threshold asymmetries were slight. Ear differences never exceeded 5 dB for any of the various combinations of target and competition. Larger asymmetries appeared only when the target and the competition were presented in opposite fields (CC mode).

In summary, when threshold measures were used to define ability to suppress auditory background, our subject showed an ear asymmetry of about 10 dB. Unwanted background was less successfully suppressed when the background competition was presented in the right auditory field and the target was presented in the left auditory field.

To measure *suprathreshold background suppression* we presented SSI sentences at various message-to-competition ratios (MCRs). There were three types of competition; white noise, multitalker babble, and single-talker continuous discourse. When the target was presented via the right loudspeaker the competition was presented via the left loudspeaker and vice versa. Figure 11 summarizes the results of these measures. Percent correct sentence identification is plotted against MCR for each of the three types of background competition. When the

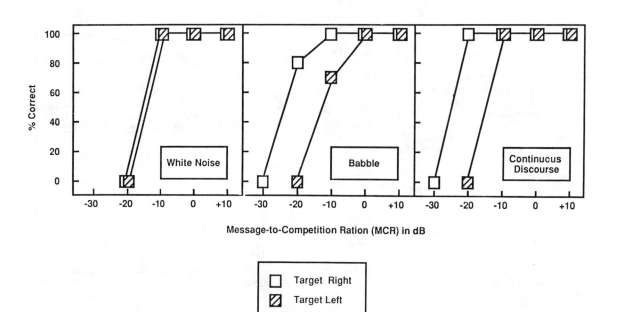

Figure 11   Suprathreshold SSI scores as a function of MCR, in the presence of three types of contralateral competition.

competition was white noise, there was no difference between sides. But when the competition was either multitalker babble or single-talker continuous discourse, performance was better when the target was presented from the right side than from the left side. In terms of MCR the difference was about 10 dB. In other words, in order to achieve equivalent performance, the MCR had to be made more favorable by about 10 dB when the target was presented in the left field. And, again, such asymmetry did not appear in any of the conditions of ipsilateral competition. The fact that white noise, as competition, did not produce the performance asymmetries that were observed for the threshold measures may be related to the fact that the data of Figure 11 represent only the effects of competition on suprathreshold synthetic sentence identification scores. Previous research (Carhart and Tillman, 1970) has demonstrated that, in this paradigm, noise is a less effective source of competition than is actual speech.

For the *cued target task* we employed the instrumentation already illustrated in Figure 8. This paradigm[11] represents, for the subject, a relatively difficult case of foreground-background differentiation. The subject must attend to continuous discourse lateralized to one side of the head while simultaneously suppressing noncoherent continuous discourse lateralized to the other side of the head. Then, when a signal light cues the opposite side, the subject must redefine foreground as the discourse coming from the new side, and redefine background as the signal previously defined as foreground. Throughout this alternate cueing, the subject must also suppress the additional background represented by the multitalker babble from above.

In spite of the complexity of this task our subject completed it successfully. She complained, however, that it was more difficult when the left side was cued than when the right side was cued. She volunteered that, "When the babble comes on, the sound from the left loudspeaker gets fainter." Figure 12 plots percent error scores from each side, both without babble and at various target-to-babble ratios. Whenever the babble was present, the left side showed more errors than the right side, and the magnitude of the difference increased as the target-to-babble ratio became less favorable.

ELECTROPHYSIOLOGIC STUDIES

We studied hearing function in a non-behavioral context by means of three different types of electrophysiologic response: (1) acoustic reflexes, (2) auditory evoked potentials, and (3) otoacoustic emissions.

Acoustic Reflex

The morphology of the acoustic reflex was examined by means of special laboratory ap-

---

[11] The subject was seated in the sound-treated room equidistant between the right and left loudspeakers. The third loudspeaker was mounted on a stand immediately above, and slightly behind the subject's head. Directly in front of the subject, at eye level, were mounted two lights, one labeled "left" and the other "right." A stereo tape recording was played to both the right and left loudspeakers. One channel of the tape contained 20 min of continuous discourse, a male talker with General American dialect reading an adventure story written in the first person. The second channel contained the same recording but offset by about 2 min relative to the first channel. Thus the identical discourse was recorded on both channels, but at any moment in time different parts of the story appeared on the 2 channels. When both loudspeakers were activated, therefore, the continuous discourse was "noncoherent" in the sense that different speech messages were directed to each ear. A trial, or cued listen interval was defined by one of the two lights directly in front of the subject. During the time that one or the other light was illuminated, the subject must attend to the discourse from the side indicated by the signal light. The subject's task, during this cued interval, was to press a response button each time she heard the personal pronoun "I" from the cued direction. During each cued interval, anywhere from 0 to 12 "I's" were presented from the cued side. An error was scored if the subject failed to respond when an "I" was presented, or if she responded when an "I" had not been presented. In order to manipulate the difficulty of the task, continuous multitalker babble was played from a second tape recorder through the loudspeaker mounted above the subject's head. The presentation level of the continuous discourse containing the "I" targets was 60 dB SPL. The intensity level of the multitalker babble was varied to produce target-to-babble ratios of -10 dB, -15 dB and -20 dB. In addition, there was a "no babble" condition.

The subject's performance was based on responses during 48 cued intervals, 12 intervals at each of four competing babble conditions. At each condition six intervals were cued to the loudspeaker on the right side, and six were cued to the loudspeaker on the left side. The sequence in which sides were cued was quasi-random, with the constraint that the right and left sides be cued an equal number of times. The total number of target presentations for a given competing babble condition varied between 78 and 81 per condition across the four conditions. The total number of targets presented over all conditions was 319 of which 161 were presented to the right side, and 158 to the left side. From these raw data percent error scores were computed for right and left sides at each MCR condition.

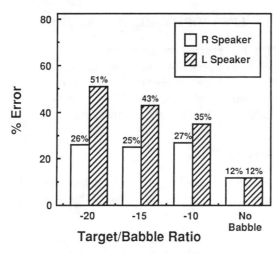

Figure 12 Cued target task. Percent errors versus target/babble ratio for cueing of right and left loudspeakers.

paratus described elsewhere (Stach and Jerger, 1984). Using dual acoustic probes, both ears are measured simultaneously, yielding averaged reflex waveforms (n=8) for the right crossed and uncrossed, and the left crossed and uncrossed reflex waveforms. For the present study we presented 500 msec reflex-eliciting signals at levels ranging from 90 to 110 dB SPL. Test signals were either tone bursts at frequencies of 500, 1000, 2000, or 4000 Hz, or burst of white noise.

In general reflex morphology was normal for all eliciting signals. All amplitude and latency measures were within normal limits. We did observe, however, that reflex amplitude growth functions tended to be smaller for reflexes elicited by sound to the left ear than for sound to the right ear. Figure 13 illustrates such amplitude growth functions for the 2000-Hz eliciting signal, where the ear difference was most prominent. In both the crossed and uncrossed modes, reflex amplitude was slightly greater when signals were presented to the right ear than to the left ear. Similar differences were observed for all other eliciting signals.

Auditory Evoked Potentials

We measured early (ABR), middle (MLR), late (LVR), and long-latency task-related (LLTRR) auditory evoked potentials by means of conventional averaging procedures.[12]

In general ABR, MLR, LVR, and LLTRR waveforms were well-formed and within normal

ranges for absolute latencies, interpeak latencies, and amplitudes. It was the case, however, that both the N_a - P_a amplitude of the MLR, and the N_1 - P_2 amplitude of the LVR were smaller with left ear stimulation than with right ear stimulation. Figure 14 shows representative waveforms, and their replicates, for ABR, MLR, and LVR auditory evoked potentials. Figure 15 shows LLTRR waveforms for both right ear and left ear stimulation. Included, also, in Figure 15 is an averaged electro-oculographic response (EOG) from electrodes monitoring eye movement. In the case of LLTRR the displayed waveform is the difference between a baseline condition, in which the frequent signal occurred 100 percent of the time, and the experimental condition, in which the frequent signal occurred 80 percent of the time and the rare signal occurred 20 percent of the time. This algorithm effectively cancels out the LVR, which occurs in both conditions. Thus the difference waveform reflects only the response to the rare event. The LLTRR waveform shows the expected positive peak in the vicinity of 300 msec (sometimes referred to as P_3 or P_{300}), indicating a normal task-related potential.

Otoacoustic Emissions

Is it possible that our subject's auditory problem stems from a subtle cochlear defect not revealed by the conventional pure-tone audiogram? Could the left ear deficit revealed by the various speech audiometric procedures derive

---

[12] The active electrode at C_z was referred to the ipsilateral earlobe, for ABR, MLR, and LVR, and referred to linked earlobes for the LLTRR. EEG preamplifiers were Grass P 511, with filters set from 300 to 3000 for ABR, 3 to 300 for MLR, and 1 to 100 for LVR and LLTRR. Filter slope was 6 dB/octave. For ABR we averaged 2560 signals, for MLR 1280 signals, for LVR 160 signals, and for LLTRR 128 signals. For ABR the stimulus was a 100-microsecond, alternating-polarity click. For MLR the stimulus was a 1000 Hz tone pip (2-1-2 configuration) with a total duration of 5 msec. For LVR the signal was a 1000 Hz tone burst with a 5 msec rise-decay time and a total duration of 500 msec. For LLTRR we used the "oddball" paradigm. The frequent stimulus was the 1000 Hz tone burst used for LVR; the rare stimulus was a 500 Hz tone burst of equal duration. Rare stimuli were randomly interspersed among frequent stimuli, except that two rare stimuli were not permitted to occur successively. The *a priori* probability of a rare stimulus was 0.20. Stimulus rate was 24/sec for ABR, 2.1/sec for MLR, and 0.5/sec for LVR and LLTRR. For ABR the epoch was 15 msec, for MLR 100 msec, for LVR 800 msec, and for LLTRR 1200 msec following a 100 msec, pre-stimulus baseline.

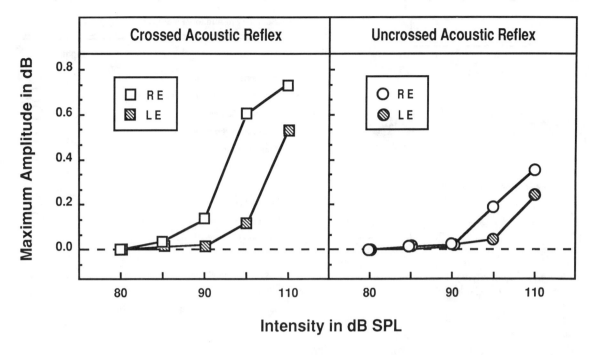

Figure 13   Amplitude growth functions for both crossed and uncrossed suprathreshold acoustic reflex waveforms.

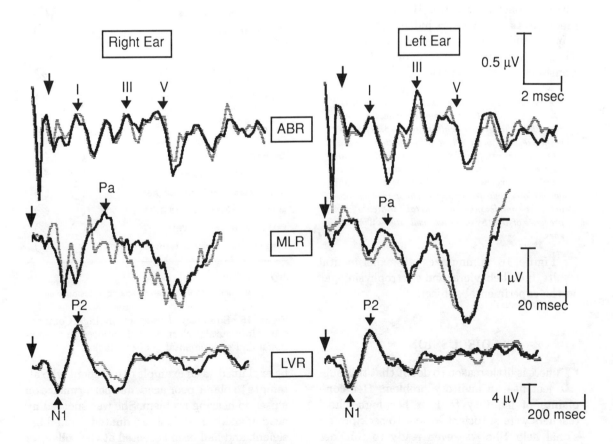

Figure 14   Early, middle, and late averaged auditory evoked potentials.

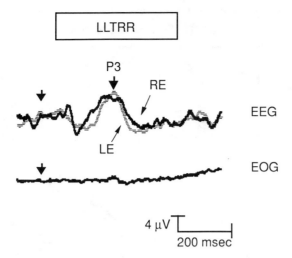

Figure 15 Long-latency, task-related averaged potentials generated by "oddball" paradigm.

from left-sided hair cell damage which in some way alters normal speech perception without, at the same time, impacting pure-tone sensitivity? In an attempt to answer this question, we studied transiently-evoked and distortion-product otoacoustic emissions. These measurements were carried out in the laboratory of Dr. Brenda Lonsbury-Martin, Baylor College of Medicine, to whom we are indebted for the otoacoustic emission data and their interpretation. The following summary is condensed from Dr. Lonsbury-Martin's report:

> *Transiently evoked emissions were examined in both ears. Each ear emitted a healthy emission, with the left ear exhibiting a slightly larger response...A complete test of distortion-product emission growth functions was accomplished for both ears. These emissions, in general, tended to be slightly larger than normal, except for the right ear at one test frequency...The patient's otoacoustic emissions, in general, indicate the presence of healthy outer hair cell function in both ears.*

Figure 16 summarizes all experimental results, both behavioral and electrophysiologic, on the experimental subject.

DISCUSSION

There is little reason to doubt that this subject has an auditory problem. Her complaints of inability to hear her high-school teachers were sufficient for her to seek professional help. She was even ready to consider using a hearing aid. Nor could her complaints

Summary of Auditory Findings

	Right	Left
Pure-tone audiogram	○	○
Monosyllabic word recognition (PB)	○	○
Synthetic Sentence Identification (SSI)	○	○
Masking level difference (MLD)	○	
Tympanogram	○	○
Acoustic reflex thresholds	○	○
Temporal order	○	○
Voice-onset time	○	○
Duration discrimination	○	⊘
Interaural intensity difference detection	○	○
Interaural temporal difference detection	○	○
Speech with Alternating Masking (SWAMI)	○	
Serial recall		○
Staggered Spondee Words (SSW)	○	○
Competing Environmental Sounds (CES)	○	○
Dichotic Sentence Identification (DSI)	○	⊘
Absolute azimuth localization	○	○
Relative azimuth localization	○	○
Soundfield thresholds in ipsilateral vs contralateral competition	○	⊘
Soundfield speech with contralateral competition	○	⊘
Cued target task	○	⊘
Otoacoustic emissions	○	○
Acoustic reflex amplitudes	○	⊘
Auditory brainstem response (ABR)	○	○
Middle latency response (MLR)	○	⊘
Late vertex response (LVR)	○	⊘
Long latency task-related response (P-300)	○	○

Key to symbols:

○ = normal   ⊘ = reduced compared to opposite ear

Figure 16 Summary of auditory findings. Comparison of interaural performance differences on conventional and experimental auditory tasks.

be explained as an example of a student who attempts to blame poor academic performance on a pseudo-hearing problem. She was succeeding academically, had just graduated from high school, and had been accepted at the college of her choice. She was seeking help, not to justify past failure, but to forestall any problems that might jeopardize her future academic performance.

Could her problems be explained by a cognitive deficit in attention, memory, or speed of mental processing? Several lines of evidence argue against an attentional or memory deficit. First, the relatively robust LLTRR potential in the "oddball" paradigm (see Fig. 15) shows that the subject was able to perform satisfactorily in an auditory-monitoring task requiring sustained attention. Second, the neuropsychologic examination showed that, on visual-motor tasks requiring attention and memory, our subject performed in the supranormal range. Further evidence arguing against a memory deficit is the fact that the subject scored normally on the Wechsler Memory Scale and on the Digit Span subtest on the Wechsler Adult Intelligence Scale. Serial recall for lists of digits (see Figs. 5 and 6) also showed normal modality, recency, and speech suffix effects, hallmarks of normal short-term auditory memory. Finally, efforts to manipulate DSI scores by varying cognitive demands on memory and attention (see Fig. 7) were not successful. The fact that performance was 100 percent on both ears in the double sequential condition shows that the ability to remember two sentences long enough to report both sentences was not at issue. In addition, further argument against an attentional problem was the fact that the DSI asymmetry was the same whether the subject was asked to report only what was heard from one pre-cued ear, to report what was heard in both ears, or to report what was heard in an ear that was cued only after the paired sentences had been presented. The constancy of the performance deficit, in the face of variation in attentional and memory demands, argues against a cognitive deficit in either attention, or memory as a viable explanation for the asymmetry in DSI performance.

Finally, evidence against a deficit in speed of mental processing includes the observations that intelligence, visual-spatial organizational abilities, and simple and choice reaction times (see Table 2) were all either in the normal or the supranormal range.

What, then, is the evidence for an auditory-specific, as opposed to an extra-auditory deficit? Perhaps the most persuasive argument lies in the asymmetry of auditory abnormalities. On DSI, and on all soundfield tasks involving a target in one field and speech competition in the other field, the left ear was consistently poorer than the right ear. It is difficult to hypothesize an extra-auditory deficit capable of producing such an interaural asymmetry.

Is it necessary to invoke a central mechanism to explain the abnormality? Could the basis for the left ear deficit be a subtle unilateral cochlear defect? Two lines of evidence argue against this hypothesis. First there is no audiometric evidence, in either the pure-tone audiograms or the conventional speech audiometric results, of a left peripheral disorder. Indeed, pure-tone sensitivity and conventional speech audiometric scores were, if anything, slightly poorer on the right ear. Second, examination by otoacoustic emissions, an exceedingly sensitive measure of inner ear integrity, failed to disclose asymmetry in hair cell function.

These various lines of evidence seem to converge on a central, specifically auditory, deficit involving sound input to the left ear. What can we say about the nature of this central auditory deficit? First, it does not appear to be a problem in rapid temporal analysis. The subject performed normally on tests involving the temporal ordering of pure tones and the perception of voice onset time. In addition the subject performed normally on a variety of measures requiring the processing of small interaural time and intensity differences. Furthermore, all neuropsychologic tests with a time component were in the superior range. Second, it does not appear to be a problem in azimuth localization. The subject had no difficulty in the absolute localization of clicks or in the relative localization of pure tones from either auditory field.

The test procedures in which the subject did have difficulty were; (1) DSI, (2) threshold and suprathreshold measures of speech understanding in the presence of various types of contralateral competition, and (3) the cued target task in the presence of speech competition. Each of these results seems to suggest a fundamental weakness in the processing of targets delivered to the left ear when an interfering background sound was directed to the right ear. Whenever the experimental structure directed a speech target to one ear, and some form of competition either to the other ear or to both ears, our subject did less well when the left ear was targeted. The deficit does not appear to be a problem in the suppression of background competition, *per se*, since there was no asymmetry in performance when the competing message was delivered ipsilaterally (see Fig. 10). Nor does the deficit appear to be a processing disorder for all inputs to the left ear, since there were many experimental conditions, involving relatively difficult listening tasks, in which the left ear performed as well as the right ear (see Fig. 16).

In summary, the present data suggest that this subject has an asymmetric disorder in the processing of binaural, noncoherent signals. When auditory space was structured such that the target was directed to the left ear, and the competition to the right ear, unwanted background was less successfully suppressed than when the physical arrangement was reserved.

Acknowledgments. We are grateful to Rose Chmiel, Gloria Delgado-Vilches, Craig Jordan, Henry Lew, Brenda Lonsbury-Martin, Terrey Penn, Brad Stach, and Debra Wilmington for their assistance in the completion of this project.

REFERENCES

Annett M. (1970). A classification of hand preference by association analysis. *Br J Psychol* 61:303–321.

Barr D. (1972). *Auditory Perceptual Disorders.* Springfield, IL: Charles C Thomas.

Beasley D, Freeman B. (1977). Time-altered speech as a measure of central auditory processing. In: Keith R, ed. *Central Auditory Dysfunction.* New York: Grune & Stratton, 129–176.

Berlin C, Lowe-Bell S, Janneta P, Kline D. (1972). Central auditory deficits after temporal lobectomy. *Arch Otolaryngol* 96:4–10.

Bloom L, Lahey M. (1978). *Language Development and Language Disorders.* New York: John Wiley & Sons.

Calearo C, Antonelli A. (1968). Audiometric findings in brain stem lesions. *Acta Otolaryngol* 66:305–319.

Campbell T, McNeill M. (1985). Effects of presentation rate and divided attention on auditory comprehension in children with acquired language disorder. *J Speech Hear Res* 28:513–520.

Carhart R, Jerger J. (1959). Preferred method for clinical determination of pure-tone thresholds. *J Speech Hear Disord* 24:330–354.

Carhart R, Tillman T. (1970). Interaction of competing speech signals with hearing losses. *Arch Otolaryngol* 91:273–279.

Cohen R. (1980). Auditory skills and the communicative process. *Semin Speech Lang Hear* 1:107–115.

DeMarco S, Harbour A, Hume W, Givens G. (1989). Perception of time-altered monosyllables in a specific group of phonologically disordered children. *Neuropsychologia* 27:753–757.

Egan J. (1948). Articulation testing methods. *Laryngoscope* 58:955–991.

Fifer R, Jerger J, Berlin C, Tobey E, Campbell J. (1983). Development of a dichotic sentence identification test for hearing impaired adults. *Ear Hear* 4:300–305.

Gerber S, Mencher G. (1980). *Auditory dysfunction.* Houston: College-Hill Press.

Gascon G, Johnson R, Burd L. (1986). Central auditory processing and attention deficit disorders. *J Child Neurol* 11:27–33.

Hirsh I. (1959). Auditory perception of temporal order. *J Acoust Soc Am* 31:759–767.

Hirsh I, Sherrick C. (1961). Perceived order in different sense modalities. *J Exp Psychol* 62:423–432.

Jerger J. (1960). Audiological manifestations of lesions in the auditory nervous system. *Laryngoscope* 70:417–425.

Jerger J, Jerger S. (1974). Auditory findings in brain stem disorders. *Arch Otolaryngol* 99:342–350.

Jerger J, Jerger S. (1975). Clinical validity of central auditory tests. *Scand Audiol* 4:147–163.

Jerger J, Jerger S, Oliver T, Pirozzolo F. (1989). Speech understanding in the elderly. *Ear Hear* 10:79–89.

Jerger J, Mier M, Boshes B, Canter G. (1960). Auditory behavior in parkinsonism. *Acta Otolaryngol* 52:541–550.

Jerger J, Speaks C, Trammell J. (1968). A new approach to speech audiometry. *J Speech Hear Disord* 33:318–328.

Jerger S, Johnson K, Loiselle L. (1988). Pediatric central auditory dysfunction: comparison of children with confirmed lesions versus suspected processing disorders. *Am J Otol* 9 (Suppl):63–71.

Jerger S, Martin R, Jerger J. (1987). Specific auditory perceptual dysfunction in a learning disabled child. *Ear Hear* 8:78–86.

Jerger S, Watkins M. (1988). Evidence of echoic memory with a multichannel cochlear prosthesis. *Ear Hear* 9:231–236.

Kalikow D, Stevens K, Elliott L. (1977). Development of a test of speech intelligibility in noise using sentence materials with controlled word predictability. *J Acoust Soc Am* 61:1337–1351.

Katz J. (1962). The use of staggered spondaic words for assessing the integrity of the central auditory nervous system. *J Audit Res* 2:327–337.

Katz J. (1985). *Competing Environmental Sounds Test.* Vancouver, WA: Precision Acoustics.

Katz J, Illmer R. (1972). Auditory perception in children with learning disabilities. In: Katz J, ed. *Handbook of Clinical Audiology.* Baltimore: Williams & Wilkins, 540–563.

Keith R. (1981). Tests of central auditory function. In: Roeser R, Downs M, eds. *Auditory Disorders in School Children.* New York: Thieme-Stratton, 159–173.

Knox C, Roeser R. (1980). Cerebral dominance in auditory perceptual asymmetrics in normal and dyslexic children. *Semin Speech Lang Hear* 1:181–194.

Lasky E. (1983). Parameters affecting auditory processing. In: Lasky E, Katz K, eds. *Central Auditory Processing Disorders: Problems of Speech, Language, and Learning.* Baltimore: University Park Press, 11–29.

Levitt H. (1971). Transformed up-down methods in psychoacoustics. *J Acoust Soc Am* 49:467–477.

Liden G, Korsan-Bengtsen M. (1973). Audiometric manifestations of retrocochlear lesions. *Scand Audiol* 2:29–40.

Lubert N. (1981). Auditory perceptual impairments in children with specific language disorders: a review of the literature. *J Speech Hear Disord* 46:3-9.

Lynn G, Benitez J, Eisenbrey A, Gilroy J, Wilner H. (1972). Neuro-audiological correlates in cerebral hemisphere lesions. *Audiology* 11:115-134.

Lyon R. (1977). Auditory perceptual training: the state of the art. *J Learn Disabil* 10:564-572.

Musiek F. (1989). Personal communication.

Musiek F, Gollegy K, Baran J. (1984). Myelination of the corpus callosum and auditory processing problems in children: theoretical and clinical correlates. *Semin Hear* 5:231-241.

Musiek F, Guerkink N. (1980). Auditory perceptual problems in children: considerations for the otolaryngologist and audiologist. *Laryngoscope* 90:962-971.

Rampp D. (1979). Hearing and learning disabilities. In: Bradford L, Hardy W, eds. *Hearing and Hearing Impairment*. New York: Grune & Stratton, 381-389.

Rees N. (1973). Auditory processing factors in language disorders: the view from Procrutes' bed. *J Speech Hear Disord* 38:304-315.

Rees N. (1981). Saying more than we know: is auditory processing disorder a meaningful concept? In: Keith R, ed. *Central Auditory and Language Disorders in Children*. Houston: College Hill Press, 94-120.

Robin D, Tomblin J, Kearney A, Hug L. (1989). Auditory temporal pattern learning in children with speech and language impairments. *Brain Lang* 36:604-613.

Schow R, Tannahill J. (1977). Hearing handicap scores and categories for subjects with normal and impaired hearing sensitivity. *J Am Audiol Soc* 3:134-139.

Sloan C. (1980). Auditory processing disorders in children. In: Levinson P, Sloan C, eds. *Auditory Processing and Language: Clinical and Research Perspectives*. New York: Grune & Stratton, 101-115.

Speaks C, Gray G, Miller J, Rubens A. (1975). Central auditory deficits and temporal lobe lesions. *J Speech Hear Disord* 40:192-205.

Stach B, Jerger J. (1984). Acoustic reflex averaging. *Ear Hear* 5:289-296.

Tallal P. (1980). Auditory processing disorders in children. In: Levinson P, Sloan C, eds. *Auditory Processing and Language: Clinical and Research Perspectives*. New York: Grune & Stratton, 81-100.

Tallal P, Stark R, Mellitus D. (1985a). Identification of language-impaired children on the basis of rapid perception and production skills. *Brain Lang* 25:314-322.

Tallal P, Stark R, Mellitus D. (1985b). The relationship between auditory temporal analysis and receptive language development: evidence from studies of developmental language disorder. *Neuropsychologia* 23:314-322.

Willeford J. (1985). Assessment of central auditory disorders in children. In: Pinheiro M, Musiek F, eds. *Assessment of Central Auditory Dysfunction: Foundation and Clinical Correlates*. Baltimore: Williams & Wilkins, 239-255.

Scand Audiol 1992; 21: 187–194

PHASE COHERENCE OF THE MIDDLE-LATENCY RESPONSE IN THE ELDERLY

Ali A. Ali and James Jerger

From the Division of Audiology and Speech Pathology, Baylor College of Medicine, Houston, Texas, USA

ABSTRACT

Phase coherence of the middle-latency response in the elderly.
Ali, A.A. and Jerger, J. (Division of Audiology and Speech Pathology, Baylor College of Medicine, Houston, Texas, USA).
Scand Audiol 1992; 21: 187–194.

We compared phase coherence of the auditory-evoked, middle-latency response (MLR) and the 40-Hz steady-state evoked potential (SSEP) in two groups of elderly listeners, matched for degree of audiometric hearing sensitivity loss. In group A, speech understanding was appropriate to the degree of audiometric sensitivity loss. In group B, speech understanding was disproportionately poor in relation to the degree of loss. In both modes of measurement (MLR and SSEP) phase coherence was significantly poorer in group B than in group A. In the case of MLR, maximum phase coherence was observed at the expected 40 Hz in group A, but at 30 Hz in group B. In the case of SSEP, maximum phase coherence was observed at 40 Hz in both groups but was poorer at almost all Fourier components in group B.

Key words: aging, elderly, 40 Hz, MLR, phase coherence, SSEP

INTRODUCTION

In view of the hypothesis that some of the speech understanding problems of the elderly may be related to changes in the central auditory system rather than to changes in the auditory periphery (Baran et al., 1986; Musiek, 1986; Jerger et al., 1989; Gatehouse, 1991), it is of interest to ask to what extent such central changes might be reflected in the morphology of the middle-latency response MLR. Previous studies of the general effect of aging on the MLR have not yielded a clearcut picture. Woods & Clayworth (1986) reported that the effect of intensity on response parameters in the elderly was similar to the effect in younger subjects. They did observe, however, enhancement of the amplitude and delay in the latency of the positive peak (P_a) in the elderly subjects. Similarly, Martini et al. (1991) have reported changes in the first negative peak (N_a) of the MLR in elderly females. Finally, Lenzi et al. (1989) reported poor definition of positive peaks P_o

and P_b of the MLR, and increased variability of P_a (dome shaped or rounded) with poor reproducibility in the elderly, although they did conclude that the differences in latency and amplitude were difficult to interpret due to the high inter-subject variability. Other recent studies have reported no significant changes in either the amplitude or the latency of peak P_a in the elderly (Jerger & Chmiel, 1991; Martini et al., 1991; Paludetti et al., 1991). Moreover, Paludetti et al. (1991), using conventional response parameters, found no relationship between speech understanding ability and MLR in elderly people.

It may be that a more sensitive index of MLR abnormality may yield less ambiguous findings in the elderly. Such an index might be derived from the variability of the latency of successive samples of the MLR waveform over time. Such 'sequential variability' might be affected by aging in spite of the absence of clear aging effects on either the amplitude or the latency of a single, averaged waveform.

Objective methods for calculating sequential variability, based on spectral analysis, have been developed by a number of investigators (Sayers et al., 1974, 1979; Beagley et al., 1979; Jervis et al., 1983). These methods are based on the variance of phase angles of a given spectral component across a sequence of individual sweeps. The principal problem with the application of these measures to individual sweeps, however, is that the signal-to-noise ratios of individual sweeps are poor and the variability in phase angle is correspondingly large. In 1982 Fridman et al. applied this sequential-variability model to the auditory brain-stem response (ABR), but used averaged waveforms instead of individual sweeps. In this technique, phase variability is calculated for a sequence of averaged waveforms rather than for a sequence of individual sweeps. Two years later, Fridman and his colleages (1984) claimed clinical value for the quantification of sequential variability in patients with tumors of the posterior fossa. Other investigators used sequential variability to evaluate the effect of sleep on the 40-Hz variant of MLR, the steady-state evoked potential (SSEP; Stapells et al., 1984; Linden et al., 1985; Jerger et al., 1986). They reported that, although amplitude of the SSEP decreased significantly in the sleeping state, sequential variability was not altered. A year later, two more studies demonstrated the advantage of sequential variability for evaluating the SSEP (Picton et al., 1987; Stapells et al., 1987). Recently, Harada (1990) studied the sequential variability of 30-, 40- and 50-Hz components of the MLR and the 40-, 80- and 120-Hz components of the SSEP in patients with central nervous system disorders. He reported that sequential variability was more useful than other parameters of the MLR for the detection of such disorders.

This finding suggests the possibility that central aging may impact sequential variability of the MLR even though neither the amplitude nor the latency of a conventional averaged waveform are significantly altered. The literature, however, shows a lack of studies of sequential variability for either the MLR or the SSEP in elderly subjects. The present study was designed, therefore, to evaluate the extent to which sequential variability of either the MLR or the SSEP might be related to differences in speech understanding among elderly subjects.

METHODS

The MLR can be studied in two modes, at relatively slow (conventional) and at relatively high stimulus rates. In the conventional mode the response is evoked by stimulus presentation rates in the range from one to 12 stimuli per second. In the high-rate mode the response is evoked by stimulation at the relatively rapid rate of about 40 stimuli per second (Galambos et al., 1981). The waveform evoked by stimulation at such high rates has been called the steady-state evoked potential (SSEP). In the present study, elderly subjects were examined in both modes. For the conventional MLR the stimulus rate was 9/s. For SSEP the stimulus rate was 39/s.

To measure sequential variability, 10 averaged waveforms were obtained successively. Each average was based on 128 sweeps. All averaged waveforms were stored in digital form for subsequent off-line analysis. Each averaged waveform was subjected to fast Fourier transform (FFT) spectral analysis to extract the amplitude and phase angle of the Fourier components at 10-Hz intervals from 20 to 150 Hz. The sequential variability of each such component was quantified by a phase coherence (PC) measure defined by the equation:

$$PC = [(1/n \Sigma \cos\phi_i)^2 + (1/n \Sigma \sin\phi_i)^2]^{1/2}$$

where ϕ_i is the phase angle of the Fourier component of the ith sample, and n is the number of samples. Phase coherence

varies between 0 and 1, and is directly proportional to variability.

Subjects

Twenty elderly subjects were selected from a pool of paid volunteers, all of whom had participated in a previous study of hearing in aging (Jerger et al., 1989). Subjects were selected according to the following criteria:

(1) Chronological age in the range 65–90 years.
(2) Ambulatory, in good general health, and without history or evidence of neurologic disease.
(3) No more than a mild hearing sensitivity loss. Pure-tone threshold hearing levels averaged across 500, 1 000 and 2 000 Hz (PTA_1) could not exceed 40 dB HL in either ear. Pure-tone threshold hearing levels averaged across 1 000, 2 000 and 4 000 Hz (PTA_2) could not exceed 50 dB HL in either ear.
(4) Inter-aural symmetry: the sensitivity difference between the two ears of a given subject, for either PTA_1, PTA_2, or the threshold at 1 kHz, could not exceed 14 dB.

The 20 subjects were divided into two groups of 10 subjects each according to their speech understanding ability. This categorization was based on speech audiometric scores available from each subject's previous participation in our aging research program. Scores were available for PB words in quiet, synthetic sentence identification (SSI) against a background of continuous discourse (MCR = 0 dB), SPIN sentences against a background of multi-talker babble (talker-to-babble ratio = +8 dB), and the dichotic sentence identification test (DSI). On the basis of these scores subjects were categorized as normal or abnormal according to available norms (Fifer et al., 1983; Bilger et al., 1984; Jerger et al., 1989). A subject was categorized as abnormal if his performance on either ear fell below the norm on one or more of three speech understanding measures; the PB–SSI difference; the relation between SPIN scores for high- and low-context items; and the DSI scores. In this paper the two groups will be referred to as group A, with 'normal' speech understanding ability (i.e. appropriate to audiometric sensitivity loss), and group B, with 'abnormal' speech understanding ability (i.e. poorer than would be expected on the basis of audiometric sensitivity loss). The average age of subjects in group A was 72.3 years (SD 4.8 years) and in group B 73.9 years (SD 4.9 years). Table I summarizes mean hearing threshold levels (HTL) and SD of three measures of audiometric status, PTA_1 (average of HTLs at 500, 1 000 and 2 000 Hz), PTA_2 (average of HTLs at 1 000, 2 000 and 4 000 Hz) and the HTL at 1 000 Hz, for both groups of elderly subjects. Figure 1 shows average hearing threshold levels, and their SD at each of the audiometric frequencies from 250 to 8 000 Hz, for both groups of elderly subjects.

Apparatus

The eliciting signal was a 1 000-Hz tone pip with a total baseline duration of 5 ms. To generate this tone pip, the output from an audio generator (Hewlett–Packard, model 311) was gated by an electronic switch, triggered by a timer (Grason–Stadler, series 1 200). The '2-1-2' tone-pip configuration was used. Thus for the 1 000-Hz test signal, rise and decay times were 2 cycles (2 ms) and duration at plateau was 1 cycle (1 ms) for a total baseline duration of 5 ms. The gated output was amplified, attenuated and delivered to a pair of matched dynamic earphones (TDH-39), mounted in circumaural cushions (Zwislocki, CZW-6). Tone-pip signal level was calibrated in dB nHL by determining the behavioral

Table I. *Comparison of various measures of hearing sensitivity loss in groups A and B. Means (SD) of hearing threshold levels for PTA$_1$, PTA$_2$ and threshold at 1 000 Hz*

Measure	Right ear (Group)		Left ear (Group)	
	A	B	A	B
PTA$_1$	19.5 (7.74)	20.2 (8.24)	20.7 (9.54)	17.9 (9.8)
PTA$_2$	25.6 (9.63)	27.1 (9.33)	27.5 (9.63)	25.2 (10.64)
1 kHz	19.0 (10.49)	17.5 (8.25)	23.5 (9.73)	15.6 (9.77)

thresholds for this signal on a jury of 11 young adult listeners with normal hearing.

EEG was recorded from scalp electrodes located at vertex, Cz (active, non-inverting), earlobes, A1 and A2 (reference, inverting), and forehead (ground). EEG activity was pre-amplified (Grass, P511) for a voltage gain of 100 000:1 and band-pass, analog-filtered from 10 to 300 Hz (6 dB/octave skirt). The amplified EEG activity was signal averaged (Nicolet 1174) and then stored on a microcomputer (Macintosh SE) for off-line spectral analysis and calculation of phase coherence.

Procedure

The subject was seated in a sound-treated room and instructed to relax while EEG activity was being monitored. Tone-pip signals were then presented at 80 dB nHL for right and left ear stimulation, and at 75 dB nHL for the binaural condition. Ten successive samples, 128 sweeps/sample each, were recorded for each test condition. The order of test conditions was as follows: right SSEP, left SSEP, left MLR, right MLR, binaural MLR and binaural SSEP. A control (sound inaudible) condition was run at −10 dB nHL at the end of the test. The entire experimental session lasted about 2 h.

In all subsequent data analysis statistical significance was evaluated at an alpha level of 0.05.

RESULTS

Waveforms

Figure 2 shows the overall grand-averaged waveforms recorded from both groups of elderly subjects in response to 1 000-Hz, tone-pip stimulation at presentation rates of 39/s (SSEP) and 9/s (MLR) for right, left and binaural stimulation. Each curve represents the average of 12 800 sweeps (10 Ss × 10 averages/ S × 128 sweeps/average) at the same test condition (ear and stimulus presentation rate). In general these grand-averaged waveforms agree well with previously published data on both the conventional MLR and the SSEP. Table II summarizes average values for all of the conventional parameters of MLR and SSEP in both groups.

In the case of MLR, group differences were small. The P$_a$ peak was slightly delayed and somewhat broader in group B, and the slight P$_b$ peak evident in group A was missing in group B, but overall, the waveforms were similar for right ear, left ear and binaural stimulation. In the case of the SSEP, however, a clear degradation in the quality of the averaged waveform was evident in group B.

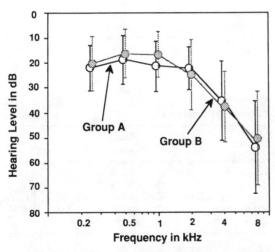

Fig. 1. Average hearing threshold levels (SD) at each of the audiometric frequencies from 250 to 8 000 Hz for both groups of elderly subjects.

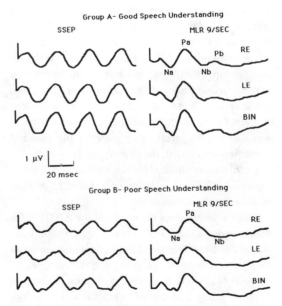

Fig. 2. Grand-average waveforms for the two groups under the two modes of measurement.

Table II. *Summary of average values for all of the conventional parameters of MLR and SSEP in both groups*

	Group A			Group B		
	RE	LE	Bin	RE	LE	Bin
Pa latency (ms)	29.2	29.5	29.5	31.7	31.8	31.7
Na–Pa amp. (μV)	1.48	1.57	1.91	1.30	1.74	1.61
Phase angle (°)	−0.9	−5.2	17.9	33.0	23.4	36.5
SSEP amp. (μV)	1.37	1.55	1.80	1.12	1.10	1.12

Analysis of conventional parameters

In order to analyze conventional latency and amplitude parameters of the MLR and the SSEP we derived a single-averaged waveform for each subject under each condition by summing across the 10 samples available for that condition. We then computed, for the MLR, the latency of P_a and the N_a–P_a amplitude, and, for the SSEP, the phase angle of the 40-Hz sinusoid and its peak-to-peak amplitude. These data were then subjected to mixed-design analyses of variance. There was one between-groups factor (group A vs group B), and one within-groups factor (right ear vs left ear vs binaural). Table III summarizes this analysis for the P_a latency of the conventional MLR. There was no significant effect due to ear of stimulation, and there was no significant effect due to the interaction between ear of stimulation and group, but there was a significant group effect ($p = 0.027$). Table IV presents a similar analysis for the N_a–P_a amplitude of the conventional MLR. Here there was no significant group effect, and no significant interaction between group and ear of stimulation, but there was, not unexpectedly, a significant main effect due to ear of stimulation. In order to demonstrate that this effect was due to the greater amplitude of the binaural response, we carried out a new analysis with the binaural data removed. This new analysis, confined to right and left ear stimulation only, failed to demonstrate a significant ear effect.

Table V summarizes the results of the ANOVA for phase angle of the SSEP. There were no significant effects due either to group, to ear of stimulation, or to their interaction. In the case of SSEP amplitude, however (Table VI), there was a significant interaction between group and ear of stimulation. It was not possible, therefore, to evaluate the significance of the main effects of either group or ear of stimulation.

Table III. *Results of analysis of variance for Pa latency of the conventional MLR*
*Statistically significant

	df	Sum of squares	F	p
Group (A vs B)	1	80.435	5.784	0.027*
Subjects	18	250.308		
Ear (R vs L vs Bin)	2	0.413	0.143	0.848
Ear × group	2	0.176	0.061	0.941
Ear × subjects	36	51.996		

Table IV. *Results of analysis of variance for Na–Pa amplitude of the conventional MLR*
*Statistically significant

	df	Sum of squares	F	p
Group (A vs B)	1	0.154	0.172	0.683
Subjects	18	16.085		
Ear (R vs L vs Bin)	2	1.394	3.799	0.032*
Ear × group	2	0.595	1.623	0.215
Ear × subjects	36	6.604		

Table V. *Results of analysis of variance for phase angle of SSEP*

	df	Sum of squares	F	p
Group (A vs B)	1	9.157	0.764	0.393
Subjects	18	11.981		
Ear (R vs L vs Bin)	2	3.863	1.444	0.249
Ear × group	2	0.623	0.233	0.794
Ear × subjects	36	2.676		

Table VI. *Results of analysis of variance for SSEP amplitude*
*Statistically significant

	df	Sum of squares	F	p
Group (A vs B)	1	3.194	7.032	0.016*
Subjects	18	8.175		
Ear (R vs L vs Bin)	2	0.462	3.792	0.032*
Ear × group	2	0.237	3.898	0.029*
Ear × subjects	36	2.192		

Reference to Table II, however, shows that SSEP amplitude was considerable larger in the binaural condition than in either monaural condition, and that

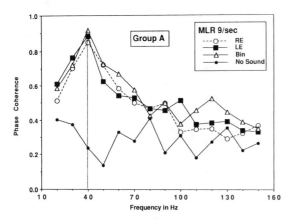

Fig. 3. Phase coherence as a function of Fourier-component frequency for the MLR of group A (good speech understanding).

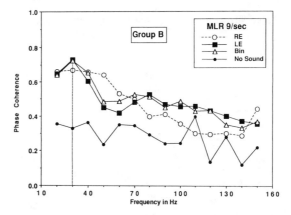

Fig. 5. Phase coherence as a function of Fourier-component frequency for the MLR of group B (poor speech understanding).

this difference was especially evident in group A. When the data for binaural stimulation were removed from the analysis, there were no significant effects for group, ear of stimulation or the interaction between the two main effects.

In summary, statistical analysis of the latency and amplitude data summarized in Table II showed a difference between groups A and B for P_a latency, but for no other conventional measure of either MLR or SSEP.

Sequential variability
Figure 3 shows phase coherence, as a function of frequency, for the MLR recorded from group A. Figure 4 shows an analogous function for the SSEP in

group A. Figure 5 shows the phase-coherence function for the MLR in group B, while Fig. 6 shows the analagous phase-coherence function for the SSEP in group B. Figures 3 and 4 show that, in the case of group A, maximum PC was observed at the 40-Hz Fourier component irrespective of the test mode. In the case of group B, however (Figs. 5, 6), while maximum PC was observed at the 40-Hz component for SSEP, the conventional MLR results showed maximum phase coherence over a broad peak encompassing both 30 and 40 Hz.

Table VII summarizes the result of the statistical analysis of these data for the phase coherence at 40 Hz, a mixed-design analysis of variance with one between-subjects factor (group) and two within-subjects factors

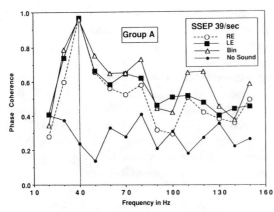

Fig. 4. Phase coherence as a function of Fourier-component frequency for the SSEP of group A (good speech understanding).

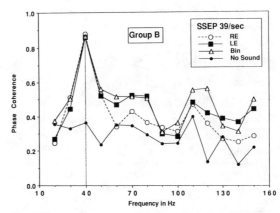

Fig. 6. Phase coherence as a function of Fourier-component frequency for the SSEP of group B (poor speech understanding).

Table VII. *Analysis of variance comparing group, ear and mode effects on phase coherence at 40 Hz*
* Statistically significant

Factor	Mean square	df	F	p
Group (A vs B)	0.683	1	11.60	0.003*
Between subjects	0.059	18		
Ear (R vs L vs Bin)	0.004	2	0.22	0.801
Ear × subjects	0.019	36		
Mode (MLR vs SSEP)	0.540	1	15.70	0.001*
Mode × group	0.090	1	2.62	0.123
Mode × subjects	0.034	18		
Ear × group	0.006	2	0.32	0.726
Ear × mode	0.008	2	1.11	0.340
Ear × mode × group	0.009	2	1.14	0.330
Within subjects	0.008	36		

(ear and mode). Neither the third-order nor any of the second-order interactions reached statistical significance; nor was there a significant ear effect. Both group and mode effects, however, were significant. Phase coherence at 40 Hz was significantly lower in group B than in group A, and significantly lower in the MLR than in the SSEP mode.

In order to determine whether the significant group effect was common to both modes of stimulation (MLR and SSEP), we carried out separate analyses of variance for each mode. For these analyses, however, we pooled ear data (right, left and binaural) since this effect had not been significant in the first analysis, and added a Fourier component factor (30 vs 40 vs 50 Hz). Thus each analysis (MLR or SSEP) was a mixed-design ANOVA with one between-subjects factor (group) and one within-subjects factor (Fourier component). Table VIII summarizes selected F ratios and p values for these two analyses. In both cases (MLR and SSEP) there was a significant group effect and a significant effect due to Fourier component. There

Table VIII. *Selected results from analyses of variance comparing group- and Fourier-component effects on phase coherence of MLR and SSEP*
* Statistically significant

	MLR		SSEP	
Factor	F	p	F	p
Group (A vs B)	5.60	0.029*	9.81	0.006*
Component (30 vs 40 vs 50 Hz)	5.50	0.008*	71.76	0.0001*
Group × component	1.50	0.236	2.17	0.129

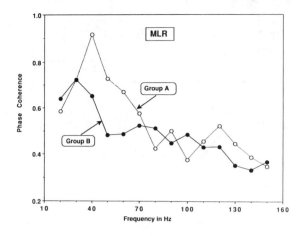

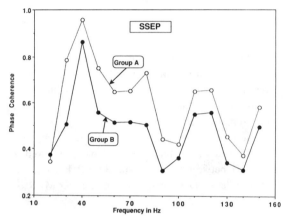

Fig. 7. Comparison of phase coherence functions of groups A and B under binaural stimulation. (*a*) MLR; (*b*) SSEP.

was, however, no significant group × component interaction.

Figure 7 compares phase coherence functions for groups A and B in the binaural condition. Results for right ear and left ear stimulation are omitted since the analysis of variance failed to reveal a significant effect on phase coherence due to ear of stimulation. Figure 7a compares the two groups in the MLR mode. It is clear that the major difference between the two groups is a decline in phase coherence at 40, 50 and 60 Hz in group B. Figure 7b compares the two groups in the SSEP mode. Here the relation to frequency is similar in the two groups, but group B shows substantially less phase coherence than group A at virtually every Fourier component frequency. Indeed, the absolute difference in phase coherence between the two groups is somewhat less at 40 Hz than at many other Fourier component frequencies.

DISCUSSION

The present results show a significant difference in sequential variability of the middle-latency, auditory-evoked response between elderly subjects with speech understanding appropriate to their audiometric losses (group A) and elderly subjects with inappropriately poor speech understanding (group B). The difference was present whether the response was measured in the conventional MLR mode or in the SSEP mode, and was characterized by poorer phase coherence in the group with poorer speech understanding.

Could this difference be related to greater hearing sensitivity loss in group B? This possibility is ruled out by the fact that average sensitivity loss (Table I) was actually somewhat less in group B than in group A. At 1 000 Hz, for example, the average HTL, collapsed across ears, was 4.7 dB less in group B. In the case of PTA_2, the loss was 0.2 dB less in group B. Similarly, in the case of PTA_1, the loss was 1.6 dB less in group B. It is not likely that hearing sensitivity differences of this magnitude will affect inter-group comparisons of either the waveform or the stability of the middle-latency response measured at a sensation level of about 60 dB. But if they do, then group B should have benefited from the difference. Yet phase coherence was actually poorer in group B despite its slightly better overall hearing sensitivity.

The basis for the poorer phase coherence in group B is unknown. We may speculate, however, that the disproportionately poor speech understanding in this group results from loss of cell population in the central auditory pathways. Decreased phase coherence of the MLR may reflect loss in synchrony resulting from such a deficit in central pathway elements. In any event, the phase coherence measure may provide an electrophysiological correlate of poor speech understanding in the elderly.

The practical significance of the present finding is that sequential variability may be a useful predictive measure for the early identification of central auditory processing disorders. In the present experiment only the latency of P_a significantly differentiated elderly subjects with good speech understanding from elderly subjects with poor speech understanding, and this difference was, on average, less than 2.5 ms. But phase coherence effectively differentiated the two groups over a range of Fourier components. It may also be noted that phase coherence is an inherently more objective measure than P_a latency since it does not

require the identification of a peak position in an often noisy waveform. The present results suggest that further research into the most effective algorithm for identifying a deficit in sequential variability of the MLR may provide a useful tool for the evaluation of auditory disorders in the elderly.

REFERENCES

Baran JA, Musiek FE, Reeves AG. Central auditory function following anterior sectioning of corpus callosum. Ear Hear 1986; 7: 359–62.

Beagley HA, Sayers B McA, Ross AJ. Fully objective ERA by phase spectral analysis. Acta Otolaryngol (Stockh) 1979; 87: 270–8.

Bilger RC, Nuetzel J, Rabinowitz WM, Rzeczkowski C. Standardization of a test of speech perception in noise. J Speech Hear Res 1984; 27: 32–48.

Fifer RC, Jerger JF, Berlin CI, Tobey EA, Campbell JC. Development of a dichotic sentence identification test for hearing-impaired adults. Ear Hear 1983; 4: 300–5.

Fridman J, John ER, Bergelson M, Kaiser J, Baird H. Application of digital filtering and automatic peak detection to brainstem auditory evoked potentials. Electro-encephalogr Clin Neurophysiol 1982; 53: 405–16.

Fridman J, Zappulla R, Bergelson M, Greenblatt E, Malis L, Morrell F, Hoeppner T. Application of phase spectral analysis for brain stem auditory evoked potential detection in normal subjects and patients with posterior fossa tumors. Audiology 1984; 23: 99–113.

Galambos R, Makeig S, Talmachoff PJ. A 40-Hz auditory potential recorded from the human scalp. Proc Natl Acad Sci USA 1981; 78: 2643–7.

Gatehouse S. The contribution of central auditory factors to auditory disability. Acta Otolaryngol (Stockh) 1991; (Suppl. 476): 182–8.

Harada J. Application of digital filtering and phase spectral analysis to middle latency response and 40 Hz event related potential in central nerve system disorders. J Otorhinolaryngol Soc Jpn 1990; 93: 1046–54.

Jerger J, Chmiel R. Effect of age on auditory evoked potentials. Paper presented at the Third Annual Convention of the American Academy of Audiology, Denver, Colorado, April 28, 1991.

Jerger J, Chmiel R, Frost JD Jr, Coker N. Effect of sleep on the auditory steady state evoked potential. Ear Hear 1986; 7: 240–5.

Jerger J, Jerger S, Oliver T, Pirozzolo F. Speech understanding in elderly. Ear Hear 1989; 10: 79–89.

Jervis BW, Nichols MJ, Johnson TE, Allen E, Hudson NR. A fundamental investigation of the composition of the auditory evoked potentials. IEEE Trans Biomed Eng 1983; 30: 43–9.

Lenzi A, Chiarelli G, Sambataro G. Comparative study of the middle latency responses and auditory brainstem responses in elderly subjects. Audiology 1989; 28: 144–51.

Linden RD, Campbell KB, Hamel G, Picton TW. Human auditory steady state potentials during sleep. Ear Hear 1985; 6: 167–84.

Martini A, Comacchio F, Magnavita V. Auditory evoked responses (ABR, MLR, SVR) and brain mapping in the elderly. Acta Otolaryngol (Stockh) 1991; (Suppl. 476): 97–104.

Musiek FE. Neuroanatomy, neurophysiology, and central auditory assessment. Part II: The Cerebrum. Ear Hear 1986; 7: 283–94.

Paludetti G, Maurizi M, D'Alatri L, Galli J. Relationships between middle latency auditory responses (MLR) and speech discrimination tests in the elderly. Acta Otolaryngol (Stockh) 1991; (Suppl. 476): 105–9.

Picton TW, Vajsar J, Rodriguez R, Campbell KB. Reliability estimates for steady-state evoked potentials. Electroencephalogr Clin Neurophysiol 1987; 68: 119–31.

Sayers B McA, Beagley HA, Henshall WR. The mechanism of auditory evoked EEG responses. Nature 1974; 247: 481–3.

Sayers B McA, Beagley HA, Riha J. Pattern analysis of auditory-evoked EEG potentials. Audiology 1979; 18: 1–16.

Stapells DR, Lindin D, Braxton J, Hamel G, Picton TW. Human auditory steady state potentials. Ear Hear 1984; 5: 105–13.

Stapells DR, Makeig S, Galambos R. Auditory steady-state responses: threshold prediction using phase coherence. Electroencephalogr Clin Neurophysiol 1987; 67: 260–70.

Woods DL, Clayworth CC. Age-related changes in human middle latency auditory evoked potentials. Electroencephalogr Clin Neurophysiol 1986; 65: 297–303.

Received August 15/Accepted November 13, 1991

Address for offprints:

James Jerger
11922 Taylorcrest Rd
Houston
Tx 77024
USA

Speech Audiometry

No one did more to advance the cause of speech audiometry than Raymond Carhart. As a captain in the Army Medical Corps at Deshon General Hospital in Butler, Pennsylvania, toward the end of World War II, Carhart virtually invented the concept of evaluating the performance of hearing aids by means of speech recognition tests. To be sure, the materials he used, spondee and PB lists, had already been developed at the Psychoacoustic Laboratory at Harvard University. The initial motivation, driven by the war effort, was to measure how well ground-to-air radio communication systems transmitted the sounds of speech. If the concept worked for radios, Carhart wondered, why wouldn't it work equally well for hearing aids. At that time, his group at Deshon was responsible for issuing hearing aids to personnel who had sustained hearing losses during their military service. Carhart adapted the spondee and PB materials to the task of determining which of several hearing aids best transmitted speech to the hearing-impaired veteran. Although these concepts were developed almost 50 years ago, they remain central to our notion of how to evaluate hearing aid performance. Carhart's specific protocol, an aided threshold for spondee words followed by a PB list at a defined sensation level, has been severely criticized, primarily on the basis of the inadequate reliability of PB scores. But the idea that you should evaluate hearing aid performance in terms of efficiency of speech communication is as viable today as it was in 1946.

Today, of course, it seems that virtually everyone who writes a paper on the real-ear measurement of hearing-aid frequency response feels compelled to motivate the effort by citing the lack of validity and reliability of Carhart's protocol and to emphasize that the procedure cannot be used to distinguish between hearing aids having similar electroacoustic characteristics.

The problem with this kind of broad generalization is that it fails to distinguish between the concept of speech recognition testing and a *particular way of carrying out* speech recognition testing. The *concept* of speech recognition testing is quite broad. It encompasses a wide variety of speech materials, testing strategies, and response measures. In particular, it includes the important notion of testing speech recognition against a background of speech competition.

In contrast, the particular way of carrying out speech recognition testing that has been so severely criticized (and quite properly, in my view) represents only a very limited subset of the possible ways that the speech recognition paradigm might be used in clinical evaluation. The inadequacy of a specific approach in no way invalidates the concept of speech recognition testing. Given the problems of the particular historical approach pioneered by Carhart, it is entirely possible to devise other ways of exploiting the concept to achieve the kind of reliable differentiation we all seek.

This is exactly what Charles Speaks and I set out to do in the early 1960s. We wanted to take a fresh approach to the problem of measuring speech recognition, guided by two considerations:

1. We wanted the speech target to be a complete sentence rather than a monosyllabic word.
2. We wanted the response to be from a closed—rather than an open—message set.

The historic problems associated with the use of sentences, of course, were (a) the fact that they were too easy because of redundancy, (b) the fact that performance was so dependent on level of linguistic competence, and (c) the fact that scoring techniques relied either on key-word identification or some form of multiple-choice answering system. The key-word approach seemed to reduce the paradigm to little more than single word recognition with an elaborate carrier, while the multiple-choice-answer approach seemed too dependent on IQ.

Our approach, presented for the first time in the 1965 paper, "Method for Measurement of Speech Identification" (*Journal of Speech and Hearing Research*, 1965) was to avoid the problems created by the varying semantic content of "real sentences" by constructing "synthetic sentences," or, more properly "synthetic syntax" sentences, using a technique in which approximations to real sentences are constructed on the basis of the transitional probabilities governing word sequence in the language. After we had constructed first, second, and third-order approximations to 5-, 7-, and 9-word sentences we settled on 7-word, third-order sentences as our test materials and constructed a number of alternative 10-sentence lists. Subsequently, we have tended to use just one of these alternative forms. These 10 sentences are the raw materials for the SSI test protocol.

To meet the problem that sentences, all by themselves, are too easy, we decided to embed the sentence "messages," or "targets," in a background competition of continuous speech. Then, by manipulating the relative intensities of the message and the competition, the message-to-competition ratio, or MCR, we could achieve any desired degree of test difficulty. In particular, we could tailor the test difficulty to the patient's range of performance capability. We recorded, for this purpose, a segment of continuous discourse taken from the Sunday supplement to the *Houston Post*, a short history of the life of Davy Crockett, an important figure in the early history of Texas and a hero of the Alamo.

We felt, from the outset, that an important feature of the new test procedure should be choice of a response from a closed, rather than an open, message set. This, we thought would help to minimize the problem of variabilty among patients in terms of previous linguistic history, competence, and general intellectual ability. So we constructed a response card with the 10 sentences listed by number. The patient's task was to listen to the continuous background competition and to respond with the appropriate number each time a sentence was presented. Scoring could be either manual or automated.

We have used the SSI testing procedure for most hearing aid evaluations at The Methodist Hospital for more than 20 years. To compare unaided with aided performance, or to compare the performance of two different amplification systems, we measure SSI performance at various MCRs, chosen in such a way that performance is sampled over the range from about 10 to 90%. In general, we have found the approach useful, both as a method for making comparisons among systems and as a basis for counseling the prospective hearing aid user.

Our early experiences with SSI as a component of the hearing aid evaluation are detailed in the paper, "Hearing Aid Evaluation: Clinical Experience with a New Philosophy" (*Archives of Otolaryngology*, 1976). We showed, in this paper, the value of being able to manipulate the test difficulty by varying the MCR. When the MCR was too favorable (e.g., +10 dB), the aided SSI score failed to distinguish among satisfied, sometimes satisfied, and not satisfied users. But when the MCR was manipulated to produce a more difficult listening task (e.g., −10 dB), the SSI score spread the three groups out over a performance range of 30%. In the same patients, the average aided PB_{max} score differed by less than 2%. In a similar survey carried out 5 years later on a larger number of hearing aid users by Hayes, Jerger, Taff, and Barber (*Ear & Hearing*, 1981), the same 30% range between "unsatisfactory" and "very helpful" ratings was observed at the −10 dB MCR condition.

One of the most interesting diagnostic applications of speech audiometry is the phenomenon of "rollover," the paradoxical decrease in the speech recognition score as signal intensity is raised beyond the point where maximum performance is reached. In effect, the performance versus intensity function reaches a maximum, then proceeds to drop off or "roll over" at higher intensities. The effect was first called to my attention by Susan Jerger who noted this unusual shape of the PI function in patients with acoustic tumor. In 1971 we published a systematic comparison of PI functions for PB words in 16 retrocochlear and 41 cochlear patients, showing that the rollover index, $PB_{max} - PB_{min}/PB_{max}$, easily differentiated patients with acoustic tumor from patients with cochlear disorder. A high point of this paper, we thought, was the rather elegant demonstration of the rollover effect for both PB words and SSI sentences and in two different languages, English and Spanish, in a bilingual patient with acoustic tumor.

The rollover effect on the PI function for speech materials has subsequently been confirmed by other investigators and has, I think, become a widely used tool of diagnostic audiometry.

The final paper in the speech audiometry section, "Norms for Disproportionate Loss in Speech Intelligibility" (*Ear & Hearing*, 1989) represents our attempt to answer the long-standing question: When is a speech recognition score so bad that you can't explain it as a simple consequence of degree of sensorineural hearing loss? In other words, when is it "disproportionately poor"? We attacked the problem by simply plotting scattergrams relating PB and SSI scores to degree of pure-tone sensitivity loss in a relatively large group (324) of patients with purely cochlear disorders. Surprisingly, the lower boundary of observed scores was a fairly linear function of pure-tone average, expressed in decibels.

This is the kind of straightforward, prosaic study that we don't do enough of in our field. The concept of "disproportionately poor" speech understanding has been with us since the initial observations of Schucknecht more than 40 years ago. It is one of the invariant signatures of retrocochlear auditory disorder. Yet few have taken the time to ask the question: "How bad does performance actually have to be before we must call it disproportionately poor?"

In summary, the papers included in this section reflect my bias that speech audiometry is now, and will continue to be, one of our most powerful clinical tools. The present trend toward minimizing its importance and its potential contributions is unfortunate. It will not be reversed, however, until we divert at least some of our attention from the fine grain of speech audiometry as a tool and begin to address some of the substantive issues that continue to plague us in our efforts to aid the hearing-impaired person.

METHOD FOR MEASUREMENT OF SPEECH IDENTIFICATION

CHARLES SPEAKS *and* JAMES JERGER

Houston Speech and Hearing Center, Houston, Texas

A new method for measuring speech identification behavior is described. Twenty-four closed-message sets representing three levels of approximation to a "real" sentence have been constructed. Each set contains 10 synthetic sentences. Sentence length and informational content are controlled. Message identification under conditions of low-pass filtering and periodic interruption was studied in 30 subjects with normal hearing. Performance varied systematically with relative informational content.

Traditional approaches to the quantitative study of speech intelligibility have employed a wide variety of verbal materials, ranging from the very analytic to reasonably synthetic. They have included nonsense syllables, phonetically balanced monosyllabic words, dissyllabic words (including both spondaic and unselected stress patterns), sentences, and continuous discourse. Much of the early work at the Bell Telephone Laboratories and at the Harvard Psycho-Acoustic Laboratory has been summarized by Fletcher and Steinberg (1929), Fletcher (1929), Miller, Weiner, and Stevens (1946), Hudgins and others (1947), and Egan (1948). The application of these techniques in the assessment of auditory function has been elaborated by Walsh and Silverman (1946), Hirsh (1952), and Silverman and Hirsh (1955).

All of these tests have one or more disadvantage for auditory research in which systematic exploration of temporal processing is desired. Interest in the time domain suggests that the verbal materials should consist of sentences of sufficient duration to permit systematic alteration of temporal characteristics of the speech message. Further, it seems desirable that the sentences be of controlled length and controllable relative informational content. "Relative information" is used here in the sense of unspecifiable variations in the amount of information conveyed in a message set as a consequence of variable sequential constraints. As Miller (1951, p. 791) emphasizes:

> Dependencies among successive words reduce the number of possible sentences and so reduce the number of alternatives that can be represented. In a very real sense, therefore, contextual restrictions reduce the amount of information that can be conveyed by a sequence of *n* symbols.

Previous lists of sentences (Fletcher and Steinberg, 1929; Hudgins, 1947; Davis and Silverman, 1960) do not appear to satisfy these criteria. We have, therefore, attempted a fresh approach to the measurement problem. The fundamental departure from traditional procedures is to require correct "identification" rather than correct "repetition" of verbal materials.

Classically, the subject either repeats aloud what he hears, or chooses the answer from among some number of alternative choices unique to the signal. In contrast, in the present paradigm, the entire set of verbal materials is available to the subject in written form. His task is to identify which of the several alternative messages was presented (House and others, 1962; House and others, 1965).

This approach to speech identification has three important advantages over classical techniques. First, the message set is always closed and of controllable size. Second, testing procedures can be easily automated, permitting acquisition of considerable data with minimal opportunity for experimenter error. Third, the effect of learning or practice for a message set can be determined with relative ease.

METHOD

Instrumentation

The instrumentation used in these experiments is shown in block diagram form in Figure 1. The subject was seated before a panel containing a row of 10 push buttons, two lights labeled "listen" and "rest" respectively, a third light labeled "correct", and an 8½″ × 11″ sheet on which was typed a list of 10 sentences comprising a message set. After each sentence of the set had been presented, the subject was given approximately seven seconds in which to identify which of the 10 typed sentences on the panel he heard and to push the corresponding button. If he identified correctly, the "correct" light automatically flashed. Correct responses were tabulated on a counter.

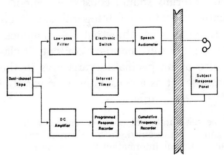

FIGURE 1. Simplified diagram of test instrumentation.

Message sets were recorded on one track of a dual-track magnetic tape recorder (Ampex, Model 351-2) and presented monaurally via earphones (Telephonic, type TDH 39) to each subject. A series of coding pulses for each message set was recorded on the second track. An automatic response recorder programmed the sequences of messages within a set, then acquired and stored data automatically. The apparatus provided instantaneous readout of the number of sentences delivered to the subject and the total number of correct responses. In addition, cumulative responses were displayed on an event recorder (Grason-Stadler, Model E3262A). This facilitated evaluation of the nature of learning or practice across successive trials for a given set of verbal materials.

After an entire message set had been presented, the apparatus could be programmed to present the same set again in a different random order, or to present a new message set.

Speech Materials

The present methodological approach imposes only minimal constraints on the nature of messages to be used. However, because of our interest in exploration of the time domain, this report is concerned only with the identification of sentences.

The nature of the sentences to be used presented several problems. In a "real" sentence, "meaning" may be conveyed by only one or two key words. Also, construction of reasonably equivalent message sets containing "real" sentences is exceedingly difficult due to the variable factors of vocabulary, word familiarity, word length, sentence length, and syntactical structure. One method for avoiding the problems inherent in "real" sentences is to use artificial sentences, constructed according to specific pre-determined rules (Fry, 1964). This avenue seemed sufficiently promising to warrant development of a series of artificial sentences.

The general procedure for constructing artificial sentences was to select each successive word for a sentence solely on the basis of the "conditional probabilities" of word sequences. Thus, each new word was conditional on the preceding word or words. Various levels, or orders, of approximation could then be constructed, depending upon whether the word sequences were based on the conditional probabilities of word-pairs, word-triplets, or longer combinations, a procedure similar to one previously employed by Miller and Selfridge (1950). The end products may be thought of as "approximations" to the "real" sentences with the advantage that relative informational content may be varied systematically. Message sets comprising three different orders of approximation were constructed. Words for all sentences were chosen from a pool of the 1 000 most common words of the Thorndike-Lorge (1944) count.

First-order approximations were constructed by choosing successive words at random from this common pool. Thus, statistical information concerning the relative frequency of occurrence provided the only constraint on word choice. All 1 000 words in the pool occur with a frequency $\geq 100/10^6$. Since no more refined statistical breakdown is available, each of the 1 000 words was considered equally probable insofar as inclusion in a sentence was concerned.

Second-order approximation sentences were constructed by choosing the first word at random from the common pool. A second word was then supplied by an individual, (A), who was instructed to supply a word (from the common pool) that could reasonably follow the first word in a declarative or imperative sentence. This second word was then given to another individual, (B), who chose the third word under the same criteria. This procedure was repeated, with a new individual used for each word, until an artificial sentence of desired length had been constructed. Thus, second-order sentences had two constraints: statistical information and the conditional probabilities of word pairs.

Third-order approximations were based on the conditional probabilities of word triplets. One of the word-pairs used in the second-order sentences was selected at random. An individual then supplied a third word to follow. Next, the last two of these three words were given to a second individual who supplied another new word, etc. Thus, all third-order sentences were characterized by the fact that the use of any word was conditional on the two words preceding it. An example of each of the three approximations is shown in Table 1.

TABLE 1. Typical examples of seven-word sentences constructed on the basis of conditional probabilities.

Order of Approximation	Example Sentence
First	Do mind instead edge drop quickly till.
Second	Laugh long name my french women laugh.
Third	Forward march said the boy had a.

In this fashion a pool of 24 10-sentence message sets has been constructed: nine first-order sets, nine second-order sets, and six third-order sets. Of the nine message sets for both first- and second-order approximations, three are five-word sentences, three are seven-word sentences, and three contain nine words. Only seven and nine-word sentences were used for third-order approximations, since shorter lengths did not permit an adequate representation of the conditional probabilities associated with third orders. Three separate forms for each sentence length were constructed. For any given number of words, sentence length was further controlled by the constraint that the number of syllables must be constant within ±1 syllable of the modal value.

Sentences were recorded by a single talker, using an Altec 682A microphone, Ampex PR-10 tape recorder, and Scotch No. 202 low-noise tape. The talker attempted to speak each sentence in as natural a fashion as possible, using a VU meter for only gross visual monitoring of overall intensity.

A series of coding pulses was recorded on the second track of the tape. For each sentence of a message set, two program-pulse instructions were recorded. The first programming instruction consisted of a single pulse, just preceding the occurrence of a sentence. This pulse set an 11-position stepping switch to a zero position. A varying series of pulses was then recorded, simultaneous with the occurrence of the sentence. The number of pulses in this series corresponded to the sentence identification number, that is, one pulse for the first sentence, two pulses for the second sentence, etc. The number of sentences presented to a subject was accumulated on one counter by totaling the number of re-set pulses that just preceded each sentence. A second counter recorded the number of times the button pushed by the subject corresponded to the number of pulses coded for the sentence; that is, correct responses.

Ten copies of each message set (10 sentences) were dubbed with a different random order for each copy. Thus, each set of sentences could be presented to a subject in 10 successive repetitions in order to establish the effect of learning or practice on performance.

EXPERIMENT I

The purpose of the first experiment was to determine the relation among orders of approximations and the nature of learning over successive trials.

Procedure

Six subjects with normal hearing listened to 10 successive repetitions of message sets (10 sentences per set) using first, second, and third orders of approximation to "real" sentences. The order of presentation of the various approximations was counter-balanced. In order to render the material sufficiently difficult for normals, the tape output was routed through a low-pass filter (Krohn-Hite, Model 330M) with a cut-off frequency of 350 cps and an attenuation rate of 24 dB/octave. Each subject was given a practice session, using a different list of sentences, to familiarize him with the task and to aid in establishing a satisfactory level of presentation. Intensity was varied, during this practice session, in order to determine a level that produced approximately 30-50% correct response. During actual test runs, all sentences were presented at this pre-determined level.

Results

Figure 2 shows the average cumulative per-cent functions generated by these six subjects for the three message sets. The ordinate represents the accumulated percentages of correct responses over successive trials. A systematic ordering of the three curves as a function of order of approximation is apparent. As the constraint on word sequence increases (from first-order to third-order), performance increases rather systematically. This effect is particularly noteworthy in view of the fact that, in all three conditions, all sentences were of equal length in terms of word and syllable count. In addition, all words were drawn from a common pool. The three conditions differed only in respect to the constraints on word sequences imposed by the conditional probabilities built into the second- and third-order approximations.

All three curves in Figure 2 show some evidence of the expected learning

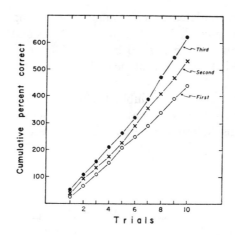

FIGURE 2. Cumulative per-cent functions over successive trials for first-, second-, and third-order approximation sentences with low-pass filtering.

TABLE 2. Mean performance on three message sets (first-, second-, and third-orders) for Trials 1 - 3, 4 - 6, and 7 - 10, 1 - 5, and 6 - 10 for the low-pass filter condition (N = 6).

			Trials		
Order	1 - 3	4 - 6	7 - 10	1 - 5	6 - 10
First	37	46	48	42	46
Second	45	52	60	46	61
Third	53	56	74	53	72

or practice effect across trials. The nature of changes in performance for the three message sets perhaps can be seen more easily in Table 2. For the first-order sentences, the greatest increase is seen between trial intervals 1 - 3 and 4 - 6. After the 6th trial very little change is apparent.

A slightly different pattern can be seen for the second-order sentences. Performance continues to increase across trials. Consequently, scores on the last half are 15% higher than on the first half.

For the third-order set, very little change is observed between trial intervals 1 - 3 and 4 - 6, but marked improvement occurs over the last four trials. Thus, scores on the last five trials are 19% higher than on the first five.

EXPERIMENT II

Until this point no attempt had been made to control the number of practice items that were given to each subject. In view of the practice effect observed, it seemed advisable to bring this variable under more precise experimental control. A second experiment was therefore performed to determine whether the effects of learning or practice would be diminished if the nature of the practice session were changed.

Procedure

All conditions were identical to those of the first experiment with two exceptions. The cut-off frequency of the low-pass filter was raised from 350 cps to 500 cps, in order to render the task less difficult, and the nature of the practice session was altered.

In the new practice session each subject was given exactly 100 items from a message set. The first five items were presented at a comfortable level (approximatly 60 dB SPL). The experimenter then determined, in a descending manner, the level at which the subject responded correctly to 40-50% of the set. This level was then used throughout all subsequent testing for a particular subject.

Eighteen subjects with normal hearing listened to 10 successive repetitions of different message sets. Six subjects listened to first-order, six to second-order, and six to third-order message sets.

Results

Figure 3 shows the average cumulative per-cent function generated by these subjects. Changes in the slope of the function, indicating the existence of a learning or practice effect, are still apparent, but the magnitude of the effect has been attenuated markedly from the changes observed in the three functions of Figure 2. A single linear function describes subject performance over the last seven trials. The function for trials one through three, although linear, has a slightly more gradual slope.

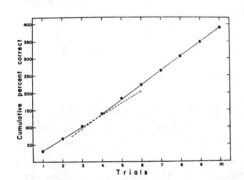

FIGURE 3. Cumulative per-cent functions over successive ·trials after systematic practice session.

Figure 4 shows individual cumulative per-cent functions for second-order sentences across 10 trials for two of the 18 subjects. Again it is apparent that the pattern of correct responses is quite stable over the last seven trials. The more carefully controlled practice session used in this experiment apparently minimized changes in performance due to learning over successive trials.

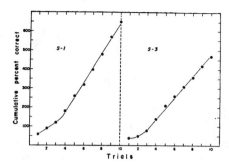

FIGURE 4. Cumulative per-cent functions over successive trials for two individual subjects after systematic practice session.

EXPERIMENT III

The purpose of the third experiment was to assess the relation among the orders of approximation to "real" sentences under a condition of periodic interruption.

Procedure

Message sets were presented monaurally to six normal-hearing subjects at approximately 58 dB SPL. Ten successive repetitions of first-, second-, and third-order sentences were presented in a counter-balanced order. Sentences were cyclically interrupted by inserting into the circuit an electronic switch (Grason-Stadler, Model 829) triggered by an interval timer (Grason-Stadler, Model 472). The interruption rate was 1.25/sec., with an on-time of 200 msec, an off-time of 600 msec, and a rise-decay time of 1 msec. Thus, speech was on only 25% of the time. Testing was preceded by a 100-item practice session in order to minimize practice effect during the experimental run.

Results

The cumulative per-cent functions for the three message sets are shown in Figure 5. The same systematic ordering as a function of order of approximation shown previously (Figure 2) is apparent. Performance improves systematically as the amount of information is decreased (from first-order to third-order) even when 75% of the message set is deleted. However, the differences observed for the periodic interruption condition are smaller than those obtained with the low-pass filter condition. Yet, some information concerning the conditional probabilities of word sequences apparently is still transmitted with only 25% of the message present.

None of the curves in Figure 5 show appreciable evidence of the practice effect observed when the messages were low-pass filtered. The stability of performance across trials is also reflected in the data of Table 3. The only obvious change occurs for the first-order sentences between the trial inter-

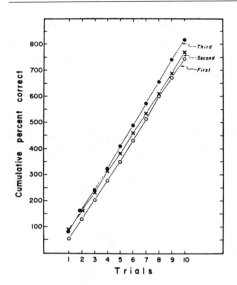

FIGURE 5. Cumulative per-cent functions over successive trials for first-, second-, and third-order approximation sentences with periodic interruption.

vals 1 - 3 and 4 - 6. For this group of sentences, scores on the last five trials are 7% higher than on the first five. Performance on second- and third-order sentences is relatively stable. The more intensive practice session used in this experiment apparently served to stabilize performance adequately.

TABLE 3. Mean performance on three message sets (first-, second-, and third-orders) for Trials 1 - 3, 4 - 6, and 7 - 10, 1 - 5, and 6 - 10 during periodic interruption (N = 6).

| Order | Trials | | | | |
	1 - 3	4 - 6	7 - 10	1 - 5	6 - 10
First	68	76	78	71	78
Second	78	76	77	77	77
Third	81	82	82	83	81

SUMMARY

This report describes a method developed for measuring speech identification. The message sets contain synthetic sentences, constructed as approximations to "real" sentences solely on the basis of the conditional probabilities of word sequences. Each message set is closed, of controlled length and controlled relative informational content. The testing procedure is automated, permitting rapid data acquisition and storage.

Thirty subjects have been tested in a variety of experimental conditions. Results show that as the amount of information in the artificial sentence decreases, subject performance improves. This relation exists both when the message is low-pass filtered and when it is periodically interrupted.

This approach to the measurement of speech identification seems promising as a tool in many experimental conditions, particularly those involving the manipulation of temporal parameters.

This investigation was supported by Public Health Service Research Grant No. NB 05044 from the National Institute of Neurological Diseases and Blindness.

REFERENCES

DAVIS, H., and SILVERMAN, S. R., *Hearing and Deafness.* Revised Ed., New York: Holt, Rinehart, and Winston, Inc. (1960).

EGAN, J. P., Articulation testing methods. *Laryngoscope,* **58,** 955-991 (1948).

FLETCHER, H., *Speech and Hearing.* New York: Van Nostrand (1929).

FLETCHER, H., and STEINBERG, J. C., Articulation testing methods. *Bell Syst. tech. J.,* **8,** 806-854 (1929).

FRY, D. B., Modifications to speech audiometry. *Int. Aud.,* **3,** 226-236 (1964).

HIRSH, I. J., *The Measurement of Hearing.* New York: McGraw-Hill Book Co., Inc. (1952).

HOUSE, A. S., STEVENS, K. N., SANDEL, T. T., and ARNOLD, JANE B., On the learning of speechlike vocabularies. *J. verb. Learn verb. Behav.,* **1,** 133-143 (1962).

HOUSE, A. S., WILLIAMS, C. E., HECKER, M. H. L., and KRYTER, K. D., Articulation-testing methods: consonantal differentiation with a closed-response set. *J. acoust. Soc. Amer.,* **37,** 158-166 (1965).

HUDGINS, C. V., HAWKINS, J. E., KARLIN, J. E., and STEVENS, S. S., The development of recorded auditory tests for measuring hearing loss for speech. *Laryngoscope,* **57,** 57-89 (1947).

MILLER, G. A., Speech and language, in, *Handbook of Experimental Psychology,* S. S. Stevens (Ed.), New York: John Wiley and Sons (1951).

MILLER, G. A., and SELFRIDGE, J. A., Verbal context and the recall of meaningful material. *Amer. J. Psychol.,* **53,** 176-185 (1950).

MILLER, G. A., WEINER, F. M., and STEVENS, S. S., Transmission and reception of sounds under combat conditions. *Summary Technical Report of Division 17, NDRC,* Washington: 3 (1946).

SILVERMAN, S. R., and HIRSH, I. J., Problems related to the use of speech in clinical audiometry. *Ann. Oto. Rhino. Laryng.,* **64,** 1234-1244 (1955).

THORNDIKE, E. L., and LORGE, I., *The Teachers Word Book of 30,000 Words.* New York: Bureau of Publications, Teachers College, Columbia University (1944).

WALSH, T. E., and SILVERMAN, S. R., Diagnosis and evaluation of fenestration. *Larygoscope,* **56,** 536-555 (1946).

Received January 4, 1965.

Diagnostic Significance of PB Word Functions

James Jerger, PhD, and Susan Jerger, MS, Houston

Performance-Intensity (PI) functions for phonetically balanced (PB) words were compared in 41 patients with presumably cochlear disorder and 16 patients with retrocochlear disorder. The PI functions of all of 10 eighth nerve disorders and three of six brain stem disorders showed a pronounced rollover phenomenon. After reaching a maximum the PI function declined substantially with further increase in speech level. Implications of the phenomenon for differential diagnosis of cochlear and retrocochlear disorders are discussed.

ALTHOUGH the measurement of "discrimination loss" for speech has been a standard audiologic procedure for many years, the diagnostic significance of speech intelligibility scores has not been fully exploited. Several investigators (Schuknecht and Woellner[1] and Crabbe[2]) have noted that the maximum score for word discrimination (PB max) is often disproportionately poor in relation to the sensitivity loss in patients with eighth nerve disorder, but the substantial overlap in the PB max scores of cochlear and eighth nerve patients (Johnson[3]) effectively limits the diagnostic value of PB max.

Recently, interest in the diagnostic significance of speech intelligibility measures has been renewed by the observation of a "rollover" phenomenon (Jerger et al; Jerger and

Accepted for publication Dec 31, 1970.

From the Department of Otolaryngology, Division of Audiology and Speech Pathology, Baylor College of Medicine, and the Methodist Hospital, Houston.

Reprint requests to 11922 Taylorcrest Rd, Houston 77024 (Dr. Jerger).

Jerger[4-6]) in the PB performance-intensity functions (PB-PI) of patients with retrocochlear disorder. As speech intensity increased, the PB score reached a maximum, then "rolled over" as intensity was increased above the maximum score, and became, paradoxically, substantially poorer as the speech level was further raised.

The present communication explores the diagnostic significance of this rollover phenomenon by comparison of the PB-PI functions of patients with both cochlear and retrocochlear disorder.

Method

Subjects.—The subjects of this investigation were 41 patients with presumed cochlear disorder and 16 patients with confirmed retrocochlear disorder.

Subjects in the presumably cochlear group met all of the following criteria: (1) bilateral sensorineural loss greater than 25 dB (I SO-64) at two or more frequencies in the range from 250 to 4,000 Hz; (2) Bekesy audiogram type I or type II; and (3) absence of positive neurological signs suggestive of retrocochlear disorder.

The 41 subjects in this group ranged in age from 19 to 78 years. The average hearing level (I SO-64) for the frequency range 500 to 2,000 Hz (PTA) ranged from 6 to 72 dB, and the PB max ranged from 24% to 100%.

Subjects in the retrocochlear group all met the criterion that site of lesion was confirmed either surgically or radiographically. Of the 16 subjects in this group, ten had surgically confirmed tumors in the cerebellopontine angle affecting the eighth nerve, and six had tumors

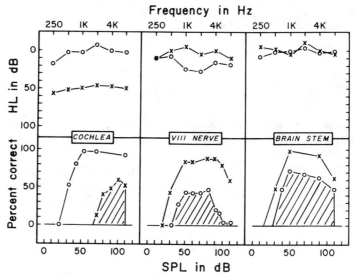

Fig 1.—Examples of PB-PI functions in three patients with unilateral disorder. Cochlear patient shows moderate sensitivity loss, marked by reduced PB max, but little rollover. Eighth nerve patient shows mild sensitivity loss, severely reduced PB max, and virtually complete rollover. Brain stem patient shows no sensitivity loss, moderately reduced PB max in ear contralateral to affected side of brain, and slight rollover.

in the brain stem. Three of the latter six tumors were confirmed surgically, the remaining three radiographically. Subjects in this group ranged in age from 6 to 63 years. PTA ranged from 0 to 70 dB, and PB max ranged from 28% to 96%.

Instrumentation and Materials.—Six NDRC PB-50 word lists (Egan 1948)[8] were recorded on magnetic tape (Ampex, 351) by a male speaker with general American dialect (JFJ). The taped lists were amplified, attenuated, and switched by means of a speech audiometer (Grason-Stadler, 162) and delivered to the patient via earphone (Telephonic, TDH-39) mounted in a circumaural cushion (CZW-6). Speech intensity was uniformly defined as the sound pressure level (SPL) in dB, of a 1,000 Hz calibration tone recorded at the average level of frequent peaks of the PB words.

Procedure. — Performance-Intensity (PI) functions for PB words were constructed by presenting half-lists (25 words) in 10 to 20 dB steps until the shape of the function was clearly defined. In general, the aim was to cover the range from that speech intensity yielding a PB score of approximately 20% up to a maximum speech intensity of 110 dB SPL. Usually six levels were sufficient to define a function. Rarely were seven or eight levels required.

Whenever the speech level to the test ear was sufficiently intense that the signal might conceivably cross over and be heard on the nontest ear, the latter was masked by white noise at a level 20 dB less than the speech presentation level on the test ear.

In one patient, a child of 6 years with a brain stem glioma, the standard test procedure was modified in order to present speech materials more appropriate to age level, and to accommodate the patient's malaise. For this patient PB-K word lists of ten words each were presented via live-voice in order to define the PI function.

Results

Figure 1 shows the audiograms and PB-PI functions of three illustrative patients; one with presumably cochlear disorder, one with eighth nerve disorder, and one with brain stem disorder. In general, the results on these three patients typify our findings.

The cochlear patient, in spite of substantially impaired sensitivity and pronounced discrimination loss, shows little or no rollover in the PB-PI function. The eighth nerve patient, with less sensitivity loss, shows an even poorer PB max and complete rollover of the PB-PI function. The function plateaus at about 44% over the range from 50 to 80 dB SPL, then drops virtually to 0% at 100 and 110 dB SPL. The brain stem patient, with no sensitivity loss, shows clearcut discrimination loss, but only slight rollover.

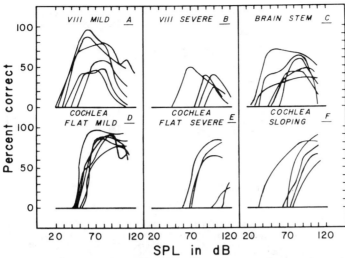

Fig 2.—Thirty-two PB-PI functions illustrating consistent rollover in eighth nerve disorders, inconsistent rollover in brain stem disorders, and lack of rollover in cochlear disorders. **A,** Eighth nerve disorders with mild audiometric loss. **B,** Eighth nerve disorders with severe audiometric loss. **C,** Brain stem disorders. **D,** Cochlear disorders with flat, mild audiometric loss. **E,** Cochlear disorders with flat, severe audiometric loss. **F,** Cochlear disorders with sloping audiometric contours.

In the cochlear and eighth nerve patients speech intelligibility was, of course, impaired in the affected ear. In the brain stem patient, however, speech intelligibility was involved in the ear contralateral to the affected side of the brain.

Figure 2 shows 32 individual PB-PI functions. Panel A shows the PB-PI functions of six eighth nerve patients with mild sensitivity loss (PTA < 35 db). Panel B shows the PB-PI functions of four eighth nerves with greater sensitivity loss (PTA [pure tone average] 35 dB). Panel C shows the PB-PI functions of all six patients with brain stem disorder. Panels D, E, and F show typical PB-PI functions of 16 cochlears, grouped according to severity and slope of loss. The six patients of panel D had relatively flat mild sensitivity loss (PTA < 45 dB). The four patients of panel E had flat but relatively more severe sensitivity loss (PTA > 45 dB). The six patients of panel F all had markedly sloping audiometric contours.

We may note that all of the patients with eighth nerve disorder (panels A and B) show pronounced rollover, but in the brain stem group (panel C) the degree of rollover is quite variable. Three patients show a substantial effect, but one shows only a slight effect, and two show no rollover at all.

The cochlear patients, in contrast, show little or no rollover irrespective of degree or slope of audiometric loss. In general, cochlears tend to reach a plateau and stay there with little or no falling off at very high speech levels.

In order to explore the diagnostic value of the shape of the PB-PI function we first plotted PB max against PTA for each of the three groups (Fig 3). In the cochlear group we have plotted the results for 54 ears of the 41 patients. The *dashed line* shows the expected relation between PB max and PTA. In the eighth nerve group we can see a tendency toward a somewhat lower PB max at small PTA than in the cochlear group; but, in general, the ranges are quite comparable, thus limiting the diagnostic value of the PB max insofar as the distinction between cochlear and eighth nerve is concerned. The brain stem patients show extremely poor PB max scores in relation to PTA, and here a strong case could be made for the diagnostic significance of a PB max below 70% when the PTA is less than 20 dB.

In order to quantify the magnitude of the rollover phenomenon, each PB-PI function was analyzed for the PB min, that is, for the lowest PB score above the PB max. The

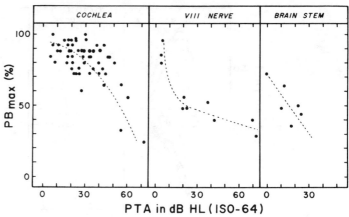

Fig 3.—PB max as a function of PTA in 54 cochlear ears, 10 eighth nerve ears, and six brain stem ears. Overlapping ranges of cochlears and eighth nerves limit diagnostic value of PB max.

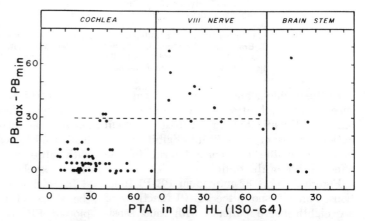

Fig 4.—Rollover (PB max-PB min) as a function of PTA in cochlear, eighth nerve, and brain stem disorders. This index shows greater diagnostic potential than PB max, but there is still some overlap between cochlears and eighth nerves.

Fig 5.—Rollover ratio (PB max-PB min/PB max) as a function of PTA. This index virtually eliminates overlap between cochlear and eighth nerve ears.

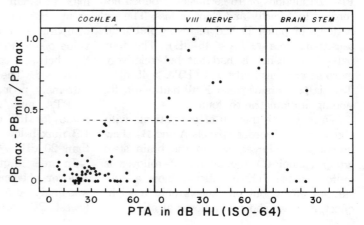

difference between these two scores, PB max minus PB min, defined degree of rollover. Figure 4 plots this rollover index as a function of PTA for each group. Here we see a considerable reduction in the overlap between cochlears and eighth nerves. Only two of the 54 cochlear ears show rollover greater than 30% whereas seven of the 10 eighth nerve ears show rollover greater than 30%. In the brain stem group there is, as expected, considerable overlap with the cochlear group.

Closer examination of the individual PB-PI functions revealed a possible basis for sharpening the diagnostic value of the rollover effect. We noted that, in the cochlear group, rollover in excess of 20% only occurred when the PB max itself was relatively high, whereas, in the eighth nerve group, rollover was less dependent on PB max. Stated differently, cochlears never showed the complete decline from PB max down to virtually zero performance as the eighth nerves so often did. In order to take this factor into account, each rollover score (PB max − PB min) was divided by PB max. The resultant index is plotted, as a function of PTA, in Fig 5. We now note the complete separation of the cochlear and eighth nerve groups. There is no overlap whatever. The highest cochlear index is 0.40 and the lowest eighth nerve index is 0.45. Again, however, the brain stem group overlaps both the cochlear and eighth nerve distributions.

In order to obtain a more detailed picture of the general nature and degree of rollover in the general population of patients with hearing disorder, the PB-PI functions of 741 ears, gathered in the routine clinical evaluation of patients referred to our audiology service, were analyzed. Figure 6 shows the distribution of rollover index (PB max-PB min/ PB max) in 218 normals, 102 conductive and mixed losses, and 421 sensorineural losses. The three distributions are remarkably similar. About 85% of ears show rollover indices smaller than 0.20; about 13% show indices between 0.20 and 0.39; only about 2% show indices greater than 0.39.

It is interesting that only nine of the 741 ears showed rollover indices of 0.50 to 0.59. Eight of these nine patients had sensorineural loss, and one was mixed. Of the nine, eight were more than 50 years old, seven were more than 60 years old, and six were more than 70 years old.

We conclude, therefore, that rollover indices as large as those observed in our eighth nerve and brain stem patients are exceedingly rare in the general population of hearing disorders. When they do occur, however, they seem to be uniquely predominant in the extremely elderly patient.

In order to study the generality of the rollover effect we compared PI functions for PB words with PI functions for synthetic sentence identification in the presence of an ipsilateral competing speech message (Jerger et al, 1968[7]). Figure 7 shows illustrative results for one patient with brain stem disorder and for two patients with eighth nerve disorder. For sentences, varying message competition ratios were deliberately chosen to highlight the fact that, in spite of varying maxima, the rollover effect is consistently observed for speech tasks involving either word repetition in quiet or sentence identification against continuous competitions.

Still another example of the generality of the rollover phenomenon is shown in Fig 8. We had the good fortune to test a patient with a left acoustic neuroma who spoke both English and Spanish fluently. Figure 8 shows PI functions for English PB words, English synthetic sentences, and analogous Spanish synthetic sentences (Benitez and Speaks[9]). Here the generality of the rollover effect is seen in two different languages.

Comment

The exact shape of the PI function for verbal materials would appear to have potential diagnostic significance. In the present study the "rollover" effect easily differentiated ten paients with eighth nerve disorder from 41 patients with cochlear disorder. A simple index of rollover, the difference between the highest point on the PB-PI function (PB max) and the lowest point above PB max (PB min) separated the two groups with only minimal overlap. A more refined index, obtained by dividing this simple index by PB max, separated the two groups without overlap. These effects were observed in spite of the fact that PB max, per se, showed substantial overlap between the two groups.

The previous literature on the rollover effect is somewhat confused and conflicting. Eby and Williams[10] described rollover in 15 of 17 cases of end-organ deafness, but not in five of six cases of nerve fiber degeneration. Huizing and Reyntjes[11] described rollover in patients with recruitment, and named the helmet-shaped articulation curve *chapeau de gendarme*. Similar findings in ears with loudness recruitment were noted by Hedgecock[12] and Schultz and Streepy.[13] On the other hand, little or no rollover was reported by Leisti,[14] Palva,[15] or Liden[16] in any type of sensorineural hearing loss. More recently Hood[17] and König[18] have described the rollover effect in both cochlear and retrocochlear disorder. Finally, Punch and McConnell[19] found no rollover at all in 24 presbycusics.

The present results are not in disagreement with previous findings of a helmet-shaped articulation function in end-organ, cochlear, or recruiting losses. As shown in Fig 6, our own data do show some rollover in many patients with cochlear hearing loss. However, large effects are quite uncommon. In contrast, our data indicate that, in retrocochlear disorder, rollover effects far in excess of those usually encountered in cochlear losses are very common indeed. It is not a difference in kind, but a difference in degree and in expected frequency of occurrence.

In view of this obvious difference it is reasonable to ask why the rollover phenomenon in retrocochlear disorder has not been more widely observed. One reason is surely the fact that clinicians, especially in the USA, seldom run PB lists at more than one level. There is a widespread implicit assumption that, if this single level is at an appropriate suprathreshold point, the PB max is guaranteed. The present data show that this is a false assumption in the case of retrocochlear disorder. The PI function is often so narrow that variation of only 10 dB above or below the actual level of PB max may change the PB score by a substantial amount. If the single standard level employed by the clinician is relatively high, eg, 40 dB SL, the resultant PB score may seriously underestimate the true PB max.

The rollover phenomenon in retrocochlear disorders has, in fact, been observed fre-

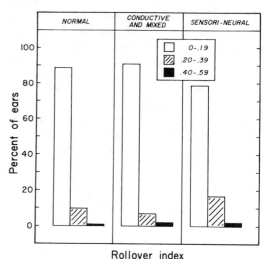

Fig 6.—Distribution of rollover index in 741 ears—218 normals, 102 conductives or mixed, and 421 sensorineurals. Note only small percentage (2%) shows index greater than 0.39.

quently by investigators who have plotted complete PI functions. Citron et al[20] found it in a case of multiple sclerosis, and Bocca and Calearo demonstrated the effect repeatedly in both brain stem and temporal lobe disease (Fig 15, 21, 22, and 23).[21]

The present results suggest that, whenever the distinction between cochlear and retrocochlear disorder is at issue, the exact shape of the PI function for PB words should be carefully defined by presenting PB lists at several suprathreshold levels up to the maximum intensity that the patient will tolerate.

It should not, however, be implied from this communication, that all patients with eighth nerve disorder will show the rollover effect. The present data suggest that, when the rollover effect is observed, the likelihood of an eighth nerve site is high. They say nothing, however, about the likelihood that patients with eighth nerve disorder may not show the effect. The present sample of ten is far too small to provide stable estimates of such probabilities. However, judging from statistics provided by Johnson[3] for other eighth nerve signs such as Bekesy type, SISI test, etc, we may anticipate that roughly 70% to 80% of eighth nerve disorders will show the effect, and the remainder probably will not. For neoplastic growths, the likelihood that a particular sign will be observed seems related, as Johnson notes, to the size of the neoplasm.

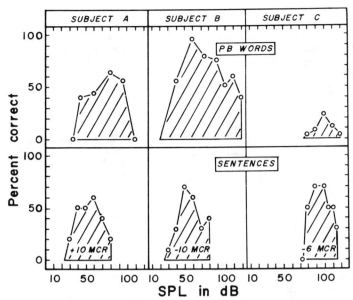

Fig 7.—Comparison of PI functions for PB words and for synthetic sentences in one patient with brain stem and two patients with eighth nerve disorder. Rollover effect is seen in both functions despite considerable differences in type of test material, method of test administration, etc.

Fig 8.—Comparison of PI functions for English PB words, English synthetic sentences, and Spanish synthetic sentences in a patient with left acoustic neuroma and bilingual facility. Rollover effect is seen despite differences in test materials and test language.

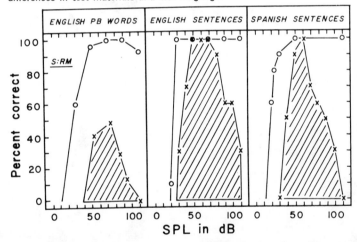

The rollover phenomenon, then, should be viewed as an additional clinical tool whose diagnostic value lies in the fact that its presence raises the strong presumption of retrocochlear disorder. It is in this sense that the effect has diagnostic significance. Its presence alerts the clinician to, or supplements other signs of, eighth nerve disorder.

We are not suggesting, however, that this is a perfect test in which all cochlears give a negative result and all eighth nerves give a positive result. Behavioral signs seldom achieve such a high degree of accuracy. They can, nevertheless, provide the clinician with valuable information.

This study was supported by Public Health Service Research grant NS 05842 from the National Institute of Neurological Diseases and Stroke.

References

1. Schuknecht H, Woellner R: An experimental and clinical study of deafness from lesions of the cochlear nerve. *J Laryng* **69**:75-97, 1955.

2. Crabbe F: Le neurinome de l'acoustique vu par l'otologiste. *Acta Otorhinolaryng Belg* **20**:33-96, 1966.

3. Johnson E: Confirmed retrocochlear lesions. *Arch Otolaryng* **84**:247-254, 1966.

4. Jerger J, Jerger S, Ainsworth J, et al: Recovery of auditory function after surgical removal of cerebellar tumor. *J Speech Hearing Dis* **31**:377-382, 1966.

5. Jerger J, Jerger S: Psychoacoustic comparison of cochlear and VIIIth nerve disorders. *J Speech Hearing Res* **10**:659-688, 1967.

6. Jerger J, Jerger S: Progression of auditory symptoms in a patient with acoustic neurinoma. *Ann Otol* **77**:230-242, 1968.

7. Jerger J, Speaks C, Trammell JL: A new approach to speech audiometry. *J Speech Hearing Dis* **33**:318-328, 1968.

8. Egan J: Articulation testing methods. *Laryngoscope* **58**:955-991, 1948.

9. Benitez L, Speaks C: A test of speech intelligibility in the Spanish language. *Int Audiol* **7**:16-22, 1968.

10. Eby LG, Williams HL: Recruitment of loudness in the differential diagnosis of end-organ and nerve fibre deafness. *Laryngoscope* **61**:400-414, 1951.

11. Huizing HC, Reyntjes JA: Recruitment and speech discrimination loss. *Laryngoscope* **62**:521-527, 1952.

12. Hedgecock LC: The measurement of auditory recruitment. *Arch Otolaryng* **62**:515-527, 1955.

13. Schultz MD, Streepy CS: The speech discrimination function in loudness recruiting ears. *Laryngoscope* **77**:2114-2127, 1967.

14. Leisti T: On speech audiograms. *Acta Otolaryng* **37**:256-260, 1949.

15. Palva T: Finnish speech audiometry: Method and clinical applications. *Acta Otolaryng* **101** (suppl):128, 1952.

16. Liden G: Speech Audiometry: An experimental and clinical study with Swedish language material. *Acta Otolaryng* **114**(suppl):145, 1954.

17. Hood JD: Speech discrimination and its relationship to disorders of the loudness function. *Int Audiol* **7**:232-238, 1968.

18. König E: Das problem des sprechaudiometrie im deutschweizerischen Sprachgebiet. *Pract Otorhinolaryng* **28**:39-63, 1966.

19. Punch J, McConnell F: The speech discrimination function of elderly patients. *J Audiol Res* **9**:159-166, 1969.

20. Citron L, Dix MR, Hallpike CS, et al: A recent clinico-pathological study of cochlear nerve degeneration resulting from tumor pressure and disseminated sclerosis, with particular reference to the finding of normal threshold sensitivity for pure tones. *Acta Otolaryng* **56**:330-337, 1963.

21. Bocca E, Calearo C: Central hearing processes, in Jerger J (ed): *Modern Developments in Audiology*. New York, Academic Press Inc, 1963.

Hearing Aid Evaluation

Clinical Experience With a New Philosophy

James Jerger, PhD, Deborah Hayes, MA

● We report a new method of hearing aid evaluation with the underlying philosophy that evaluation of hearing aid performance is not an end in itself, but an integral part of the total rehabilitation of the hearing-impaired patient. This new method uses synthetic sentences and speech competition in varying "message-to-competition ratios (MCRs)" to evaluate patient performance with hearing aids. We report six illustrative cases and a follow-up survey of patient satisfaction with recommended hearing aids to relate our experience with this technique.

(*Arch Otolaryngol* 102:214-225, 1976)

The hearing aid evaluation has been an important clinical procedure for over 20 years. It is often the only rehabilitative service the audiologist can employ in the management of the hearing-impaired patient.

The traditional method of hearing aid evaluation was originally described by Carhart almost 30 years ago.[1] This method evaluates patient performance with selected hearing aids in three ways. First, spondee

Accepted for publication Nov 26, 1975.

From the Department of Otolaryngology, Baylor College of Medicine, Texas Medical Center, Houston.

Reprint requests to Mail Station 009, the Methodist Hospital, Texas Medical Center, Houston, TX 77025 (Dr Jerger).

words are used to measure the acoustic gain of the hearing aid. Second, phonetically balanced (PB) words are used to measure the patient's ability to understand aided speech at conversational loudness in an optimum (quiet) listening condition. Finally, competing noise is added to the PB words in order to "stress" the hearing aid. The recommended aid is the instrument that gives the best acoustic gain as measured with spondees, and the best aided speech understanding as measured with PB words presented in quiet and in noise at a fixed sensation level (SL) relative to the aided speech reception threshold (SRT).

One of the most frequently cited limitations of this approach is its inability to delineate differences among hearing aids or aid arrangements. When only two conditions, PB words presented in quiet and in noise, are used to test the patient's ability to understand aided speech, substantial aid differences rarely emerge. Another frequently cited limitation is the technique's lack of face validity. Conversational speech consists of a sequence of thoughts or ideas, usually expressed by phrases or sentences, not by isolated words. Single word repetition as a method for measuring a patient's communicative impairment

would not, therefore, be a test technique of maximum validity. A patient's performance on this task, so the argument goes, can scarcely be expected to predict his communication handicap, his aided improvement, or his remaining hearing deficit. Citing these limitations, numerous investigators have questioned both the validity and the reliability of the conventional hearing aid evaluation concept.[2-5]

Our own experience with this approach has led us to the same conclusions. We have observed that both the aided and unaided PB scores are overly dependent on the amount and configuration of the patient's high-frequency hearing loss. Furthermore, the PB score does not seem to relate the patient's clinical performance to his real life experiences with amplification in a consistent fashion. In spite of negative experience, however, we have been reluctant to abandon the procedure of clinical hearing aid evaluation. For all its faults, the hearing aid evaluation concept is still a powerful tool in the rehabilitation of the hearing-impaired patient.

About three years ago, we set out to determine whether it would be possible to design a new procedure that would overcome the inherent limitations of the conventional technique.

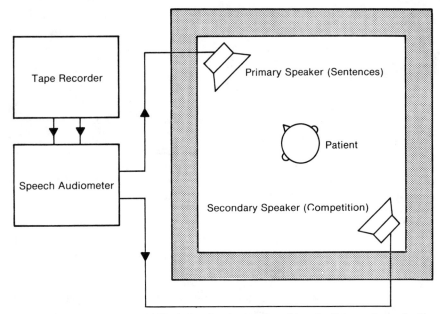

Fig 1.—Seating arrangement in test chamber for hearing aid evaluations performed with sentence identification materials.

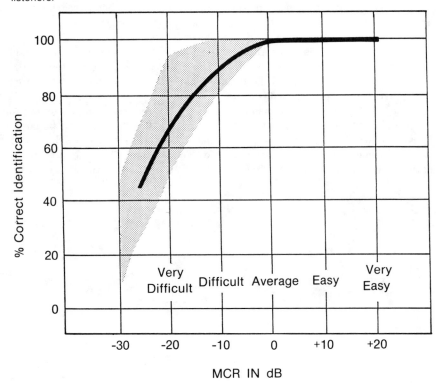

Fig 2.—Hearing aid evaluation summary form for recording patient performance with sentence identification materials. Shaded area represents performance range of normal listeners.

Our approach to a new methodology was based on the conviction that specific tests and procedures must be founded on a broad philosophical base that emphasizes evaluation of hearing aid performance not as an end in itself, but as an integral part of the total rehabilitative process. The principal limitation of the conventional method, it seemed to us, was its emphasis on the "selection" of the best hearing aid. We consider this to be one of several possible rehabilitative goals. Equally important are the goals of judging prognosis for successful hearing aid use and determining realistic expectations from amplification. In addition to fulfilling these goals, we felt that an effective hearing aid evaluation technique must delineate differences among hearing aids in a systematic manner, achieve face validity by employing test materials more closely resembling conversational speech, and be a simple procedure that utilizes standard clinical instrumentation.

We describe a new hearing aid evaluation technique designed to meet these criteria. We believe that the technique effectively avoids the shortcomings of the conventional method of hearing aid evaluation. It is directed toward the following specific goals: (1) to determine the most suitable hearing aid arrangement for the individual; (2) to define differences among arrangements in real life listening conditions; (3) to provide information on realistic expectations of hearing aid use for patient counselling; and (4) to make accountable rehabilitative recommendations to patients.

METHOD

The patient is seated in the test chamber, equidistant between two loudspeakers. Figure 1 shows this seating arrangement. The loudspeaker directly in front of the patient delivers the primary message. The loudspeaker directly behind the patient delivers the secondary message.

The primary message is a sequence of ten synthetic sentences.[6] These sentences are approximations to real English sentences, based on the transitional probabilities linking adjacent words.

The ten sentences of the primary message set are as follows.

Fig 3.—Hypothetical hearing aid evaluation summary showing concepts of "aided improvement" and "residual deficit."

1. Small boat with a picture has become
2. Built the government with the force almost
3. Go change your car color is red
4. Forward march said the boy had a
5. March around without a care in your
6. That neighbor who said business is better
7. Battle cry and be better than ever
8. Down by the time is real enough
9. Agree with him only to find out
10. Women view men with green paper should

The secondary message is continuous discourse in the form of a biographical story. This continuous discourse provides speech competition during the presentation of each test sentence.

The primary sentences and the secondary competition are recorded on dual channel magnetic tape by the same male talker. Channel 1 contains the primary

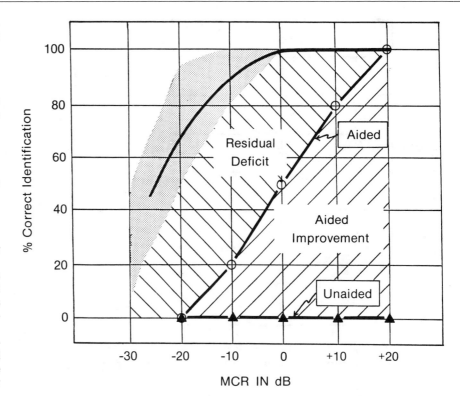

Fig 4.—Audiogram and hearing aid evaluation summary form for case 1, 76-year-old man with moderate sensorineural loss in right ear and profound loss in left ear. NR, No response. CNE, Could not evaluate.

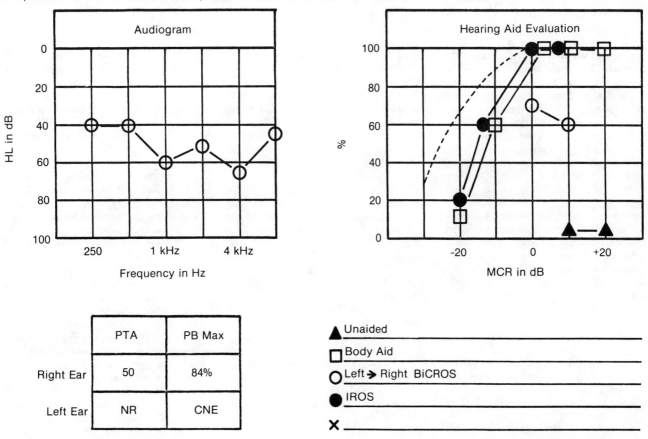

	PTA	PB Max
Right Ear	50	84%
Left Ear	NR	CNE

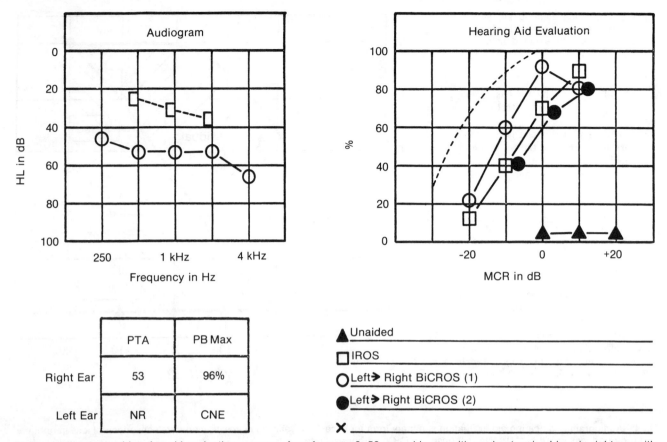

Fig 5.—Audiogram and hearing aid evaluation summary form for case 2, 56-year-old man with moderate mixed loss in right ear with patient facing primary speaker. NR, No response. CNE, Could not evaluate.

sentences. They are recorded at ten-second intervals. The same ten-sentence list is recorded in ten successively randomized blocks. These taped materials are played via a speech audiometer through the two loudspeakers in the test chamber.

The intensity of the primary sentences is set to 60 dB sound pressure level (SPL). This intensity is never varied during the evaluation procedure. The secondary speech competition, however, is varied between 40 dB SPL and 80 db SPL. At each secondary level, all ten primary sentences are presented. Throughout the evaluation procedure, the patient holds before him a large card listing the ten primary sentences. He is instructed to call out the number of each sentence as it is presented.

Each combination of intensity levels defines a "message-to-competition ratio (MCR)." A positive or negative value is assigned based on the relationship of the secondary speech competition to the primary sentences. For example, when the primary sentences are at 60 dB SPL and the secondary speech competition is at 40

dB SPL, the MCR is +20 dB. When the primary sentences are at 60 dB SPL and the secondary speech competition is at 80 dB SPL, the MCR is −20 dB. Each MCR condition corresponds to a real-life listening condition. The MCR conditions and their corresponding real-life analogues are as follows: +20 dB, very easy; +10 dB, easy; 0 dB, average; −10 dB, difficult; and −20 dB, very difficult.

The patient practices, unaided, with the primary sentences at a comfortable loudness level. The actual test procedure begins at a +20 MCR condition. The level of the primary sentences is set to 60 dB SPL, and the level of the speech competition is set to 40 dB SPL. The level of the speech competition is then varied to produce a different MCR condition. The patient's performance is tested, unaided, under the various MCR conditions.

Performance with a given hearing aid arrangement is then evaluated under the same varying MCR conditions. While the continuous discourse (speech competition) is presented at 60 dB SPL, the audiologist adjusts the acoustic gain of the hearing aid

to a comfortable loudness level for the patient. This gain setting remains constant during the subsequent testing.

At the completion of the evaluation procedure, the patient's unaided performance is retested under several MCR conditions. This allows the clinician to evaluate the "practice effect" in comparing unaided with aided performance.

The patient's unaided and aided scores at each MCR are plotted graphically in relation to the performance of normal listeners in the same condition. Figure 2 shows this graph. The abscissa represents the varying MCR conditions from −20 dB (very difficult) to +20 dB (very easy); the ordinate shows performance in percent. The patient's performance is described as his "SSI score." The shaded area of the graph represents the expected performance range of normal listeners. Figure 3 shows a hypothetical hearing aid evaluation plotted on this summary form. The solid triangles represent the patient's unaided performance and indicate that he was unable to identify any sentences in any listening condition. The open circles

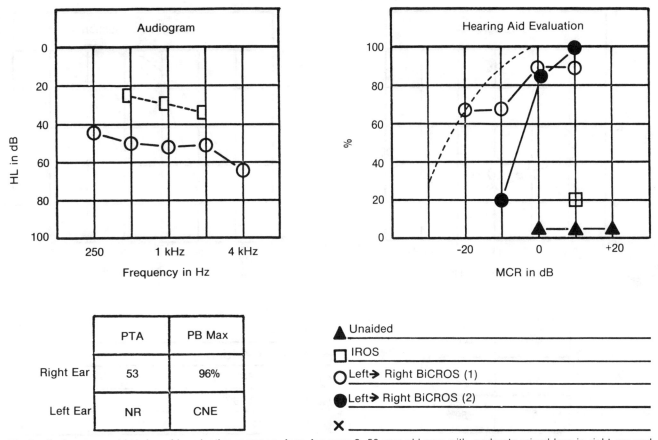

	PTA	PB Max
Right Ear	53	96%
Left Ear	NR	CNE

▲ Unaided

▢ IROS

◯ Left➔ Right BiCROS (1)

● Left➔ Right BiCROS (2)

✕

Fig 6.—Audiogram and hearing aid evaluation summary form for case 2, 56-year-old man with moderate mixed loss in right ear and profound loss in left ear. Evaluation was performed with patient's poorer, left ear facing primary speaker. NR, No response. CNE, Could not evaluate.

represent the patient's performance with a hearing aid. The difference between this patient's unaided and aided performance is considered his "aided improvement," and is easily visualized on this graph. Similarly, the difference between his aided performance and normal performance is considered the patient's "residual deficit." Both concepts, "aided improvement" and "residual deficit," are helpful in counselling the patient successfully.

REPORT OF CASES

We have been using this method of hearing aid evaluation at the Methodist Hospital for over three years. The following cases are presented to illustrate our clinical experience with this technique.

CASE 1.—A 76-year-old man had a moderate sensorineural loss in his right ear, and a profound loss in his left ear. His PB score was good (84%) in his right ear, but could not be measured in his left ear. This patient had worn a body-borne hearing aid for a number of years. Although he was satisfied with this

arrangement, he wanted to know whether an ear-level hearing aid arrangement would improve his communication ability. His audiogram and hearing aid evaluation summary form are shown in Fig 4.

Without a hearing aid, this patient was unable to identify any of the primary sentences in the very easy listening condition (+20 MCR). With his own body-borne hearing aid, his SSI score was 100% in the easy and average listening conditions (+10 MCR and 0 MCR), 60% in the difficult listening condition (−10 MCR) and 10% in the very difficult listening condition (−20 MCR). His score did not improve with the other arrangements tested, a directional microphone ear-level ipsilateral routing of sound (IROS) aid and a left-to-right contralateral routing of off-side signal with bilateral input (BiCROS) aid.

This case illustrates how the SSI procedure successfully evaluated the patient's performance with various hearing aid arrangements. Each arrangement tested was a distinct configuration of amplification. These various configurations were compared in four listening conditions by

the same test protocol. The graphic comparison of the arrangements tested quickly revealed how much aided improvement he experienced in each listening condition, which arrangement afforded him the most aided improvement, and how much residual deficit still remained. Clearly, his own body-borne hearing aid was as good as, or better than, the other arrangements tested.

CASE 2.—A 56-year-old university professor had a moderate mixed loss in his right ear and a profound loss in his left ear. His PB score in his right ear was excellent (96%), but could not be measured in his left hear. He wore a standard IROS hearing aid arrangement and found it adequate in most listening situations. He had specific difficulty, however, in conferences, when the speaker was seated on his left side. He came to the Audiology Service, therefore, to be evaluated for a BiCROS hearing aid arrangement. His audiogram and hearing aid evaluation summary form are shown in Fig 5 and 6.

In view of this patient's specific complaints, we evaluated his performance

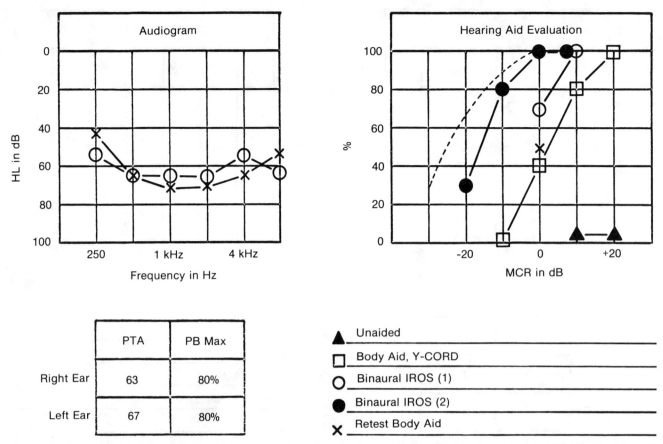

	PTA	PB Max
Right Ear	63	80%
Left Ear	67	80%

▲ Unaided

☐ Body Aid, Y-CORD

○ Binaural IROS (1)

● Binaural IROS (2)

✕ Retest Body Aid

Fig 7.—Audiogram and hearing aid evaluation summary form for case 3, an 11-year-old girl with moderate, bilateral sensorineural loss.

in two seating arrangements. First, he was seated directly facing the primary speaker so that both ears were equidistant from the primary sentence source. Second, he was seated with his poorer, left ear directly facing the primary speaker (sentences), and his better, right ear directly facing the secondary speaker (competition). In this way, we could evaluate his performance in his most difficult listening circumstances and evaluate the head-shadow effect.

Figure 5 shows his performance while facing the primary speaker. Unaided, he was unable to identify any of the primary sentences in the very easy listening condition (+20 MCR). With his own standard IROS hearing aid, his SSI score was 90% in the easy listening condition (+10 MCR), 70% in the average listening condition (0 MCR), and 40% in the difficult listening condition (−10 MCR). With the first BiCROS arrangement tested, his SSI score improved by 20% in both the average and difficult listening conditions (0 MCR and −10 MCR). His performance with the second BiCROS arrangement tested was essentially equivalent to his performance with his own IROS hearing aid.

When this patient's poorer, left ear faced the primary speaker (Fig 6), results clearly showed the inadequacy of his own IROS hearing aid. Even in the easy listening condition (+10 MCR), his SSI score was only 20%. With BiCROS 1, his SSI score was 70% to 90% in all listening conditions tested (easy, +10 MCR, to very difficult, −20 MCR). With BiCROS 2, his SSI score was 100% in the easy listening condition (+10 MCR), but only 20% in the difficult listening condition (−10 MCR). We recommended BiCROS 1 for this patient.

This case highlights the flexibility of the selection procedure. By evaluating this patient in two seating arrangements, we could not only assess his performance in the usual, forward-facing situations, we could also test him in those listening situations he found most difficult (off-side speakers near his poorer, left ear). Essentially, we were able to "tailor" the hearing aid evaluation to this patient's communication problems. This flexibility allowed us to select the most efficacious hearing aid arrangement for the patient's particular listening demands.

CASE 3.—An 11-year-old girl had a moderate, bilateral, apparently congenital hearing loss. Her PB-K (kindergarten) score

was good bilaterally (80%). Her hearing loss was identified at age 3 years, and she had worn a body-borne hearing aid with a Y-cord since that time. Her audiogram and hearing aid evaluation summary form are shown in Fig 7.

Unaided, this patient could not identify any primary sentences in the very easy listening condition (+20 MCR). With her own body-borne hearing aid, her SSI score was 80% in the easy listening condition (+10 MCR), 40% in the average listening condition (0 MCR), and 0% in the difficult listening condition (−10 MCR). With a standard binaural IROS arrangement, her score improved 20% to 30% in the easy and average listening conditions (+10 MCR and 0 MCR). Binaural IROS hearing aids with a directional microphone feature, moreover, improved her performance even further. With this arrangement, her SSI score was 100% in the average listening condition (0 MCR) and 80% in the difficult listening condition (−10 MCR). We recommended the binaural IROS arrangement with the directional microphone.

This case shows how our test procedure can successfully evaluate the audiologist's most challenging patient, the child. Ideally,

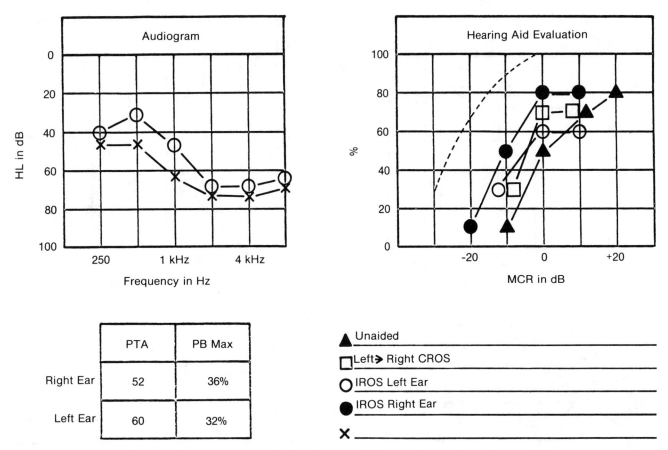

	PTA	PB Max
Right Ear	52	36%
Left Ear	60	32%

▲ Unaided

☐ Left ➤ Right CROS

○ IROS Left Ear

● IROS Right Ear

✕

Fig 8.—Audiogram and hearing aid evaluation summary form for case 4, 22-year-old man with moderate, bilateral sensorineural loss.

a hearing aid evaluation for a child should not only identify the most suitable hearing aid arrangement, but also should initiate meaningful discussion with the parents on hearing handicap and hearing aid use. This evaluation allowed us to quickly determine the most suitable hearing aid arrangement for the child. It also allowed the parents to observe their child's performance under listening conditions they could understand. This contributed to a thorough discussion of the child's hearing handicap and a consideration of realistic expectations from hearing aid use.

CASE 4.—A 22-year-old man had a moderate, bilateral sensorineural loss. The loss was reportedly progressive. His PB scores were very poor (36% in the right ear and 32% in the left ear). He had not used a hearing aid previously. Furthermore, his expectations of help from hearing aid use were quite unrealistic. He expected the aid to restore normal hearing, much as his eyeglasses restored normal vision. His audiogram and hearing aid evaluation summary form are shown in Fig 8.

Unaided, this patient's SSI score was 70% in the easy listening condition (+10 MCR), 50% in the average listening condition (0 MCR), and 10% in the difficult listening condition (−10 MCR). With all hearing aid arrangements tested, a contralateral routing of off-side signal (CROS) aid and two IROS aids, his score improved 10% to 40% in the average and difficult listening conditions (0 MCR and −10 MCR). Even with this aided improvement, however, this patient's performance implies a serious continuing communication handicap. The "residual deficit" indicates that he will continue to be a seriously hearing-impaired individual even with an aid.

This case demonstrates how this technique predicts the patient's performance with amplification in real-life listening situations. We had expected that this patient's very poor PB scores would limit his successful use of a hearing aid. In view of his unrealistic expectations of hearing aid use, however, it was crucial to demonstrate his aided performance in communication situations he routinely encountered. This test technique allowed us to do just that and led to meaningful counselling concerning the residual hearing handicap.

CASE 5.—An 88-year-old man had a mild-to-moderate sensorineural loss in his right ear, and a moderate-to-severe sensorineural loss in his left ear. The PB score was fair in the right ear (76%) but very poor in the left ear (24%). This patient had recently purchased binaural IROS hearing aids worn with solid earmolds. He was dissatisfied with this arrangement and seldom wore these aids. At his family's insistence, he sought the opinion of an audiologist. His audiogram and hearing aid evaluation summary form are shown in Fig 9.

Unaided, this patient could not identify any of the primary sentences in a very easy listening condition (+20 MCR). With his own arrangement, binaural IROS aids worn with solid earmolds, his SSI score was 100% in a very easy listening condition (+20 MCR), but only 20% in an easy listening condition (+10 MCR). With just one of these aids, worn with an open earmold in the right ear, his score was 90% in both the very easy and easy listening conditions (+20 MCR and +10 MCR) but 0% in the average listening condition (0 MCR). His performance with another aid worn with an open earmold in the right ear was even poorer. We recommended that he use his own hearing aid with an open earmold in the right ear on a part-time basis.

This case highlights how the SSI test can successfully evaluate the elderly patient

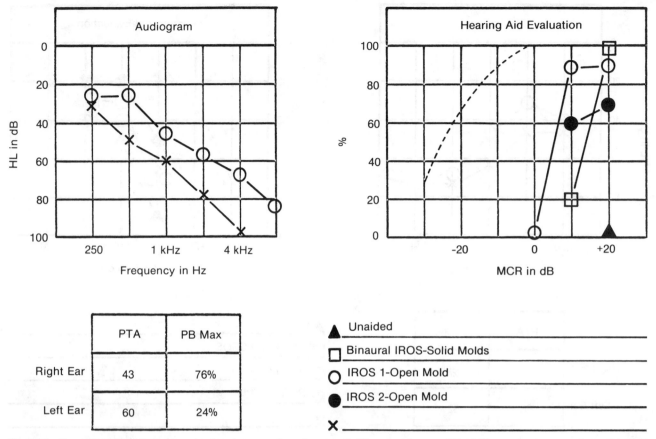

	PTA	PB Max
Right Ear	43	76%
Left Ear	60	24%

▲ Unaided

☐ Binaural IROS-Solid Molds

○ IROS 1-Open Mold

● IROS 2-Open Mold

✗

Fig 9.—Audiogram and hearing aid evaluation summary form for case 5, 88-year-old man with mild-to-moderate sensorineural loss in right ear and moderate-to-severe sensorineural loss in left ear.

and improve his family's understanding of the communication handicap. The most important aspect of this evaluation was patient and family counselling. By clinically demonstrating this patient's aided performance in average listening conditions (0 MCR), we could stress why a hearing aid was beneficial only in quiet listening conditions. This initiated timely family discussion of the problems of hearing handicap in elderly family members.

CASE 6.—A 76-year-old woman had a moderate mixed hearing loss in her right ear and a mild sensorineural loss in her left ear. Her PB score was good in the right ear (80%) and excellent in the left ear (96%). She was investigating hearing aid use for the first time. Her audiogram and hearing aid evaluation summary form are shown in Fig 10.

Unaided, this patient's SSI score was 50% in the very easy listening condition (+20 MCR), 60% in the easy listening condition (+10 MCR), and 0% in the average listening condition (0 MCR). Her performance was evaluated with two mild-gain IROS hearing aids worn with a vented earmold in her left ear. With IROS 1, her

score improved in the very easy and easy listening conditions (+20 MCR and +10 MCR), but did not improve in the average listening condition (0 MCR). With IROS 2, however, her score improved in all three listening conditions.

Figure 11 compares this patient's performance on the SSI test with the two hearing aids. It is evident that IROS 2 is better for this patient than IROS 1. In the very easy listening condition (+20 MCR), both hearing aids improved her SSI performance more than 20%. No real aid difference emerged in this condition. In the average listening condition (0 MCR), however, a substantial aid difference did emerge. The IROS 1 improved her score 10%; IROS 2 improved her score 70%. The average listening condition (0 MCR) sufficiently stressed the two hearing aids and revealed which aid was superior for this patient.

We also evaluated this patient's aided performance with PB words in quiet and in noise. With the patient facing the primary speaker, the PB words were delivered at a comfortable loudness level, 60 dB SPL. Competing noise was delivered from the loudspeaker directly behind the patient.

The competing noise was also delivered at 60 dB SPL, creating a 0 dB signal-to-noise ratio. The same two IROS hearing aids were evaluated in these conditions. Figure 12 shows the result. The unaided PB score in quiet was 16%; the unaided PB score in noise was 24%. With IROS 1, the PB score was 48% in quiet and 52% in noise. With IROS 2, the PB score was 52% in quiet and 48% in noise. Clearly, conventional PB scores did not demonstrate a substantial difference between the two hearing aids.

This case demonstrates why the SSI materials are often superior to PB Max technique. The two PB test conditions did not demonstrate a substantial difference between these two hearing aids. By this technique, in fact, it appeared that this patient received very limited benefit from amplification. The SSI test conditions, however, did demonstrate a pronounced difference between the two hearing aids. In addition, these materials indicated that the patient obtained benefit from amplification in several real-life listening conditions.

FOLLOW-UP SURVEY

In an effort to measure our success

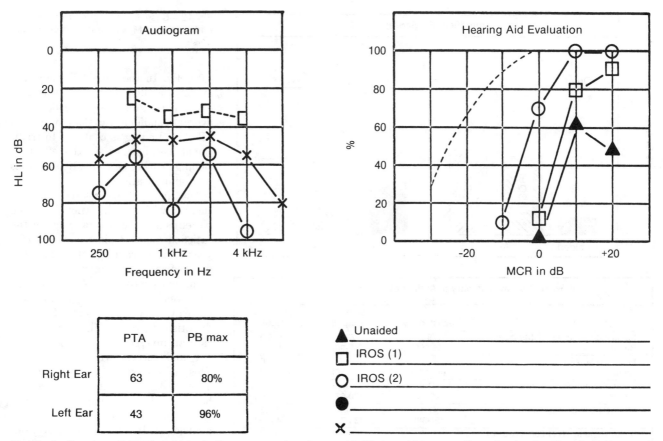

	PTA	PB max
Right Ear	63	80%
Left Ear	43	96%

▲ Unaided
☐ IROS (1)
○ IROS (2)
● ___
✕ ___

Fig 10.—Audiogram and hearing aid evaluation summary form for case 6, 76-year-old woman with moderate mixed loss in right ear and mild sensorineural loss in left ear.

in recommending satisfactory amplification to patients following evaluation by the SSI procedure, we carried out a follow-up survey.

The records of all patients who had been evaluated for hearing aid use in 1974 were reviewed. Of 135 patients evaluated by the SSI technique, 33 patients had been advised not to purchase a hearing aid, 13 patients had been advised to continue use of their present hearing aid, and 89 had been advised to purchase a specific new hearing aid. Questionnaires were mailed to these latter 89 patients. They were asked if they had purchased the recommended aid following the evaluation. They were also asked to rate their satisfaction with the recommended instrument as "satisfactory," "sometimes helpful," or "unsatisfactory."

Sixty-three (70.7%) questionnaires were returned. Of these 63 patients, 47 had purchased the recommended hearing aid. Thirty-four (72.3%) of the 47 patients who had purchased the

Fig 11.—Case 6, comparison of unaided and aided SSI performance in two MCR conditions.

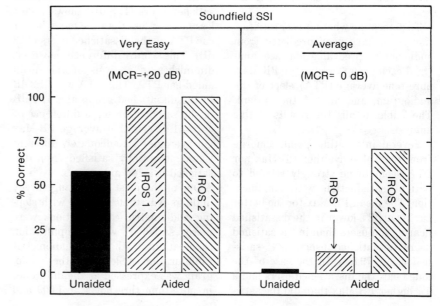

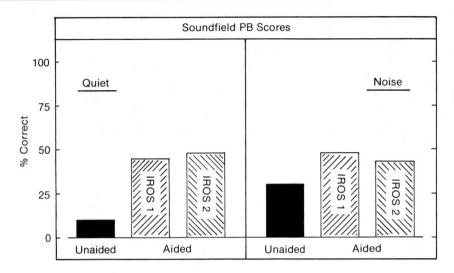

Fig 12.—Case 6, comparison of unaided and aided PB Max scores in quiet and in noise.

Follow-Up Survey Summary of Audiometric and Age Data*			
Index	Satisfactory	Sometimes Helpful	Unsatisfactory
Mean PB Max in % (better ear)	79.8	79.2	78.0
Range	(56-100)	(40-96)	(56-88)
Mean PB Max in % (aided ear)	77.0	78.4	78.0
Range	(44-100)	(40-96)	(56-88)
Mean PTA in dB HL (better ear)	41.8	49.0	49.3
Range	(20-80)	(30-67)	(37-61)
Mean PTA in dB HL (aided ear)	47.1	54.7	51.2
Range	(27-88)	(35-77)	(45-58)
Mean slope in dB (1,000-4,000 Hz)	26.9	12.6	17.2
Range	(7-50)	(0-26)	(10-35)
Mean age in yr	60.4	65.9	71.5
Range	(11-89)	(53-76)	(61-79)

* Data given for patients who rated hearing aid as "satisfactory," "sometimes helpful," or "unsatisfactory."

recommended hearing aid rated it as "satisfactory," seven (14.9%) rated the aid as "sometimes helpful," and six (12.8%) rated the aid as "unsatisfactory."

To determine whether user satisfaction could have been predicted from audiometric preevaluation, we analyzed each group by average PB Max, pure-tone average (PTA), slope of the audiogram, and age of the patient. The Table details the results of this analysis.

Several interesting points emerge from the Table. Neither PB Max nor PTA seem to be strongly related to patient satisfaction with amplification. The mean PB Max for the better ear is only 2% lower in the dissatisfied hearing aid users than in the satisfied users (dissatisfied users, 78%; satisfied users, 79.8%). In the case of the aided ear, the dissatisfied users had a 1% higher PB Max than did the satis-

fied users (dissatisfied users, 78%; satisfied users, 77%). The mean PTA shows only a slightly greater difference. The mean better ear PTA of the satisfied users (41.8 dB) shows 7.5 dB less hearing loss than the mean better ear PTA of the dissatisfied users (49.3 dB). This 7.5-dB difference, however, diminishes in analysis of the mean aided-ear PTA. This PTA was 51.2 dB in the dissatisfied group and 47.1 dB in the satisfied group, a difference of only 4.1 dB. Neither average PB Max nor average PTA adequately differentiated potentially satisfied from dissatisfied hearing aid users.

One of the most interesting survey findings was that patients with sloping audiometric configurations were more satisfied with amplification than patients with flatter audiometric configurations. Slope of the audiogram was expressed as the difference in pure-tone thresholds at 1,000 and

4,000 Hz. In the satisfied group, the average audiometric slope was 26.9 dB. In the dissatisfied group, the average audiometric slope was 17.2 dB. This finding is contrary to traditional assumptions on the effect of sloping hearing loss on patient success with amplification.

The index that related best to success with amplification was the patient's age. The average age of the satisfied hearing aid users was 60.4 years. The average age of the dissatisfied hearing aid users was 71.5 years. Sometimes-satisfied users' average age was 65.9 years, approximately halfway between the satisfied and dissatisfied groups. These data indicate an inverse relationship between age and success with amplification. This, of course, is not unexpected. That the probability of successful hearing aid use declines with age is a fact well known to every practicing audiologist. It is an important consideration in any hearing aid evaluation.

To determine whether the three groups exhibited differences in SSI performance, we analyzed patient satisfaction in relation to aided sound field SSI scores. Figure 13 shows the result of this analysis. Little difference in performance among satisfied, sometimes satisfied, and dissatisfied hearing aid users occurred in the easy listening condition (+10 MCR). In this condition, all three groups had a mean score greater than 90%. A 15% difference in performance emerged in the average listening condition (0 MCR). The satisfied users had a mean SSI score of 85%, while the dissatisfied users had a mean score of only 70%. A striking 30% difference occurred in the difficult listening conditions (−10 MCR). The satisfied hearing aid users' mean SSI score in this condition was 55%, while the dissatisfied hearing aid users' mean score was only 25%. The −10 MCR conditions of the sentence identification task seems to be a promising index of satisfaction with amplification. We believe this is related to the patient's ability to use a

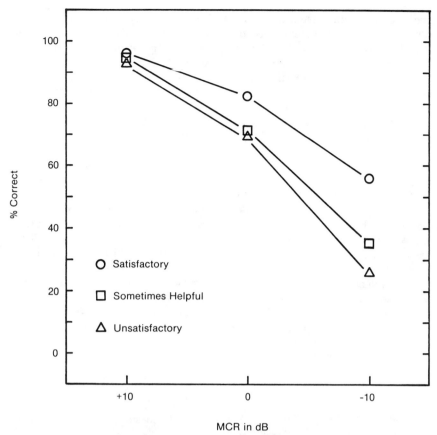

Fig 13.—Average aided SSI performance in three MCR conditions by patients who rated hearing aid use as "satisfactory," "sometimes satisfactory," or "unsatisfactory."

hearing aid successfully in "stressful" listening conditions. When the listening task was too easy (+10 MCR), it did not adequately stress the hearing aid. Both satisfied and dissatisfied hearing aid users performed equally well in this condition. As the listening task became more difficult, however, the average performance of the satisfied hearing aid users emerged as systematically better than the performance of the dissatisfied users. We consider this to be one of the most important features of this method of hearing aid evaluation. For almost any degree of hearing impairment, the listening conditions of the SSI task can provide several levels of listening difficulty to adequately stress aided performance.

COMMENT

What we have attempted to describe in this report is more than a new method of hearing aid evaluation. It is a new philosophy of rehabilitative management. We believe that the

hearing aid evaluation can be a powerful tool in the rehabilitation of the hearing-impaired patient. To develop a procedure to fulfill this role, we first reviewed our previous method of evaluation, determined its underlying assumptions and goals, and defined its limitations. We then designed an evaluation methodology to address broader and more critical rehabilitative issues. That is, we defined specific goals for the evaluation procedure in order to render the most effective management of the hearing-impaired patient.

The goal of the conventional method of hearing aid evaluation is to "select" the best hearing aid for the patient. We believe this is self-limiting as the only goal of the hearing aid evaluation, and prevents full exploitation of the technique. The new philosophy emphasizes not only determining the best hearing aid arrangement for the patient, but also defining differences among arrangements in real-life listening conditions,

providing information on realistic expectations of hearing aid use for patient counselling, and making accountable recommendations on hearing aid use to the patient.

There are several important advantages of the SSI technique. By creating more life-like listening conditions, we can determine the most suitable hearing aid arrangement for the patient. Real-life listening conditions are created by the use of sentence materials in the presence of speech competition. The use of sentences rather than single words to assess performance is based on usual real-life listening conditions. The actual seating arrangement of the test technique was also designed to approximate real-life communication. Rather than listening to an off-side primary source, the patient faces the primary speaker. This is, of course, how most conversational situations take place. This seating arrangement, however, can be easily changed to an off-side listening condition for patients with complaints in this specific listening situation.

By varying the difficulty of the listening task, we can clearly define differences among hearing aid arrangements. Two PB test conditions, presented at a fixed SL relative to the aided SRT, may not provide accurate definition of hearing aid differences. One condition may be "too easy," such that any arrangement may appear to provide benefit. The other condition may be "too difficult," such that no arrangement would be beneficial. The five potential test conditions of the new method provide a complete range of listening difficulty, from "very easy" to "very difficult." Differences among arrangements may be evident in some, but not all, listening conditions.

By quantifying patient performance, both unaided and aided, relative to normal listeners' performance, we can more realistically counsel patients on expectations of hearing aid use. The test conditions, similar to "very easy," "easy," "average," "difficult," and "very difficult" real-life listening conditions, provide a meaningful framework for interpreting test results to patients. The graphic representation of the patient's performance relative to normal listeners' performance facilitates patient understanding of both his aided improvement and his residual communication deficit.

By suggesting potential patient satisfaction with amplification in situ, this technique can help us to make more accountable hearing aid recommendations. We found, in the follow-up survey, that patients who performed best with a hearing aid in the difficult SSI condition were most satisfied with hearing aid use. It appears that the better the patient performs, aided, in difficult listening situations, the more likely he is to be satisfied with amplification. This datum can be easily supplemented with information on patient age, life-style, listening demands, and motivation to help us make more accountable recommendations for hearing aid use.

In addition to these advantages, the procedure can be used to evaluate patients with almost any degree of hearing loss. For patients with very severe hearing impairments, we might consider improvement in the very easy and easy listening conditions (+20 MCR and +10 MCR) sufficient for recommending a hearing aid. Conversely, for patients with minimal hearing loss, we might not recommend an aid unless improvement could be demonstrated in difficult and very difficult listening conditions (−10 MCR and −20 MCR). The patient's degree of hearing loss, therefore, does not limit the effectiveness of the procedure. In addition, the head-shadow effect, in evaluation of CROS and BiCROS, can be quickly assessed by changing the patient's seating arrangement in the test chamber.

The evaluation technique is also adaptable to almost any language. We routinely use Spanish synthetic sentences and discourse to evaluate our large population of Spanish-speaking patients. The examiner requires no more knowledge of the language than the recognition of the digits from one to ten.

Finally, an important consideration for future application of the technique is its open-endedness. That is, changes can easily be incorporated into the present framework to further enhance its effectiveness. We have considered, for example, adding a video portion to the evaluation to assess the effects of visual cues on aided performance. The procedure is sufficiently flexible to incorporate several such additions.

Our experience leads us to the conclusion that this technique of hearing aid evaluation is substantially better than the conventional method. It not only validly evaluates hearing-impaired patients and their performance with amplification, it also does what we have always wanted a hearing aid evaluation to do. It differentiates performance with various hearing aid arrangements, and engenders more accountable hearing aid recommendations.

This study was supported by PHS program project grant NS 10940, from the National Institute of Neurological and Communicative Disorders and Stroke.

Walt Otto assisted in data collection and analysis.

References

1. Carhart R: Selection of hearing aids. *Arch Otolaryngol* 44:1-18, 1946.

2. Davis H, Hudgins CV, Marguis RJ, et al: The selection of hearing aids. *Laryngoscope* 56:85-115, 135-163, 1946.

3. Shore I, Bilger R, Hirsh I: Hearing aid evaluation: Reliability of repeated measurements. *J Speech Hear Dis* 25:152-170, 1960.

4. Resnick DM, Becker M: Hearing aid evaluation: A new approach. *ASHA* 5:695-699, 1963.

5. Chial MR, Hayes CS: Hearing aid evaluation methods: Some underlying assumptions. *J Speech Hear Dis* 39:270-279, 1974.

6. Speaks C, Jerger JF: Method for measurement of speech identification. *J Speech Hear Res* 8:185-194, 1965.

Relation between Aided Synthetic Sentence Identification Scores and Hearing Aid User Satisfaction

Deborah Hayes, James Jerger, Janet Taff, and Bunny Barber

Baylor College of Medicine, and The Methodist Hospital, Houston, Texas

ABSTRACT

Satisfaction with hearing aid use was surveyed in 78 subjects who had been evaluated for hearing aid use by formal speech audiometric measures (synthetic sentence identification). At −10 dB message-to-competition ratio, synthetic sentence identification performance was an average 30% better in satisfied than in dissatisfied users.

The hearing aid evaluation is one of the cornerstones of clinical audiology. First proposed and elaborated by Carhart[2] more than 30 yrs ago, it has become, for many clinicians, an essential tool of aural rehabilitation. Indeed, recent surveys of audiological practices have concluded that approximately 85% of clinics administer some kind of hearing aid evaluation measure.[1, 10]

There is considerable range of opinion on the proper procedure for carrying out a hearing aid evaluation, but one fundamental assumption underlies all hearing aid evaluation techniques: namely, that how a person performs with a hearing aid in the test situation is, in some sense, predictive of successful use of the aid in everyday living. Unless this assumption is made, there can be little justification for any kind of formal comparative hearing aid testing procedure.

In spite of the crucial importance of this assumption there is remarkably little hard evidence to support it. One searches in vain for a substantial body of data showing relation between aided test scores and successful use of amplification.

Indeed, the dearth of such data prompted Harris[4] to observe that:

> Even if one has a good candidate and the theoretically ideal prosthesis for him, there is no validated way to measure, much less to predict, what that aid does in the wearer's daily life. Without such research and validated evaluation, the audiologist today is in no position to state on any basis other than his own 'clinical judgment', however good that may be, which aid is best for his client and how much good it will do. To state otherwise is to arrogate to the audiologist a level of objectivity and scientific caution which is not apparent to the scientist. (p. 5)

Or, as Carhart[3] observed:

> ...we are still awaiting a definitive validational study of the relationship between formal scores obtained via speech audiometry and work-a-day hearing aid efficiency. (p. XXIX); by permission. M. Pollack, ed. 1975. *Amplification for the Hearing-Impaired.* Grune & Stratton, New York.)

The significance of this gap between knowledge and clinical practice is highlighted by the current resurgence of interest in selective amplification.[7-9] The main thrust of these research efforts is usually related to the prediction of the very kinds of speech recognition scores whose predictive validity remains to be demonstrated.

The purpose of the present study was to attempt to relate aided performance scores to the hearing aid user's self-reported satisfaction with his aid. To this end, we developed and mailed out, to a sample of patients who had purchased hearing aids on our recommendation, a simple questionnaire probing the extent to which the individual used the aid and his relative satisfaction with it. The questionnaire was mailed to all patients to whom a hearing aid had been dispensed by our clinic during the previous 14 mos. Respondents were asked to sign the questionnaire because anonymity would have limited our ability to compare audiometric data with questionnaire results.

One can, of course, raise many objections to the use of questionnaire responses as the validating criterion for ultimate user satisfaction. The user's attitude toward the aid, at least during the first few weeks of wear, is likely to be influenced by earmold comfort, annoyance of amplified noise, personality interactions between the patient and the audiologist/dispenser, and by a host of other contaminating variables.

In the present case, however, the majority of respondents had been using their aids for at least several months before receiving the questionnaire. All but three respondents reported continuous use of their aid from dispensing to questionnaire. All three respondents who no longer used their aids attempted to adjust to amplification for periods ranging from 2 mos to 1 yr.

The actual length of prequestionnaire aid use for all subjects ranged from 2 to 14 mos. The average period was 7 mos.

PROCEDURE

The questionnaire used in the present study asked the subject to rate his satisfaction with the aid on a 4-point scale ranging from "Very helpful" to "Unsatisfactory," and to estimate his hours per day of usage of the instrument.

Questionnaires were sent to subjects who had been evaluated for hearing aid use by the synthetic sentence identification (SSI) technique. This procedure has been described previously.[5] Briefly, the subject is seated in the test chamber, between and equidistant from two loudspeakers. The loudspeaker directly in front on the subject delivers the primary message; the loudspeaker directly behind the subject delivers the competing speech discourse. The primary message is one of a closed set of 10 synthetic sentences.[11] The competing speech discourse is a biographical story. Intensity of the primary message is fixed (50 or 60 dB SPL); intensity of the competing message is varied (from 30 to 70 or 40 to 80 dB SPL). Varying the competition relative to the primary sentences results in five different message-to-competition ratios (MCR): +20 dB; +10 dB; 0 dB; −10 dB; and −20 dB. A block of 10 sentences is presented at each MCR. The subject's task is to identify each primary sentence as it is presented. At each MCR, he is tested both unaided and aided with three to five hearing aids or hearing aid arrangements.

The exact nature of the comparative evaluation necessarily varied according to the individual patient's audiometric configuration. In some cases, the comparison was among three to five different monaural aids on the same ear. In other cases, the comparison was among two to three monaural aids, followed by a monaural-binaural comparison of the most promising monaural aid. In still other cases, the basic comparison was among alternative arrangement (e.g., right ear versus left ear, contralateral routing of signals versus bilateral contralateral routing of signals) using only one or two selected aids.

In every case, an aid or pair of aids was ultimately dispensed. In most cases, the recommended aid was based on clearly superior aided performance scores (SSI difference between aids of more than 20% at two or more MCRs).

In addition to the hearing aid evaluation, most subjects had also received a basic audiometric evaluation at The Methodist Hospital. This evaluation includes routine pure-tone audiometry, diagnostic speech audiometry, and clinical acoustic immittance and acoustic reflex measures. Diagnostic speech audiometry consists of performance-intensity functions for both monosyllabic phonemically balanced (PB) words in quiet, and synthetic sentences in ipsilateral speech competition of 0 dB MCR.[6] These procedures were administered monaurally, under earphones. From each performance-intensity function, the maximum speech performance score for that material (PB max or SSI max) is extracted.

A total of 143 questionnaires was sent to adult (age 20 yrs and older) subjects. Seventy-eight subjects (54%) responded.

RESULTS

Of the 78 respondents, 38 (49%) rated hearing aid use as "Very helpful," 22 (28%) found amplification "Satisfactory," 13 (17%) rated their hearing aid as "Sometimes helpful," and five (6%) found hearing aid use "Unsatisfactory." As note earlier, the average time interval between dispensing and the questionnaire was 7 mos and

ranged from 2 to 14 mos. In order to ensure that the satisfaction rating was not influenced by this variable, we computed this interval for subjects in each rating category. There was no systematic relation between rating category and time interval between dispensing and follow-up questionnaire. In the "Very helpful" group, the interval ranged from 2 to 14 mos, the average was 6.0 mos; in the "Satisfactory" group, the interval ranged from 2 to 10 mos, with an average interval of 5.4 mos; in the "Sometimes helpful" group, the interval ranged from 4 to 11 mos, the average was 7.7 mos; and finally, in the "Unsatisfactory" group, the interval ranged from 5 to 13 mos with an average interval of 7.7 mos.

Table 1 summarizes average characteristics of the four subgroups of respondents. It shows average and range of ages, average and range of hearing levels (pure-tone average, PTA) and results of diagnostic speech audiometry (PB max and SSI max).

The table suggests several interesting characteristics of the four subgroups of respondents. First, there was little apparent relation between age of the subject and satisfaction with hearing aid use. Average age in the four subgroups varied from 58.0 yrs in the "Very helpful" subgroup to 70.0 yrs in the "Sometimes helpful" subgroup, but the age range in each subgroup was substantial and overlap was considerable. Difference in age among the four subgroups was not significant ($F = 2.50$; $p > 0.05$).

Second, neither degree of hearing loss nor unaided speech recognition scores under earphones (monaural) appeared strongly related to satisfaction with amplification. Although the subgroup which rated hearing aid use as "Unsatisfactory" had, on the average, more hearing loss than the other three subgroups (Unsatisfactory = 50.8 dB HL; Very helpful = 43.6 dB HL; Satisfactory = 39.8 dB HL; Sometimes helpful = 43.4 dB HL), the subgroup with the next greatest degree of hearing loss found hearing aid use "Very helpful." Difference in PTA among the four subgroups was not significant ($F = 1.07$; $p > 0.05$). Similarly, neither unaided PB max nor unaided SSI max revealed a specific trend related to satisfaction with hearing aid use. Difference in average maximum speech recognition scores, under earphones, for both words in quiet (PB max) and sentences in competition (SSI max) did not exceed 11% among the four subgroups, nor did the four subgroups exhibit an orderly trend in performance. Once again, these differences were not statistically significant (PB max, $F = 0.40$; $p > 0.05$; SSI max, $F = 0.56$; $p > 0.05$). Satisfaction with hearing aid use could not be readily predicted from either patient age, degree of hearing loss, or unaided, monaural speech recognition performance.

Figure 1 summarizes average aided performance of the four subgroups in the sound field. Data are shown for only three of the five MCR test conditions (+10 dB, 0 dB, and −10 dB). Two MCR conditions (+20 dB and −20 dB) did not provide useful differentiating data for the present investigation. Results at +20 dB were uniformly 100% in all groups, whereas results at −20 dB could not be obtained in all subjects.

The results summarized in Figure 1 represent sound field performance with the recommended hearing aid coupled to

Table 1. Summary of audiometric and age data for patients who rated hearing aid use, ''Very helpful,'' ''Satisfactory,'' ''Sometimes helpful,'' or ''Unsatisfactory'' (N = 78)[a]

Index	Very Helpful (N = 38)	Satisfactory (N = 22)	Sometimes Helpful (N = 13)	Unsatisfactory (N = 5)
Average age (yrs)	58.0	62.2	70.0	57.0
Range	22–90	28–96	54–89	36–76
Average PTA (dB HL)	43.6	39.8	43.4	50.8
Range	3–70	7–55	30–62	31–76
Average PB max (%)	80.1	81.5	73.4	76.0
Range	20–100	32–100	12–100	64–84
Average SSI max (%)	70.0	80.5	75.4	73.3
Range	20–100	20–100	40–100	60–90

[a] *Audiometric results are shown for the aided ear only, or, in the case of binaural fittings, for the better ear.*

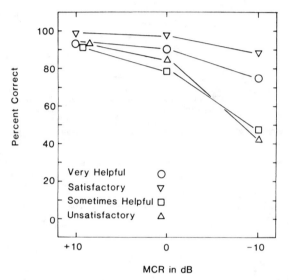

Figure 1. Average aided performance of four subgroups of hearing aid users categorized by self-reported satisfaction with amplification.

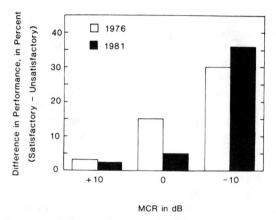

Figure 2. Comparison of difference in average aided performance at +10, 0, and −10 dB MCR of satisfied versus dissatisfied hearing aid users from two different surveys (1976 and 1981). In both surveys, difference in performance between the two subgroups increases from less than 5% at +10 dB MCR to greater than 30% at −10 dB MCR.

Table 2. Summary of analysis of variance of aided SSI scores classified by satisfaction with aid (groups) and MCR

Source	SS[a]	df	MS[b]	F
Between subjects				
Groups	11378.4	3	3792.8	4.6[c]
SWG	59570.8	73	816.0	
Within subjects				
MCRs	24127.5	2	12063.7	55.1[d]
Groups × MCRs	6359.9	6	1059.9	4.8[d]
MCR × SWG	31947.0	146	218.8	

[a] *Sum of squares.*
[b] *Mean square.*
[c] *p < 0.01.*
[d] *p < 0.001.*

the recommended, custom earmold. At + 10 dB MCR, very little difference was observed among the four subgroups; average performance for each subgroup was 94%. At 0 dB MCR, the four subgroups begin to diverge. The "Very helpful" and "Satisfactory" subgroups scored, on the average, 91% or greater and the "Sometimes helpful" and "Unsatisfactory" subgroups scored, on the average, 86% or less. Finally at −10 dB MCR, a clear difference emerged

between subjects who found hearing aid use either "Very helpful" or "Satisfactory" and those who found hearing aid use either "Sometimes helpful" or "Unsatisfactory." In this listening condition, the more satisfied hearing aid users scored, on the average, 30% better than their less satisfied counterparts (Very helpful = 76.8%; Satisfactory = 88.1%; Sometimes helpful = 47.8%; Unsatisfactory = 44.0%).

Results of a two-factor analysis of variance performed on these data are summarized in Table 2. For this analysis the significance of the "groups" effect was evaluated using the "subjects within groups" (SWG) variance as the error term, but the significance of the MCR effect, and the groups × MCR interaction were evaluated using the MCR × SWG interaction as the error term because the MCR factor represents repeated measures on the same subjects. Significant differences were observed for both main effects, groups (p < 0.01) and MCRs (p < 0.001), and for the groups × MCR interaction (p < 0.001). These results confirm a significant relation between aided performance in the sound field and satisfaction with amplification.

The 30% difference in aided performance at −10 dB MCR between satisfied and dissatisfied hearing aid users is quite similar to results obtained in an earlier survey of user satisfaction.[5] These results are compared to the present data in Figure 2 (subgroups "Very helpful" and "Satisfactory" of the present survey are collapsed in this figure to provide direct comparison to the data from 1976). The figure shows difference in performance between the "Satisfactory" and "Unsatisfactory" subgroups by MCR. Note that, in both surveys, difference in performance between the two subgroups at +10 dB MCR was less than 5%, increased to 6 to 17% at 0 dB MCR, and averaged more than 30% at −10 dB MCR.

COMMENT

We believe that results of this preliminary study are encouraging. They indicate that it is possible to design a formal hearing aid evaluation measure which is, in fact, related to user satisfaction.

The ultimate hearing aid evaluation must take into account a number of important variables in addition to aided performance measures. Such variables include patient motivation and life-style, and family interest and support. The present data bear on only one aspect of the total evaluation, aided performance for speech materials in a controlled environment. Within this context, the SSI measure at −10 dB MCR shows an orderly relation to user satisfaction.

Can this finding be generalized to other speech materials and speech recognition tasks? The question can only be answered by further research. A key guideline for future research appears to be use of speech competition as a means of manipulating degree of difficulty of the speech task. We believe that degree of listening difficulty must be manipulated over a substantial range such that the speech task is neither too easy nor too difficult to reveal important performance differences. We suggest that the failure to relatively simple speech materials (i.e., monosyllabic words in quiet) to reveal these differences is related to the fact that degree of listening difficulty cannot be easily manipulated over a wide range.

To us, the practical significance of the present data is the implication that at least some kinds of aided speech recognition measures can, indeed, tell us something about "... what that aid does in the wearer's daily life."[4] (p. XIX) We offer this observation as a first step toward the development of a comparative hearing aid evaluation procedure which will ultimately place the testing, fitting, and dispensing of hearing aids on a fully objective and scientifically verifiable basis.

References

1. Burney, P. 1972. A survey of hearing aid evaluation procedures. Asha **14**, 439–444.
2. Carhart, R. 1946. Selection of hearing aids. Arch Otolaryngol. **44**, 1–18.
3. Carhart, R. 1975. Introduction. p. XXIX. *in* M. Pollack, ed. *Amplification for the Hearing-Impaired.* Grune & Stratton, New York.
4. Harris, J. 1976. Introduction. p 5. *in* M. Rubin, ed. *Hearing Aids: Current Developments and Concepts.* University Park Press, Baltimore.
5. Jerger, J., and D. Hayes. 1976. Hearing aid evaluation: clinical experience with a new philosophy. Arch. Otolaryngol. **102**, 214–225.
6. Jerger, J., and D. Hayes. 1977. Diagnostic speech audiometry. Arch. Otolaryngol. **103**, 216–222.
7. Miller, J., A. Niemoeller, D. Pascoe, and M. Skinner. 1980. Integration of the electroacoustic description of hearing aids with the audiologic description of clients. pp. 355–378. *in* G. Studebaker, and I. Hochberg, eds. *Acoustical Factors Affecting Hearing Aid Performance.* University Park Press, Baltimore.
8. Pascoe, D. 1975. Frequency responses of hearing aids and their effects on speech perception of hearing-impaired subjects. Ann. Otol. Rhinol. Laryngol. Suppl. (23) **84**, 5.
9. Skinner, M., D. Pascoe, J. Miller, and G. Popelka. 1981. Measurements to determine the optimal placement of speech energy within the listener's auditory area: a basis for selecting amplification characteristics. Paper presented at A Working Conference on Amplification for the Hearing Impaired: Research Needs, Nashville, June 7–10.
10. Smaldino, J., and J. Hoene. 1981. The nature of common hearing aid fitting practices. Hear. Instrum. Jan–Feb.
11. Speaks, C., and J. Jerger. 1965. Method for the measurement of speech identification. J. Speech Hear. Res. **8**, 185–194.

Address reprint requests to Deborah Hayes, Ph.D., Otorhinolaryngology, Baylor College of Medicine, 1200 Moursund Avenue, Houston, TX 77030.

Received August 10, 1981; accepted December 21, 1982.

Norms for Disproportionate Loss in Speech Intelligibility*

M. Wende Yellin,† James Jerger, and Robert C. Fifer‡

Baylor College of Medicine, Houston, Texas

ABSTRACT

The audiometric records of 324 subjects with sensorineural hearing loss, presumed to be cochlear, were analyzed in order to develop norms for "disproportionate loss" in speech intelligibility. From the scatterplot relating PB_{max} to PTA_2 (average of HTLs at 1000, 2000, and 4000 Hz), and the scatterplot relating SSI_{max} to PTA_1 (average of HTLs at 500, 1000, and 2000 Hz), linear boundaries were constructed encompassing approximately 98% of observed values. A speech intelligibility score (PB or SSI) may be considered "disproportionately poor" if it falls below this empirically derived boundary.

The concept of "disproportionately poor" speech understanding in the hearing impaired dates from 1948, when John Gaeth observed that some elderly patients seemed to show much poorer scores on conventional tests of monosyllabic word intelligibility than one would expect from their audiograms. Shortly thereafter, Schuknecht and Woellner (1955) made the same observation in patients with VIIIth nerve disorders. Conventional speech intelligibility scores were often severely depressed in spite of normal, or near-normal pure-tone sensitivity levels on the affected ears. The phrase disproportionately poor came to be associated with this combination of results. In subsequent years the reality of these early observations has been repeatedly confirmed. Indeed, the combination of relatively normal pure-tone sensitivity level and depressed speech intelligibility is increasingly recognized (Jerger & Hayes, 1977; Jerger & Jerger, 1974; Noffsinger & Kurdziel, 1979) as the audiologic signature of a retrocochlear auditory disorder.

When the audiogram is normal, and the speech intelligibility score is 40%, the notion of "disproportionately poor" is easily understood. Such a combination of results is relatively unambiguous. But when the audiogram is at the 50 dB level, and the speech intelligibility score is 40%, it is not always clear whether such a score should be regarded as disproportionately poor or whether it is consistent with the severity of the peripheral hearing loss. Thus, it is important to know what is "proportionately poor" speech intelligibility, that is, the lower boundary of the range of speech intelligibility scores associated with a particular degree of cochlear loss.

The purpose of the present study was to provide such "normative values" for two specific speech intelligibility measures; (1) the PB_{max}, or maximum of the performance versus intensity (PI) function for monosyllabic phonemically balanced (PB) words; and (2) the SSI_{max} or maximum of the PI function for synthetic sentences.

METHOD

Subjects and Procedures

We analyzed, retrospectively, the audiometric records of all patients with sensorineural hearing loss who had been evaluated by the Audiology Service of the Methodist Hospital, Houston, TX in the years 1981 and 1982. From this pool we extracted a sample of 324 patients who met the following criteria: (1) age less than 56 years; (2) no medical evidence of active otologic disease; (3) no medical evidence of active neurologic disease; (4) no medical or audiologic evidence of retrocochlear disorder; (5) either hearing loss or tinnitus as the referring complaint.

The age restriction was imposed to eliminate the potentially confounding effects of age, and possible concomitant cognitive decline, on the speech audiometric measures. Audiologic evidence of retrocochlear disorder was operationally defined by the difference between the PB_{max} and the $SSI_{max(reference)}$, and by abnormal "rollover" (Jerger & Jerger, 1971) of either PI function. If the PB-SSI difference exceeded 20%, on either ear, or if rollover exceeded 20% on either PI function of either ear, then the patient was excluded. This criterion was applied without regard for the absolute performance levels on either test. The application of these relatively rigid criteria undoubtedly resulted in the exclusion of some "false positives," that is, patients with cochlear loss who, in spite of failing these criteria, did not, in fact, have retrocochlear disorder. We regarded this as a conservative exclusion strategy in the sense that we were more concerned to avoid

* This project was carried out at the Baylor College of Medicine and The Methodist Hospital, Houston, TX and was supported in part by USPH grant NS10940.

† Present address: University of Texas Southwestern Medical Center, Dallas, TX 75235.

‡ Present address: Carle Clinic Association, Urbana, IL 61801.

the erroneous inclusion of a retrocochlear in the study sample than to avoid the erroneous exclusion of an actual cochlear from the sample.

The final study sample included 236 males and 88 females, ranging in age from 8 to 55 years. The overall mean age was 43.7 years. In order to ensure the statistical independence of data we included the results from only one, randomly selected, ear of each of the 324 patients.

All patients had been evaluated on a battery of conventional audiometric measures, including immittance audiometry, pure-tone audiometry by both air and bone conduction, and speech audiometry. The latter included performance versus intensity (PI) functions for PB words (NDRC, PAL-PB 50; Egan, 1948) and for SSI sentences (Speaks & Jerger, 1965). All speech audiometric materials were presented via magnetic tape. Both PB words and SSI sentences had been previously recorded by a male talker with general American dialect.

For both the PB and SSI materials the maximum score was defined as the highest point on the PI function. Typically, a PI function was obtained first for the SSI materials. After presenting one 10-sentence block at an initial, easily audible level, the intensity level of subsequent blocks was varied, usually in steps of 10 dB, up to a maximum level of 100 dB SPL. A typical PI function for SSI was defined by percent correct scores at 4 to 5 suprathreshold intensities. PB words were presented in 25-word blocks. In most cases, the initial test level for a block of PB words was the presentation level at which maximum SSI performance had been observed. Ordinarily, the word presentation level was then increased to 100 db SPL for the next block of words. Thus, in most cases, performance for PB words was defined by results at just two presentation levels. In some cases, however, a more complete function, at 4 to 5 suprathreshold levels, was defined.

RESULTS

In order to define the most appropriate measures of hearing sensitivity loss against which to compare the two speech intelligibility scores we first examined the correlation matrix among the following variables:

PB_{max}—the maximum of the PI function for PB words.
SSI_{max}—the maximum of the PI function for SSI sentences.
PTA_0—the average of the pure-tone hearing threshold levels at 250, 500, and 1000 Hz.
PTA_1—the average of the pure-tone hearing threshold levels at 500, 1000, and 2000 Hz.
PTA_2—the average of the pure-tone hearing threshold levels at 1000, 2000, and 4000 Hz.
Slope 0.5–4k—the difference between the pure-tone hearing threshold levels at 500 and 4000 Hz.
Slope 1k–4k—the difference between the pure-tone hearing threshold levels at 1000 and 4000 Hz.
Slope 2k–4k—the difference between the pure-tone hearing threshold levels at 2000 and 4000 Hz.

Table 1 summarizes relevant Pearson product-moment coefficients of correlation among these variables. Two conclusions seem appropriate. First, the various PTAs, measuring degree of loss, correlate better with the two speech measures than any of the three measures of slope of the audiometric configuration. Second, PB_{max} correlates

best with PTA_2 ($r = 0.668$), while SSI_{max} correlates best with PTA_1 ($r = 0.665$). Based on these findings we elected to display the effect of PTA_2 on the PB_{max}, and of PTA_1 on the SSI_{max}.

Figure 1 shows the actual scatterplot of all 324 PB_{max} scores as a function of PTA_2. As expected, the lower boundary of the scatterplot declines systematically with increasing hearing sensitivity loss. Inspection of the actual distribution of points suggested to us that a meaningful empirical boundary could be constructed by simply drawing a straight line along the lower edge of the data points in such a way that approximately 98% of the points lie above the line. Figure 1 shows such a linear boundary. It encompasses all but five of the 324 PB_{max} scores. Thus, the boundary formed by this empirically derived straight line defines the lower limit of the range of PB_{max} scores to be expected as a result of any particular degree of cochlear hearing sensitivity loss. Any PB_{max} score falling below this boundary may be considered, with high probability (98%) to be disproportionately poor. Thus, for example, if the PTA_2 is 50 dB, then any PB_{max} below 38% must be considered outside the range of expectation for cochlear hearing loss. Table 2 presents this lower boundary in tabular form for ease of clinical use. Figure 2 and Table 3 present analogous data for PTA_1 and the SSI_{max}. Again the lower boundary defines the 98% range of SSI_{max} scores to be expected, as a function of audiometric level.

It should be emphasized that these normative boundaries apply only to the specific recordings and materials used in this study (i.e., PAL-PB 50 words and SSI sentences). Analogous normative boundaries for other popu-

Table 1. Correlation coefficients among PB_{max}, SSI_{max}, three pure-tone averages and three audiometric slope measures in 324 subjects with cochlear hearing loss.

	PTA_0	PTA_1	PTA_2	Slope (0.5–4k)	Slope (1k–4k)	Slope (2k–4k)
PB_{max}	−0.490	−0.656	−0.668	−0.024	0.100	0.262
SSI_{max}	−0.619	−0.665	−0.558	0.191	0.277	0.313

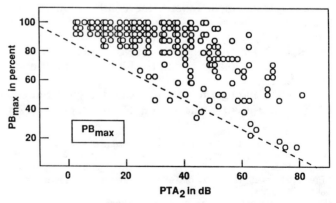

Figure 1. Scatterplot relating PB_{max} score to PTA_2 in 324 subjects with cochlear hearing loss. Linear boundary encompasses 98% of observed points.

Table 2. Lower boundary of PB$_{max}$ score as a function of PTA$_2$. For any given value of PTA$_2$, any score below the tabled value of PB$_{max}$ must be considered disproportionately poor.

PTA$_2$	PB$_{max}$ (%)	PTA$_2$	PB$_{max}$ (%)	PTA$_2$	PB$_{max}$ (%)
0	89	31	57	61	26
1	88	32	56	62	25
2	87	33	55	63	24
3	86	34	54	64	23
4	85	35	53	65	22
5	84	36	52	66	21
6	83	37	51	67	20
7	82	38	50	68	19
8	81	39	49	69	18
9	80	40	48	70	17
10	79	41	47	71	16
11	78	42	46	72	15
12	77	43	45	73	14
13	76	44	44	74	13
14	75	45	43	75	12
15	74	46	42	76	11
16	73	47	41	77	10
17	72	48	40	78	9
18	71	49	39	79	8
19	70	50	38	80	7
20	69	51	37	81	6
21	68	52	36	82	5
22	67	53	35	83	4
23	65	54	34	84	3
24	64	55	32	85	2
25	63	56	31	86	1
26	62	57	30		
27	61	58	29		
28	60	59	28		
29	59	60	27		
30	58				

Table 3. Lower boundary of SSI$_{max}$ score as a function of PTA$_1$. For any given value of PTA$_1$, any score below the tabled value of SSI$_{max}$ must be considered disproportionately poor.

PTA$_1$	SSI$_{max}$ (%)	PTA$_1$	SSI$_{max}$ (%)	PTA$_1$	SSI$_{max}$ (%)
0	86	31	55	61	25
1	85	32	54	62	24
2	84	33	53	63	23
3	83	34	52	64	22
4	82	35	51	65	21
5	81	36	50	66	20
6	80	37	49	67	19
7	79	38	48	68	18
8	78	39	47	69	17
9	77	40	46	70	16
10	76	41	45	71	15
11	75	42	44	72	14
12	74	43	43	73	13
13	73	44	42	74	12
14	72	45	41	75	11
15	71	46	40	76	10
16	70	47	39	77	9
17	69	48	38	78	8
18	68	49	37	79	7
19	67	50	36	80	6
20	66	51	35	81	5
21	65	52	34	82	4
22	64	53	33	83	3
23	63	54	32	84	2
24	62	55	31	85	1
25	61	56	30		
26	60	57	29		
27	59	58	28		
28	58	59	27		
29	57	60	26		
30	56				

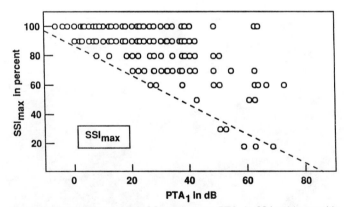

Figure 2. Scatterplot relating SSI$_{max}$ score to PTA$_1$ in 324 subjects with cochlear hearing loss. Linear boundary encompasses 98% of observed points.

lar speech materials (e.g., NU No. 6, W-22, SPIN) remain to be developed.

SUMMARY

The audiometric records of 324 subjects with sensorineural hearing loss, presumed to be cochlear, were ana-

lyzed in order to develop norms for disproportionate loss in speech intelligibility. From the scatterplots relating PB$_{max}$ to PTA$_2$ (average of HTLs at 1000, 2000, and 4000 Hz), and SSI$_{max}$ to PTA$_1$ (average of HTLs at 500, 1000, and 2000 Hz) linear boundaries were constructed encompassing approximately 98% of observed speech intelligibility scores. A speech intelligibility score (PB or SSI) may be considered disproportionately poor if it falls below this empirically derived boundary.

References

Egan J. Articulation testing methods. Laryngoscope 1948;58:955–991.
Gaeth JH. A study of phonemic regression in relation to hearing loss. Unpublished Doctoral Dissertation. Northwestern University, 1948.
Jerger J and Brown D. Effect of peripheral hearing loss on the interpretation of ABR results. In Starr A, Rosenberg C, Don M, Davis H, Eds. Sensory Evoked Potentials. International Conference on Standards and Auditory Brain Stem Response (ABR) Testing. Milan: Amplifon, 1984.
Jerger J and Hayes D. Diagnostic speech audiometry. Arch Otolaryngol 1977;103:216–222.
Jerger J and Jerger S. Auditory findings in brain stem disorders. Arch Otolaryngol 1974;99:342–350.

Jerger J and Jerger S. Diagnostic significance of PB word functions. Arch Otolaryngol 1971;93:573–580.

Noffsinger PD and Kurdziel SA. Assessment of central auditory lesions. In Rintelmann WF, Ed. Hearing Assessment. Baltimore: University Park Press, 1979: 351–377.

Schuknecht H and Woellner R. An experimental and clinical study of deafness from lesions of the cochlear nerve. J Laryngol 1955;69:75–97.

Speaks C and Jerger J. Method for measurement of speech identification. J Speech Hear Res 1965;8:185–194.

Address reprint requests to James Jerger, Ph.D., Division of Audiology, Department of Otolaryngology and Communicative Sciences, Baylor College of Medicine, Houston, TX 77030.

Presented at the annual convention of the American Speech-Language-Hearing Association, Cincinnati, November 18, 1983.

Received December 2, 1988; accepted January 19, 1989.

IV

Impedance Audiometry

In 1960, I was invited to present a paper at the International Congress of Audiology in Bonn, West Germany. This was my first contact with the great names of European audiology, and I was duly impressed. I met Luscher of Switzerland; Langenbeck of Germany; Ewertsen and Bentzen of Denmark; Liden, Klockhoff, and Barr of Sweden; Hood of the United Kingdom; and a host of others. It was a heady experience.

After the Congress I spent a few weeks visiting audiology centers in Denmark and Sweden. In Copenhagen, Professor Ewertsen and his group showed me a new electroacoustic gadget they were trying out in the clinic. They called it an "impedancemeter" since it measured impedance characteristics of the middle ear. Another Dane, Otto Metz, had already pioneered the measurement of the acoustic stapedius reflex, by means of a mechanical bridge, during and after World War II. This new device carried the concept a few steps further. In addition to the bridge circuitry necessary to detect stapedius muscle contraction, it had additional circuitry making it possible to measure the absolute static impedance of the middle ear system. In fact, you could measure two dimensions of the static impedance: (1) the vector magnitude, or real component, and (2) the phase angle, or imaginary component. Finally, by means of a calibrated air pump, you could study the way in which the middle-ear impedance changed under conditions of both positive and negative air pressure. A graph of these changes they called a "tympanogram." The new sys-

tem had been designed by Terkildsen and Scott-Nielsen and fabricated by Madsen Electronics. They called it the model ZO-60.

When I returned to Evanston, I was invited to give a presentation to our department, reporting on what I had seen and heard. In that talk I described the Madsen "impedancemeter" and predicted that it would probably have a very significant impact on audiometric evaluation. I don't think that anyone took me very seriously on that occasion. They all nodded agreeably but didn't quite see what middle-ear impedance had to do with audiograms. If you wanted to know about the middle ear, after all, you simply tested by bone conduction.

A year later, in 1961, I left Northwestern and moved to Washington, D.C. Here I was associated with both Gallaudet College and the Audiology outpatient clinic of the Veteran's Administration (now the Department of Veteran's Affairs). While at the VA, I ordered a Madsen "impedancemeter," now the model ZO-61. It was, I believe, the first Madsen bridge in the USA. But I didn't get to use it very much before I was off again, this time to Houston.

Late in 1962, I joined the Houston Speech and Hearing Center as Director of Research. By this time, Grason-Stadler had come out with the Zwislocki mechanical bridge and, in a colossal demonstration of bad judgment, I bought one of these instead of another Madsen. I still have a photograph of that hardy band of pioneers who traveled to Syracuse in 1963 to take the first course in how to use the new bridge. Alan Feldman was our patient tutor. He told us everything we had to know about the bridge—except that you needed at least three arms and four hands to operate it. I was constantly reminded of Charlie Chaplin on the assembly line in "Modern Times."

The Zwislocki bridge was, of course, very good at measuring both the reactive and resistive components of static impedance. It turned out, however, that this middle ear measure was far less interesting than two other measures, the tympanogram and the acoustic reflex, neither of which could easily be assessed with the Zwislocki bridge.

In 1968 I moved again, this time to Baylor College of Medicine as Professor of Audiology. We set up a small audiology clinic in the basement of The Methodist Hospital and began to see patients from the Otolaryngology Service headed by Dr. Bobby Alford. That summer, a very fine gentleman named Jimmy Brown, then the local Madsen representative, came by to show us a new instrument. Madsen Electronics had redesigned the old ZO-61 impedancemeter. The new model, called the ZO-70, eliminated the phase-angle measure and had improved sensitivity for acoustic reflex detection. It was just beginning to appear in the USA. I wanted one desperately but didn't have anything like the money to buy it. Jimmy sensed, however, that I would put it to good use and graciously loaned me an instrument.

We did indeed put it to good use. Throughout 1969, we used it to test every patient coming through our audiology clinic. After seeing the results of what came to be called "impedance audiometry" (still later, the more politically correct "immittance audiometry") in a consecutive series of about 400 patients, we thought we had a pretty good grasp of the clinical value of tympanograms, acoustic reflex thresholds, and the static impedance measures. We detailed our experience in a 1970 paper, "Clinical Experience with Impedance Audiometry," which was widely read and quoted. The importance of this paper was that it showed how the three components of impedance audiometry, the tympanogram, the static impedance, and the acoustic reflex could be diagnostically effective if used as a total test battery. Previous investigators had studied one or another component and found it unimpressive as a precise diagnostic tool. The 1970 paper reached the same conclusion about the individual components, but showed, paradoxically, that results across the three components fell into distinct categories that could be very useful diagnostically.

As it turned out, this has been a fruitful approach to a number of other test paradigms for diagnostic evaluation. Although some researchers continue to seek one ideal measure of a phenomenon, usually with only limited success, others have exploited the test battery/distinctive pattern approach to better advantage. Some examples are the use of auditory evoked potentials at various latencies rather than the ABR alone, the use of speech audiometric materials sampling a continuum of linguistic complexity rather than intelligibility for monosyllabic (PB) words alone, and the interpretation of evoked otoacoustic emissions within the context of the total audiometric evaluation rather than in relation to audiometric thresholds alone.

Throughout the 1970s, our group continued to gather clinical impedance data. Susan Jerger, Larry Mauldin, Phyllis Segal, and Lois Anthony analyzed this growing database. In a series of three papers in the *Archives of Otolaryngology*, we presented data from over 1,800 children and adults. In the first paper, "Studies in Impedance Audiometry: I. Normal and Sensorineural Ears" (1972), we confirmed, on a relatively large sample ($n = 1,133$), observations by a number of previous investigators that in normal hearers the average sensation level of the acoustic reflex threshold is just about 85 dB; that acoustic reflex thresholds are normally distributed on a log intensity (dB) scale; that static impedance is normally distributed on a log compliance scale; that there is a gender difference in static impedance; that there are age effects for both the static impedance and the acoustic reflex; and that, as degree of sensorineural loss increases, the sensation level of the acoustic reflex threshold declines systematically, and with unit slope, down to a limiting sensation level of 25 dB. We also demonstrated that, although there were no differences in frequencies across the range from 500 to 2000 Hz, the frequency of 4000 Hz was clearly aberrant in both normal ears and ears with sensorineural losses. Why this should be so has never been satisfactorily explained.

Perhaps our most important observation, in this series of 1,133 patients, was the relatively high prevalence of impedance abnormalities in ears without audiometric air-bone gaps. Even using a fairly lax set of criteria of impedance abnormality, 8% of this sample still showed either type B or C tympanograms and/or absent acoustic reflexes at frequencies other than 4000 Hz. Many audiologists still have not absorbed the significance of this observation. They continue to view bone-conduction thresholds as the "gold standard" of the middle-ear disorder. But we have known for 20 years that impedance measures are considerably more sensitive.

In the second paper, "Children Below Six Years Old" (1974), we attempted to show how well impedance audiometry could be carried out in this difficult-to-test age range (77%) and how results could be used to supplement conventional behavioral observations. Again, we showed that, although no single impedance measure was uniformly effective, the overall pattern on the three-test battery could be quite helpful, especially when conventional audiometric data could not be obtained. The advent of pediatric ABR in the late 1970s has attenuated somewhat the immediate clinical need for impedance measures, but we still find them useful, especially in children with atypical reactions to sedation.

The third paper, "Middle Ear Disorders" (1974), shows how the impedance battery can supplement the air- and bone-conduction audiograms to paint a more detailed portrait of the nature and extent of the conductive loss. We noted, for example, that, in spite of the considerable ambiguity and overlap of the individual components, the combination of air-bone gap, shallow type A tympanogram, less than average static impedance, and absent acoustic reflexes leads to the strong presumption of ossicular chain fixation, although the tympanogram alone, the static impedance alone, or the reflex absence alone would not be unique to fixation.

The concluding sentence of this paper might serve as a metaphor for virtually all diagnostic audiometric evaluation:

> ". . . the key to the successful application of impedance measurement in the clinical evaluation of middle ear disorder is to minimize the fine detail of individual measures and to attach considerable significance to the overall configuration of results on the complete test battery." (p. 171)

I have never felt that the last paper in this section, "Inter- Versus Intrasubject Variability in Acoustic Immittance" (*Ear and Hearing*, 1980), written in collaboration with Bill Keith, has received the attention it deserves. It speaks to an important issue in experimental design, the relative magnitudes of the variability within the same subject (error of measurement) and the variability among different subjects (true individual differences). If true individual differences are small and error of measurement is large, then it makes sense to test a small number of subjects, but to test each exhaustively to reduce measurement error. If, on the other hand, it is known that true individual differences are large and error of measurement is small, then it is essential to test a relatively large number of subjects to be sure that the sample mean accurately represents the population mean.

Many investigators have approached impedance measures (and a number of other audiologic measures, for that matter) from the point of view that it is appropriate and desirable to test a small number of subjects with exceeding care. There has been the implicit assumption that such studies are more "rigorous" than large-scale clinical surveys. But Keith and I showed that, in the case of static immittance, the ratio of inter- to intra-subject variability was an astonishing 10 to 1. That is, variability due to true individual differences was 10 times larger than variability due to error of measurement. If, therefore, you want to look at something like age effects or gender differences, it makes more sense to examine clinical data taken on large samples than laboratory data, however carefully taken, on relatively small samples.

Those who make it their business to ponder things may want to ponder whether such considerations might explain why traditional psychoacoustic studies of persons with hearing impairment have so consistently failed to explain very much about the problems such persons have in understanding real speech in the real world.

Clinical Experience With Impedance Audiometry

James Jerger, PhD, Houston

Impedance audiometry was performed as part of the routine clinical examination in a consecutive series of more than 400 patients with various types and degrees of hearing impairment. An electroacoustic bridge (Madsen, ZO 70) was used to carry out the measurement of tympanometry, acoustic impedance, and threshold for the acoustic reflex. Results indicate that, while individual components of the total impedance battery lack diagnostic precision, the overall pattern of results yielded by the complete battery can be of great diagnostic value, especially in the evaluation of young children.

THE development of impedance audiometry during the past decade has added new scope and dimension to clinical audiology. Based on the pioneering efforts of Metz,[1] subsequent workers have refined instrumentation, technique, and interpretation to produce an invaluable tool for differential diagnosis.

The development of contemporary instrumentation for impedance audiometry has, in the main, followed two essentially parallel paths. In the United States, Zwislocki and his colleagues[2-6] developed an electromechanical bridge. In Europe, Thomsen, Terkildsen, Møller, and others,[7-10] pioneered the application of the electroacoustic approach, culminating in the present commercially available electroacoustic bridge.

The present paper reports our clinical experience with the latter instrument based on its routine administration to well over 400 successive patients over a one-year period. Our aim was to assess the efficacy of the electroacoustic approach as a routine clinical procedure and to evaluate its diagnostic value in a typical audiologic case load.

In general we found that the testing procedure was easily mastered, even by audiologically unsophisticated personnel, that valid and meaningful results could be obtained for almost every patient, and that, with certain reservations, the data of impedance audiometry constitute extremely valuable diagnostic information.

Subsequent sections present statistical information when patients are grouped according to age and type of hearing loss, and individual case reports illustrating the diagnostic value of impedance audiometry.

Method

Apparatus.—Impedance audiometry was carried out by means of an electroacoustic impedance bridge (Madsen, type ZO-70) and an associated pure-tone audiometer (Beltone, type 10D). Figure 1 shows a schematic diagram of the principal components of the impedance bridge.

A probe tip containing three tubes is sealed in the external meatus, forming a closed cavity bounded by the inner surface of the probe tip, the walls of the external meatus, and the tympanic membrane. One tube is used to deliver, into this closed cavity, a probe tone generated by a 220-hertz oscillator driving a miniature receiver. The second tube is connected to a miniature probe microphone which monitors the sound pressure level of the 220-Hz probe tone in the closed cavity and delivers the transduced voltage through an amplifier to a bridge circuit and balance meter. The balance meter is nulled by an SPL of exactly 95 dB in the closed cavity. A potentiometer on the output of the 220-Hz oscillator permits variation of the SPL over a range corresponding to a compliance variation (equivalent volume) of 0.2 to 5.0 cc. The third tube is connected to an airpump which permits variation in air pressure in the closed cavity over a range of ±400 mm (water). Air pressure is read on an electromanometer.

Accepted for publication June 19, 1970.

From the Department of Otolaryngology, Baylor College of Medicine, and the Audio-Vestibular Laboratory, the Methodist Hospital, Houston.

Reprint requests to 11922 Taylorcrest, Houston 77024.

The receiver and probe microphone are contained in a small housing mounted at the end of a conventional headband. They are connected to the probe tip by small rubber hoses. A third rubber hose delivers air to the probe tip. At the opposite end of the headband a conventional earphone is mounted. When connected to a suitable sound source it delivers signals to the ear opposite the one in which the probe tip is sealed, in order to measure threshold for the acoustic reflex. In our project the sound source was a standard clinical audiometer (Beltone, type 10D) feeding an earphone (Telephonic TDH-39) mounted in a cushion (M X 41/AR). When the headband is positioned on the patient's head, the earphone cushion covers one ear and the probe tip, attached to the housing on the headband by the three rubber hoses, may be conveniently sealed in the external meatus of the opposite ear.

With this instrumentation the three basic components of impedance audiometry—tympanometry, acoustic impedance, and acoustic reflex threshold—may be carried out.

Tympanometry.—Tympanometry describes how eardrum compliance changes as air pressure is varied in the external canal. The basic datum is the pressure-compliance function, a graph relating compliance change to pressure variation. The shapes of pressure-compliance functions fall into three basic types—A, B, and C. The three types are illustrated, in idealized form, in Fig 2.

The type A function is characterized by a relatively sharp maximum at or near 0 mm. Type A functions are found in normal and otosclerotic ears. The type B function shows little or no maximum. Compliance remains essentially unchanged over a large range of pressure variation. Type B functions are found in ears with serous or adhesive otitis media.

In the type C function the maximum is shifted to the left of zero by negative pressure in the middle ear. Slight negative pressure is quite common in many otherwise normal ears, but when the maximum equals or exceeds approximately 100 mm (water) significant negative pressure in the middle ear may be presumed.

Lidén[11,12] describes a fourth type of function characterized by a double maximum at or near 0 mm. Such functions are found, according to Lidén,[12] in cases with discontinuity of the ossicular chain. In our experience with the bridge we have never encountered this function. All of our cases of ossicular chain discontinuity show relatively deep type A functions, indicating considerable compliance change, but we have not observed the double maximum

described by Lidén. This discrepancy is undoubtedly due to the difference in probe frequency used in tympanometry. Lidén has used a probe frequency of 800 Hz, whereas the bridge we employ uses a probe frequency of 220 Hz. Indeed, in recent still unpublished work by Lidén, Peterson, and Björkman (made available to us by Dr. John Peterson, Louisiana State University School of Medicine) the authors demonstrate, in a case of hypermobile tympanic membrane that whereas a probe frequency of 800 Hz shows a clearly defined Lidén function, the double maximum is greatly attenuated by changing the probe frequency to 625 Hz and entirely abolished by shifting to 220 Hz. It is not surprising, therefore, that one does not observe Lidén's function with the bridge we use. Instead, cases of ossicular discontinuity typically show exceedingly deep type A functions.

In the unit we employ acoustic impedance is derived from two input potentiometer settings, Z_1 and Z_2 (expressed in equivalent air volume or acoustic ohms). Z_1 is obtained by introducing a positive air pressure of 200 mm and adjusting the probe tone oscillator potentiometer until the balance meter is nulled. Z_2 is obtained by setting the air pressure to the value which yields maximum compliance and rebalancing the meter.

Impedance, in acoustic ohms, is given by the relation:

$$Z = \frac{Z_1 \, Z_2}{Z_1 - Z_2}.$$

Acoustic Reflex Threshold.—In the measurement of the acoustic reflex threshold the electroacoustic bridge is used only to show relative changes in impedance. The balance meter is first nulled to zero. Then an acoustic signal is introduced to the opposite ear. If the signal is sufficient to elicit the bilateral acoustic reflex, the resulting contraction of the stapedius muscle in the ear containing the probe tip will increase the impedance at the eardrum, resulting in an upward deflection of the balance meter. In order to determine the reflex threshold the tester varies the signal level until he has identified the lowest level capable of eliciting an observable deflection of the balance meter.

Procedure.—The bridge we employ was used to carry out impedance audiometry as a routine procedure on virtually every patient tested by the Audiology Service of the Methodist Hospital during 1969. Of the more than 400 patients on whom the procedure was attempted, successful results were obtained in approximately 96% of the cases. The primary reason for failure was inability to achieve a lasting airtight seal of

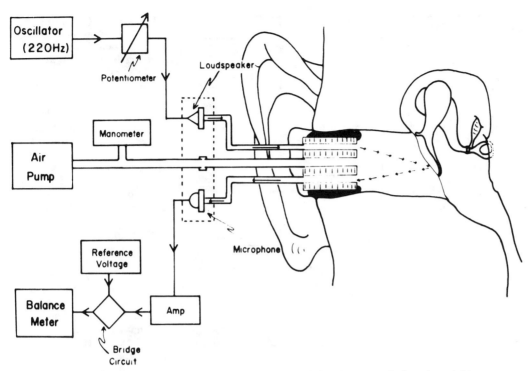

Fig 1.—Schematic diagram of principal components of the electroacoustic impedance bridge.

the probe tip in the external canal. This problem could undoubtedly have been overcome, in this small number of cases, by special measures, such as inflatable cuffs, custom molding, or extraordinary sealing procedures, but our purpose was to evaluate the efficacy of the test as a routine clinical procedure. From this standpoint it is noteworthy that in the overwhelming majority of patients (96%) an airtight seal was achieved without particular difficulty.

The second most common reason for failure arose from very young children who could not maintain the requisite degree of immobility for a period sufficient to obtain complete data (usually five to ten minutes). Some of these children were retested under sedation (chloral hydrate), usually with successful results.

In order to carry out impedance audiometry, the patient was seated in a comfortable chair and the headband was carefully positioned so that the test earphone covered one ear. The probe tip was then sealed into the external canal of the opposite ear by means of an ear tip. During the first six months of the project we used the hard rubber ear tips supplied with the instrument. More recently, however, we have abandoned the hard rubber tip in favor of a tip made from a silicone material. We have found that the latter greatly facilitates the establishment of an adequate seal.

Fig 2.—The three types of tympanometry curves (pressure-compliance functions): Type A curves are found in normal and otosclerotic ears; type B curves are found in serous and adhesive otitis. type C curves are due to negative pressure in the middle ear.

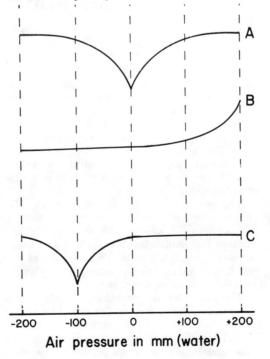

Air pressure in mm (water)

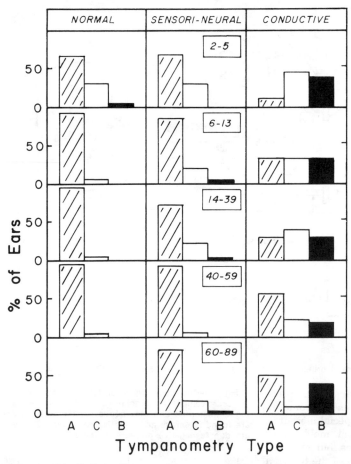

Fig 3.—Distributions of types of tympanometry curves as functions of age and type of audiometric configuration.

The intensity of the pure tone was varied until the tester had identified the lowest hearing level (HL) at which a deflection of the balance meter, synchronous with the onset and offset of the tone (making suitable allowance for the latency of the reflex response), could be observed. This level was recorded as the acoustic reflex threshold HL. In this fashion reflex thresholds were measured for signals of 500, 1,000, 2,000 and 4,000 Hz.

It should be noted that the acoustic reflex phase of the total procedure tests the ear opposite to the ear in which tympanometry and impedance measures have been carried out. For tympanometry and impedance the left ear is tested by inserting the probe tip in the left ear. For reflex thresholds, however, the left ear is tested by introducing sound to the left ear while the probe tip is inserted in the right ear.

As a result of this reversal there is some confusion in the literature over the appropriate symbol to indicate that sound is presented to one ear and the reflex is detected in the contralateral ear. Some investigators[13] feel that they are testing the right ear when the bridge is connected to the right ear and sound is introduced to the left ear. Others[14] feel that they are testing the right ear when sound is introduced to the right ear and the bridge is connected to the left ear.

The present paper conforms to the latter convention. The symbol "O" indicates the lowest hearing level at which sound presented to the right ear elicited an acoustic reflex as detected by the bridge in the left ear. The symbol "X" indicates the lowest hearing level at which sound presented to the left ear elicited an acoustic reflex as detected by the bridge in the right ear.

When testing had been completed on the first ear, headband, earphone, and probe tip were reversed, and the entire procedure was repeated on the opposite ear. Typically the entire procedure on both ears required five to ten minutes of testing time. Longer testing time

After the adequacy of the seal had been verified by the introduction of positive air pressure in the external canal, the tester proceeded to plot the pressure-compliance function (tympanometry). Compliance, in arbitrary units, was plotted as a function of varying air pressure. The latter was varied in steps of 10 to 20 mm (water) until the shape of the pressure-compliance function, and the position of its maximum, had been defined.

The second step in the examination was the measurement of acoustic impedance. Compliance values, in acoustic ohms, necessary to balance the null meter, first with air pressure at +200 mm (Z_1), then with air pressure at the maximum value of the pressure-compliance function (Z_2), were determined.

The final step in the examination was the measurement of the acoustic reflex. With the balance meter set to maximum sensitivity and nulled to zero, pure tones were introduced to the opposite ear by means of the audiometer.

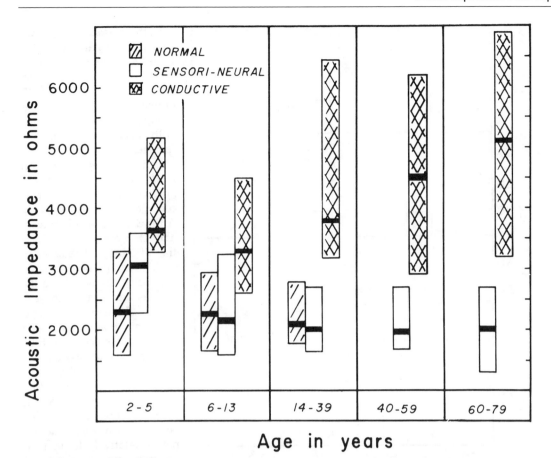

Fig 4.—Distributions (median and semi-interquartile ranges) of acoustic impedance as functions of age and type of audiometric configuration.

was occasionally required when an adequate seal could not be readily obtained on one or both ears.

Subjects.—The total group of patients tested constituted a relatively representative sampling of a typical hospital audiologic case load. Patients ranged in age from 10 months to 81 years, and included virtually every type and degree of loss. Approximately 32% of the total sample showed a purely sensorineural audiometric configuration. Conductive and mixed patterns accounted for 28% and 22% respectively. The remaining 18% showed normal sensitivity.

Results

Results are presented in two sections. The first section summarizes statistical data on the distribution of the various measures of impedance audiometry. The second section presents a series of case reports illustrating the diagnostic value of impedance audiometry.

Distributions.—In order to analyze distributions as functions of age and type of loss, a subsample was formed from the total sample according to the following criteria: (1) age greater than 2 years; (2) audiometric pattern consistent with normal hearing, pure conductive loss (excluding ossicular discontinuity), or pure sensorineural loss; and (3) no history of middle ear surgery.

Patients with either suspected or confirmed retrocochlear disorder and patients with either suspected or confirmed functional hearing problems were excluded from the analysis. These criteria yielded usable data for 554 ears of 316 patients. Table 1 summarizes the breakdown of these subjects and ears by age and type of loss.

Tympanometry.—Figure 3 shows the percent of ears in each age and type-of-loss category yielding either type A, B, or C pressure-compliance functions.

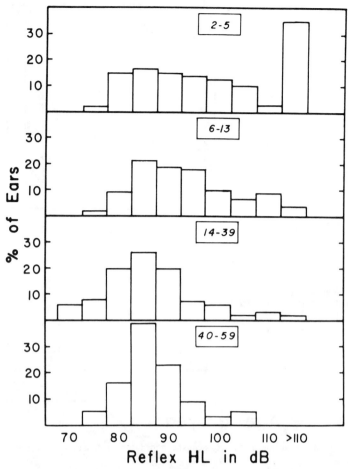

Fig 5.—Distributions of acoustic reflex threshold hearing levels as function of age in subjects with normal hearing.

In the sensorineural group, like the normal group, the type A function predominates, but the type C curve occurs in an alarming 31% of ears in the 2 to 5 age group. This percentage gradually declines with increasing age.

In the conductive group it is interesting to observe a gradual increase in the percentage of ears showing type A functions as age increases. This change perhaps reflects the differing distributions of middle ear pathological abnormality characterizing the various age groups. In very young children one might anticipate that otitis media and faulty eustachian tube function would account for the majority of middle ear problems, thus accounting for the predominance of types B and C. In adults, however, one would anticipate a relatively lower incidence of such problems but a relatively higher incidence of stapes fixation due to otosclerosis. Hence, the increase in the type A curve and the decrease in the B and C curves is not unexpected.

Impedance.—Figure 4 shows the distribution of acoustic impedance values for the various groups. The solid horizontal bar in each vertical box is the median value. The box itself encompasses the semi-interquartile range or middle 50% of the impedance distribution.

No data are shown for normal groups in the age categories of 40 to 59 and 60 to 79 years, since we have not tested numbers of patients with truly normal sensitivity in these age categories sufficient to ensure stable medians and semi-interquartile ranges.

The primary message of Fig 4 is a point made by previous investigators,[9,15] namely that there is considerable overlap between the impedance distributions of normal and disordered middle ears. As a very rough rule

Roughly, the distributions in Fig 3 are according to expectation. In ears with either normal or sensorineural audiometric patterns, the type A curve predominates. In ears with conductive audiometric findings, however, types B and C curves predominate. It is instructive, however, to study the distributions in the age category of 2 to 5 years. Here we observe that, in both the normal and sensorineural groups, there appears to be a higher incidence of types B and C patterns than would be predicted from the distributions for older children and adults. This is especially true of the children from 2 to 5 years with normal audiograms. The appearance of some B and a fair number of C curves in this group suggests the presence of undetected middle ear problems in children without obvious audiometric evidence of a conductive component.

of thumb, one might say that the highest 20% of normals overlap the lowest 20% of conductives. This overlap limits the diagnostic value of the impedance score when viewed in isolation. As we shall attempt to show in subsequent sections, however, the impedance may have substantial diagnostic value when considered within the framework of complete impedance audiometry.

It is also interesting to note, in Fig 4, that, in the 2 to 5 age group both the normal and sensorineural distributions are displaced upward relative to the adult distributions. The shift is especially obvious in the sensorineural group. These shifts are consistent with the high incidence of types B and C tympanometry functions noted earlier, and furnish added evidence of middle ear problems in these very young children.[16]

Using the distributions of the normal and sensorineural ears in the 14 to 39 age group as a standard we can form the rough rule of thumb that most normal middle ears will yield impedance scores in the range from 1,000-3,000 ohms, but that occasionally scores as low as 800 or as high as 4, 200 ohms can be expected.

Acoustic Reflex.—Figure 5 shows the distribution of the hearing level necessary to elicit the acoustic reflex. The analysis is limited to ears with normal audiometric configurations. Data for all four frequencies—500, 1,000, 2,000, and 4,000 Hz— have been pooled, since preliminary analysis failed to suggest a significant frequency effect.

Three significant factors emerge from Fig 5. First, the modal reflex HL is 85 dB in all

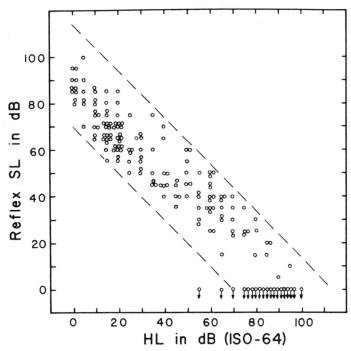

Fig 6.—Relation between reflex SL and degree of hearing loss in patients with sensorineural (presumably cochlear) loss.

SEROUS OTITIS MEDIA

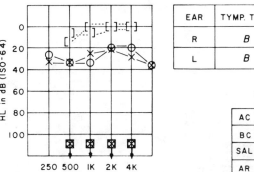

EAR	TYMP. TYPE	IMPEDANCE
R	B	7500 Ω
L	B	11667 Ω

	R	L
AC	○	×
BC	[	]
SAL	⊢	⊣
AR	⧄	⧅

Fig 7.—Impedance audiometry in a 7-year-old boy with serous otitis media. Note type B tympanometry curves, very high acoustic impedance scores, and bilateral absence of acoustic reflex.

age groups. Second, the distribution is about 40 dB wide. Third, there is a fairly high incidence of ears in which the reflex could not be elicited (>110 dB) in the 2 to 5 age group. This is consistent with the previous findings of Robertson et al.[17] The distributions exhibit two relatively systematic trends with age. First, there is a tendency toward narrowing and sharpening of the distribution as age increases. Second, there

OTOSCLEROSIS

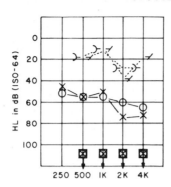

EAR	TYMP. TYPE	IMPEDANCE
R	A	4680 Ω
L	A	5525 Ω

	R	L
AC	○	×
BC	[	]
SAL	⊱	⊣
AR	▢	⊠

Fig 8.—Impedance audiometry in a 54-year-old man with otosclerosis. Note type A curves, relatively high impedance scores, and bilateral absence of acoustic reflex.

LABYRINTHINE HYDROPS

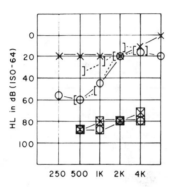

EAR	TYMP. TYPE	IMPEDANCE
R	A	844 Ω
L	A	1784 Ω

	R	L
AC	○	×
BC	[	]
SAL	⊱	⊣
AR	▢	⊠

Fig 9.—Impedance audiometry in a 59-year-old woman with labyrinthine hydrops. Note type A curves, normal impedances, and reduced reflex SL at 500 and 1,000 Hz on right ear (due to loudness recruitment).

RIGHT ACOUSTIC NEURINOMA

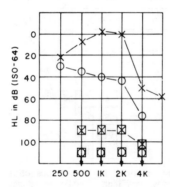

EAR	TYMP. TYPE	IMPEDANCE
R	A	4125 Ω
L	A	2250 Ω

	R	L
AC	○	×
BC	[	]
SAL	⊱	⊣
AR	▢	⊠

Fig 10.—Impedance audiometry in a 60-year-old man with a right acoustic neurinoma. Note type A curves. Impedance is high (4,125 ohms) on the right ear but is still within the normal range. Absence of reflexes on the right ear indicates that recruitment is not present.

is a decreasing incidence of ears that fail to show a reflex response. These trends could be interpreted to support a hypothesis of maturation of the reflex arc, up to perhaps early adulthood. On the other hand, one cannot exclude the possibility that the high incidence of no-response in the 2 to 5 age group merely reflects the middle ear problems suggested by the B and C tympanometry types and shifted impedance distributions noted earlier.

Although the acoustic reflex to pure tones occurs at a sensation level of approximately 85 dB in the average normal ear, the reflex SL is reduced by the presence of loudness recruitment.[13,18-21] This occurs because the reflex is apparently mediated by the loudness of the sound signal. In the normal ear this loudness level is reached for pure tones at sensation levels of 70 to 100 dB.[13] In the ear with loudness recruitment, however, the loudness level required to elicit the reflex

TOTAL LEFT FACIAL PARALYSIS — BELL'S PALSY

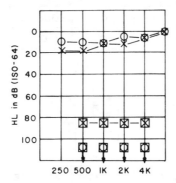

Fig 11.—Impedance audiometry in a 22-year-old woman with left-sided facial paralysis. Absence of reflexes on right ear is due to loss of innervation to left stapedius muscle.

EAR	TYMP. TYPE	IMPEDANCE
R	A	2338 Ω
L	A	2057 Ω

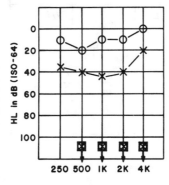

Fig 12.—Impedance audiometry in a child of 37 months. Type B curve, higher impedance on left than on right ear, and bilateral absence of acoustic reflex indicate conductive loss on left ear.

EAR	TYMP. TYPE	IMPEDANCE
R	C	1737 Ω
L	B	3619 Ω

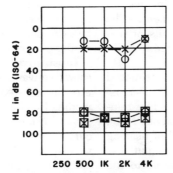

Fig 13.—Impedance audiometry in a child of 27 months. Type A curves, normal impedances, and normal acoustic reflexes confirm behavioral impression of normal hearing.

EAR	TYMP. TYPE	IMPEDANCE
R	A	1710 Ω
L	A	1636 Ω

Table 1.—No. of Subjects and Ears by Age and Type Categories

Age (yr)	Type Category					
	Normal		Sensorineural		Conductive	
	Subjects	Ears	Subjects	Ears	Subjects	Ears
2-5	19	35	22	41	15	27
6-13	25	49	25	44	19	33
14-39	19	38	25	47	30	43
40-59	10	20	22	41	30	47
60-89	—	—	35	61	20	28
Total	73	142	129	234	114	178

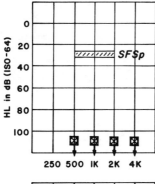

EAR	TYMP. TYPE	IMPEDANCE
R	C	6000 Ω
L	C	2150 Ω

	R	L
AC	O	X
BC	[	]
SAL	>-	-/
AR	☐	☒

EAR	TYMP. TYPE	IMPEDANCE
R	C	2000 Ω
L	C	2111 Ω

	R	L
AC	O	X
BC	[	]
SAL	>-	-/
AR	☐	☒

Fig 14.—**Top,** Impedance audiometry carried out under sedation in a child of 10 months. Behavioral observation suggests relatively normal sensitivity, but high impedance (6,000 ohms) and bilateral absence of acoustic reflex suggest conductive loss on right ear. **Bottom,** Same child two months later after medical treatment for otitis media. Decrease of impedance from 6,000 to 2,000 ohms and appearance of acoustic reflex bilaterally indicate that middle ear problem has been resolved.

will be reached at a much lower level above the impaired threshold.

Figure 6 shows how the reflex SL declines as a function of increasing hearing loss in patients with loudness recruitment. The data are taken from the test results of sensorineural patients in the age range from 14 to 59 years.

Figure 6 shows that, as sensorineural hearing loss increases, the reflex SL decreases in regular, one-to-one fashion. The relationship is linear and of unit slope. Note, also, that for any particular level of hearing loss, the range of variability among patients is about 40 dB, a range comparable to the distribution of reflex levels in normal ears.

Analysis of the trend in Fig 6 suggests two conclusions. First, when the reflex SL is less than 60 dB, the presence of loudness recruitment may be reasonably inferred. Second, most sensorineural losses with recruitment should yield reflex responses until the hearing level exceeds about 80 dB. This means that, when a reflex is observed at a particular frequency, the hearing level at that frequency must lie somewhere between 0 and 80 dB. Eighty decibels is, to be sure, a fairly substantial range, and well illustrates

the principle that the reflex threshold level cannot be used to predict the absolute threshold level with any degree of precision. Nevertheless, the rule that reflex response means a hearing level of 80 dB or better can be extremely useful in the evaluation of very young children.

Illustrative Case Reports.—Figure 7 shows conventional and impedance audiometry in a 7-year-old boy with serous otitis media. Results are consistent with mass lesions in the middle ears. Tympanometry curves are type B, impedance values are well above the normal range of 1,000 to 3,000 ohms, and acoustic reflexes cannot be elicited.

Figure 8 shows results in a 54-year-old man with bilateral otosclerosis. Tympanometry curves are type A, impedance scores are above the normal range, and acoustic reflexes are absent.

Figure 9 shows results in a 59-year-old man with a unilateral loss due to endolymphatic hydrops. Tympanometry curves are type A, and impedance values are within normal limits on both ears. In this case acoustic reflexes occur at the expected normal hearing levels on both ears. The reduced sensation levels at which the reflex occurs on the right ear at 500 and 1,000 Hz are due to the loudness recruitment phenomenon.

Figure 10 summarizes results in a 60-year-old man with a right acoustic neurinoma. As expected, tympanometry curves are type A in both ears, and impedance values are within the normal range. The value of 4,125 ohms on the right ear is high, but, as noted earlier, a very small number of normal ears may show impedances as high as 4,200 ohms. On the left ear, reflexes are observed at the expected sensation levels of 85 to 90 dB, except at 4,000 Hz where loudness recruitment due to the high-frequency cochlear loss causes the reflex to appear at a sensation level of only 50 dB. On the right ear reflexes are absent at all frequencies. Since eighth nerve disorders, such as acoustic neurinoma, are not accompanied by loudness recruitment, sounds presented to this patient's right ear never attain sufficient loudness to elicit the reflex.

Figure 11 shows how facial nerve lesions central to the branch supplying the stapedius muscle abolish the acoustic reflex.[19] The patient had a left facial nerve paralysis due to Bell's palsy. When sound was presented to the left ear, and the probe tip was sealed in the uninvolved right ear, reflexes appeared at normal levels. However, when sounds were presented to the right ear, and the probe tip was sealed in the left ear, reflexes were not observed because the left stapedius muscle could not contract.

Figure 12 illustrates the value of impedance audiometry in very young children. The audiogram of this 3-year-old child suggested a mild unilateral loss. Properly masked bone conduction thresholds were difficult to obtain because of the child's age. Impedance audiometry clearly demonstrated, however, the conductive basis for the reduced sensitivity on the left ear. The left tympanometry curve was type B and the impedance on the left side was more than double the impedance on the right. This finding illustrates the diagnostic value of the absolute impedance score in spite of the overlap problem described earlier. Here the value of 3,619 ohms is within the normal range, but the fact that it is so much larger

than the right ear value of 1,737 ohms adds support to the overall picture of left middle ear involvement suggested by the type B tympanometry function. Finally, the fact that acoustic reflexes are absent in both ears yields still more support for a left middle ear disorder. Failure to elicit reflexes when sound is introduced to the left ear results from the fact that the conductive loss attenuates the loudness of the input signal to such an extent that, even at the maximum output of the audiometer, 110 dB HL, the loudness is not sufficient to trigger the reflex. Failure to elicit reflexes when sound is presented to the normal right ear results from the fact that, even though the loudness in the right ear is sufficient to elicit a reflex, the probe tip in the left ear will fail to detect the contraction because of the middle ear disorder.

This particular configuration of results has considerable diagnostic value. It means, in effect, that the combination of unilateral loss and bilateral absence of the acoustic reflex can only mean unilateral middle ear disorder. In unilateral cochlear disorder one would always see the reflex on the good ear and, if the loss did not exceed 80 dB, on the bad ear as well. In unilateral eighth nerve disorder one would at least see the reflex on the good ear. Only unilateral middle ear problems abolish the reflex bilaterally.

In the case of this 3-year-old boy the results of impedance audiometry pointed unequivocally to a unilateral conductive problem. Subsequent medical examination and treatment confirmed the accuracy of this conclusion.

The value of impedance audiometry in this patient lay in the fact that it led to an unequivocal diagnosis of conductive impairment without the need for bone conduction audiometry. The clinician who has attempted to measure bone conduction thresholds on children in this age range, while simultaneously masking the ear not being tested, will, perhaps, appreciate the value of such diagnostic support.

Figure 13 shows the result of impedance audiometry in a child of 27 months. The audiogram suggested reasonably normal sensitivity in both ears, but, again, one does not always feel comfortable about the validity of

Table 2.—Showing How Results of Impedance Audiometry Help to Confirm Audiometric Impression in the Evaluation of Young Children

Tympanometry	Impedance	Acoustic Reflex	Confirm Behavioral Audiometric Impression of
A in both ears	Normal in both ears	Normal bilaterally	Bilateral normal hearing or bilateral mild-moderate sensorineural loss or unilateral mild-moderate sensorineural loss
A in both ears	Normal in both ears	Absent bilaterally	Severe bilateral sensorineural loss
A in one ear; B or C in other ear	Normal in A ear; high in B or C ear	Absent bilaterally	Unilateral conductive loss
B or C in both ears	High in both ears	Absent bilaterally	Bilateral conductive loss

threshold estimates in children so young. In this case impedance audiometry served to confirm the impression of normal hearing. The fact that all results were normal gave, at least to us, valuable confirmation of our impression that the child suffered no significant ear pathological abnormality.

Figure 14, *top* and *bottom*, illustrates how impedance audiometry can be carried out under sedation in the very young child. Figure 14, *left*, shows the result of our first examination of a child of 10 months. Orienting responses to familiar speech sounds in a sound field (SFSP) suggested a threshold sensitivity level of about 30 dB. Impedance audiometry, carried out under chloral hydrate sedation, showed type C tympanometry functions in both ears. On the left ear impedance was well within the normal range (2,150 ohms), but on the right ear a value of 6,000 ohms, well above the normal range, was noted. In addition, there was no reflex bilaterally. We interpreted these findings to indicate a right middle ear disorder. After two months of medical treatment the child was retested (Fig 14, *right*). The speech awareness level had improved only slightly, to 15 dB, but changes in impedance audiometry were dramatic. Although the tympanometry curve was still type C, indicating continuing negative pressure, the impedance had dropped from 6,000 to 2,000 ohms on the right ear. Impedance was unchanged on the left ear. In addition, reflexes could be elicited from both ears at expected levels.

This case illustrates the value of impedance audiometry in detecting middle ear problems in the child too young for conventional play audiometry.

Comment

In our experience, impedance audiometry represents an invaluable diagnostic tool in clinical audiology. It has become, in our clinic, a routine part of the audiologic assessment of every patient. We frankly wonder how we ever got along without it.

Equally clear, however, is the fact that the technique is useful only as a complete battery and that diagnostic judgments must be based on the overall configuration of tympanometry, acoustic impedance, and the acoustic reflex.

Tympanometry alone is useful only to a limited degree. Types B and C curves strongly suggest middle ear disorder but, as illustrated in Fig 3, type A curves also occur in a large percentage of conductive losses, especially in older adults.

The acoustic impedance score, per se, is simply too variable for accurate diagnosis. As shown in Fig 4, there is an overlap of about 20% between normals and conductives. An impedance in the vicinity of 4,000 ohms is quite ambiguous. It may be normal or it may indicate a considerable increase in a patient whose impedance is normally less than 2,000 ohms.

Of the three measures the acoustic reflex thresholds are probably most useful individually. But here, again, there may be ambiguity. Absence of the reflex may be due to conductive loss, to cochlear loss greater than 80 dB, to eighth nerve loss at virtually any level, or to a facial nerve lesion.

Individually, then, each measure has serious limitations. In combination, however, they yield patterns of great diagnostic value.

In unilateral conductive loss, for example, we have noted the recurrence of the following pattern: (1) tympanometry of types B or C on the bad ear; (2) impedance higher than normal on the bad ear; and (3) acoustic reflex absent in both ears.

This pattern points, unequivocally, to the presence of middle ear disorder on the bad ear. There are only two common exceptions to this pattern. Otosclerotics will usually give a type A function rather than a B or C. Cases of ossicular discontinuity may give unusually deep type A functions and lower than normal impedance. Also, in the latter group, there may be an observable acoustic reflex at high levels when sound is introduced to the good ear.

In unilateral cochlear loss with loudness recruitment the following pattern recurs: (1) tympanometry of type A on both ears; (2) impedance normal on both ears; and (3) acoustic reflex elicited at normal HL in both ears (ie, at reduced SL in the bad ear).

The only common exception to this pattern occurs when the loss on the bad ear exceeds about 80 dB. Then the reflex is absent on the bad ear, but still present on the good ear.

In unilateral eighth nerve loss the following pattern recurs: (1) tympanometry of type A on both ears; (2) impedance normal on both ears; and (3) acoustic reflex elicited at normal HL on the good ear, but absent on the bad ear.

The only exception to this pattern occurs when the loss on the bad ear is very mild. Under this circumstance the sound may reach a loudness sufficient to elicit a reflex at a normal or greater than normal SL on the bad ear. Under this circumstance the reflex amplitude decay test of Anderson et al[14] may be applied for further confirmation of the retrocochlear site.

Using these recurring patterns as a frame of reference, we have employed the results of impedance audiometry to great advantage diagnostically. It must be reemphasized, however, that there will always be exceptions to the expected outcomes of individual components of the impedance battery. As illustrated in Fig 3, some normals and many sensorineurals will give type C tympanometry functions. And, as we have emphasized earlier, acoustic impedance values may be difficult to interpret unless they easily exceed the normal range. Finally, there is a very small percentage of otherwise normal individuals who simply do not show the acoustic reflex at any level.[17]

Nevertheless, the expected patterns recur with sufficient regularity so that we find them distinctly advantageous in clinical work. They are especially useful in the evaluation of very young children. Here we find that impedance audiometry is valuable in either confirming or denying the diagnostic impressions gained from observation and behavioral audiometry.

Table 2 shows how the overall pattern of impedance data can be helpful in confirming the tester's clinical impression based on behavioral observation. Table 2 is also useful in denying the likelihood that one's clinical impression is correct. If, for example, one cannot observe response to sound at any level, yet acoustic reflexes occur at normal levels bilaterally, it is unlikely that the behavioral impression of total deafness is correct. One must then seek other reasons for the child's failure to respond behaviorally. Similarly, if the child seems to be responding behaviorally at moderate sound levels, yet the reflex is bilaterally absent in spite of normal impedance and type A tympanometry, then the validity of the behavioral responses is rendered suspect. Finally, the results of impedance audiometry can be extremely valuable in identifying middle ear disorders in children whose bone conduction levels cannot be validly measured either because of age and cooperation factors or because the sensorineural loss is too severe.[22-24] In our clinical experience the combination of play or conditional orienting reflex (COR) audiometry and impedance audiometry yields a reasonably accurate estimate of both degree and type of loss in all but a small percentage of the children referred to our service.

Many studies published in the American literature[3,4,6] have dwelt on the value of impedance audiometry in distinguishing between stapes fixation and ossicular discontinuity. As a result, there is a feeling in many quarters that this is the principle application of impedance audiometry. Otologic surgeons have, therefore, questioned whether the results of impedance audiometry are of more than academic interest since surgical intervention is indicated in either event.

Our own experience certainly concurs with the results of previous investigators in demonstrating that the distinction between fixation and discontinuity is dramatically revealed in both the pressure-compliance function and the acoustic impedance. We have, however, purposely avoided extensive discussion of this issue in the present paper in order to emphasize, to the clinician, that impedance audiometry has far broader implications for the diagnostic evaluation of hearing disorder.

This study was supported by grant FR-05425 from the Public Health Service.

Mrs. Phyllis Segal, supervising audiologist, the Methodist Hospital, Houston, assisted in the collection of data.

References

1. Metz O: The acoustic impedance measured on normal and pathological ears. *Acta Otolaryng*, suppl 63, 1946.

2. Zwislocki J: Acoustic measurement of the middle ear function. *Ann Otol* **70**:1-8, 1961.

3. Feldman A: Impedance measurements at the eardrum as an aid to diagnosis. *J Speech Hearing Res* **6**:315-327, 1963.

4. Feldman A: Acoustic impedance measurements as a clinical procedure. *Int Aud* **3**:1-11, 1964.

5. Feldman A: Acoustic impedance studies of the normal ear. *J Speech Hearing Res* **10**:165-176, 1967.

6. Zwislocki J, Feldman A: *Acoustic Impedance of Pathological Ears,* technical report LSC-S-5 of the Laboratory of Sensory Communication. Syracuse, NY, Syracuse University, 1969.

7. Thomsen K: Employment of impedance measurement in otologic and oto-neurologic diagnostics. *Acta Otolaryng* **45**:159-167, 1955.

8. Terkildsen K: Movements of the eardrum following intra-aural muscles reflexes. *Arch Otolaryng* **66**:484-488, 1957.

9. Terkildsen K, Nielsen SS: An electroacoustic impedance measuring bridge for clinical use. *Arch Otolaryng* **72**:339-346, 1960.

10. Møller A: Improved technique for detailed measurements of the middle ear impedance. *J Acoust Soc Amer* **32**:250-257, 1960.

11. Lidén G: The scope and application of current audiometric tests. *J Laryng* **83**:507-520, 1969.

12. Lidén G: Tests for stapes fixation. *Arch Otolaryng* **89**:215-219, 1969.

13. Jepsen O: Middle-ear muscle reflexes in man, in Jerger J (ed): *Modern Developments in Audiology.* New York, Academic Press Inc, 1963, pp 193-239.

14. Anderson H, Barr B, Wedenberg E: Intra-aural reflexes in retrocochlear lesions, in Hamberger C, Wersall J (eds): *Disorders of the Skull Base Region.* Stockholm, Almqvist & Wiksell, 1969.

15. Bicknell M, Morgan N: A clinical evaluation of the Zwislocki acoustic bridge. *J Laryng* **82**:673-691, 1968.

16. Brooks D: The use of the electro-acoustic impedance bridge in the assessment of middle ear function. *Int Aud* **8**:563-569, 1969.

17. Robertson E, Peterson J, Lamb L: Relative impedance measurements in young children. *Arch Otolaryng* **88**:70-76, 1968.

18. Metz O: Threshold of reflex contractions of muscles of middle ear and recruitment of loudness. *Arch Otolaryng* **55**:536-543, 1952.

19. Ewertsen H, Filling S, Terkildsen K, et al: Comparative recruitment testing. *Acta Otolaryng* **140**(suppl):116-122, 1958.

20. Klockhoff I: Middle ear muscle reflexes in man: A clinical and experimental study with special reference to diagnostic problems in hearing impairment. *Acta Otolaryng*, suppl 164, 1961.

21. Lamb L, Peterson J, Hansen S: Application of stapedius muscle reflex measures to diagnosis of auditory problems. *Int Aud* **7**:188-199, 1968.

22. Farrant R, Skurr B: Measuring the acoustic impedance of severely deaf ears to test for conductive component. *J Otolaryng Soc Aust* **2**:49-53, 1966.

23. Brooks D: An objective method of detecting fluid in the middle ear. *Int Aud* **7**:280, 1968.

24. Djupesland G: Use of impedance indicator in diagnosis of middle ear pathology. *Int Aud* **8**:570-578, 1969.

Studies in Impedance Audiometry

I. Normal and Sensorineural Ears

James Jerger, PhD; Susan Jerger, MS; and Larry Mauldin, Houston

Results of impedance audiometry were analyzed in 1,133 consecutive patients with either normal or sensorineural audiograms. The static compliance of the normal middle ear varies uniquely with both the age and sex of the patient. In the normal ear, the threshold of the stapedial reflex to pure tones is normally distributed around a mean of approximately 85 dB hearing threshold level (ISO-64) with a standard deviation of 8 dB. In the ear with sensorineural hearing loss, the sensation level (SL) of the stapedial reflex declines in proportion to increasing hearing loss to a limiting (SL) of approximately 25 dB. The frequency of 4,000 hertz appears to be atypical. Absent reflexes at this frequency do not necessarily have pathological significance.

A previous report from this laboratory[1] summarized our experience with impedance audiometry in a successive series of 400 patients tested during 1969. The present series of papers extends these observations to a consecutive series in excess of 2,000 patients tested during 1970 and 1971. This larger series reveals the fine grain of individual differences in middle ear function. In addition, we feel that we are now in a better position to delineate norms for the technique and to define, with some precision, the likelihood of abnormal findings as a function of type of audiometric configuration.

The present paper details results found in older children (6 years or older) and adults with either normal hearing or sensorineural hearing loss. Subsequent papers in this series will consider results found in young children (less than 6 years) and in adults with conductive hearing loss.

Methods

Subjects.—The subjects of the present paper were 1,133 patients with either normal hearing or sensorineural hearing loss seen for routine audiometric examination by the Audiology Service of the Methodist Hospital, Texas Medical Center, Houston, during 1970 and 1971. The entire age range is represented with the single exception that children less than 6 years old

Accepted for publication April 20, 1972.
From Baylor College of Medicine, Texas Medical Center, Houston.
Reprint requests to Mail Station 009, Methodist Hospital, Houston 77025 (Dr. Jerger).

are excluded; they will be the subject of a later communication.

All of the 1,133 patients had either normal or sensorineural audiograms. A normal audiogram was defined as one in which no threshold, on either ear, exceeded 25 dB (ISO-64) over a range from 250 to 4,000 Hertz. Of the total group, 382 had normal audiograms.

A sensorineural audiogram was defined as one which did not demonstrate a significant conductive component on either ear. This decision was made primarily on the basis that air and bone, or air and sensorineural acuity level (SAL), thresholds were essentially interwoven across the range of frequencies tested (500 to 4,000 Hz). Sensorineural audiograms occurred in 751 patients.

The total sensorineural group was divided into two subgroups on the basis of hearing threshold level (HTL). Group A consisted of 511 patients in whom no threshold on either ear exceeded 70 dB (ISO-64) over a 500 to 4,000 Hz range. Group B consisted of the remaining 240 patients in whom at least one threshold in this range exceeded 70 dB. The purpose of this subdivision was to define a group of sensorineural subjects (group A) who would be expected to show the stapedial reflex across the 500 to 4,000 Hz range, provided that no significant middle ear problem existed in either ear.

Finally, no patient was included in the present study if retrocochlear disorder was either suspected or confirmed. Thus, no member of the present series of 1,133 patients showed any retrocochlear symptoms on history, physical, audiometric, or radiographic examination.

Apparatus and Procedure.—Complete impedance audiometry was done on each patient as part of his routine audiometric examination.

An electroacoustic impedance bridge (Madsen, model ZO-70) was used to obtain tympanogram on each ear, the static compliance (sometimes called "absolute impedance"), and the threshold of the stapedial reflex for pure tones of 500, 1,000, 2,000, and 4,000 Hz. Auditory signals for the stapedial reflex measures were provided by a standard audiometer (Beltone, model 10D) calibrated to the ISO-1964 standard.

Tympanograms were defined by a relative rather than an absolute procedure. That is, only relative changes in compliance were recorded as a function of positive and negative air-pressure changes in the external-ear canal.

Static compliance was measured by subtracting the air volume of the external canal from the equivalent volume of the external canal and middle ear system combined. The difference defined the equivalent volume or "compliance" of the middle ear in the plane of the eardrum. This compliance value can be expressed either in ohms or in cubic centimeters of equivalent volume. The present paper adheres to the latter convention. The electroacoustic bridge used in this study measures compliance for a single probe-tone frequency of 220 Hz.

The stapedial-reflex threshold was defined as the lowest HTL (ISO-64) that produced reliable, detectable changes in compliance when the pure-tone signal was presented to the ear opposite the ear containing the probe tip of the impedance bridge.

Results

Incidence of Abnormality.—As a necessary first step in the definition of a subgroup of patients with unequivocal evidence of normal middle ear function, the impedance data of all 1,133 patients were analyzed for evidence of abnormality in either the tympanogram or the stapedial reflex. All tympanograms were categorized as either type A, B, or C.[1] Type A tympanograms showed a well-defined compliance maximum at or around an air-pressure differential of 0 mm H_2O; as long as the maximum did not exceed -100 mm H_2O, the tympanogram qualified as type A. Type B tympanograms failed to demonstrate any well-defined compliance maximum at any air pressure; they showed a characteristic flat or gradually rising shape. Type C tympanograms showed a well-defined compliance maximum, but it was shifted significantly in the negative direction (greater than -100 mm H_2O). Stapedial-reflex data were surveyed to detect instances in which no detectable reflex could be observed at one or more test frequencies.

Normal Audiograms.—Analysis of the tympanograms and stapedial-reflex thresholds of the 382 patients with normal audiograms revealed that 67 (18%) showed some abnormality in either the tympanogram, the stapedial reflex, or both. The exact distribution of abnormality is shown in Table 1; of the 67 patients, 35 (52%) showed some abnormality in the tympanogram of one or both ears. In most of these 35 patients the stapedial reflex was also abnormal at one or more test frequencies. Many tympanograms were either type B or type C. Others were categorized as abnormal even though they were type A if, in our clinical judgment, they seemed either unusually shallow (A_S) or unusually deep (A_D) for otherwise normal ears. It is certainly possible that in rejecting type A tympanograms on this basis, we may have excluded what were perfectly normal middle ears. If we have so erred it has been on the side of caution, since our ultimate purpose was to define a subgroup of normals for whom we could reasonably infer lack of any significant middle ear pathology.

In any event, the application of this very strict interpretation of normality reveals that 9% of the total group with normal audiograms showed some abnormality on the tympanogram of one or both ears. An additional seven patients (2%) of the total group had facial-nerve disorder on one side, a condition that could account for stapedial-reflex abnormality.

Thus, of the original 67 patients with abnormal impedance data, abnormal stapedial-reflex results could be explained either by an abnormal tympanogram or by a facial nerve disorder in 42 patients. This left 25 patients with otherwise apparently normal middle ears, but with absent stapedial reflex at one or more frequencies in at least one ear. Table 2 shows the incidence of various outcomes in this subgroup of 25 patients; we note that in 14 of these 25 patients (56%) the reflex was only absent at a single frequency (4,000 Hz) in a single ear. In an additional seven subjects (28%) the reflex was absent in both ears, but only at 4,000 Hz. Thus, in 84% of the patients in this group, reflex abnormality was confined exclusively to 4,000 Hz; in only one patient was the reflex unexplainably absent at all test frequencies in both ears. This last finding corresponds to an incidence of approximately three in every 1,000 patients with normal audiograms.

There are some who would argue that even this incidence is too high; that the absence of the stapedial reflex can only mean middle ear disorder. We cannot argue the point here; we can only note that we could find no corroborating evidence of middle ear disorder in any of these 25 patients. The history and physical examinations were negative, the audiogram was normal, and the tympanogram passed a relatively stringent test of normality. In spite of these criteria there are at least two other possible explanations for the absent reflexes. One is the possibility of a congenitally absent stapedial tendon; we cannot completely reject this explanation, but it seems unlikely that such a situation would not be revealed, at least as a very deep tympanogram. A second explanation is that the absent reflexes are due to an undetected central-auditory disorder; we cannot completely reject this explanation either. It remains a distinct possibility, certainly worthy of further investigation.

Sensorineural Audiograms.—The 751 patients with sensorineural audiograms were considered in two groups: group A included 511 patients with an HTL of 70 dB or better at all frequencies from 250 to 4,000 Hz; group B was composed of the remaining 240 patients with thresholds greater than 70 dB at one or more frequencies in the test range.

Of the 511 patients in group A, 35 (7%) had either type B or type C tympanograms. An additional 91 patients (18%) had what we considered to be either too shallow (A_S) or too deep (A_D) tympanograms. The remaining 385 patients were considered to have completely normal tympanograms. Analyses of stapedial-reflex results in these 385 patients revealed that reflexes were present at 500, 1,000, and 2,000 Hz in both ears of every patient. In 83 patients (22%), however, the reflex was absent in one or both ears at 4,000 Hz. We attributed this finding to the fact that hearing loss was maximal at 4,000 Hz so that, in many patients, a sensation level (SL) sufficient to elicit the reflex could not be reached. Although the requirement that no HTL exceed 70 dB guaranteed a

minimum SL of 40 dB, even at 4,000 Hz, the not inconsiderable variability of the stapedial-reflex HTL in normal ears supports the possibility that a SL of 40 dB may be insufficient in some patients with sensorineural loss in the absence of significant middle ear disease. Furthermore, results on normals (Table 2) suggest that 4,000 Hz is an atypical frequency for stapedial-reflex measurement. There is a low, but real, probability that the reflex will not appear even though no other objective evidence of middle ear disorder can be demonstrated. We chose, therefore, to disregard the absence of the stapedial reflex at 4,000 Hz in some patients in this group. All 385 were considered to have normal middle ears on the basis that the tympanogram passed a stringent test of normality and that the stapedial reflexes were present at 500, 1,000, and 2,000 Hz in both ears of all patients.

Of the 240 patients in group B, an alarm-

Table 1.—Incidence of Abnormal Impedance Findings in Subgroup of Patients With Normal Audiograms

	No.	% of Subgroup (No.=67)	% of Total Group (No.=382)
Abnormal tympanogram	35	52	9
Facial-nerve disorder	7	11	2
Abnormal stapedial reflex	25	37	7
Total, subgroup	**67**	**100**	**18**

Table 2.—Incidence of Stapedial-Reflex Abnormalities*

Reflex Absent at	No.	% of Subgroup (No.=25)	% of Total Group (No.=382)
4K, one ear only	14	56	3.7
4K, both ears	7	28	1.8
2K & 4K, one ear only	1	4	0.3
2K & 4K, both ears	1	4	0.3
500, 1K, 2K, and 4K, one ear only	1	4	0.3
500, 1K, 2K, and 4K, both ears	1	4	0.3
Total, subgroup	**25**	**100**	**6.7**

*In subgroup of patients with normal audiograms and tympanograms.

ing 48% (115) had abnormal tympanograms; this left only 125 with normal tympanograms. Because of the severe losses in this group, the presence or absence of the stapedial reflex could not be used to infer middle ear disorder.

As a result of these selective processes, we emerged with a total of 825 patients whose middle ears could reasonably be classified as normal. The 315 patients with normal audiograms all had normal tympanograms and stapedial reflexes at all four test frequencies on both ears. The 385 patients with sensorineural audiograms of 70 dB or less all had normal tympanograms and stapedial reflexes at 500, 1,000, and 2,000 Hz in both ears. The 125 patients with sensorineural audiograms greater than 70 dB all had normal tympanograms. All subsequent analyses of static compliance and stapedial-reflex data are based solely on these 825 patients.

Static Compliance.—The term "static" compliance is used here to contrast this measurement with the "dynamic" compliance measurements exemplified by the tympanogram and the stapedial reflex. In the previous literature this measure has often been referred to as either "impedance" or "absolute impedance." Strictly speaking, these terms are not correct since the compliance is related only to the reactive component of impedance and does not consider the resistive component. Impedance may be inferred from compliance only if the resistive component of impedance is assumed to be either constant or negligible.

In the electroacoustic bridge used in this study, static compliance is measured at the point of maximum compliance of the tympanogram. In the case of normal middle ears this point occurs at or near an air-pressure differential of 0 mm H_2O, but is usually slightly in the negative direction. The average effect is small (-20 to -30 mm H_2O) but, in individual patients, negative displacements as large as -60 to -80 mm H_2O occur. Maximum static compliance will only

Table 3.—Distribution of Static Compliance*

Study	Type of Bridge[†]	No.	Percentile				
			2.5	10	50	90	97.5
Present study	A	825	0.30	0.39	0.67	1.30	1.65
Brooks (1971)[2]	A	697	0.35	0.42	0.70	1.05	1.40
Rose & Keating (written communication, Nov 8, 1971)	A	50	0.32	0.43	0.63	1.07	1.35
Bicknell and Morgan (1968)[3]	M	39	0.30	...	0.63	...	1.00
Feldman (1967)[4]	M	33	...	0.45	0.65	0.90	...
Burke et al (1970)[5]	M	25	...	0.45	0.65	1.00	...

* Static compliance, in cc, as reported by various investigators for 220 or 250 Hz probe tone.
† Type of bridge: A—electroacoustic (Madsen, ZO-70) 220 Hz probe tone; M—electromechanical (Zwislocki, E8872A) 250 Hz probe tone.

appear when this static-negative pressure is taken into account.

In the case of an electromechanical bridge such as the Zwislocki model E8872A, there is no provision for making this pressure compensation. Thus, compliance can only be measured at atmospheric air pressure. If a static-negative pressure exists in particular patients, the maximum compliance will be slightly underestimated by this technique since maximum compliance can be measured only by compensating for the static-negative pressure in the middle ear.

For this reason, compliance measures obtained by an electroacoustic bridge such as the Madsen Z070, and an electromechanical bridge such as the Zwislocki E8872A, are not directly comparable. Unless negative pressure is taken into account, both the central tendency and the variability of compliance measures will be underestimated. The effect, to be sure, will be small in normal ears, but we emphasize the point since it can help to account for discrepancies among published distributions of compliance obtained by various investigators using both electroacoustic and electromechanical bridges. Furthermore, the effect could be substantial in middle-ear disorders, especially otitis media.

Figure 1 shows the distribution of the static compliance (in cubic centimeters of equivalent volume) for the three groups of patients defined above; the total number of patients is 825. The static compliance of each patient is the average compliance of his two ears. Two observations may be made: first, we note that compliance is normally distributed when

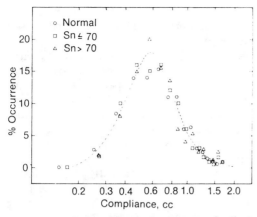

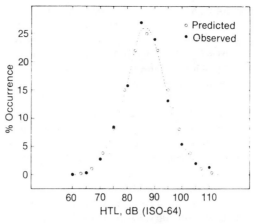

Fig 1.—Static compliance in three groups of patients (presumably normal middle ears); data from both ears of 825 subjects (315 normal, 385 sensorineural (SN) ≤ 70 dB, 125 sensorineural > 70 dB).

Fig 3.—Stapedial reflex in normal ears; data from both ears of 315 normals at 500, 1,000, 2,000, and 4,000 Hz.

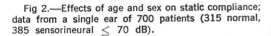

Fig 2.—Effects of age and sex on static compliance; data from a single ear of 700 patients (315 normal, 385 sensorineural ≤ 70 dB).

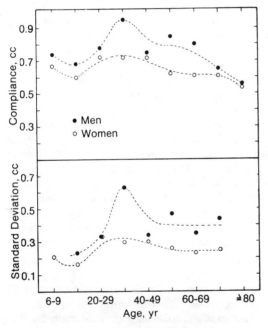

the volume, in cubic centimeters, is represented logarithmically; second, there are no systematic differences among the three groups. This implies that our selection procedure was effective in ruling out middle ear problems in the two groups with sensorineural audiograms, in spite of the fact that stapedial-reflex data were incomplete—especially in the group with loss greater than 70 dB. Since the latter group was chosen

solely on the basis of the tympanogram, the findings lend support to the belief that in the absence of stapedial-reflex data the tympanogram alone is an effective screen for middle ear disorder.

The distributions shown in Fig 1 indicate considerably greater variance in static compliance than one would infer from previous studies. Table 3, for example, compares the present distribution with percentile values obtained in five previous studies[2-5] (Rosen D., and Keating L., written communication, Nov 8, 1971). These six studies represent data from both electroacoustic and electromechanical bridges, and represent a fairly wide range in sample size, from a low of 25 in the study of Burke et al[5] to a high of 825 in the present study. The electroacoustic-bridge studies used a probe tone of 220 Hz, whereas the electromechanical-bridge studies used a probe tone of 250 Hz. The slight difference is probably of no significance since compliance does not seem to change appreciably between 250 and 125 Hz.[6]

Several noteworthy observations may be made from the data in Table 3. First, results generally conform to classic principles of mathematical statistics relating to the estimation of population parameters from small samples. There is very good agreement among the six studies on the 50th percentile (the median), and values range from 0.63 cc to 0.70 cc. This confirms the hypothesis that stable estimates of the central tendencies of populations can be obtained from very small random samples of the population. It is interesting to note, however, that the weighted average of the three estimates obtained with the mechanical bridge (0.64 cc) is 0.04 cc lower than the weighted average of the three estimates obtained with the acoustic bridge (0.68 cc). This is exactly the direction of difference that would be expected from the fact that the mechanical bridge fails to take slight, negative air pressure into account and, therefore, slightly underestimates the maximum compliance of the average, normal middle ear. In any event, there is good agreement among the six studies on the 50th percentile.

Agreement becomes poorer, however, as we consider percentiles closer to the extreme margins of the distribution. In general, the results conform to statistical expectation. Small samples can be expected to underestimate the true population variance because they are insensitive to those rare probabilistic events that occur at the tails of the distribution.[7] We may expect that the larger the sample size the larger will be its estimate of the population variance. The data conform to this expectation remarkably well. If, for example, we study the 10th and 90th percentiles, we may discern a slight but consistent trend toward greater variance as sample size increases from 25 to 825. Similar conclusions hold for the 2.5th and 97.5th percentiles. There is only one apparently contradictory finding: the sample size of Brooks[2] was 697, a value so close to 825 that we would not anticipate significant discrepancies between variance estimates obtained in the two studies. Yet, the present results clearly show greater variability than Brooks's results. However, this discrepancy is consistent with, and exactly predicted by, the relation between the variability of compliance measures and the age range of the sample studied. Brooks's 697 subjects were confined entirely to the 4 to 11 year age range; but in the present study, patients range in age from 6 to 90 years. As subsequent sections will show, the age range of a sample, as well as its sex distribution, exerts a profound influence on the sample variance when compliance is the variable under study.

Effects of Age and Sex on Static Compliance.—In order to study the variables of age and sex, 700 patients (the normals and group A sensorineurals) were divided by sex and by age decades. For each sex at each age decade both the mean and standard deviation of the compliance were computed. The number of patients per cell ranged from 15 to 63. For this analysis only one ear per patient was used; the right ear was arbitrarily selected. Figure 2 shows how both the mean compliance and its variance change as a function of both age and sex. We note, first, that women consistently show a lower average compliance and less variance than men at all ages. Second, there is a very pronounced age effect: both sexes, but especially men, show a well-defined maximum in both mean and variance in the age decade 30 to 39 years. Above this age decade the average compliance declines relatively systematically with increasing age for both sexes.

The sex difference is not unexpected. Both Zwislocki and Feldman[6] and Bicknell and Morgan[3] noted that women seemed to show lower compliance than men. Bicknell and Morgan also noted that women seemed to show a narrower compliance range. Neither study, however, provided quantitative data on sex difference.

Figure 2 eloquently explains the difference in variability between the present study and the previous study of Brooks (Table 3). We may note that, in the age range studied by Brooks (4 to 11 years), variability is at its absolute minimum in both sexes. Since the present study included the entire age range from 6 to 90 years, greater variability must necessarily appear.

We are at a loss to explain the curious maximum in both the average compliance and its standard deviation for men aged 30 to 39 years. We considered the possibility that greater noise exposure of men in this age range might fatigue the intra-aural muscles, thereby increasing compliance; but a comparison of noise-exposed with non-noise exposed men in this age decade failed to demonstrate a compliance difference sufficient to explain the age effect. The average compliance differed by only 0.04 cc in the two groups.

Stapedial Reflex.—The threshold of the stapedial reflex is the lowest sound intensity capable of eliciting a detectable contraction of the stapedial muscle. In electroacoustic bridges this contraction is, of course, detected by the decrease in compliance resulting from the stiffened ossicular chain. If sound intensity is represented logarithmically (eg, on a decibel scale) then the threshold of the stapedial reflex is normally distributed.

Figure 3 shows the distribution of reflex thresholds in the previously defined 315 patients with normal audiograms and normal impedance findings. Results for four test frequencies, 500, 1,000, 2,000, and 4,000 Hz, on both ears have been pooled to produce this single distribution of 2,520 reflex thresholds. Also shown, for comparison, is the distribution predicted by the normal equation:

$$y = \frac{1}{\sigma\sqrt{2\pi}} e^{-1/2 \left(\frac{x-\mu}{\sigma}\right)^2}$$

The actual distribution fits the prediction quite well.

The central tendency of this distribution can be variously described depending on how one defines the class interval represented by a 5 dB audiometric step. If each 5 dB step is considered as the midpoint of a 5 dB interval extending 2.5 dB on either side of it (eg, 85 dB is considered to be the midpoint of the interval from 82.50 to 87.49 dB), then the mean of the distribution is 86.8 dB. It seems more reasonable, however, to consider each 5 dB step as the upper limit of a 5 dB class interval (eg, 85 dB is considered to be the upper limit of the interval from 80.01 to 85 dB). In other words, an observed reflex threshold of 85 dB means that the true reflex threshold must lie somewhere above 80 dB but cannot exceed 85 dB. If the class interval is thus defined, then the mean of the distribution is 84.3 dB.

The standard deviation of the distribution is 8.04 dB. We may therefore infer, from properties of the normal distribution, that 95% of normal reflex thresholds will be encompassed between hearing levels of 70 and 100 dB, and 99% of reflex thresholds between 65 and 105 dB.

One of the most important clinical applications of the stapedial reflex is its use as an objective test for loudness recruitment.[8-9] Since the stapedial reflex is based on the apparent loudness of the eliciting sound, an abnormally rapid growth of suprathreshold loudness will cause the reflex to appear at a smaller-than-normal SL. Indeed, in patients with loudness recruitment the SL of the reflex declines in a one-to-one relationship with hearing loss. Figure 4 shows this relation at each test frequency. Data were obtained from the 515 sensorineural patients with normal impedance findings. Figure 4 shows how the median-reflex SL declines as the hearing loss increases. With the exception of 4,000 Hz, all functions are, at their upper ends, reasonably linear and of unit negative slope. In other words, every decibel of hearing loss reduces the reflex SL by that amount. It is intuitively obvious, however, that the functions must eventually level off. If they were to continue descending in linear fashion, we should eventually have the impossible result that at some hearing loss the reflex SL was 0 dB. As hearing loss continued beyond this point, we should have to address ourselves to the equally impossible concept of a negative-reflex SL.

Clearly there must exist some minimal SL, below which there will never be enough loudness to elicit the reflex no matter how much loudness recruitment is present. Figure 4 shows that this minimal SL is approximately 25 dB. At about this SL the descending functions level off and remain relatively constant with increasing hearing loss. The functions must necessarily end in the hearing loss region of 80 to 90 dB. If the upper audiometric limit is 110 dB, and if there must be a minimal SL of 25 dB, then 85 dB is the maximum hearing loss for which a reflex can be observed. Of course, this value of 85 dB, so derived, is only an average since it is based on median SL of 25 dB.

In order to determine the effect of variability in the reflex threshold on this upper limit, we tabulated, for all 515 sensorineurals, the incidence of reflex absence as a function of hearing loss (Fig 5). The frequencies of 500, 1,000, and 2,000 Hz yield similar results. At levels of hearing loss less than 60 dB, the percentage of absent reflexes is quite low, only about 5%. As hearing loss increases above 60 dB, however, the incidence of reflex absence increases proportionately. Exactly as predicted from Fig 4, the hearing loss corresponding to 50% reflex absence is 85 dB. At 4,000 Hz, the pattern is similar to the other three frequencies, but the function is displaced to the left so that a 50% reflex absence corresponds to a hearing loss of only 75 dB. On the basis of the percentages in Fig 5, we can adopt the rough rule of thumb that, so long as the sensorineural hearing loss does not exceed 60 dB, there is a 90% likelihood (70% at 4,000 Hz) that a patient with loudness recruitment will demonstrate a stapedial reflex at the frequency under test. As the hearing loss increases above 60 dB, the likelihood of a reflex becomes increasingly smaller: at 85 dB, the likelihood is only 50%; at 100 dB, the likelihood is only about 5% to 10%.

Finally, the fact that 4,000 Hz is slightly different from the lower frequencies is not unexpected in view of the high incidence of absent reflexes in otherwise normal ears at this frequency, (Table 2).

Effects of Age and Sex on Stapedial Reflex.—In view of the dramatic age and sex effects previously demonstrated for the static-compliance measure (Fig 2), it is of interest to ask whether similar effects characterize the stapedial-reflex thresholds.

A systematic age effect has, of course, already been demonstrated by Jepsen.[10] He showed that in a series of 91 normals of various ages, the sound intensity required to elicit stapedial reflex declined systematically with increasing age.

Figure 6 shows this effect for both normal (No. = 315) and sensorineural (No. = 385) ears; the average stapedial-reflex threshold and its corresponding auditory threshold are plotted by age decade for each of the four test frequencies. Like Jepsen, we found no significant frequency effect. At all test frequencies there is a gradual and systematic decline in the HTL required to elicit the reflex.

The curious age effect shown in Fig 2 for the static compliance measure is not evident in Fig 6. We can discern nothing unusual about the 30 to 39 year decade or any other single decade; the decline seems uniform with age.

The possibility of a sex difference in stapedial reflex was explored by computing the average reflex thresholds for men and women separately. For this analysis all four test

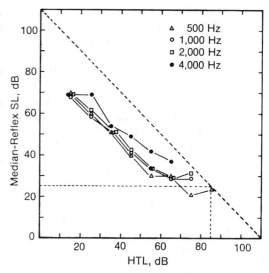

Fig 4.—Reflex SL and degree of hearing loss (in HTL) in 515 patients with sensorineural loss.

Fig 5.—Incidence of reflex absence and degree of hearing loss in 515 patients with sensorineural loss.

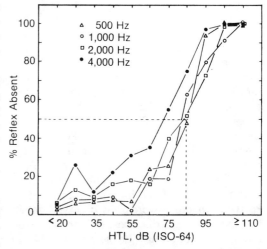

frequencies were pooled, but the results were entirely negative. Neither the normals nor the sensorineurals showed the kind of systematic sex difference evident in Fig 2.

In summary, there is an age effect on stapedial reflex, but it is unlike, and probably unrelated to, the age effect seen in static compliance. Nor is the sex difference, so evident in static compliance, reflected in the stapedial reflex.

Reliability.—Twenty-four patients were retested on at least once. All met the criterion that the tympanogram results were normal on all tests. Figure 7 shows the distribution of test-retest difference scores for both static compliance and stapedial-reflex thresholds. Data from both ears of each subject are included in the distributions. In the case of static compliance, test-retest differences in excess of 0.30 cc are relatively uncommon; the standard deviation of the distribution is 0.22 cc.

The coefficient of correlation between test and retest scores is largely irrelevant to the issue of the reliability of the static compliance measures, since it merely indicates the extent to which individuals preserve their rank orders in the group from test to retest. In the clinical application of impedance audiometry, the individual patient's rank order in the group is ordinarily of little interest. We ask only whether his score lies within or without the expected range of normal scores. It is of interest, however, to note that the coefficient computed from the present data (r = .79) is in good agreement with the previous results of Tillman et al[11] who used an electromechanical bridge to obtain test-retest compliance measures on 30 normals. Coefficients of correlation were computed separately for each of three examiners; for 250 Hz, probe-tone coefficients ranged from .73 to .86.

Figure 7 also shows the distribution of test-retest differences for stapedial-reflex thresholds at the four test frequencies. Reliability is similar for all frequencies. Test-retest differences greater than 15 dB are uncommon; the standard deviation of the distribution is 6.4 dB.

Comment

The age and sex effects illustrated in Fig 2 and 6 must necessarily direct us to be extremely cautious in any attempt to construct norms for impedance audiometry; this is especially true of the static compliance measure. Norms for this measure will be more or less inaccurate to the extent that they fail to take both age and sex into account. The concept of a compliance "norm"[12] based on

Fig 6.—Reflex threshold, auditory threshold, and age in 315 normals and 385 sensorineurals; intensity required to elicit reflex declines as age increases, especially in normal group.

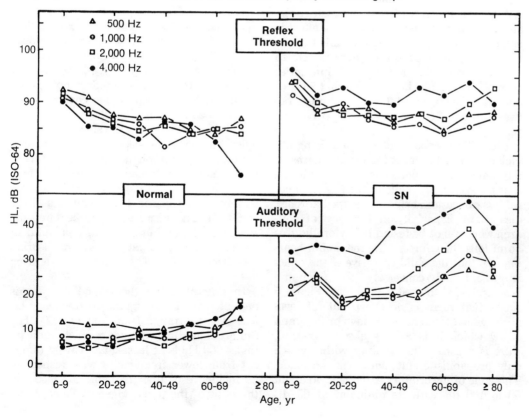

a small sample (25 to 50 cases) composed of both men and women of various ages is of questionable value. If the static compliance measure is ever to achieve its maximum diagnostic potential, both the age and sex distributions of the specific patients under study must be taken into account.

These curious age and sex differences are certainly worthy of further exploration. We have scrutinized our data thoroughly, seeking some clue to the differences, but a satisfactory explanation eludes us. Our fruitless pursuit of the noise-exposure variable was based on the premise that it is the men who are diverging from a stable age trend exemplified by the women. This seems a reasonable assumption in view of the apparently aberrant data for men in the 30 to 39 year decade, both in average compliance and variability around the average value. We cannot, however, categorically dismiss the alternative possibility that it is the women who are, in fact, diverging from nature's plan. Of particular interest would be a systematic study of possible age-related anatomical and physiological differences, or both, between the sexes in relation to middle ear function.

Although the stapedial reflex also shows an age change, the magnitude of the effect is not sufficient to cause serious difficulty. In general, we must expect younger people to show slightly higher threshold intensities than older patients, but the rule that 95% of normal reflexes will fall in the range between 70 and 100 dB HTL should be universal.

From the viewpoint of the practicing clinician, one of the most important norms in impedance audiometry is the maximum hearing loss that a patient with sensorineural loss can sustain before the stapedial reflex disappears. Especially in the case of children who cannot be tested behaviorally, this norm tells the clinician the maximum hearing loss that the child can have if the reflex is present and, conversely, the minimum hearing loss if the reflex is absent. Figure 5 shows that there is no sharp cut off level above which the reflex is always present and below which it is always absent. Instead, there is a zone of uncertainty within which only probabilistic statements can be made. This zone of uncertainty extends from about 60 to 100 dB with its midpoint at 85 dB

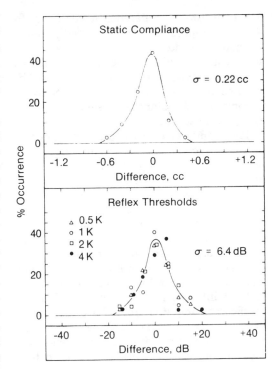

Fig 7.—Test-retest differences in static compliance and stapedial reflex threshold; data from both ears of 24 patients tested on two separate occasions.

(4,000 Hz excepted). The practical implications of this uncertainty zone are as follows:

1. If the patient shows a stapedial reflex at a particular test frequency, there are five chances in ten that the loss does not exceed 85 dB, and there is only one chance in ten that it is as much as 100 dB.

2. If the patient does not show a stapedial reflex (in the presence of normal tympanograms, normal compliance, and intact facial-nerve innervation) then there are 5 chances in ten that the loss exceeds 85 dB, and there is only one chance in ten that it is as little as 60 dB. These ranges are, to be sure, distressingly broad, but they can be helpful in differentiating moderate or severe hearing loss from profound sensorineural hearing loss.

In general, when the stapedial reflex is present there is no significant frequency effect over the range from 500 to 4,000 Hz. But accumulating evidence seems to indicate that 4,000 Hz is at least qualitatively different from lower frequencies with respect to its incidence of unexplainable absence. On the basis of the percentages in Table 2 and

Fig 5, we strongly suspect that the absence of stapedial reflex at 4,000 Hz need not have pathological significance. Its unexplained absence in many otherwise normal ears, and its greater incidence of absence in sensorineural loss of given magnitude, leads us to extreme caution in the interpretation of its absence in a particular ear. It would be unwise to discard 4,000 Hz as a test frequency, since the presence of the reflex can have considerable diagnostic value in spite of the ambiguity of its absence.

At first glance, the apparent incidence of middle ear disorders in this series of 1,133 patients seems alarmingly high (308 or 27%), especially since there was no audiometric evidence of a conductive component in any patient. It must be reemphasized, therefore, that we have purposely applied exceedingly stringent criteria to both tympanograms and stapedial-reflex data in order to insure a subsample uncontaminated by middle ear problems. In ruling out either very shallow or very deep tympanogram configurations, we have undoubtedly eliminated many perfectly normal middle ears. Similarly, in ruling out normals with the reflex missing only at 4,000 Hz, we have probably excluded more normal ears.

If we consider only type B and C tympanograms, and reflex abnormalities only at frequencies lower than 4,000 Hz, then the incidence of abnormal findings drops to 92 patients (8%). Although this is considerably lower than the 27% incidence, the fact remains that, in this series of 1,133 patients without audiometric evidence of conductive component, eight out of every 100 patients showed significant impedance abnormality. This is one of the several reasons why we believe that impedance audiometry should be carried out as an integral and routine part of every audiometric examination.

References

1. Jerger J: Clinical experience with impedance audiometry. *Arch Otolaryngol* 92:311-324, 1970.
2. Brooks D: Electroacoustic impedance bridge studies on normal ears of children. *J Speech Hear Res* 14:247-253, 1971.
3. Bicknell M, Morgan N: A clinical evaluation of the Zwislocki acoustic bridge. *J Laryngol Otol* 82:673-691, 1968.
4. Feldman A: Acoustic impedance studies of the normal ear. *J Speech Hear Res* 10:165-176, 1967.
5. Burke K, Nilges T, Henry G: Middle ear impedance measurements. *J Speech Hear Res* 13:317-325, 1970.
6. Zwislocki J, Feldman A: Acoustic impedance of pathological ears, in *Special Report, Laboratory of Sensory Communication.* Syracuse, NY, Syracuse University, 1969, Fig 6, p 22.
7. Guilford J: *Fundamental Statistics in Psychology and Education.* New York, McGraw-Hill Book Co Inc, 1950, p 89.
8. Metz O: Threshold of reflex contractions of muscles of middle ear and recruitment of loudness. *Arch Otolaryngol* 55:536-543, 1952.
9. Ewertsen H, Filling S, Terkildsen K: Comparative recruitment testing. *Acta Otolaryngol (Suppl)* 140:116-122, 1958.
10. Jepsen O: Middle-ear muscle reflexes in man, in Jerger J (ed.): *Modern Developments in Audiology.* New York, Academic Press Inc, 1963, pp 193-239.
11. Tillman T, Dallos P, Kuruvilla T: Reliability of measures obtained with the Zwislocki acoustic bridge. *J Acoust Soc Am* 36:582-588, 1964.
12. Burke K, Nilges T: A comparison of three middle ear impedance norms as predictors of otosclerosis. *J Audiol Res* 10:52-58, 1970.

Studies in Impedance Audiometry

II. Children Less Than 6 Years Old

Susan Jerger, MS; James Jerger, PhD; Larry Mauldin; Phyllis Segal, MS, Houston

Results of impedance audiometry were analyzed in 398 consecutive children less than 6 years of age seen for routine audiologic evaluation. Ages ranged from 3 to 71 months. Complete impedance results were obtained from 308 children (77%) during the initial audiologic evaluation. In contrast, only 219 children (55%) yielded satisfactory audiograms on the first visit.

Impedance results offered supplementary information not available from conventional behavioral audiometric findings in approximately 67% of children. In general, maximum compliance values were the least useful of the three impedance measures in providing auxiliary diagnostic information. In a subgroup of 82 children with presumably normal middle ear function, stapedius reflex threshold hearing levels changed as a function of age.

This is the second in a series of three papers concerning impedance audiometry results from approximately 2,000 consecutive patients. The initial paper[1] dealt exclusively with results in older children and adults with either normal hearing or sensorineural hearing loss. The present paper is limited to impedance results in children less than 6 years of age. The third paper will summarize results in adults with middle ear disorder. In this report, we attempt to describe the degree to which impedance audiometry supplements conventional behavioral audiometry in young children and to define the likelihood of abnormal impedance results in relation to audiometric findings.

Method

Subjects.—Subjects were 398 children less than 6 years of age seen consecutively for audiologic evaluation at the Methodist Hospital during 1970 and 1971. Ages ranged from 3 to 71 months.

Of the 398 children, relatively complete air- and bone-conduction audiograms were obtained from 219 (55%). Of these audiograms, 17% were normal, 44% showed a conductive impairment, and 39% showed a sensorineural configuration.

Conventional audiograms could not be obtained in the remaining 179 children. However, 157 of these 179 children (39% of the total group) did yield useful soundfield audiometric data. Results in these children were usually limited to head-orienting responses to noise-makers, live-voice, or frequency-modulated (warbled) pure-tone signals. Rarely, however, we did obtain conditioned, overt responses to pure-tone signals and/or speech reception thresholds in the soundfield.

Finally, there were 22 children (6%) that could not be tested by any behavioral technique. This percentage was significantly decreased by additional test sessions. In the present paper, however, we have limited data to results obtained on the child's first visit to the Audiology Service.

Apparatus and Procedure.—Impedance audiometry was attempted on all children as part of the routine audiometric examination. Measurements were carried out as described in our first communication of this series.[1]

In brief, an electroacoustic bridge (Madsen, model ZO-70) was used to obtain three impedance measurements on each ear: (1) the tympanogram, (2) the maximum static compliance, and (3) the threshold of the stapedius reflex for pure tones of 500, 1,000, 2,000, and 4,000 Hz. Auditory signals were generated by a standard audiometer (Beltone, model 10D) calibrated to the ISO-1964 standard.

Results

Probability of a Successful Test.—The Table summarizes the success with which impedance audiometry could be carried out in the 398 children. Results are categorized according to whether the outcome was successful or unsuccessful. A successful result was defined as a test yielding all three impedance measures on both ears: the tympanogram, the maximum static compliance, and sta-

Impedance Audiometry In 398 Children Less Than Six Years Old		
Test Outcome	No. of Children	Percent of Children
Successful result	308	77.4
Unsuccessful result	90	22.6
Earphones not tolerated	35	8.8
Sedative ineffective	10	2.5
No seal	7	1.8
Uncooperative	12	3.0
Incomplete results	26	6.5

Accepted for publication Sept 27, 1972.

From Baylor College of Medicine and the Methodist Hospital, Texas Medical Center, Houston.

Reprint requests to Mail Station 009, Methodist Hospital, Houston, TX 77025 (Dr. J. Jerger).

pedius reflex thresholds. Taken as a whole, completely successful results were obtained from 308 children (77%) during the first audiologic evaluation. This percentage is especially meaningful in relation to the fact that only 219 of the 398 children (55%) yielded conventional audiograms on the first visit.

The Table also summarizes unsuccessful results, broken down according to reason for failure, in the 90 children (22.6%) who could not be successfully tested by impedance audiometry. In this group, findings were limited by the following factors: earphones not tolerated, sedative ineffective, no seal, uncooperativeness, or incomplete data (eg, tympanogram only).

These same data are shown as a function of age in Fig 1. The number of children in each age group ranged from a low of 18 in the 0 to 11 months group to a high of 121 in the 60 to 71 months group. As in the Table, data are categorized according to whether results were successful or unsuccessful. Several interesting observations emerge from Fig 1. First, the percentage of successful results steadily increases with age, from approximately 40% good results in children less than 12 months to approximately 90% good results in children 60 to 71 months. In fact, we begin to see good results in almost all children at approximately age 3. The categories of "incomplete results" and "earphones not tolerated" decrease, as expected, with age. We see approximately 20% of children in each of these two categories in the age range 0 to 11 months. However, only about 5% remain in each category by age 3. The problem of obtaining a seal also decreases with age, from approximately 10% at the earliest ages to only 1% in the oldest age group. The percentage of children that could not be tested due to ineffective sedation is also shown in Fig 1. However, this percentage can only be interpreted within a given age category since sedation was not attempted on all children. For example, lack of data in the 0 to 11 months category does not imply that children can be more effectively sedated in this age group.

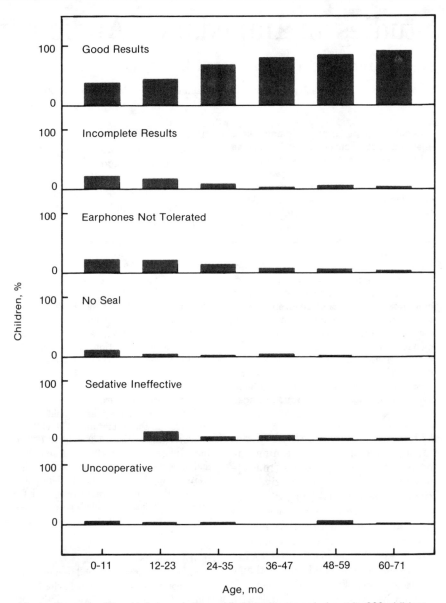

Fig 1.—Success with which impedance audiometry was carried out in 398 children grouped according to age. Unsuccessful results were due to uncooperativeness, ineffective sedation, inadequate seal, earphones not tolerated, or incomplete data such as tympanometry only.

Rather, lack of a significant percentage simply reflects the small number of children on whom sedation was attempted. Therefore, we can only conclude from our data in this area that both the need for and the ineffectiveness of sedation decrease as children become older. Finally, Fig 1 also shows that the number of uncooperative children (approximately 5%) is relatively constant, regardless of age.

Figure 2 shows the distribution of impedance findings in a single age category, the 57 children in the crit-

ical period from 24 to 35 months. Note, again, the high percentage of satisfactory results (70%) in this young, often difficult, age group. Unsuccessful results in these children were primarily due either to rejection of earphones or to an unwillingness to remain quiet long enough to obtain complete results.

In summary, there were only 90 children (22.6%) out of a total group of 398 that could not be successfully tested by impedance audiometry. Of these 90 children, we could not obtain

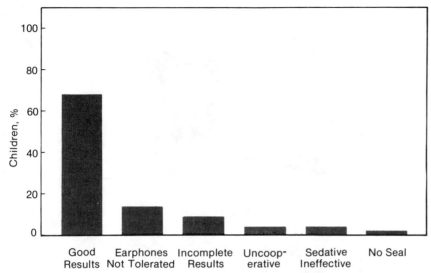

Fig 2.—Distribution of impedance findings in 57 children between 24 to 35 months of age.

audiograms on 82%. Since subsequent data analysis in this subgroup must necessarily be limited, we confine further discussion to those 308 children with complete impedance data.

Contribution of Impedance Results to Audiometric Findings.—Our next step was to examine the clinical value of impedance results in the 308 children with complete impedance data. The number of children remaining in each age group ranged from a low of 7 in the 0 to 11 months group to a high of 108 in the 60 to 71 months group.

Children were categorized into four groups on the basis of audiometric findings. Three groups (204 children) were formed according to type of audiogram: (1) *normal*, hearing levels on both ears less than 25 dB (ISO 1964) at all frequencies between 250 to 4,000 Hz (N = 31); (2) *conductive* or *mixed*, significant air-bone gap (10 dB or greater) at any frequency between 500 to 4,000 Hz (N = 92); and (3) *sensorineural*, hearing level greater than 20 dB at any frequency between 250 to 4,000 Hz but no significant air-bone gap (N = 81). The remaining 104 children were categorized into a "no audiogram" group. Findings for this group were either "no audiometric data" or "soundfield results only."

Analysis of impedance data and audiometric findings was limited to only one ear of each child. For the 204 children with audiograms, impedance data and audiometric results were analyzed on the same ear. For the 104 children with no audiogram, impedance results for one ear were randomly selected.

In order to determine the extent to which impedance results contributed to the diagnostic decision in these children, we categorized results as to whether they supplemented, confirmed, or disagreed with audiometric findings. Rules for determining whether or not impedance results supplemented audiometric findings were difficult to construct since any result is supplementary to the extent that it increases the probability of making a correct diagnostic decision. However, for this specific purpose, "supplementary" was defined by the rule that any of the following conditions held for a particular child: (1) There were no behavioral audiometric data at all. (2) There were soundfield results only. (3) Unmasked bone conduction showed an air-bone gap, nonspecific to either ear. (4) Impedance audiometry indicated a middle ear disorder that was not discerned audiometrically either because the air-conduction audiogram was normal or because it showed a profound sensitivity loss.

The rule for deciding that impedance results "confirmed" audiometric findings was that both tests yielded the same finding, either normal or ab-

normal middle ear condition. The rule for deciding that results "disagreed" was that one test indicated normal middle ear function and the other test indicated abnormal function.

Figure 3 shows the relation between impedance results and audiometric results for the 308 children categorized by audiometric findings.

In children with normal audiograms, impedance results confirmed audiometric findings in 84% of cases and supplemented audiometric findings in 16%. The number of children in the supplementary category highlights the difficulty of defining "normal" hearing on the basis of sensitivity measures alone. In these children we found normal sensitivity and no behavioral audiometric evidence of conductive pathology, yet impedance findings indicated abnormal middle ear function.

In children with conductive audiograms, impedance findings supplemented audiometric results in 75% of children, confirmed results in 16%, and disagreed in 9%. Impedance results were supplementary rather than confirmatory in most children to the extent that the tympanogram suggested a particular type of middle ear abnormality, eg, serous otitis, ossicular chain fixation, discontinuity, on a specific ear. For the children in the "disagree" category, we obtained audiograms with a consistent air-bone gap between 500 and 4,000 Hz, yet all impedance measures were normal. Since impedance audiometry argued against the existence of any middle ear abnormality, we concluded that the air-bone gap in these children was invalid.

For children with sensorineural audiograms, impedance results confirmed audiometric findings in 73% of cases and supplemented audiometric findings in 27%. In other words, approximately one fourth of children with sensorineural audiograms had concomitant middle ear disorder not revealed by conventional audiometric testing. Bone-conduction scores did not reveal conductive impairment in these children primarily because of the profound extent of the sensorineural hearing component.

Finally, all impedance results in the

no-audiogram group were supplementary by our criteria.

In summary, impedance data supplemented audiometric findings in approximately 67% of children less than 6 years of age. The most useful assistance, in our opinion, occurred for children with either no behavioral audiometric data at all or with soundfield results only. This group represented approximately one third of all children in the total group with impedance results.

Distribution of Impedance Measures.—Impedance measures in these children included tympanometry, maximum static compliance, and stapedius reflex thresholds for pure tones of 500, 1,000, 2,000, and 4,000 Hz. Each measure has been described in detail in our previous communication.[1] In order to determine the distributions of these three impedance measures in children with common audiometric findings, we again analyzed results in the 308 children with complete impedance data. However, for this analysis, we eliminated 17 children with either mixed hearing losses or unilateral conductive losses (opposite ear normal) and nonspecific bone-conduction scores. The remaining 291 children were grouped into five audiometric categories. Only one ear of a child was used in each category. However, if the child's other ear qualified for a different audiometric category, then both ears of that child were included. This resulted in data on 305 ears of 291 children, as follows: (1) normal or sensorineural audiogram less than 70 dB (ISO 1964) at all frequencies from 250 to 4,000 Hz (N = 50); (2) conductive audiogram (N = 68); (3) sensorineural audiogram greater than 70 dB (N = 69); (4) soundfield result less than 70 dB (N = 73); (5) soundfield result greater than 70 dB (N = 21); or (6) no audiometric data (N = 24).

Tympanometry.—All tympanograms were categorized as either type A, B, or C.[2] Type A tympanograms were defined as showing a definite, well-defined compliance maximum around an air-pressure differential of 0 mm/ H_2O. Type B tympanograms were characterized by a flat or gradually falling shape. They consistently

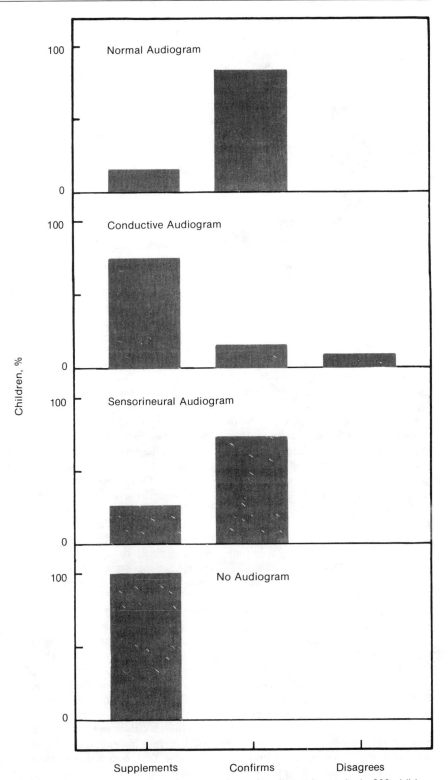

Fig 3.—Relation between impedance results and audiometric results in 308 children grouped according to audiometric findings. Data were categorized as "supplements" when impedance results indicated middle ear disorder that could not be discerned audiometrically.

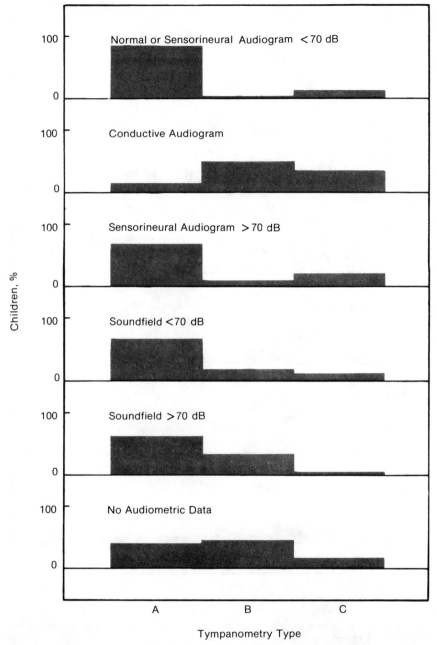

Fig 4.—Distribution of tympanometry results in 305 ears of 291 children grouped according to audiometric findings. Tympanograms classified as A (normal), B (flat), or C (negative pressure).

failed to demonstrate a well-defined compliance maximum at any air pressure. Type C tympanograms showed a well-defined compliance maximum but at a negative air pressure greater than -100 mm/H_2O.

Figure 4 shows the distribution of tympanometry types as a function of audiometric findings. In ears with either normal or sensorineural (<70 dB) audiometric patterns, type A tym-

panograms predominate. Type A curves were obtained in 86% of children. The incidence of type B and C patterns is 14%, again indicating the presence of undetected middle ear problems in children without audiometric evidence of conductive disorder.

In children with conductive audiograms, tympanometry results are as expected. Of children with audio-

metric evidence of middle ear disorder, 85% show type B or C curves. The low incidence of type A patterns is probably due to the nature of the abnormality accounting for the majority of middle ear dysfunction in this age group, namely otitis media and faulty eustachian tube function.

In children with severe sensorineural impairment (sensorineural >70 dB), we find an alarming 30% of children with type B and C tympanograms. This incidence of middle ear disorder is in close accord with our previous data[2] on children between 2 and 5 years of age and with Brooks'[3] results on 1,053 school children between 4 and 11 years of age.

A high incidence of type B and C tympanograms is also observed for children with soundfield audiometric results. In this group, only 65% of all children had type A tympanograms by our criteria. Additionally, Fig 4 indicates that children with more severe hearing impairments, audiogram (sensorineural >70 dB) or soundfield (>70 dB), seem to have more middle ear problems. In both groups, we see 10% to 15% more type B and C tympanograms than in the matching audiometric group with less hearing loss. Finally, an unusually large percentage of children with no behavioral audiometric results had tympanograms reflecting middle ear disorder. We obtained type B or C tympanograms in 63% of these children.

Maximum Static Compliance.—Figure 5 shows the distribution of maximum static compliance measures as a function of audiometric findings. Compliance is expressed in cubic centimeters (equivalent volume of air).

The most distressing feature of Fig 5 is the extensive overlap among groups. There are simply no great differences among distributions for children with normal, sensorineural, or conductive audiograms. In general, we found that absolute compliance data were the least useful of the three impedance measures in providing supplemental diagnostic information. The median maximum static compliance value for the children with normal or sensorineural (<70 dB) audiograms was 0.55 cc. This value is in good agreement with our previous finding[2] for children between 2 and 5 years of age but is lower than averages describing other age groups.[3,4]

Stapedius Reflex.—Figure 6 shows the distribution of hearing levels (HL) necessary to elicit the stapedius reflex. Results were pooled across frequencies of 500, 1,000, 2,000, and 4,000 Hz. Several interesting observations emerge. First, almost all children with normal or sensorineural (<70 dB) audiograms show a stapedius reflex to sound. Only 4% (8 out of 200) of all reflexes in this group were absent. Closer inspection of the missing reflexes reveals that one child accounted for four out of the eight missing reflexes. He had absent reflexes at all four test frequencies, and even though sensitivity was presently within the normal range on both ears, this child presented a history of otitis media. Also, on this visit, he showed abnormal tympanograms on both ears.

All other absent reflexes in this group occurred at only one frequency. Three children had normal sensitivity, type A tympanograms, and absent reflex at 4,000 Hz only. One child had normal sensitivity, type C tympanogram, and absent reflex at 1,000 Hz only.

Results for stapedius reflex threshold measures in the conductive and sensorineural (>70 dB) groups are as expected. Reflex contractions could not be elicited or observed in most children in these groups.

Distributions of stapedius reflex thresholds in children with soundfield results are essentially identical to complementary distributions for children with complete audiometric data. The only exception is the somewhat higher incidence of missing reflexes in the soundfield (<70 dB) group. In general, we felt that soundfield behavioral observations on these children were considerably strengthened by stapedius reflex data, particularly when coupled with tympanometry results. Certainly the fact that all reflexes were missing in children with soundfield results (>70 dB) was, to us, reassuring.

Approximately 80% of reflexes were absent in children with no audiometric data. This result is not unexpected since approximately 65% of these children had type B or C tympanograms.

Effect of Age on Stapedius Reflex Threshold.—In order to examine the effect of age on stapedius reflex thresholds, we formed a subgroup of 82 children for whom we could reasonably infer lack of significant middle ear abnormality. In order to form this subgroup, we first selected the 50 children with normal or sensorineural (<70 dB) audiograms and the 73 chil-

dren with soundfield results (<70 dB). Children with soundfield results were included in order to extend the age range down to the earliest months. Children with sensorineural losses greater than 70 dB were not included since the minimal loudness level necessary to elicit reflex contraction could not be obtained in these patients.

Our next step was to eliminate all children in this subgroup with type B or C tympanograms. Only those children with well-defined type A tym-

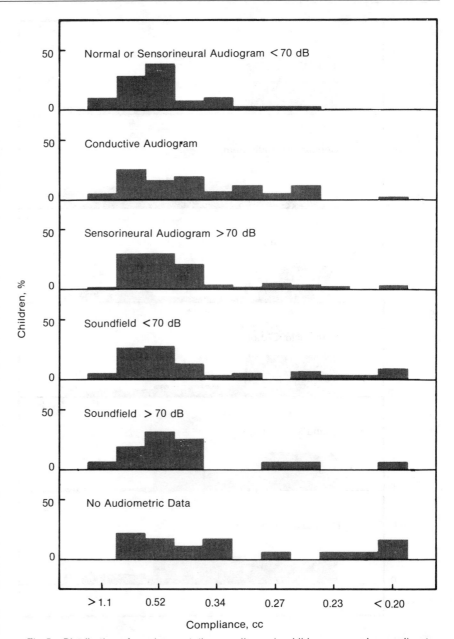

Fig 5.—Distribution of maximum static compliance in children grouped according to audiometric findings.

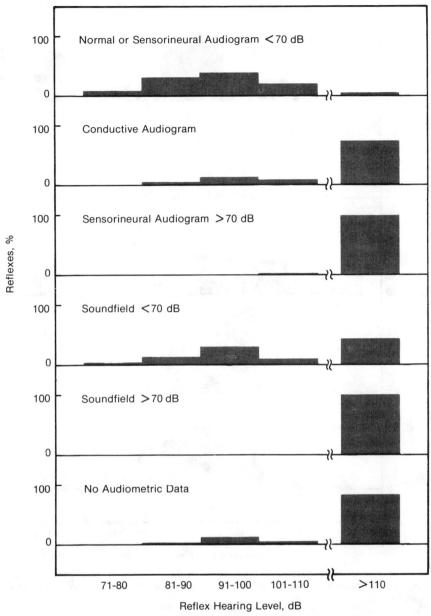

Fig 6.—Distribution of hearing levels necessary to elicit stapedius reflex in children grouped according to audiometric findings. Data pooled across frequencies of 500 to 4,000 Hz.

incidence of absent reflexes (>110). The number of missing reflexes decreases from 20% at ages 0 to 35 months to only 5% at ages 60 to 71 months. This relatively systematic decrease in the number of absent reflexes with increasing age is consistent with the findings of Robertson et al[5] for 40 children less than 4 years old. There are at least two possible explanations for the absence of reflexes in young children with apparently normal middle ear function. One explanation is that the reflex arc undergoes maturation during the early years of childhood. A second possibility is that the reflex arc is complete in the neonate but that there is a relatively high incidence of undetected middle ear abnormality in very young children. Our own experience tends more and more to the latter explanation.

In this group of 82 young children, for example, reflexes were inexplicably absent at one or more frequencies in 20 children, but in 12 of these 20 children, reflexes were absent at 4,000 Hz only, a finding which seems to have no pathological significance.[1]

In the remaining eight children, reflexes were absent at all four test frequencies. There was no obvious age correlation in this group. Two children were less than 24 months; one was between 24 and 35 months; three were between 36 and 47 months; and two were between 48 and 59 months. In five cases, close inspection revealed what were, in our opinion, unusually shallow type A tympanograms. In addition, six of the eight children had type C tympanograms on the opposite (nontest ear) suggesting at least faulty eustachian tube function and a possible past history of middle ear infection. Otologic examination did, in fact, indicate otitis media in five of the eight children. Indeed, seven of these eight children presented a history of multiple problems such as convulsive disorder, mental retardation, microcephaly, and hyperactivity. The only one of these eight children without obvious physical or mental handicap was an infant of 9 months with a history of multiple episodes of otitis media due to an allergic condition noted at age 2 months.

panograms were accepted. We realized that this relatively stringent criterion could possibly reject some children with normal middle ear function. Yet, we preferred to err on the side of caution in order to maintain a strict definition of normalcy. At this point, we had a final subgroup of 82 children with presumably normal middle ear function. Only one ear of each child was used in subsequent data analysis.

Figure 7 shows the distribution of reflex threshold HL as a function of age for these 82 children. Data were pooled across frequencies of 500, 1,000, 2,000, and 4,000 Hz. Two systematic changes with age are observed. First, there is an increasing number of reflexes at lower HL as age increases. For example, at 90 dB HL, the incidence of reflexes increases from only 7% at ages 0 to 35 months to 33% by ages 60 to 71 months. The second systematic change with age is a decrease in the

These observations strengthen our conviction that the presence of the stapedius reflex should be expected as the rule rather than the exception in even very young children and that failure to elicit the reflex at any test frequency should lead to the presumption of aural abnormality.

Figure 7 also shows the distribution of reflex thresholds for the total group of 82 children. The distribution is approximately 40 dB wide with a modal value of 95 dB and a median value of 93.8 dB. Although the modes of the distributions for each age group shown in Fig 7 did not change significantly with age, the median reflex HL changed approximately 6 dB as age increased up to 6 years. Figure 8 shows median reflex HL for these 82 children and for 315 adults with normal audiograms and normal impedance findings. Data for adults are from part I (normal and sensorineural ears) of this series.[1] Median reflex HLs are plotted at one-year intervals for children less than 6 years and by decade intervals for patients from 6 to 79 years. Results were pooled across frequencies of 500, 1,000, 2,000, and 4,000 Hz. For these data each HL was considered as the upper limit of a 5-dB class interval (eg, 85 dB was considered the upper limit of the interval from 80.01 to 85 dB). In other words, a reflex threshold of 85 dB means that the true reflex value exceeds 80 dB but cannot exceed 85 dB.

Figure 8 shows that the reflex HL decreases from approximately 96 to 84 dB as a function of age from infancy to 80 years. A decline in reflex threshold levels with age is consistent with the observation of Jepsen[6] on 91 normal subjects from 10 to 80 years of age. However, the present data indicate that the decrement in reflex HL does not progress at an even rate. Approximately one half of the total decline occurs between infancy and 6 years. Median reflex HL changes from 95.5 dB at ages less than 3 years to 89.5 dB at age 5 years. The second half of the total decline occurs between 6 and 30 years. After age 30, median reflex HL does not show further change. Thresholds remain at approximately 85 dB from 30 to 80 years of age.

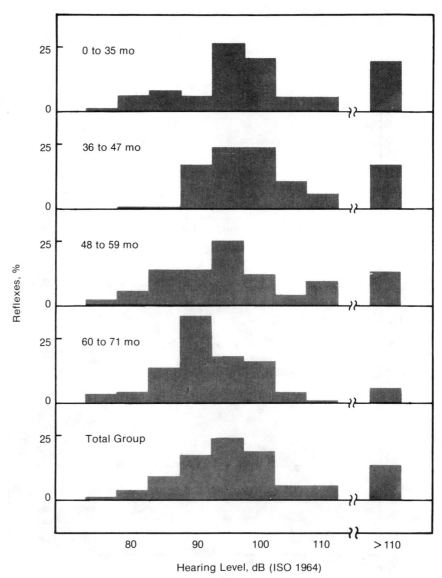

Fig 7.—Distribution of stapedius reflex threshold hearing levels as function of age in 82 children with presumably normal middle ears. Data pooled across frequencies of 500 to 4,000 Hz.

Comment

Impedance audiometry yielded relatively successful results in this sample of children less than 6 years of age. There were only 90 children (22.6%) who would not tolerate the procedure sufficiently well for us to obtain the tympanogram, maximum static compliance, and stapedius reflex thresholds on both ears. Unsuccessful results were generally found in children less than 3 years of age who could not be tested either by impedance audiometry or conventional behavioral audiometric techniques.

In those children who could be tested, impedance audiometry offered supplementary information not available from conventional behavioral audiometric findings in a large percentage. In general, we felt that impedance results offered the greatest assistance for children with either no audiometric data or soundfield behavioral results only. However, for all children at all ages, the combination of impedance results and conventional behavioral audiometric findings offered valuable information that could not be obtained from either test procedure alone.

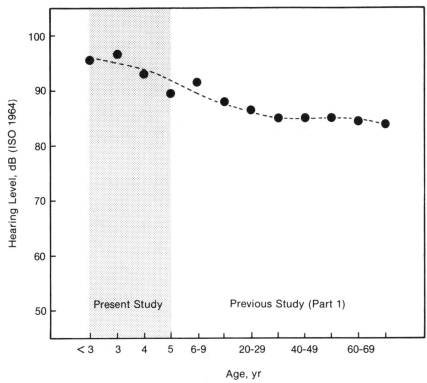

Fig 8.—Median reflex hearing levels for 82 children with presumably normal middle ears and 315 adults with normal audiograms and normal impedance findings. Data for adults obtained from part I (normal and sensorineural ears) of this series on impedance audiometry.[1] Results pooled across frequencies of 500 to 4,000 Hz.

Some specific examples of this interaction are as follows:

The behavioral audiogram suggests a unilateral loss by air conduction. Here impedance audiometry easily differentiates between a conductive and a sensorineural loss without the need for bone-conduction thresholds. If tympanograms are type A and reflexes are present in both ears or at least in the good ear, the loss is sensorineural. If, on the other hand, the tympanogram is A in the good ear, but B or C on the bad ear and reflexes are absent from both ears, then the loss must be conductive. In very young children, the capacity to make this distinction without recourse to masked bone-conduction audiometry can be of some value.

Behavioral results suggest a severe bilateral loss. The child seems to respond only to very intense signals. Here impedance audiometry confirms the picture if tympanograms are A and reflexes are bilaterally absent.

Behavioral results suggest normal or near-normal hearing. The child

seems to respond to familiar sounds at 20 to 30 dB HL. Here impedance audiometry confirms the picture if tympanograms are type A and reflexes are present bilaterally. If, however, tympanograms are B or C on at least one ear and reflexes are absent at all test frequencies from one or both ears, then a mild conductive loss must be considered likely.

Behavioral results suggest reasonably good levels (20 to 30 dB HL), but the parents report a great deal of fluctuation in sensitivity. Here type B or C tympanograms and absent reflexes confirm the picture of recurrent otitis media.

Behavioral results suggest reasonably good sensitivity to familiar environmental sounds (20 to 30 dB HL), but the parents report that the child seems to hear some sounds more consistently than others. Some parents may phrase this as, "He hears what he wants to hear. Sometimes he doesn't seem to hear us at all." Here type A tympanograms combined with reflexes at 500 Hz and possibly 1,000

Hz but absent reflexes at 2,000 and 4,000 Hz confirm the picture of a steeply sloping high-frequency loss.

Behavioral results suggest a total loss. The child fails to respond to sound at any level. If tympanograms are type A and reflexes are absent, the impression of total deafness is confirmed. If, however, reflexes are present at normal levels, an alternative explanation for the behavioral observation must be sought (ie, retardation, autism).

The behavioral audiogram shows an air-bone gap of 15 dB but results of otologic examination were normal. Here type A tympanograms and bilateral reflexes confirm the results of otologic examination and argue that the air-bone gap is invalid. On the other hand, abnormal tympanograms and absent reflexes support results of the audiogram and indicate that the otologic examination failed to detect significant middle ear disorder.

These are just some of the many ways in which we have found impedance audiometry useful as a supplement to conventional behavioral audiometry in the evaluation of young children. On the basis of our experience we consider impedance audiometry to be the single most powerful tool at our disposal in pediatric evaluation. It cannot, however, stand alone. It can be interpreted successfully only in combination with some independent assessment of sensitivity level. When this condition is met, the combination leads to a significant advance in the sophistication of pediatric audiologic assessment.

References

1. Jerger J, Jerger S, Mauldin L: Studies in impendance audiometry: I. Normal and sensorineural ears. *Arch Otolaryngol* 96:513-523, 1972.

2. Jerger J: Clinical experience with impedance audiometry. *Arch Otolaryngol* 92:311-324, 1970.

3. Brooks D: Electroacoustic impedance bridge studies on normal ears of children. *J Speech Hear Res* 14:247-253, 1971.

4. Brooks D: The use of the electro-acoustic impedance bridge in the assessment of middle ear function. *Int Aud* 8:563-569, 1969.

5. Robertson E, Peterson J, Lamb L: Relative impedance measurements in young children. *Arch Otolaryngol* 88:162-168, 1968.

6. Jepsen O: Middle-ear muscle reflexes in man, in Jerger J (ed): *Modern Developments in Audiology.* New York, Academic Press Inc, 1963, pp 193-239.

Studies in Impedance Audiometry

III. Middle Ear Disorders

James Jerger, PhD; Lois Anthony, MA;
Susan Jerger, MS; Larry Mauldin, Houston

Results of impedance audiometry were analyzed in 454 consecutive patients with conductive hearing loss. Completely successful results were obtained on 428 patients (94%).

Tympanometry results indicated that type A patterns were usually associated with otosclerosis or other ossicular chain fixations and type B and C patterns were usually found in otitis media. Maximum static compliance values had only limited diagnostic value due to overlap between conductive and normal groups. Stapedial reflex could not be elicited in most patients. When reflexes were observed in otosclerotic ears, an unusual pattern characterized by negative deflections at onset and termination of a sound appeared. In a subgroup of 154 patients with unilateral conductive loss, results showed that amount of AC-BC gap necessary to abolish stapedial reflex was approximately 25 dB with sound in bad ear and approximately 5 dB with probe-tip in bad ear.

This is the third, and final, report on the application of impedance audiometry to clinical evaluation. Part I of this series described results in 1,133 patients with either normal hearing or sensorineural hearing loss. Part II summarized findings in 398 children less than 6 years of age. The present report, part III, details impedance findings in 454 patients with middle ear disorder.

Methods

Subjects.—The experimental group consisted of 454 subjects with some degree of either unilateral or bilateral conductive

Accepted for publication Feb 19, 1973.
From Baylor College of Medicine and the Methodist Hospital, Houston.
Reprint requests to Department of Otolaryngology, Baylor College of Medicine, Houston, TX 77025 (Dr. Jerger).

hearing loss as manifested by an air-bone or air-sensorineural acuity level (SAL) gap on the pure-tone audiogram. Patients ranged in age from 3 to 79 years. The number of patients by type of middle ear disorder is as follows:

Otosclerosis	60
Otitis media	62
Cholesteatoma	20
Scarred or thickened tympanic membrane	12
Ossicular discontinuity	18
Chronic mastoiditis	4
Unknown	278
Total	454

In all cases, the type of disorder was defined either by otolaryngologic diagnosis or by surgical findings.

Procedure.—All patients were tested by both conventional and impedance audiometry as a routine part of their clinical evaluation by the Audiology Service, the Methodist Hospital, Texas Medical Center, during all of 1970 and the first six months of 1971. Impedance audiometry was carried out by means of a single electro-acoustical impedance bridge (Madsen, type Z070). Exact procedures for obtaining the tympanogram, the maximum static compliance, and thresholds of the stapedial reflex are detailed in an earlier report.[1]

Results

Incidence of Successful Results.— Since all patients had been evaluated consecutively over an 18-month period, it is of some interest to ask with what success impedance audiometry could be carried out in each patient. Of the total of 454 patients on whom impedance audiometry was attempted, completely successful results were obtained in 428 cases (94%). In the remaining 26 cases, complete results could not be obtained because, in 8 (32%) of the 26 patients, the ear canal was too tender to tolerate the probe-tip. In another eight (32%), the canal could not be sealed, usually because of excessive cavity size due to previous middle ear surgery, in the remaining ten (36%), the procedure could not be carried out for a variety of miscellaneous reasons, such as draining ear.

Otosclerosis.— The 60 patients diagnosed as otosclerotic ranged in age from 7 to 70 years. The average age was 43.8 years. Results were available on 95 ears of the patients in this group. The distribution of tympanogram types[6] in these 95 ears conformed closely to expectation.[2,3] The type A shape was observed in 95% of the ears, the type B shape in 1%, and the type C shape in 4%. Figure 1 compares the average tympanogram of the 95 otosclerotic ears with the average tympanogram of 73 normal ears chosen at random from the normal pool summarized in part I (normal and sensorineural ears) of this series. While the otosclerotic tympanogram is, expectedly, slightly shallower than the normal tympanogram, the difference is not dramatic. In addition, the overlap between the distributions of tympanograms for these two groups is so great that one cannot readily differentiate the otosclerotic tympanogram from the normal tympanogram.[3] To be sure, otosclerosis produces a progressive diminution of the

maximum compliance of the middle ear system and, therefore, a progressively more "shallow" tympanogram, but the effect is small in comparison with the considerable intersubject variability of the maximum compliance in any large group of patients.

The extent of this overlap is best illustrated by comparing the distributions of maximum static compliance in the two groups. Table 1 presents the 10th, 50th, and 90th percentiles of the otosclerotic group and, for comparison, analogous percentiles of the distribution of normal maximum static compliance described in part I of this series. While the median (50th percentile) shows the expected reduction in the otosclerotic group, the overlap with the normal group is so great that only a small percentage of the otosclerotic ears falls substantially below the lower boundary of the normal group. This finding is in agreement with the observation of several previous investigators[4-6] (Jerger and van Dishoeck, unpublished data).

The stapedial reflex (to sound presented to the test ear) could not be elicited about 80% of the time in the otosclerotic group. Exact percentages ranged from 77% at 1,000 Hz to 83% at 4,000 Hz. This failure to observe the reflex at maximum audiometric level (110 dB, ISO-1964) is always ambiguous in bilateral conductive loss since reflex absence can be due to either or both of two possible reasons: (1) the sound never can get loud enough in the test ear due to the attenuation caused by the conductive loss, or (2) the change in impedance caused by stapedial contraction cannot be observed due to the middle ear disorder in the nontest ear (ie, the ear containing the probe-tip of the impedance bridge). The 80% figure, therefore, reflects the presence of either or both of these factors. In the remaining 20% of cases, however, a stapedial reflex could be elicited at some audiometric level.

About one half of these reflexes seemed to be quite normal in shape and form. In the other one half, however, we observed a pronounced biphasic pattern in which the reflex

showed a brief negative deflection at both the onset and the termination of the sound. Djupesland[7,8] and Terkildsen et al[9] have recently described this phenomenon in detail. It seems to be a predictable stage in the progressive change of the stapedial reflex of the otosclerotic ear. In some 20% of our observed reflex responses, there was, in fact, no positive component to the reflex at all. The response consisted solely of negative deflections (ie, decrease in impedance) at the onset and termination of the sound. This is a phenomenon that, in our opinion, warrants further intensive study.

In summary, the otosclerotic ear shows a distinctive pattern on impedance audiometry. The tympanogram is type A, the maximum static compliance is decreased, and the stapedial reflex is likely to be absent. Looking at the picture under higher magnification, we can note that the tympanogram should be somewhat more shallow than normal but that variability in maximum static compliance is so great that the overlap between normals and otosclerotics precludes the effective diagnostic use of any absolute datum for an individual patient. The stapedial reflex probably undergoes a progressive change with time in the otosclerotic ear. In the first stage, a slight negative deflection is noted at both the beginning and the end of the sound. In the second stage, the main body of the reflex, the positive deflection (ie, increased impedance) disappears and only the negative deflections (ie, decreased impedance) remain. In the third stage, even the negative deflections disappear, and no response whatever can be elicited.

Otitis Media.— The 62 patients diagnosed as having otitis media in one or both ears ranged in age from 6 to 79 years. The average age was 22.2 years. Results were available on 118 ears of the patients in this group. Type B or type C tympanograms occurred in 90% of ears. The remaining 10% were type A. Of the 90% who conformed to expectation,[9] 43% were type B, and 47% were type C. Since tympanograms were about equally distributed between B and C types, it is of interest to ask whether the pres-

Table 1.—Distribution of Maximum Static Compliance
in Normal and Otosclerotic Ears

| Percentile | Maximum Static Compliance, cc | |
	Otosclerotic (N = 95*)	Normal (N = 825*)
10	0.10	0.39
50	0.35	0.67
90	1.01	1.30

* Numbers of ears.

Table 2.—Distribution of Tympanogram Types in 172 Patients
With Various Types of Middle Ear Disorder

| Group | No. | | Tympanogram Type, % | | |
	Subjects	Ears	A	B	C
Otosclerosis	60	95	95	1	4
Otitis media	62	118	10	43	47
Cholesteatoma	20	30	4	54	42
Scarred or thickened tympanic membrane	12	20	45	15	40
Discontinuity	18	19	100	...	...

Table 3. Distribution of Maximum Static Compliance in 172 Patients
With Middle Ear Disorder and 825 Normals

| Group | No. | | Percentiles, cc | | |
	Subjects	Ears	10th	50th	90th
Normal	825	...	0.39	0.67	1.30
Otosclerosis	60	95	0.10	0.35	1.01
Otitis media	62	118	0.06	0.29	0.81
Cholesteatoma	20	30	0.04	0.16	0.44
Scarred or thickened tympanic membrane	12	20	0.04	0.37	2.83
Discontinuity	18	19	0.76	1.93	>3.66

Table 4.—Absence of Stapedius Reflex in 172 Patients
With Middle Ear Disorder

| Group | No. | | Percent Each Frequency | | | |
	Subjects	Ears	500 Hz	1,000 Hz	2,000 Hz	4,000 Hz
Otosclerosis	60	95	81	77	79	83
Otitis media	62	118	92	91	90	91
Cholesteatoma	20	30	86	82	82	86
Scarred or thickened tympanic membrane	12	20	55	55	55	55
Discontinuity	18	19	47	53	53	58

ence of fluid in the middle ear space was associated with a greater incidence of either the B or C shape. Fluid was present in 88% of ears in the total group. In the subgroup with fluid, type B tympanograms were observed in 44%, type C in 45% and type A in 11%. In the subgroup without fluid (12% of the total group), type B tympanograms occurred in 38% of ears, type C in the remaining 62%. Apparently, tympanogram shape (B or C) is not strongly associated with presence or absence of fluid in the middle ear, probably because of the multiplicity of other factors influencing the shape of the tympanogram in this group of patients.

The maximum static compliance was low in this group, in accord with Brooks'[10] previous observations on patients with otitis media. The median was 0.29 cc. The 10th and 90th percentiles were 0.06 and 0.81 cc, respectively. This distribution is shifted downward considerably in comparison with the normal values and is even somewhat below comparable percentiles for otosclerosis (Table 1). Nevertheless, there is still considerable overlap among these three groups. Again, therefore, it must be concluded that the maximum static compliance, per se, has only limited diagnostic significance.

The stapedial reflex (to sound presented to the test ear) could not be elicited about 91% of the time in the otitis media group. Exact percentages ranged from 90% at 2,000 Hz to 92% at 500 Hz. Those ears in which a stapedial reflex could be elicited usually showed relatively small air-conduction, bone-conduction (AC-BC) gaps. Approximately 40% of reflexes were observed at AC-BC gaps of less than 10 dB, and 90% at AC-BC gaps of less than 20 dB. In this group, we observed no abnormalities of the stapedial reflex comparable to the negative deflection noted earlier in otosclerosis. In ears with otitis media, the reflex was usually absent. On those rare occasions when it could be elicited, however, it seemed to be of normal shape and form.

Cholesteatoma.—The 20 patients with cholesteatoma varied in age from 7 to 67 years. Data were available on 30 ears. Tympanograms in this group were typically type B (54%) or type C (42%). Only 4% were type A. The median static compliance was 0.16 cc, with the 10th and 90th percentiles at 0.04 and 0.44 cc, respectively. The stapedial reflex was absent 82% to 86% of the time. In those rare cases where the reflex was observed, the AC-BC gap averaged 24 dB.

In general, the pattern of impedance findings in this group was determined by the manner in which the cholesteatoma had influenced middle ear function. In some cases, the cholesteatoma exerted only slight pressure on the intact ossicular chain, producing minimal impedance abnormalities. At the other extreme, the cholesteatoma may have destroyed the entire chain and replaced it as the sound-conducting mechanism. Here we typically observed the impedance pattern associated with a substantial increase in the mass of the vibratory system, ie, a type B tympanogram and a very low static compliance.

Scarred or Thickened Tympanic Membrane.—Twelve patients, ranging in age from 61 to 69 years, showed scarred or thickened drums without evidence of active otitis media. Data were available on 20 ears in this group. The tympanogram was usually type A (9, 45%) or type C (8, 40%), rarely type B (3, 15%). The median maximum static compliance was 0.37 cc, with the 10th and 90th percentiles at 0.04 and 2.83 cc, respectively. The stapedial reflex was absent 55% of the time. When present, however, the AC-BC gap averaged only 14 dB.

Ossicular Discontinuity.—The 18 patients with ossicular discontinuity ranged in age from 3 to 67 years. The average age was 39 years. Results indicated that these patients are easily differentiated from other middle ear disorders on the basis of a unique configuration of deep, type A tympanogram and relatively high maximum static compliance. All patients showed the deep type A tympanogram (probe frequency, 220 Hz). The maximum static compliance varied from 0.64 to > 3.66 cc.

Tables 2, 3, and 4 summarize data on distributions of tympanogram types, maximum static compliance,

and absence of stapedial reflex in the five groups discussed above. Tables 2 and 3 illustrate the fundamental conclusion that neither the tympanogram nor the maximum static compliance, by itself, has unambiguous diagnostic significance for the individual patient. There is simply too much overlap among groups.

Table 4 reemphasizes the observation that the stapedial reflex is rarely observed in conductive hearing loss.[11] When it does appear at all, one can be confident that two factors coexist. First, the AC-BC gap on the test ear (ear to which sound is being delivered) is quite small, and second, the ear containing the probe-tip has a virtually normally functioning middle ear. These concepts are discussed in greater detail in the following section.

Stapedial Reflex in Unilateral Conductive Loss.—Patients with unilateral conductive loss provide a unique opportunity to study the effect of size of conductive component on the stapedial reflex. In patients with bilateral conductive loss, failure to observe the reflex is always ambiguous. Reflex absence could be due simply to attenuation of loudness in the ear to which the acoustic signal is presented. On the other hand, even if the acoustic signal can attain a loudness sufficient to elicit the reflex, the impedance bridge may fail to detect the impedance change as a result of the middle ear disorder in the ear containing the probe-tip.

In the case of unilateral conductive loss, however, one can investigate the influence of each factor separately. When sound is presented to the bad ear, failure to observe the reflex can only be due to attenuation of loudness by the conductive component on the bad ear. Conversely, when sound is presented to the good ear, failure to observe the reflex can only be due to the middle ear disorder in the ear containing the probe-tip.

The present series included 154 patients with unilateral conductive loss, as defined by the following criteria: (1) The bad ear showed a consistent AC-BC gap and an abnormal tympanogram. (2) The good ear showed no significant AC-BC gap, the tym-

panogram was normal, and AC thresholds in the range from 250 to 4,000 Hz did not exceed a hearing level of 25 dB (ISO-1964). Stapedial reflex data were analyzed separately for (1) sound presented to the good ear and (2) sound presented to the bad ear. At each test frequency (500, 1,000, 2,000, and 4,000 Hz), the distribution of reflex responses was tabulated. No significant frequency effect was noted. The data for the four frequencies were, therefore, combined to form a single distribution of reflex response as a function of the size of the AC-BC gap in the bad ear. Figure 2 shows the results of this analysis. Percent reflex absence is plotted as a function of the AC-BC gap in the bad ear.

The data for sound presented to the bad ear (filled circles) show the effect of loudness attenuation by the conductive loss. Here the probe-tip is in the normal ear. Failure to observe the reflex must, therefore, be attributed to insufficient loudness in the ear with the conductive loss. The likelihood of observing a reflex decreases systematically as the size of the AC-BC gap increases. When the AC-BC gap is 10 dB, for example, the reflex is absent in only 15% of cases. When the AC-BC gap is 50 dB, however, the reflex is absent in almost 90% of cases. We can predict, on theoretical grounds, that the AC-BC gap yielding a 50% likelihood of reflex absence should be somewhat more than 25 dB (ie, distance between median normal reflex hearing level of 85 dB and audiometric ceiling of 110 dB). The actual value, interpolated from the function of Fig 2 is, in fact, 27 dB.

The data for sound presented to the good ear (triangles) show the effect of the middle ear disorder on the side containing the probe-tip. Here, the acoustic signal, presented to the normal ear, can evoke sufficient loudness to elicit the reflex. Failure to observe the reflex, therefore, must be attributed to the middle ear disorder on the bad side. Under this circumstance, even a very small AC-BC gap is sufficient to reduce, substantially, the likelihood of observing the stapedial reflex. When the AC-BC gap is only 10 dB, for example, the likelihood of

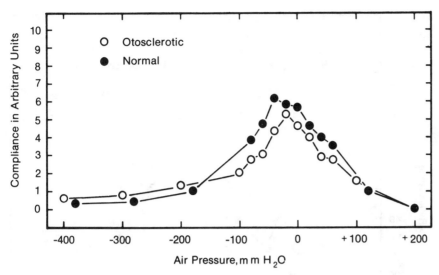

Fig 1.—Comparison of mean tympanograms on normal (N = 73) and otosclerotic (N = 95) ears.

Fig 2.—Percent of reflex absence as function of AC-BC gap in unilateral conductive losses.

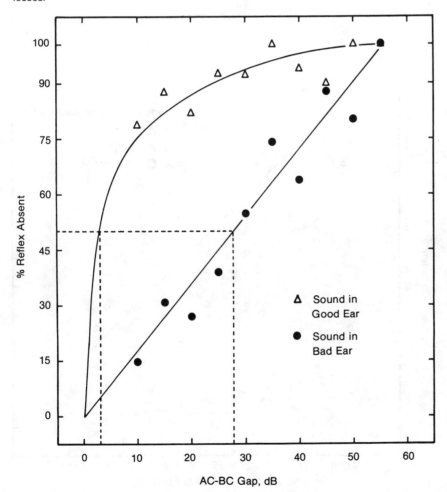

observing a reflex is less than 25%. Extrapolation of the observed function downward to an AC-BC gap of 0 dB, produces a function in which the 50% likelihood of reflex absence coincides with an AC-BC gap of less than 5 dB. This finding is the basis for an extremely sensitive diagnostic application of impedance audiometry. In the case of mild unilateral conductive loss, the reflex may be present when sound is presented to the bad ear but will usually be absent when sound is presented to the good ear, no matter how small the AC-BC gap on the bad ear. This fact can be especially useful when valid BC thresholds are difficult to obtain from the bad ear.

Figure 3 shows the relation between the stapedial reflex and the static compliance of the bad ear in the same 154 patients. We see the expected trends. As static compliance decreases (ie, impedance increases), the likelihood of observing a reflex decreases systematically. Again, we see the extreme sensitivity of the sound-in-good-ear probe-tip-in-bad-ear combination. As static compliance on the bad ear decreases toward, .00 to .09 cc, the likelihood of not observing a reflex to sound in the good ear rapidly approaches 100%.

Relation Between Static Compliance and AC-BC Gap.—Since conductive loss modifies both static compliance and AC-BC gap, it is of some interest to examine the relationship between these two variables. To this end, data from 425 patients (617 ears) were analyzed. Figure 4 shows median maximum static compliance as a function of AC-BC gap (averaged across the 500-2,000 Hz interval) for each of the three tympanogram types. All three subgroups show the expected trend: static compliance decreases as AC-BC gap increases. It is interesting to note, however, that the rate of change (slope) is much greater in the group with type A tympanograms than in either of the other groups. Rate of change is similar for type B and C tympanograms, but the absolute values for the type B are considerably less than for the type C.

These various trends are basically consistent with the abnormalities underlying various tympanogram types.

Fig 3.—Percent of reflex absence as function of static compliance in unilateral conductive losses.

Otosclerosis, or other ossicular chain fixation, undoubtedly accounts for the majority of type A tympanograms. What we see, in Fig 4, then, is the progressive decline in maximum static compliance as fixation increases from an essentially normal value at very small AC-BC gaps to a minimum of about 0.10 to 0.20 at a maximum AC-BC gap of 50 to 60 dB.

The majority of type B and C tympanograms, on the other hand, are due to otitis media. The type C tympanogram represents a stage in which negative middle ear pressure and tympanic membrane retraction are the predominant conditions. Under these conditions even a very small AC-BC gap is accompanied by a substantial reduction in the maximum static compliance (about 0.35 cc). As AC-BC gap increases, however, there is only a small additional reduction in maximum static compliance.

The type B tympanogram usually represents a stage of otitis media in which the ossicular chain has been so immobilized that even rather substantial changes in air pressure in the external canal have little effect on the middle ear system. Under this circumstance, even very small AC-BC gaps are accompanied by severe reduction in the maximum static compliance (about 0.15 cc). As AC-BC gap increases, static compliance expectedly declines even further almost to absolute zero compliance at an AC-BC gap of 50 to 60 dB.

Comment

In spite of the frequent ambiguity of the various individual impedance measures, the overall pattern of results, interpreted in relation to other relevant audiometric data, can have considerable diagnostic significance. For example, the combination of a small audiometric AC-BC gap, a shallow type A tympanogram, and maximum static compliance in the lower portion of the normal range leads to

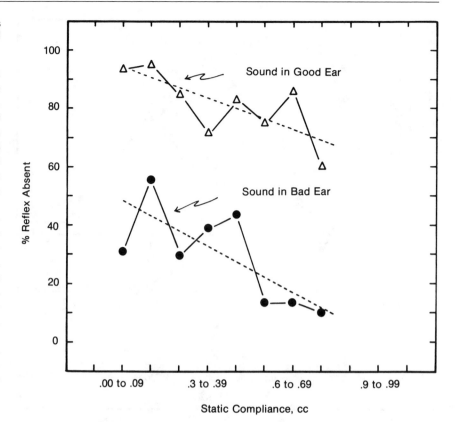

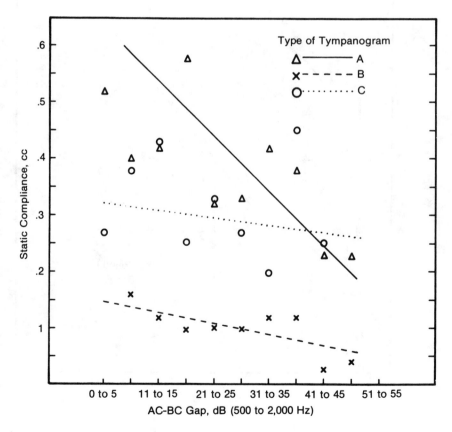

Fig 4.—Median maximum static compliance as function of AC-BC gap for type A, B, and C tympanograms.

the strong presumption of ossicular chain fixation. Conversely, the combination of large AC-BC gap, very deep type A tympanogram, and maximum static compliance in or above the high side of the normal range should lead to the strong presumption of ossicular discontinuity. Similarly, the combination of a moderate AC-BC gap, a type B tympanogram, and very low maximum static compliance is the typical configuration for otitis media. One of the most useful applications of impedance audiometry occurs in the case of mild unilateral conductive loss. Here the configuration of stapedial reflex results helps to quantify the AC-BC gap in the bad ear. If reflexes are absent from both ears, the AC-BC gap is probably greater than 25 dB. If reflexes are absent only to sound in the good ear, then the AC-BC gap in the bad ear is in the 10-25 dB range. If reflexes are present on both ears, the AC-BC gap in the bad ear is probably less than 10 dB. These are, of course, predictions made on the basis of the average performance of patients with conductive loss and assume an upper audiometric limit of 110 dB.

In the evaluation of impedance audiometric results in patients with conductive loss, one must always consider the possibility of multiple abnormalities. In this circumstance, the impedance results will reflect the abnormalities that have the most immediate effect on the tympanic membrane. A patient with stapes fixation may, for example, also have a disarticulation of the incudostapedial joint. This discontinuity will dominate the results in spite of the stapes fixation. Similarly, if the ear canal is blocked with wax, impedance results will show a type B tympanogram and low static compliance no matter what the actual state of the middle ear mechanism.

In our experience, the key to the successful application of impedance measurement in the clinical evaluation of middle ear disorder is to minimize the fine detail of individual measures and to attach considerable significance to the overall configuration of results on the complete test battery.

References

1. Jerger J, Jerger S, Mauldin L: Studies in impedance audiometry: I. Normal and sensorineural ears. *Arch Otolaryngol* 96:513-523, 1972.

2. Lidén G: Tests for stapes fixation. *Arch Otolaryngol* 89:399-403, 1969.

3. Lidén G, Peterson J, Björkman G: Tympanometry. *Arch Otolaryngol* 92:248-257, 1970.

4. Bicknell M, Morgan N: A clinical evaluation of the Zwislocki acoustic bridge. *J Laryngol Otol* 82:673-691, 1968.

5. Alberti P, Kristensen R: The clinical application of impedance audiometry: A preliminary appraisal of an electroacoustic impedance bridge. *Laryngoscope* 80:735-746, 1970.

6. Jerger J: Clinical experience with impedance audiometry. *Arch Otolaryngol* 92:311-324, 1970.

7. Djupesland G: Middle ear muscle reflexes elicited by acoustic and nonacoustic stimulation. *Acta Otolaryngol*, suppl 188, pp 287-292, 1963.

8. Djupesland G: Use of impedance indicator in diagnosis of middle ear pathology. *Int Aud* 8:570-578, 1969.

9. Terkildsen K, Osterhammel P, Bretlau P: Acoustic middle ear muscle reflexes in patients with otosclerosis. *Arch Otolaryngol* 98:152-155, 1973.

10. Brooks D: An objective method of detecting fluid in the middle ear. *Int Aud* 7:280-286, 1968.

11. Klockhoff I: Middle ear muscle reflexes in man: A clinical and experimental study with special reference to diagnostic problems in hearing impairment. *Acta Otolaryngol*, suppl 164, pp 1-92, 1961.

Inter- Versus Intrasubject Variability in Acoustic Immitance

James Jerger and William Keith

Baylor College of Medicine, Houston, Texas

ABSTRACT

To compare inter- versus intrasubject variability of static acoustic immitance, 10 normal subjects were tested on 10 separate occasions. The ratio of intersubject to intrasubject standard deviations was approximately 10 to 1. These results argue for large sample clinical surveys rather than small sample laboratory studies when one seeks to explore trends in static acoustic immitance as functions of other variables.

One of the most important factors determining the choice of a research design is the ratio of inter- to intrasubject variance (13). In general, the ratio of variance due to true differences among subjects to variance due to error of measurement[1] determines optimal design (Ref. 6, p. 62; Ref. 13, pp. 65–88). If true differences among subjects are small, relative to error of measurement, then the optimal research design is usually the small-sample laboratory experiment emphasizing the careful, repeated testing of relatively small numbers of subjects under controlled laboratory conditions. Error variance is minimized by careful and repeated testing of each subject, and a large number of subjects is not critical because intersubject variability is not great.

If, on the other hand, variability among subjects is relatively large and error variance is comparatively small, then the large sample clinical survey is the more appropriate approach. The importance of a large sample size for obtaining unbiased estimates of population parameters grows as a function of population variance (2, 5, 8, 9). If population variance is substantial, then statistics based on small samples may yield unstable estimates of population parameters.

Studies of the volume-equivalent static acoustic immitance (Ve) of the human middle ear as a function of other variables (e.g., age and sex) well illustrate these principles. They can be divided into 2 general categories: large sample clinical surveys (e.g., 1, 7, 11) and small sample laboratory experiments (e.g., 3, 4, 14). The former have stressed trends observed on large numbers of patients using data gathered in the clinical setting. The latter have emphasized the careful, repeated testing of relatively small numbers of subjects under controlled laboratory conditions.

Proponents of large-sample clinical surveys stress the not inconsiderable intersubject variability of static immitance, hence the need for large samples to estimate population parameters adequately. Advocates of small-sample laboratory studies, on the other hand, distrust the precision of clinical data. They prefer to minimize error variance by careful attention to detail and technique of measurement.

In choosing an appropriate design for estimating changes in average acoustic immitance as a function of other variables, then, it is important to consider whether the underlying population is characterized by substantial intersubject variability and how this variability compares with variability due to measurement error.

In the present study, we attempted to illuminate this question by carrying out serial measures of acoustic immitance. Ten subjects were tested on each of 10 successive trials. Results provide an estimate of the ratio of variability due to individual differences with variability due to measurement error in the assessment of volume-equivalent static acoustic immitance.

METHOD

Subjects

Ten young adults with normal hearing and normal middle ear function served as the subjects of this experiment. Nine were female; one was male. They ranged in age from 23 to 33

---

[1] In this paper, "error of measurement" is used in the sense of all possible factors which may affect the measurement, known and unknown, exclusive of true individual differences. They are assumed to vary in random and unpredictable fashion from trial to trial. Such factors typically include fluctuations in the measuring instruments, changes in subject state, motivation and attention, momentary fluctuations in sensitivity of the sensory system, etc. The effects of all such factors are assumed to be random, independent, and additive.

years. Middle ear function was evaluated by conventional impedance audiometry. In all cases, tympanograms at 220 Hz were judged to be of normal shape.

Apparatus

Ve measures were obtained on a commercially available instrument, the Amplaid model 702 Impedance Audiometer.[2] The instrument was calibrated according to manufacturer's instructions. Air pressure, varied by a motor-driven pump, changed at the rate of 25.25 deka Pascals/sec. Tympanograms were graphically displayed, by means of an X-Y plotter, on a calibrated form. Volume-equivalent static acoustic immitance was always defined as the difference, in ml between the immitance measured at +200 deka Pascal air pressure and the immitance measured at the air pressure corresponding to the peak of the tympanogram. Probe-tone frequency was 220 Hz.

Procedure

Each subject was tested on 10 separate occasions, usually on successive days. The minimum interval between successive tests was 8 hr, and the maximum was 72 hr.

At each test session, a single tympanogram was executed. At each subject's initial test session, an airtight seal of the probe was achieved, and the exact size of the soft-rubber ear tip was noted. This tip size was used on all subsequent sessions for this subject.

Tympanograms were executed by a single examiner in a manner consistent with good clinical practice. Beyond this, however, no further attempt was made to minimize error of measurement. The intent was to obtain 10 successive tympanograms using a technique characterizing the gathering of such data in the clinical situation.

RESULTS

The data take the form of a 10 x 10 matrix of Ve values, with the 10 subjects defining one dimension of the matrix (subjects) and the 10 replications defining the other dimension (trials). If we compute the mean and standard deviation of the 10 trial values for a given subject, then the sample mean estimates the true value of Ve for that subject, and the standard deviation estimates variability due to error of measurement

If, on the other hand, we compute the mean and standard deviation of the 10 subject scores for a given trial, then the sample mean estimates the population mean for Ve, and the standard deviation estimates variability due to intersubject differences.

Table 1 shows the means and standard deviations computed for the 10 subjects across trials. We note that there is a considerable range of means for the 10 subjects (intersubject variability), but that the standard deviations for individual subjects across the 10 trials (intrasubject variability) are relatively small.

Table 2 shows means and standard deviations for each of the 10 trials computed across subjects. We note that the means are quite familiar (intertrial trend) and that the standard deviations across subjects (intersubject variability) are quite large.

These results indicate that, at 220 Hz, human acoustic immitance is characterized by relatively greater intersubject than intrasubject variance. It is a situation in which true individual differences are large, and error of measurement is small. The standard deviation for intrasubject variability ranged, over the 10 trials, from 0.02 to 0.10. The median of the 10 values was 0.05. The standard deviation for intersubject variability ranged from 0.48 to 0.53. The median of the 10 values was 0.50. From these data, we can estimate the ratio of inter- to intrasubject standard deviations at approximately 10 to 1.

Another estimate of this ratio may be obtained from the coefficient of correlation between immitance values obtained from the same subjects on 2 different instruments on a single trial (see Footnote 2). As noted above, this coefficient was $r = 0.987$. Rounding to 0.99, and

Table 1. Means and standard deviations[a] of Ve in ml computed across 10 trials for each of 10 subjects

Subject	Mean	S.D.
1	0.48	0.04
2	1.00	0.06
3	0.49	0.03
4	0.38	0.03
5	1.47	0.10
6	0.81	0.06
7	0.59	0.02
8	0.74	0.05
9	0.54	0.03
10	1.92	0.06

[a]*Unbiased estimate of population standard deviation.*

Table 2. Means and standard deviations[a] of Ve in ml computed across 10 subjects for each of 10 trials

Trial	Mean	S.D.
1	0.82	0.48
2	0.86	0.50
3	0.85	0.51
4	0.85	0.49
5	0.84	0.52
6	0.80	0.49
7	0.85	0.49
8	0.84	0.53
9	0.86	0.51
10	0.84	0.48

[a] *Unbiased estimate of population standard deviation.*

---

[2] Comparable data were also obtained on a Grason-Stadler model 1723 Otoadmittance Meter. On this instrument, air pressure changed at the rate of 50.50 deka Pascals/sec. The Pearson-product-moment coefficient of correlation between immitance values for the 2 instruments on a single trial was 0.987. For subject data averaged over the 10 trials, the coefficient of correlation was 0.99.

substituting in the equation

$$\sigma_e/\sigma = \sqrt{1 - r}$$

$$\text{or: } \sigma/\sigma_e = 1/\sqrt{1 - r}$$

where: σ_e is the standard error of estimate, σ is the intersubject variance, and r is the Pearson product-moment coefficient of reliability we obtain

$$\sigma/\sigma_e = 10$$

DISCUSSION

The data on variability summarized above argue for large sample rather than small sample testing when the investigator seeks to estimate parameters of the distribution of volume-equivalent static acoustic immitance (e.g., the mean). In a situation where intersubject differences are so great, reliance on the means of small samples may lead to erroneous conclusions. This point is especially critical in studies attempting to assess changes in acoustic immittance as functions of age, sex, etc. In such situations, where trends in the mean are likely to be small in comparison to intersubject variability, small sample means, due to their instability, may not reveal trends shown by studies with larger samples. A case in point is the apparent disagreement between the results of Thompson et al. (14) and Jerger et al. (11) relative to an age effect on static immitance. Thompson et al. (14) compared the mean Ve of 60 female subjects, 10 in each of the 6 age decades from 20 to 79 years, and found no significant age effect. However, Jerger et al. (11) examined trend in age effect over 9 age decades ($N = 700$) and found an average age effect for females between 20 and 79 years of 0.11 ml. This apparent disparity could be the result of insufficient sample size in the study of Thompson et al. The minimum sample size per age decade for such an experiment can be estimated (Ref. 10, p. 148; Ref. 12, p. 39) from the equation

$$w = 2Z\alpha\sigma/\sqrt{N} \tag{1}$$

or, solving for N

$$N = \sqrt{2Z\alpha\sigma/w} \tag{2}$$

where w is the desired confidence interval, σ is the population standard deviation, $Z\alpha$ is the normal deviate for given α error (type I or error of the first kind), and N is the sample size.

If we take 0.11 as the desired sensitivity, then for a 2-tailed test

$$w = 2 \times 0.11 = 0.22$$

From the present data we have estimated that

$$\sigma = 0.50$$

Using these values to solve equation 2 for N, we find

$$N = 79, \text{ for } \alpha = 0.05$$

$$N = 137, \text{ for } \alpha = 0.01$$

It is not surprising, therefore, that Thompson et al. (14), using sample sizes of only 10 per age decade, failed to observe a significant age effect.

It is illusory to expect in this situation that laboratory precision in measurement technique will counteract the detrimental effects of small sample size. As shown in Tables 1 and 2, the intrasubject variability characterizing standard clinical technique is already small, relative to true individual differences. Reducing it even further by careful and repeated testing of a comparatively small sample in no way circumvents the problem that when intersubject variability is substantial, the population mean may be seriously misrepresented by the mean of a small sample, no matter how precisely the data on that small sample are gathered.

References

1. Alberti, P., and R. Kristensen. 1972. The compliance of the middle ear—its accuracy in routine clinical practice. *in* D. Rose and L. Keating, eds. pp. 159–167. *Impedance Symposium.* Mayo Clinic, Rochester, Minnesota.
2. Arkin, H., and R. R. Colton. 1961. pp. 114–117. *Statistical Methods.* Barnes and Noble, New York.
3. Beattie, R. and D. Leamy. 1975. Otoadmittance: normative values, procedural variables, and reliability. J. Am. Aud. Soc. **1,** 21–27.
4. Blood, I., and H. Greenberg. 1976. Acoustic admittance of the ear in the geriatric individual. Paper presented at the annual convention American Speech and Hearing Association, Houston.
5. Cohen, J. 1969. pp. 6–7. *Statistical Power Analysis For The Behavioral Sciences.* Academic Press, Inc., New York.
6. Federer, W. T. 1955. pp. 61–62. *Experimental Design: Theory and Application.* MacMillan Co., New York.
7. Hall, J. W. 1979. Effects of age and sex on static compliance. Arch. Otolaryngol. **105,** 153–156.
8. Hill, A. B. 1971. *Principles of Medical Statistics, 9th Edition.* Chap. 9. Oxford University Press, New York.
9. Hill, A. B. *A Short Textbook of Medical Statistics, 10th Edition.* Chap. 12. J. B. Lippincott Co., Philadelphia.
10. Huntsberger, D. V., and P. Billingsley. 1973. pp. 148–149. *Elements of Statisitcal Inference, 3rd Edition.* Allyn and Bacon, Inc., Boston.
11. Jerger, J., S. Jerger, and L. Mauldin. 1972. Studies in impedance audiometry. I. Normal and sensori-neural ears. Arch. Otolaryngol. **96,** 513–523.
12. Mendenhall, W., L. Ott, and R. Scheffer. 1971. pp. 39–49. *Elementary Survey Sampling.* Duxbury Press, Belmont, CA.
13. Silverman, F. H. pp. 65–88. *Research Design in Speech Pathology and Audiology.* Prentice-Hall, Inc., Englewood Cliffs, NJ.
14. Thompson, D., J. Sills, K. Recke and D. Bui. 1979. Acoustic admittance and the aging ear. J. Speech Hear. Res. **22,** 29–36.

Address reprint requests to James F. Jerger, Ph.D., 11922 Taylorcrest, Houston, TX 77024.

Received April 30, 1980; accepted July 29, 1980.

V

The
Acoustic
Reflex

The acoustic reflex, or contraction of the stapedius muscle elicited by intense acoustic stimulation, has turned out to be a surprisingly versatile measure. The six papers in this section illustrate how the acoustic reflex (AR) has been used to predict degree of sensorineural hearing loss, differentiate cochlear from retrocochlear site of disorder, and estimate the useful range of electrical stimulation by a cochlear implant.

A German colleague, Wolf Niemeyer, was the first to suggest that the bandwidth effect (i.e., the fact that broad-band signals elicit the AR at lower signal levels than narrow-band signals) could be used to predict degree of sensorineural hearing loss. If frequency resolution declines as sensorineural hearing loss advances, then the advantage enjoyed by broad-band signals in the normal ear should systematically decline as cochlear loss increases. Niemeyer showed that this was indeed the case. The difference between acoustic reflex threshold (ART) levels for single component and multi-component tones was largest in the normal ear and declined progressively as degree of sensorineural loss increased. We spent a lot of time in our laboratory exploring this band-width effect. We defined a measure sensitivity prediction from acoustic reflex (SPAR) as the difference between the ART for white noise and the ART for pure tones averaged over 500, 1000, and 2000 Hz test frequencies. We found that the technique worked, but that there were serious problems confronting its successful clinical use. As noted in the first paper in this section, "Predicting Hearing Loss from the Acoustic Reflex" (*Journal of Speech*

and Hearing Disorders, 1974), consistent physical calibration of the broad-band signal levels from one instrument to the next turned out to be an impossible problem. We ended up recommending a physiological or biological calibration, but such techniques have their own sets of problems. Further, as data began to come in from other investigators, it was clear that there was too much error in the ART measures to make them useful for individual prediction. Too many serious errors of prediction were being made. These kinds of problems have greatly attenuated our initial enthusiasm for the technique. We still find it useful, however, in two kinds of patients: (1) in difficult-to-test children and (2) in patients with functional loss. In either case, a normal SPAR lends strong confirmation to the impression of normal hearing.

The next three papers are all concerned with differentiating cochlear from retrocochlear disorder. The first paper, "The Acoustic Reflex in Eighth-Nerve Disorders" (*Archives of Otolaryngology*, 1974), shows the sensitivity (87%) of the elevated threshold and decay characteristics of the reflex. The second paper, "Latency of the Acoustic Reflex in Eighth-Nerve Tumor" (*Archives of Otolaryngology*, 1983), addresses the latency question. Is the reflex onset delayed in retrocochlear disorder? Here we show that the apparent latency delay is simply an aritifact of the strong relation between reflex amplitude and reflex latency.

The third paper, "Signal Averaging of the Acoustic Reflex" (*Scandinavian Audiology*, 1982), is one that I have always liked. It illustrates an approach to reflex analysis that

I don't think has ever been satisfactorily exploited. We tried to show in this paper that: (1) you could record all four reflexes, the two crossed and the two uncrossed, simultaneously, (2) you could clean up the waveforms very nicely by simple signal averaging, and (3) you could then apply some very simple analytic techniques to extract useful diagnostic information from the reflex array. This is a straightforward and powerful technique. The only problem is that there is still no commercial equipment available to do it. All of our work was necessarily done with software designed for other applications and with a very complicated homemade apparatus that tied up much expensive equipment. I have tried to get manufacturers of immittance instrumentation interested in the problem but, so far, to no avail.

The last two papers in this section are concerned with the application of stapedius muscle contraction to the problem of mapping the electrodes in a cochlear implant. The original idea came from Dianne Mecklenburg, who was then with Cochlear Corporation but has since moved to Switzerland. Bob Fifer, then a graduate student at Baylor, was instrumental in our first efforts to show that the stapedius muscle would contract to the electrical stimulation of auditory nerve provided by the multi-channel Nucleus cochlear implant. In subsequent work, Rose Chmiel and I measured electrically elicited reflexes in a series of adults and children with cochlear implants. We were able to show that the dynamic range of the reflex generally overlapped the preferred listening level, leading to a simple algorithm for the initial mapping of electrodes in young children.

These six papers are just a sampling of the many clinical applications of the versatile acoustic reflex. Like so many other tools in our field, the full exploitation of this one awaits the availability of suitable commercial equipment, in this case apparatus capable of sophisticated measurement of suprathreshold waveforms, simultaneous measurement from both ears, and signal averaging.

The Acoustic Reflex in Eighth Nerve Disorders

James Jerger, PhD, Houston; Earl Harford, PhD, Evanston, Ill;

Jack Clemis, MD, Chicago; Bobby Alford, MD, Houston

Acoustic reflex data were analyzed in 30 patients with surgically confirmed retrocochlear disorder, primarily acoustic neurilemoma. Results confirm the reality of both elevated reflex thresholds and reflex decay as diagnostic signs of retrocochlear disorder. The acoustic reflex was present and normal in 7 patients, present and abnormal in 4 patients, but absent at all test frequencies in 19 of the 30 patients. Results support the diagnostic value of the acoustic reflex test in the evaluation of suspected eighth nerve disorders.

Of the many diagnostic applications proposed for the acoustic reflex, one of the most interesting from the standpoint of both its practical and theoretical implications is the reflex decay test recently proposed by Anderson et al.[1] These investigators studied the time course of the acoustic reflex in 17 patients with surgically-confirmed retrocochlear le-

Accepted for publication July 10, 1973.

From the Department of Otolaryngology, Baylor College of Medicine, Houston (Drs. Jerger and Alford), and the departments of communicative disorders and otolaryngology and maxillofacial surgery, Northwestern University, Evanston, Ill (Drs. Harford and Clemis).

Reprint requests to Mail Station 009, The Methodist Hospital, Texas Medical Center, Houston TX 77025 (Dr. Jerger).

sions. In seven of these 17 patients no reflex could be elicited at the equipment limit (120 dB HL). In the remaining ten patients, however, reflexes could be observed at some test frequencies, although the reflex threshold was abnormally elevated. In all ten patients, Anderson et al[1] observed marked reflex decay. Under prolonged stimulation at a reflex sensation level of 10 dB, reflex amplitude declined to less than one half of its initial value in less than five seconds. Anderson et al[1] emphasized the important implications of this finding for the early detection of small acoustic tumors. Because of the comparative ease with which the reflex decay test can be administered clinically, and the short time required, this approach promises good efficiency as a screening technique for detecting the relatively infrequent occurrence of acoustic tumor.

The present study reports our experience with acoustic reflex measurement in 30 consecutive cases of surgically-confirmed retrocochlear disorder. We have attempted to relate the two phenomena described by Anderson et al,[1] elevated reflex threshold and reflex decay, to conventional audiometric indices of sensitivity, speech intelligibility and abnormal adaptation.

Material and Method

Eighteen of the 30 patients with retrocochlear lesion were tested by the Audiology Service, The Methodist Hospital, Houston. The remaining 12 patients were tested at Northwestern University, Evanston and Chicago, Ill. Twenty-four patients had acoustic neuroma, the remaining six had other tumors in the cerebellopontine angle. In all 30 patients, site and nature of the auditory disorder were confirmed surgically.

In both test locations, acoustic reflex threshold and reflex decay procedures were carried out during routine diagnostic audiometric testing. In both locations measurements were made with an electroacoustic impedance bridge (Madsen, type ZO-70). At test frequencies of 500, 1,000, 2,000, and 4,000 Hz, signal intensity was varied until the reflex threshold had been defined or until the absence of response was noted at 110 dB HL (ISO-64). If the reflex threshold was noted at 100 dB or less at 500 or 1,000 Hz, the test signal (either 500 or 1,000 Hz) was presented at a reflex sensation level of 10 dB for at least ten seconds, and reflex amplitude was carefully monitored. If amplitude declined to less than one half of its initial magnitude in less then ten seconds (criterion of Anderson et al[1]) abnormal reflex decay was considered to have occurred. Otherwise reflex amplitude was considered to have a normal time course. No effort was made to measure reflex decay at test frequencies higher than 1,000 Hz in view of the considerable decay occurring at 2,000 Hz and 4,000 Hz in many normal ears.[1,2]

It is important to note that, before any reflex measurements were attempted on the suspect ear, the examiner verified the presence of a normal tympanogram (type A) on the opposite ear. This precaution was taken to ensure that failure to observe an acoustic reflex on the suspect ear could not be attributed to undetected middle ear disorder on the ear to which the probe tip of the impedance bridge was coupled.

Bekesy audiograms were all obtained on the type E-800 Bekesy audiometer (Grason-Stadler). Speech intelligibility scores for phonetically balanced (PB) monosyllabic words were always based on recorded materials. In Houston, six PB-50 word lists[3] were recorded on magnetic tape by a male speaker (JFJ) and presented to the test ear in blocks of 25 words at 10 to 20 dB intervals until the complete performance intensity function of PB words (PI-PB) had been defined. The maximum PB score (PBmax) was defined as the maximum of the PI-PB function. At Northwestern, a single 50 word modified CNC list (NU No. 6)[4] was presented at a level of 40 dB above the spondee threshold.

Results

The total group of 30 patients was first divided into three subgroups on the basis of the acoustic reflex.

Group A: Reflexes Present With no Decay.—Group A consisted of seven patients in whom acoustic reflexes were present at either 500 or 1,000 Hz and showed a normal time course. All seven patients had acoustic neurilemoma. In two of these patients, reflexes were noted at all four test frequencies. In one patient, the pure tone audiogram was virtually normal, but in the other a flat loss of about 45 dB was noted.

In two other patients of this group, reflexes were noted at 500, 1,000, and 2,000 Hz, but not at 4,000 Hz. In one of these two, the auditory threshold at 4,000 Hz was 80 dB, but in the other, threshold sensitivity at 4,000 Hz was unimpaired (0 dB HL).

In one other patient of subgroup A, reflexes were noted at 500 and 1,000 Hz only. Auditory thresholds at 2,000 and 4,000 Hz, where reflexes were absent, were 40 and 65 dB respectively.

Finally, the remaining two patients in this group yielded reflexes at 500 Hz only. In one, auditory thresholds were 45 dB at 1,000 Hz, 95 dB at 2,000

Summary of Selected Variables for the Three Subgroups		
	Group A (No. = 7)	**Group B** (No. = 4)	**Group C** (No. = 19)
Age			
Mean	31.4	48.8	40.8
Range	12-47	25-62	13-67
PTA			
Mean	27.1	48.8	39.0
Range	2-52	39-67	6-85
PBmax			
Mean	85.1	41.5	38.2
Range	54-96	16-74	0-96
Bekesy			
I or II	7	4	5
III or IV	0	0	14

Hz, and not measurable at 4,000 Hz. In the other patient, however, losses were not severe; 35 dB at 1,000 Hz, 50 dB at 2,000 Hz, and 60 dB at 4,000 Hz. In none of these seven patients of subgroup A could we observe abnormal reflex decay at either 500 or 1,000 Hz. In all patients reflex amplitude did not decline to less than one half of its initial value in less than ten seconds. In point of fact, little decay at all was observed over the ten-second test interval.

It would not be appropriate to conclude, however, that all seven of these patients would have been misdiagnosed by the acoustic reflex test. In three of these seven patients, the absence of reflexes at 110 dB HL at 1,000 or 2,000 Hz in spite of only moderate sensitivity loss (less than 70 dB), would have led to a retrocochlear interpretation. In the other four patients, however, the presence of retrocochlear disease was reflected in neither an abnormal reflex threshold nor abnormal reflex decay.

The most interesting observation we can make about this subgroup is that although 60% of the total group of 30 patients was seen in Houston, 100% of subgroup A was seen at Northwestern. All seven patients showing reflexes with normal time course were seen in Evanston, Ill, or Chicago, none in Houston. This fact probably reflects an earlier detection program for acoustic tumors in the former location. As we shall see in subsequent sections, this subgroup was characterized by the least audiometric loss, the best PB scores, and the youngest age.

Group B: Reflexes Present But With

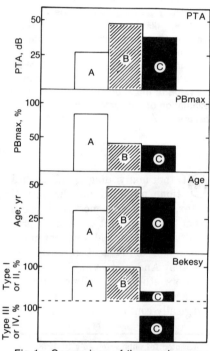

Fig 1.—Comparison of three subgroups of 30 patients with retrocochlear disorder. Average trends for PTA, PBmax, age, and Bekesy audiogram. Group A, reflexes present and normal in form; group B, reflexes present but showing abnormal temporal decay; and group C, reflexes absent at all frequencies.

Abnormal Decay.—Group B consisted of four patients in whom reflexes at 500 or 1,000 Hz were accompanied by abnormal decay of reflex amplitude. Three of the four patients had acoustic neurilemoma. The fourth had a meningioma in the cerebellopontine angle. One patient yielded reflexes at all four test frequencies, but, in the remaining three patients, reflexes could be elicited at 500 and 1,000 Hz

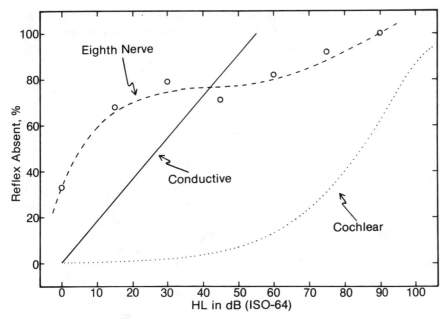

Fig 2.—Relation between degree of hearing loss and likelihood of reflex absence in conductive, cochlear, and eighth nerve disorder.

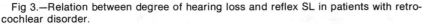

Fig 3.—Relation between degree of hearing loss and reflex SL in patients with retrocochlear disorder.

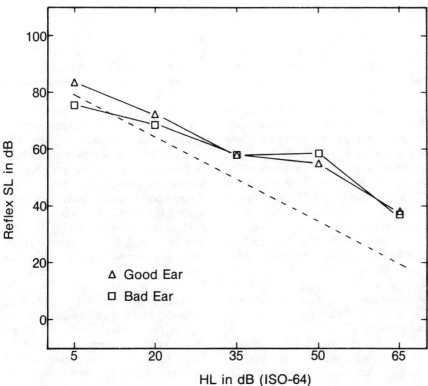

only. In all patients, abnormal reflex decay was noted at either 500 Hz or 1,000 Hz or both test frequencies. Three of the four patients in this group were tested in Houston, the fourth in Chicago.

Group C: No Reflexes at Any Frequency.—Group C consisted of 19 patients in whom no acoustic reflex could be elicited at any test frequency at 110 dB HL. Fourteen had acoustic neurilemoma, the remaining five had other cerebellopontine angle tumors. Fifteen were tested in Houston, and four in Chicago.

Comparison of Groups.—The Table summarizes selected variables for the three groups. The mean and range of age, average pure tone hearing level (PTA), PBmax, and the type of Bekesy audiogram are tabulated for each group. Group A has the lowest mean age (31.4 years), but the range (12 to 47 years) shows considerable overlap with groups B and C. Group A also shows the least PTA sensitivity loss (27.1 dB), but again, there is generous overlap with the other two groups. The PBmax shows the expected trend. Group A has the highest mean score (85.1%), followed by group B (41.5%), and group C (38.2%), but again, overlap among groups is substantial.

All 11 of the patients in groups A and B showed type I or type II Bekesy audiograms. In group C, however, 14 of the 19 patients yielded type III or type IV tracings. Here we see the strongest relationship between reflex abnormality and a related retrocochlear symptom. Except for the five patients in reflex group C with type I or II Bekesey audiograms, there is a well-defined transition from negative Bekesy findings in groups A and B, to a positive Bekesy result in group C.

These average trends are graphically illustrated in Fig 1. Note that, in terms of average performance, group A is differentiated from groups B and C by PTA, PBmax, and age, whereas there is little basis on which to differentiate group B from group C. In the case of Bekesy type, however, group C is differentiated and groups A and B are similar.

Relation of Reflex Threshold to De-

gree of Hearing Loss.—In order to determine the relation between the presence or absence of an acoustic reflex and the amount of hearing loss in eighth nerve disorder, we analyzed, at each test frequency, the percentage of patients who failed to demonstrate an acoustic reflex as a function of the auditory threshold at that test frequency, then pooled results across test frequencies. Figure 2 shows that the resulting function (eighth nerve) has the expected shape. At minimal sensitivity loss, there is only a small probability that the reflex will be absent. As hearing threshold level increases, however, the likelihood that the reflex will not be observed increases rapidly. When the sensitivity loss is only 30 dB, for example, there is a greater than 70% probability that the reflex will be absent. Thereafter, the probability of reflex absence increases slowly to 100% at about 90 dB HL.

In marked contrast, Fig 2 shows analogous functions for conductive loss[5] and for cochlear loss.[2] For any given degree of hearing loss the probabilities are quite different except in the region of 40 dB where the conductive and eighth nerve functions intersect.

The fact that the eighth nerve function climbs more rapidly than the conductive function in the region from 0 to 25 dB HL is a manifestation of the phenomenon of elevated reflex threshold (ie, larger than normal reflex sensation level [SL]), as described by Anderson et al.[1]

If this penomenon had not occurred, then the eighth nerve and conductive functions should have been identical as both reflected the fact of increasing "loudness loss" in ears without loudness recruitment. We note, however, that at comparable levels of loss in the 0 to 25 dB range, the probability of reflex absence is uniformly higher in the eighth nerve group, implying greater than normal reflex SL (ie, the "elevated reflex threshold" concept of Anderson et al[1]).

Why, then, does the eighth nerve function intersect and then fall below the conductive function at hearing loss levels above 40 dB? We believe that this is probably related to concomitant cochlear disorder in most, if not all, patients with acoustic tumors. As further shown in Fig 2, cochlear disorders have the opposite effect of reducing the reflex SL to an abnormally low value. If enough patients with acoustic tumor have related cochlear disorder, and if the cochlear disorder is not masked by the eighth nerve disorder, then the shape of the eighth nerve function in Fig 2 would be explained as the net result of two quite dissimilar hypothetical functions, one reflecting the pure effect of elevated reflex SL (due to the eighth nerve disorder), the other reflecting the pure effect of reduced reflex SL (due to the concomitant cochlear disorder).

For comparison, the conductive function in Fig 2 serves as a yardstick against which to gauge these opposing effects, since it presumably represents the pure effect of sensitivity loss without significant modification of the reflex SL in either direction. Further evidence for concomitant cochlear disorder in these patients is addressed in the next section where the SL of the observed reflexes are analyzed.

Relation of Reflex Sensation Level to Degree of Hearing Loss.—In those patients, and at those test frequencies, where a reflex was observed, we calculated the SL of the acoustic reflex threshold (ie, the difference, in decibels, between auditory threshold and acoustic reflex threshold). This analysis was carried out on both ears, the suspect or "bad" ear, and the opposite or "good" ear. The resulting functions are shown in Fig 3. In the good ear, we note the expected decline in reflex SL as HL increases. This decline in SL as a function of HL merely reflects the presence of probably unrelated cochlear loss in the good ear. The dashed line in Fig 3 is, in fact, the theoretically expected relation between HL and reflex SL based on the assumption of a purely cochlear loss with complete loudness recruitment. The actual function for the good ear departs only slightly from theoretical expectation at high HL (above 40 dB). Of paramount interest, however, is the fact that the analogous function for the bad ear is virtually indistinguishable from the good ear. In other words, when reflexes are observed in ears with retrocochlear disorder, they are observed as reflex SL entirely consistent with a cochlear disorder. This was an unexpected finding. We had anticipated that the commonly observed absence of loudness recruitment in retrocochlear disorder would be reflected in greater reflex SL on the bad ear than on the good ear. Such was not the case, however. Reflex SL was, on the average, consistent with cochlear (ie, recruitment) rather than retrocochlear (ie, no recruitment) disorder, a finding consistent with the explanation of the curves in Fig 2, as described in the previous section.

Comment

The present findings certainly confirm the reality of the twin phenomena of elevated reflex threshold and reflex decay, as described by Anderson et al.[1] In our series, the former seemed to play a more dominant role than the latter. We found reflex decay to be a relatively rare entity. Whereas Anderson et al[1] observed it in ten of 17 patients (59%), we found it in only four of 30 patients (13%). One possible explanation for this discrepancy is the fact that Anderson et al[1] limited their study population to patients whose pure-tone loss did not exceed 60 dB (PTA), whereas in the present series we have included losses up to 85 dB. In fact, however, only four of our patients exceeded the 60 dB criterion. Three of these were in group C (no reflexes at any frequency), but the fourth was in group B (abnormal reflex decay). Significantly, no patient in group A (reflexes normal and without decay) exceeded the 60 dB criterion.

It seems entirely likely that the relative incidence of the various acoustic reflex findings in acoustic tumor will ultimately relate closely to the stage at which the tumor is detected. At those centers where very early detection is emphasized, we can expect the highest incidence of reflexes with a normal time course. Conversely, at those centers where patients are not usually seen until the tumors are larger, we may anticipate the highest incidence of totally absent reflexes.

One of the most striking findings in our present series of patients is the high success ratio of the acoustic reflex test in identifying retrocochlear site. Whereas the conventional Bekesy audiogram, for example, correctly identified only 14 of the 30 patients (47%) the acoustic reflex test correctly identified 26 of the 30 cases (87%). The 47% figure for the Bekesy audiogram is quite consistent with the previous findings of Johnson,[6] but the 87% figure exceeds even their best prediction based on two or more conventional tests.

Interestingly, of the four patients undetected by the acoustic reflex test, neither the PBmax score nor the threshold tone decay test (TDT) was diagnostic, but the SISI test correctly identified two of the four.

In connection with the PBmax score, it is, perhaps, appropriate to stress the extraordinary variability of this measure in the present series and the consequent limitation on its diagnostic significance. We believe that many clinicians have developed a faulty concept of the importance of the maximum speech discrimination score as an early retrocochlear sign. A review of The Table shows that in our group C (no reflexes at any frequency), the average PBmax was 38.2%, certainly a low value, but scores in this group ranged from 0% to 96%. Furthermore, there were so many other retrocochlear signs in these 19 patients that the observation of an extraordinarily low PB score, when it occurred, was seldom of unique value.

The diagnostic challenge in retrocochlear disorders is best represented in our group A where hearing loss was slight and retrocochlear signs were rare. In this group, the acoustic reflex test was positive in three of the seven patients and the TDT (Carhart method) in one of the seven. The PBmax score, however, could not be considered as abnormally low in any of the seven patients. In five patients, the PBmax ranged from 84% to 96%. In one patient, the PBmax was only 54%, but this score was entirely consistent with a very sharply sloping audiometric loss above 500 Hz. In the seventh patient, the PBmax was 76% in the presence of a gradually sloping audiometric contour and a PTA of 35 dB. In this case, the 76% max score would have to be regarded as suspicious but hardly definitive.

Recent evidence does suggest that the shape of the PI-PB function is a valuable early diagnostic sign,[7] but our present experience indicates that the PBmax or the PB score at a single level assumed to be at maximum is of only limited diagnostic value.

Although the acoustic reflex test failed to identify four of our 30 patients with retrocochlear, one cannot help but be impressed by its relatively high success ratio. While we are slightly less optimistic than Anderson et al[1] about the efficacy of the reflex decay test, per se, in view of its limited incidence in our series, we can certainly concur with their general conclusion that measurement of the acoustical reflex adds an extremely valuable weapon to the clinician's armamentarium.

This investigation was supported by research grants NS-08542 and NS-07791 from the National Institute of Neurological Diseases and Stroke, US Public Health Service. Susan Jerger, Wayne Olsen, and Douglas Noffsinger assisted throughout this project.

References

1. Anderson H, Barr B, Wedenberg E: Intra-aural reflexes in retrocochlear lesions, in Hamberger C, Wersall J (eds): *Nobel Symposium 10: Disorders of the Skull Base Region*. Stockholm, Almqvist and Wiskell, 1969, pp 49-55.
2. Jerger J, Jerger S, Mauldin L: Studies in impedance audiometry: I. Normal and sensorineural ears. *Arch Otolaryngol* 96:513-523, 1972.
3. Egan J: Articulation testing methods. *Laryngoscope* 58:955-991, 1948.
4. Tillman T, Carhart R: *An Expanded Test for Speech Discrimination Utilizing CNC Monosyllabic Words*, technical report SAM-TR-66-55. USAF School of Aerospace Medicine, June 1966.
5. Jerger, et al: Studies in impedance audiometry: III. Middle ear disorders. *Arch Otolaryngol*, to be published.
6. Johnson E: Auditory findings in 200 cases of acoustic neuromas. *Arch Otolaryngol* 88:598-603, 1968.
7. Jerger J, Jerger S: Diagnostic significance of PB word functions. *Arch Otolaryngol* 93:573-580, 1971.

PREDICTING HEARING LOSS
FROM THE ACOUSTIC REFLEX

James Jerger, Phillip Burney, Larry Mauldin, and

Betsy Crump

Baylor College of Medicine, Houston, Texas

Acoustic reflex thresholds for pure tones and white noise were used to predict severity of audiometric loss in 1043 ears with sensorineural hearing loss. Both severity and slope of loss were predicted in an additional 113 ears. Prediction was usually quite accurate. Serious errors occurred in only 4% of cases. These findings have important implications for the auditory evaluation of babies and young children.

In a recent communication, Niemeyer and Sesterhenn (1972) proposed that hearing threshold levels could be predicted from a consideration of the relation between acoustic reflex thresholds for pure tones and broad-band noise. In a series of 223 ears with varying degrees of sensorineural hearing loss, they showed that the average hearing threshold level over the range from 500 to 4000 Hz could be predicted from the difference between reflex threshold levels for white noise and for pure tones (averaged from 500 to 4000 Hz) with an accuracy of ±10 dB in 73% of patients and at least ±20 dB in 100% of patients.

The basis for this phenomenon seems to be a change in the critical band width for loudness summation in the ear with sensorineural hearing loss. Flottorp, Djupesland, and Winther (1971) have demonstrated the existence of such critical bands for the acoustic reflex. The abnormal widening of these bands, coupled with the loss in high-frequency sensitivity so characteristic of sensorineural hearing loss, would have a substantially greater effect on the total loudness of a broad-band noise than on the loudness of individual sinusoids within the band. The result would be a reduction in the loudness advantage enjoyed by broad-band noise in the normal ear. These concepts are illustrated, in highly schematized form, in Figure 1. It is hypothesized that, in the normal ear, reflex threshold is reached when any signal exceeds a critical loudness (L). The word *loudness* is used here in the sense of that neural activity which bears a one-to-one correspondence with a human listener's loudness experience. We assume that the reflex mechanism

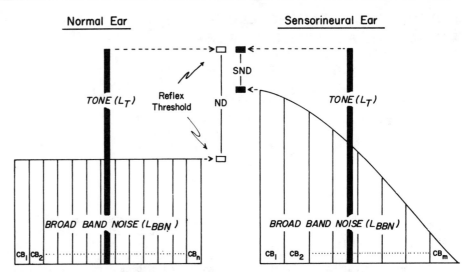

Figure 1. Hypothetical explanation for the phenomenon that the normal difference between tone and noise reflex thresholds is reduced in ears with sensorineural hearing loss.

operates on that parameter of neural activity to which human listeners typically assign the psychological construct "loudness." This critical value is labelled L_T, for the pure tone and L_{BBN}, for the noise. By definition, then, $L_T = L_{BBN}$. The loudness, L_{BBN}, is conceived to be the sum of the loudnesses contributed by the critical bands CB_x. Because the pure tone is confined to a single critical band, but the noise derives loudness from n critical bands, it takes less noise intensity than tone intensity to produce a reflex-eliciting signal (Deutsch, 1972). This is symbolized, in Figure 1, by the difference ND.

In the case of sensorineural hearing loss, however, it is hypothesized that, due to widening of critical bands, the number available for loudness summation is reduced from n to m. In addition, the sloping frequency response characteristic of the sensorineural ear greatly attenuates the relative loudness contributions of critical bands in the high-frequency region. The net result is a noise-tone reflex threshold difference (SND) much smaller than the normal difference (ND).

The potential value of this approach for the evaluation of hearing in babies and other difficult-to-test patients prompted us to attempt to follow up the work of Niemeyer and Sesterhenn in a larger series. The present report is based on the administration of their technique to a total of 1156 patients with either normal hearing or varying degrees of sensorineural hearing loss.

METHOD

Data were collected at three locations within the Texas Medical Center—the Audiology Service of the Methodist Hospital, the Audiology Service of the

Ben Taub General Hospital, and the Audiology Research Laboratory of the Division of Audiology and Speech Pathology, Baylor College of Medicine.

At the Methodist Hospital (TMH) a Madsen Z072 electroacoustic impedance bridge was used to collect data on 722 consecutive patients with either normal hearing or sensorineural hearing loss. Patients ranged in age from three to 91 years. Forty-five percent were female.

At the Ben Taub General Hospital (BTGH) a second Madsen Z072 bridge was used to test 321 patients ranging in age from three to 83 years. Fifty-seven percent were female.

At the Baylor Auditory Research Laboratory (BARL) a specially constructed electroacoustic bridge, utilizing computer-averaging techniques, was used to gather data on 113 patients ranging from six to 79 years of age. Fifty-one percent were female. At this location additional data on low-pass and high-pass filtered noise reflex thresholds were also obtained.

At the two hospital locations reflex thresholds for broad-band white noise (BBN) and for pure tones of 500, 1000, and 2000 Hz were obtained as part of the routine audiologic assessment of each patient. In all cases the reflex threshold was defined as the lowest sound level producing an observable deflection of the balance meter of the impedance bridge. At TMH, testers usually used a sensitivity setting of 3 to define reflex threshold. At BTGH, however, testers usually used the 1 setting of the sensitivity control. As subsequent sections will demonstrate, this difference had no observable effect on predictive accuracy.

At BARL, the reflex response was signal-averaged (Nicolet, 1010) and read out on a strip chart recorder (Hewlett-Packard, 322 A). Responses to eight successive acoustic signals were averaged. The signal-averaging procedure produced slight improvement in absolute reflex threshold levels, but did not effect an observable change in predictive accuracy.

To attempt prediction of slope of loss, additional reflex thresholds for both low-pass and high-pass filtered noise were gathered on the 113 patients tested at BARL. The output from a noise generator (Grason-Stadler, 1285) was either low-pass or high-pass filtered at 2600 Hz by an active network filter (Krohn-Hite, 3500 R) with a 24 dB per octave slope characteristic.

A total of 1156 patients, ranging in age from three to 91 years, was tested at the three locations.

PREDICTIVE CRITERIA

Sensitivity Loss

We did not attempt to predict sensitivity loss in decibels, for two reasons. First, as already noted by Niemeyer and Sesterhenn, such predictions are affected by the slope of the audiometric contour. Second, in the area of predicting the hearing status of babies, where one can visualize maximum usefulness for this technique, such accuracy is unnecessary. It is usually sufficient to place the child into one of four general sensitivity categories: grossly normal, mild-moderate loss, severe loss, or profound loss. If some estimate of the slope of the audiometric configuration can also be made, the basic extent of the child's hearing status has usually been adequately defined until an accurate behavioral audiogram can be obtained. We feel that any procedure capable of making this kind of prediction of degree and slope of sensorineural hearing loss in babies, with acceptable false-positive and false-negative rates, is one giant step forward from our present position.

Accordingly, in the present study we attempted to predict only four degrees of sensitivity loss. The basis for this prediction was a combination of (1) differences between reflex thresholds for pure tones and noise and (2) the absolute SPL of the reflex threshold for noise.

We defined a difference score, D, as the average of three separate differences as follows:

Let a = reflex threshold SPL for 500 Hz
b = reflex threshold SPL for 1000 Hz
c = reflex threshold SPL for 2000 Hz
$d = a + b + c\,/\,3$
e = lowest reflex threshold SPL among a, b, and c
f = reflex threshold SPL for BBN
$\ell = d - f$ (PTA-BBN)
$m = a - f$ (500-BBN)
$n = e - f$ (PT-BBN)

$$D = \frac{\ell + m + n}{3}$$

The value D is, in effect, the average difference between the reflex threshold for noise and three different weightings of the reflex thresholds for pure tones in the 500-2000 Hz range. In the first (ℓ) the three reflexes are weighted equally. In the second (m) 500 Hz is emphasized, and in the third (n) the best of the three (lowest reflex threshold SPL) is highlighted.

In general, we predicted normal hearing if D exceeded 20 dB, a mild-to-moderate loss if D fell between 10 and 19 dB, and a severe loss if D was less than 10 dB. The exact prediction was modified, however, by the absolute level of the reflex threshold for BBN. If the BBN SPL was 80 dB or less, it offset a D in the 15–19 range. Similarly if BBN SPL was 89 dB or less, it offset a D below 10 dB. The actual combinations of predictive criteria are shown in Table 1. The basic concepts are that decreasing D means increasing loss and increasing BBN SPL means increasing loss. The particular way in which we have combined them is entirely pragmatic, based on our own accumulating clinical experience. To evaluate the predictive accuracy of this scheme, the patients audiograms were categorized according to the criteria outlined in Table 2.

In the 113 patients tested at BARL, slope of loss was predicted from the

TABLE 1. Criteria for prediction of sensitivity loss (all locations).

D	*If* BBN SPL	Prediction
20 or larger	anywhere	normal
15-19	80 dB or less	normal
15-19	81 dB or more	mild-moderate
10-14	anywhere	mild-moderate
less than 10	89 dB or less	mild-moderate
less than 10	90 dB or more	severe
reflexes not observed		profound

TABLE 2. Criteria for categorizing audiograms according to PTA (all locations).

Category	Criteria
Normal	PTA less than 20 dB HL
Mild-Moderate	PTA 20 to 49 dB HL inclusive
Severe	PTA 50 to 84 dB HL inclusive
Profound	PTA 85 dB HL or more

difference between reflex thresholds for low-pass filtered (LPFN) and high-pass filtered (HPFN) noise. The filter cut-off frequency of 2600 Hz had been originally selected on the basis that it produced approximately equal threshold levels for high- and low-pass bands in normal listeners. Accordingly, audiometric contour was predicted on the basis of the difference LPFN − HPFN. If this difference was zero or positive, a flat configuration was predicted. If the difference was in the range from −1 to −5 inclusive, a gradual slope was predicted, and if the difference exceeded −5, a steep slope was predicted. In comparing prediction with actual audiometric slope the difference between auditory thresholds at 1 k Hz and 4 k Hz was the criterion. If this difference was less than 5 dB, the audiometric contour was considered flat. Differences in the region from 6 to 40 dB were considered "gradual" slopes, and differences greater than 40 dB were categorized as "steep" slopes.

RESULTS

Results are presented in the form of matrices comparing predictions with actual audiometric findings. At TMH and BTGH only severity of loss could be predicted. Table 3 compares predictions and actual audiograms in the 722 patients tested at TMH. Prediction is encouragingly good. Of the 287 ears predicted to have normal sensitivity, for example, 228 had normal audiograms, 55 had mild-moderate audiometric configurations, and only four (0.6% of the total group) actually had severe losses. Results were least satisfactory when severe loss was predicted. Of the 96 ears in this category, only 31 actually had

TABLE 3. Prediction of severity of loss from TMH data ($N = 722$).

Actual	Normal	Predicted Mild-Moderate	Severe	Profound
Normal	228	79	10	0
Mild-Moderate	55	74	19	0
Severe	4	23	31	1
Profound	0	1	1	74
Total	287	264	96	75

severe losses. Thirty-eight fell into the mild-moderate category, and 26 actually had reasonably normal hearing. Results were best when profound loss was predicted. Of the 75 ears in this category, 74 were, in fact, profound losses, and one ear had a severe audiometric level.

Table 4 shows analogous results for the 321 ears tested at BTGH. Findings

TABLE 4. Prediction of severity of loss from BTGH data ($N = 321$).

Actual	Normal	Predicted Mild-Moderate	Severe	Profound
Normal	121	78	9	0
Mild-Moderate	20	50	13	0
Severe	2	12	14	0
Profound	0	1	1	0
Total	143	141	37	0

are quite similar. Of the 143 ears predicted to have normal sensitivity, 121 had reasonably normal audiograms, 20 had mild-moderate audiograms, and only two (0.6% of the total group) actually had severe losses. Of the 37 ears predicted to be in the severe category, only 14 actually were severe. Thirteen were mild-moderate, and nine were normal.

In view of the good agreement between results at the two hospital locations, the data were pooled to form a total group of 1043 ears. Results for the pooled group are shown in Table 5. Prediction is best in the case of either normal

TABLE 5. Prediction of severity of loss from pooled TMH and BTGH data ($N = 1043$).

Actual	Normal	Predicted Mild-Moderate	Severe	Profound
Normal	349	206	35	0
Mild-Moderate	75	162	51	0
Severe	6	36	46	1
Profound	0	1	1	74
Total	430	405	133	75

hearing or profound loss, least successful when mild-moderate or severe loss was predicted.

Table 6 summarizes the distribution of the predictive errors reflected in Table 5. Errors were categorized into three types. If prediction and actual result agreed perfectly there was no error. If prediction and actual result diverged by only one scale position (for example, prediction normal but actual result mild-moderate, or prediction severe but result mild-moderate) then the error was considered "moderate." If prediction and actual result diverged by two or more scale positions (for example, prediction severe but actual result normal) then the error was considered "serious." Table 6 shows that, in the 1043 ears of Table 5, prediction was perfect in 60% of cases. The errors were moderate in 36% of ears and serious in only 4%. Figure 2 shows the distribution of these errors in graphic form.

Table 7 shows the prediction of severity of loss for the 113 ears tested by the computer-averaging technique at BARL. Again results are best when normal hearing is predicted and least satisfactory when severe loss is the prediction.

TABLE 6. Distribution of predictive errors; prediction of severity of loss from clinical data (N = 1043).

Type of Error	Number of Ears	Percentage
None	631	60
Moderate	369	36
Serious	42	4

TABLE 7. Prediction of severity of loss (PTA) from BARL data (N = 113).

Actual	Normal	Predicted Mild-Moderate	Severe
Normal	34	39	3
Mild to Moderate	0	16	12
Severe	0	1	8
Total	34	56	23

TABLE 8. Prediction of slope of loss (4K − 1K) from BARL data (N = 113).

Actual	Flat	Predicted Gradual	Steep
Flat	36	5	4
Gradual	23	13	9
Steep	1	3	19
Total	60	21	32

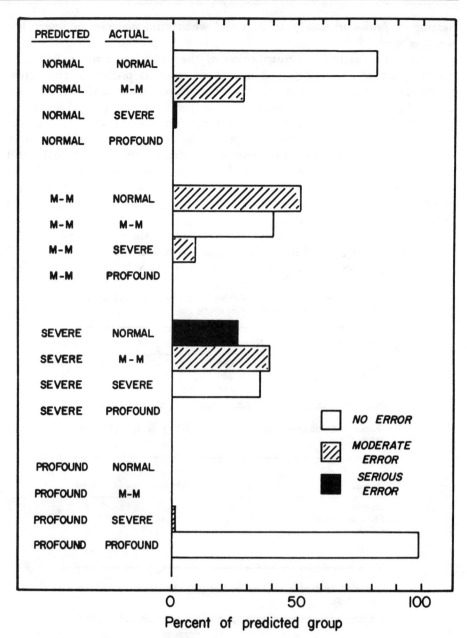

Figure 2. Distribution of predictive errors according to category of prediction (N = 1043).

In general, results are quite similar to data obtained at the two hospital locations.

Table 8 shows the prediction of slopes of audiometric configuration from the BARL data. Interestingly, predictive accuracy is about the same (60% correct) whether the prediction of configuration is flat, gradual, or steep.

When the BARL predictions of both severity and slope are combined, the result is an expected slight improvement in the fine detail of the prediction. Results of the joint prediction are summarized in Table 9.

TABLE 9. Prediction of both severity (PTA) and slope (4K $-$ 1K) of loss from BARL data ($N = 113$).

Actual	Normal	Normal (Sloping)	Mild to Moderate	Mild to Moderate (Sloping)	Severe	Severe (Sloping)
Normal	26	3	12	4	0	1
Normal (Sloping)	2	3	8	15	0	2
Mild to Moderate	0	0	8	5	1	1
Mild to Moderate (Sloping)	0	0	0	3	0	10
Severe	0	0	1	0	4	3
Severe (Sloping)	0	0	0	0	0	1

DISCUSSION

We think that the predictive accuracy of this technique is amazingly good. Serious errors (that is, divergence of two or more categories between prediction and result) occurred in only 4% of our series. Further analysis of the 41 ears in this group (see Table 5) shows that 35 were cases in which the prediction was "severe" and the actual result was "normal." In only six ears (0.6% of the total group of 1043) was the prediction normal in the case of actual severe loss. This latter error is the most serious that the audiologist can make in the evaluation of young children. It is, indeed, unfortunate when a child who was thought to have a severe hearing loss turns out to have normal hearing, but an error of far more serious consequence occurs when a child with a severe loss is called normal. In the former case, subsequent recognition of the error can usually undo most of the harm done by the erroneous fitting of an aid, mislabeling, parental trauma, and similar mistakes. In the latter case, however, the error can have much more serious and permanent consequences. Failure to detect a severe loss can result, at the very least, in irreversible delay in the acquisition of fundamental language skills and consequent educational retardation. It is encouraging, therefore, that this kind of predictive error is relatively unlikely.

We have the feeling that, in the case of very young children, predictive accuracy may be even better than we have demonstrated in this series of adults. Variables such as advancing age, collapsing ear canals, variation in the magnitude of various ear canal dimensions, and very high-frequency sensori-neural losses seem to introduce a variability in adult data that does not seem as prominent in small children. To date we have applied the technique to babies as young as three weeks of age. We are impressed with the agreement between reflex results and behavioral indices of hearing status, but long-term validation data are, of course, still lacking.

There can be no doubt that this technique shares with its behavioral and bioelectric cousins a certain likelihood of being wrong. We have found it most useful, therefore, when employed in conjunction with some other independent assessment of the child's hearing status. We are impressed with how often the combination of, for example, behavioral observation and reflex data leads to a clear-cut and consistent picture not evident from a unitary approach to testing.

The technique is especially useful to us in confirming the presence of normal hearing in babies who, because of high risk or some other factor, have raised considerable apprehension in the mother. When a normal configuration of results emerges from the reflex threshold analysis, we can assure the parent, with considerable confidence, that a significant hearing loss need not be feared. The fact that this can be done with a child of virtually any age, with or without sedation, in 5–10 minutes with a minimum of difficulty, recommends the technique highly to those clinicians who are concerned with the accurate assessment of babies and small children.

Obviously, the technique can be expected to work only if both middle ears are normal. The best evidence for this is a normal tympanogram in each ear. If there is any abnormality in either tympanogram, then the absence of reflexes becomes ambiguous. At this point, the examiner can only refer the child for medical evaluation of the possible middle ear condition, and no prediction of either severity or slope should be attempted. It is certainly true that the combination of normal-shaped tympanograms and absent reflexes can occur as a result of ossicular chain fixation. This is not an extraordinarily common condition in young children, but the possibility must be recognized as a potential source of error in predicting severity of loss. Again, however, the error is less serious than it might at first seem, since congenital ossicular fixation is usually accompanied by substantial, if not profound, sensitivity loss. The erroneous prediction of profound loss would have the positive value of alerting all concerned parties to the need for an accurate audiogram at the earliest possible time.

Another factor limiting the generality of the test is the possibility that brain injury may affect the central reflex arc. In a small number of children with strong histories suggesting brain injury at birth we have failed to demonstrate an acoustic reflex in spite of apparently normal hearing. This is, of course, a problem common to behavioral and electrophysiologic approaches as well. In the case of the acoustic reflex, however, it may be possible to overcome the central problem, at least in some cases, by ipsilateral rather than contralateral elicitation of the reflex.

To us, the most distressing aspect of this technique, from the point of view of its widespread clinical application, has been the problem of physical calibration of the intensities of the various reflex-eliciting signals. We have found that slight errors in calibration accuracy of the pure tone, attenuator non-linearities, differences in the way various sound-level meters read the SPL of broad-band noise, and differences in earphone frequency response can introduce individually slight but cumulatively large errors that seriously compromise the value of physical calibration. As a result, we urgently recommend that anyone attempting to use this technique clinically should disregard the physical calibration of his apparatus and perform a "physiologic" calibration. This can be easily accomplished by measuring reflex thresholds for the various pure tones and noise signals on 10 young normals (10–30 years) and averaging the results. To predict severity of loss, subtract the average reflex threshold for broad-band noise from the average reflex threshold for the three pure tones of 500, 1000, and 2000 Hz. This is the norm for your equipment. If you want to relate your findings to the results in the present paper you have only to subtract your norm from our norm (25 dB) to arrive at a suitable correction factor. If this correction factor is applied to your data you can then interpret your results according to our predictive criteria. For example, if your average threshold for noise is 80 dB and your average threshold for tone is 95 dB, then your norm is $95 - 80 = 15$ dB. If you subtract your norm (15) from our norm (25) the difference is 10. If this correction factor is added to your findings on a particular patient you can interpret the results according to the predictive criteria shown in our Table 1. For example, if the patient's result is a noise-tone difference of 15, adding your correction factor of 10 gives you a corrected difference of $15 + 10 = 25$. According to our Table 1 this would result in a prediction of normal hearing. You must still take into account the absolute level of the noise in the prediction, but for this purpose minor calibration errors are not a serious problem. To predict slope, a similar physiologic calibration should be carried out on the low- and high-pass noise bands. Note also that if the physiologic approach is taken the actual scale on which the physical calibration is carried out (that is, SPL vs HTL) is irrelevant. It is necessary only to determine what is the normal difference on your apparatus, to compare this difference with our difference (25), and subsequently to apply the proper correction to your data. The broad-band noise, however, should be calibrated in SPL for maximum ease of application of the absolute level subcriterion.

Our own experience with various forms of the instrumentation necessary to carry out these measures leads us to the firm belief that much needless confusion and disagreement among future investigators will be avoided if physiologic calibration is used in preference to physical calibration.

In summary, we have demonstrated, in 1156 ears with either normal hearing or sensorineural hearing loss, that gross audiometric level and configuration can be predicted, with reasonable success, from a consideration of reflex thresholds for pure tones, broad-band noise, and appropriately filtered noise. Regrettably, this necessarily colorless presentation of the experimental data fails to convey the mounting sense of excitement felt by each one of us as the results took shape and we began to discern the implications of these findings for the evaluation of babies and young children. We were able to confirm, in addition to their experimental findings, the impressive contribution of Niemeyer and Sesterhenn to pediatric audiology.

ACKNOWLEDGMENT

This investigation was supported by Public Health Service Program Project grant NS 10940 from the National Institute of Neurological Diseases and Stroke. Portions of this paper were presented at the Second International Symposium on Impedance Measurement, Houston, Texas, September 14, 1973. The authors are affiliated with the Division of Audiology and Speech Pathology, Department of Otorhinolaryngology and Communicative Sciences, at the Baylor College of Medicine. Philip A. Burney is also affiliated with Ben Taub General Hospital and Betsy Ann Crump with the Methodist Hospital. Requests for reprints should be addressed to James Jerger, Department of Otorhinolaryngology and Communicative Sciences, Baylor College of Medicine, Houston, Texas 77025.

REFERENCES

DEUTSCH, L., The threshold of the stapedius reflex for pure tone and noise stimuli. *Acta Otolaryng.*, 74, 248-251 (1972).

FLOTTORP, G., DJUPESLAND, G., and WINTHER, F., The acoustic stapedius reflex in relation to critical bandwidth. *J. acoust. Soc. Amer.*, 49, 457-461 (1971).

NIEMEYER, W., and SESTERHENN, G., Calculating the hearing threshold from the stapedius reflex threshold for different sound stimuli. Paper presented at the 11th International Congress of Audiology, Budapest, Hungary (1972).

Received October 22, 1973.
Accepted October 24, 1973.

Latency of the Acoustic Reflex in Eighth-Nerve Tumor

James Jerger, PhD, Deborah Hayes, PhD

● We evaluated acoustic reflex morphologic features in four subjects with confirmed, unilateral acoustic neuroma. All four subjects showed marked reduction in absolute reflex amplitude and alteration in the reflex amplitude-intensity function in the ear with eighth-nerve disorder. The early, fast-rising component of the normal reflex was also typically absent in the ears with tumor. Interaural latency comparisons were made in three ways. At equal reflex sensation levels and equal reflex sound pressure levels, latency was substantially delayed in the ear with the eighth-nerve disorder. At equivalent reflex amplitudes, however, latency was equivalent in normal ears and ears with eighth-nerve disorder. Results suggest that delayed onset of the acoustic reflex in subjects with eighth-nerve disorder may reflect amplitude and wave-form morphologic effects rather than a latency prolongation per se.

(*Arch Otolaryngol* 1983;109:1-5)

Recently, several investigators have suggested that latency of the acoustic reflex (AR) is a sensitive indicator of eighth-nerve disorder. Specifically, Clemis and Sarno[1,2] and Mangham et al[3] evaluated latency of

Accepted for publication July 21, 1982.

From the Department of Otorhinolaryngology and Communicative Sciences, Division of Audiology and Speech Pathology, Baylor College of Medicine, Houston.

Portions of this study were presented at the First International Workshop "Otology Today," Riva del Garda, Italy, April 22, 1982.

Reprint requests to Department of Otorhinolaryngology and Communicative Sciences, Division of Audiology and Speech Pathology, Baylor College of Medicine, Houston, TX 77030 (Dr Jerger).

the AR in subjects with eighth-nerve tumors. They reported that onset of the AR in the ear with the eighth-nerve disorder was significantly delayed relative to the contralateral ear. In patients with suspected eighth-nerve disorder, but normal roentgenographic studies, however, significant delay was not observed. Furthermore, examination of patients with well-documented unilateral cochlear disorder failed to demonstrate significant difference in AR latency between the ears with cochlear disorder and normal-hearing ears. Based on these results, both Clemis and Sarno and Mangham et al encourage the use of AR latency as a sensitive and specific indicator of eighth-nerve disorder.

Measurement of latency of the AR is complicated, however, by three factors. First, latency is strongly related to intensity of the reflex-eliciting signal.[4] In the case of unilateral hearing loss, a persistent issue is what shall be the basis for interear comparisons. Should the two ears be compared at equivalent physical intensities (equal sound pressure levels [SPLs]), at equivalent sensation levels (equal SLs), or at levels yielding equivalent reflex amplitudes? To our knowledge, there are no systematic data comparing these three potential bases of interear comparison with respect to the AR.

Second, latency is strongly related to absolute reflex amplitude. A principal effect of eighth-nerve disorder is to reduce AR amplitude.[3] In this circumstance, evaluation of interaural latencies is complicated by reduction in absolute AR amplitude and alteration of the amplitude-intensity function in the affected ear.

A third complicating factor is temporal distortion of the reflex wave form measured with commercial acoustic immittance devices.[5-7] These devices typically employ band-pass filtering to reduce background noise inherent in measurement of acoustic immittance. In most cases, filtering distorts the temporal characteristics of reflex activity. Furthermore, this filtering artifact interacts with differences in the wave form of the AR from the two ears.

In this study, we report results of an investigation in which we evaluated interaural latency differences of the AR in four patients with surgically confirmed acoustic neuromas. In all subjects, we attempted to control for differences in reflex amplitude between the normal and affected ears, and to minimize the problem of temporal distortion of reflex characteristics.

METHOD
Instrumentation

Acoustic reflex measurements were carried out on a specially designed laboratory apparatus. Figure 1 shows a simplified block diagram of the measurement system. An acoustic probe assembly is sealed into each of the subject's two ear canals. Timing circuits key two electronic switches such that a reflex-eliciting signal is alternated between the two ears. The electrical output of each probe assembly is routed through a lock-in amplifier (Princeton Applied Research, 129A) to the analog-

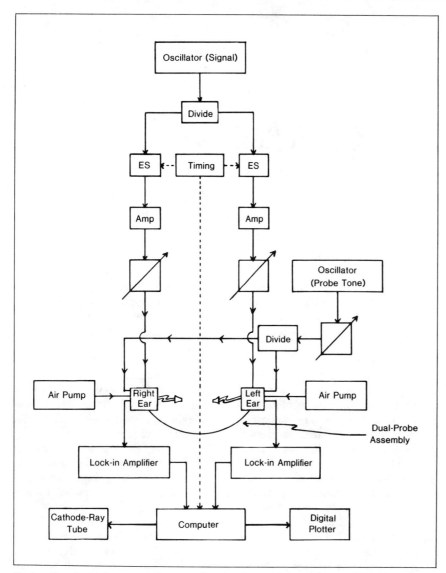

Fig 1.—Experimental apparatus for measuring signal-averaged acoustics reflex to both crossed and uncrossed stimulation. ES indicates electronic switch; Amp, amplifier.

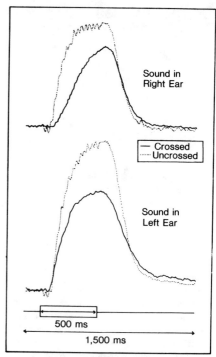

Fig 2.—Illustrative recordings of four acoustic reflex wave forms recorded by experimental apparatus in a normal subject. Stimulus frequency, 2,000 Hz; intensity, 100-dB sound pressure level.

to-digital converter of a laboratory minicomputer (Digital Equipment Corp, Lab 8E). The lock-in amplifiers are adjusted to yield a 10-ms time constant. The computer is programmed to assign inputs to one of four memory locations, to perform a signal-averaging operation on all four inputs, and to recall the four averaged wave forms to a cathode-ray tube screen and an XY plotter (Houston Instruments, HI-PLOT) on the same time base. This arrangement of alternating inputs to the dual-probe assembly, and storage in four memory locations, permits the recording of all of the following four possible reflexes: right uncrossed, right-to-left crossed, left-to-right crossed, and left uncrossed.

For this investigation, the probe tone was a 400-Hz sinusoid adjusted to 85-dB

SPL in a 2.0-mL hard-walled cavity.

Frequency of the reflex-eliciting signal varied depending on preservation of reflex activity in the affected ear of each subject. Two subjects were tested using a 500-Hz, reflex-eliciting signal, one with an 800-Hz signal and one with a 2,000-Hz signal. Probe tone interaction with the 500-Hz, reflex-eliciting signal precluded measurement of the uncrossed AR in those experimental subjects (N = 2).

Duration of the reflex-eliciting signal was 500 ms; rise-fall time was 5 ms. At each intensity tested, responses to eight signals presented to each ear were averaged to obtain a single reflex wave form for each of the four possible reflex conditions (right uncrossed, right crossed, left crossed, and left uncrossed). A pre-

stimulus interval of 150 ms was averaged to provide a prestimulus baseline. Total signal averaged epoch was 1,500 ms.

For each subject, reflex activity was measured in 5- or 10-dB steps from reflex threshold (defined as the lowest intensity that yielded an identifiable deviation from prestimulus baseline) to either 110- or 115-dB SPL. Amplitude of each reflex at each intensity was quantified as the decibel change in SPL of the probe tone (ie, the difference, in decibels, between the SPL of the probe tone at baseline immittance, and the SPL of the probe tone at the point of maximum immittance change due to stapedius muscle contraction).

Latency of the AR was measured for crossed reflexes only. This measure was defined as latency from signal onset to the first deviation of the averaged response from prestimulus baseline, irrespective of the direction of the change in acoustic immittance (either increase or decrease in acoustic immittance).

Subjects

Four patients, three men and one woman, served as experimental subjects. Ages ranged from 30 to 48 years. All subjects had surgically confirmed, unilateral acoustic neuromas.

Hearing level in the affected ear ranged

from normal (pure-tone average [PTA] of 500, 1,000, and 2,000 Hz, of 4-dB hearing level [HL]) to severely impaired (PTA, 56-dB HL). In two of the four patients, auditory brain-stem response (ABR) was positive for eighth-nerve site (prolonged absolute latency of wave V and prolonged interwave intervals). In the other two patients, ABR audiometry was ambiguous for site of disorder due to severity of the peripheral hearing loss.[8,9]

Representative AR

Figure 2 shows a typical wave form of the four signal-averaged reflexes obtained from a normal subject. Figure 2 demonstrates two aspects of normal AR amplitude characteristics. First, as noted by previous investigators,[10,11] amplitude of the uncrossed AR is slightly greater than amplitude of the companion crossed AR in each ear. Second, amplitude of the reflex pairs is relatively symmetric. There is no remarkable asymmetry of reflex amplitude between the right and left ears.

The figure also shows the presence of inevitable artifact in the uncrossed recording condition during stimulus presentation, a problem limiting our ability to measure latency in the uncrossed condition. Note, however, that maximum reflex amplitude can be measured quite unambiguously, even in the uncrossed condition, after cessation of the reflex-eliciting signal. Because of confounding acoustic artifact during uncrossed signal presentations, reflex amplitude in both uncrossed and crossed recording conditions was defined as the highest point in the reflex trace immediately following offset of the reflex-eliciting signal.

The reflexes shown in Fig 2 also demonstrate that normal reflex morphologic features are characterized by two phases of activity, a rapid initial onset response followed by a relatively more gradual rise in amplitude. We shall see later that, in patients with eighth-nerve tumor, this normal, dual-phase response may be substantially altered.

RESULTS
Amplitude-Intensity Functions

Amplitude-intensity functions for the four experimental subjects are shown in Fig 3. All four functions show the expected effect of eighth-nerve disorder on reflex amplitude. When the eliciting signal is presented to the ear with eighth-nerve disorder, amplitude is substantially reduced relative to amplitude on the normal ear. Note that this reduction in reflex amplitude appears on both the crossed

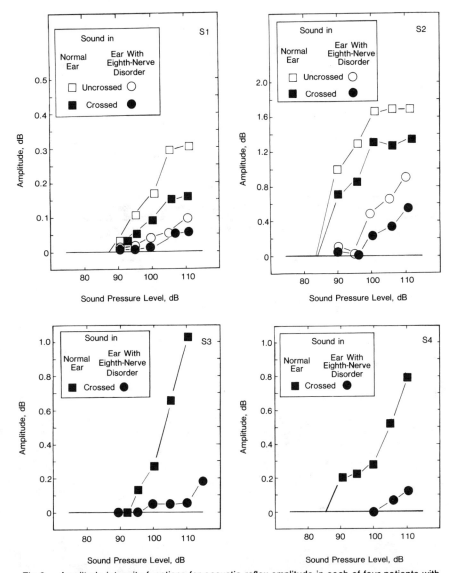

Fig 3.—Amplitude-intensity functions for acoustic reflex amplitude in each of four patients with acoustic tumor. Note substantial changes in reflex amplitude in spite of relatively minimal changes in reflex threshold. Stimulus frequencies were as follows: S1, 800 Hz; S2, 2,000 Hz; S3, 500 Hz; and S4, 500 Hz.

and uncrossed recording conditions with sound presented to the ear with eighth-nerve disorder, indicating an afferent effect.[12,13] In three of the four cases (S1, S3, and S4), maximum amplitude of the reflex in the ear with eighth-nerve disorder reached less than 25% of the maximum reflex amplitude in the normal ear. In the fourth case (S2), maximum reflex amplitude in the ear with eighth-nerve disorder reached approximately 55% of the maximum reflex amplitude demonstrated on the normal ear.

This amplitude effect appears to be independent of reflex threshold. Note

that, in cases S1, S2, and S3, reflex thresholds in the two ears were nearly equivalent (± 5 dB). However, slopes of the amplitude-intensity function in the two ears (eighth-nerve disorder v normal) were markedly different. Reduction in the slope of the amplitude-intensity functions characterized results from all four subjects, and represents, in our experience, a principal effect of eighth-nerve disorder on the AR.

Reflex Latency

Table 1 summarizes results of comparison of reflex latency between the ears with eighth-nerve disorder and

Subject	Ear	Equal SL (+10 dB)	Equal SPL (100 dB)	Equivalent Reflex Amplitudes
S1	Eighth-nerve tumor	150	60	90
	Normal	45	30	75
S2	Eighth-nerve tumor	280	120	120
	Normal	130	40	130
S3	Eighth-nerve tumor	180	405	220
	Normal	75	45	205
S4	Eighth-nerve tumor	150	150	150
	Normal	60	45	130

Table 1.—Comparison of Latency of Acoustic Reflex Between Normal Ear and Ear With Tumor*

*Four subjects with surgically confirmed, unilateral acoustic neuroma. Comparison was made in three ways: (1) at equal sensation levels (SL) (+10-dB SL), (2) at equal physical intensities (100-dB sound pressure level [SPL]), and (3) at equivalent reflex amplitudes. Values are shown in milliseconds.

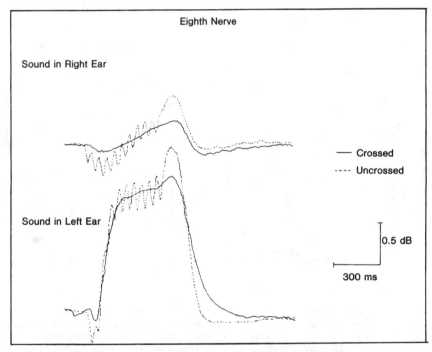

Fig 4.—Acoustic reflex wave forms for patient S2. Note marked alteration in wave-form morphologic features for reflexes elicited with sound in right ear. Maximum amplitude is decreased, early fast component of reflex wave form is absent, but latency is not substantially altered. Stimulus frequency, 2,000 Hz intensity, 100-dB sound pressure level.

normal ears for each of the four experimental subjects. Comparisons were made in the following three different ways: (1) at equal reflex SLs (+10 dB), (2) at equal reflex SPLs (110 dB), and (3) at equal reflex amplitudes. In all cases, reflex latency was measured from stimulus onset to the first deviation in acoustic immittance from prestimulus baseline, irrespective of the direction of acoustic immittance change.

Table 1 shows that interaural differences in latency vary depending on whether the latency measurement is made at equal reflex SLs, equal signal SPLs, or equal reflex amplitudes. Note that, for both equal reflex SLs and equal signal SPLs, latency of the reflex with sound presented to the ear with eighth-nerve disorder is substantially prolonged relative to latency with sound presented to the normal ear. However, at equal reflex amplitudes, latency of the reflex with sound presented to both the ears with eighth-nerve disorder and normal ears is similar. In patient S1, for example, at equal reflex SLs, latency of the AR with sound presented to the ear with eighth-nerve disorder is approximately three times longer than latency with sound presented to the normal ear (150 v 45 ms). At equal signal SPLs for this same patient, latency in the ear with eighth-nerve disorder is twice as long as latency in the normal ear (60 v 30 ms). At equal reflex amplitudes, however, difference in latency between the ears with eighth-nerve disorder and normal ears is only 15 ms (90 v 75 ms). This pattern is seen for all four patients. Significant differences in latency can emerge simply from the selection of how to equate the two ears.

Reflex Wave Form

The selection of a level at which to measure reflex latency is further complicated by possible differences in reflex wave forms between the two ears. Figure 4 illustrates this point. The figure shows two pairs of reflexes (right crossed and uncrossed and left crossed and uncrossed) from patient S2. The reflexes represent averaged activity to eight signal presentations at 110-dB SPL in each ear. The wave forms of the AR differ substantially between the ear with eighth-nerve disorder (right) and the normal ear (left). With sound presented to the ear with eighth-nerve disorder, the reflex shows only slow increase in acoustic immittance. In contrast, with sound presented to the normal ear, the reflex shows an initial rapid rise followed by a more gradual increase to maximum reflex amplitude. This difference in AR wave-form characteristics between the two ears could result in an artifactual difference in reflex latency. If, for example, we measured latency from stimulus onset to some criterion increase in acoustic immittance, then latency of the two reflexes displayed in Fig 4 would be quite different. Even if we attempted to control for differences in absolute AR amplitude by measurement to some criterial percentage increase in acoustic immittance, we would still measure an artifactually delayed onset of the right AR. Essentially, slope of the rising phase of the reflex would determine the measured value.

Sound Pressure Level, dB	Latency Criterion			
	First Deviation From Baseline		First Positive Deviation From Baseline	
	Experimental	Commercial	Experimental	Commercial
80	52	72	200	204
90	24	56	124	168
100	24	56	84	112
110	16	48	64	112

Table 2.—Comparison of Latency of Acoustic Reflex*

*Measured from records obtained from the present experimental apparatus and from a commercial acoustic immittance bridge. Latencies are expressed in milliseconds. Results are for a single normal subject.

COMMENT

These results illustrate the complexity of interpretation of reflex latency. It appears that in ears with eighth-nerve dysfunction, the AR may be modified in two ways; first, by a reduction in maximum amplitude of the AR, and, second, by alteration of reflex wave-form morphologic features. In the second effect, the entire reflex morphologic features may be determined by the relatively slowly rising, late phase of the AR.

What has been interpreted as a prolonged latency of the AR may very well be an artifact of the dynamic interaction between these two changes in reflex characteristics and the problems of signal-to-noise resolution, and temporal fidelity, of the instrumentation used to record reflex activity.

To highlight the importance of this concept, we compared AR latency measured by our experimental apparatus with AR latency measured via a commercially available immittance device (Madsen, ZO 72) in a single normal subject. Output of the commercial instrument was routed through a strip chart recorder (Hew-lett Packard, 322) with a paper speed of 120 mm/s. For both experimental and commercial apparatus, the right-to-left crossed AR was elicited by a 500-ms (5-ms rise-fall), 2,000-Hz pure tone presented at 80-, 90-, 100-, and 110-dB SPL (TDH 49 earphone; MX 41 AR cushion). Table 2 summarizes comparison of latency measured from the strip chart recording of the commercial bridge and from the XY plot of the experimental apparatus. This table shows AR latency calculated at the four SPLs by two different criteria: (1) from stimulus onset to first deviation from baseline, irrespective of direction of change in acoustic immittance, and (2) from stimulus onset to first positive change from baseline (increase in acoustic immittance). Note that the measurements differ by more than 40 ms in some conditions between the two reflex-measuring instruments. In all cases, latencies measured from the commercial bridge were substantially longer than latencies measured from the experimental apparatus. The fact that the measured results are so discrepant emphasizes the fact that latency of the AR is greatly influenced by the amplitude resolution and the temporal distortion of the measurement system.

We can see little evidence in our data to support the concept that there is any change in actual onset of reflex activity in ears with acoustic neuroma. There are, however, distinct changes in reflex morphologic features that can be easily measured and can provide useful diagnostic distinctions.

In spite of these observations, it could be argued, on a purely pragmatic level, that whatever the basis for the effect, latency, as measured on present commercial bridges, does indeed differentiate unilateral eighth-nerve from unilateral cochlear disorder. If the test works, why not use it? To this argument we would reply that if the observed latency differences between normal ears and ears with eighth-nerve disorder do indeed reflect a dynamic interaction between reflex wave-form morphologic features and the amplitude and temporal resolution characteristics of the recording instrumentation, then the test will work less well as instrumentation becomes more sophisticated and, ultimately, will fail altogether. We suggest that it may be more advantageous to measure details of suprathreshold amplitude and wave-form characteristics, and to abandon the difficult concept of latency of the AR.

This study was supported in part by Public Health Service research grant NS-10940 from the National Institute of Neurological and Communicative Diseases and Stroke.

Larry Mauldin provided the instrumentation design, Janet Taff, MA, assisted in data collection, and William Keith, PhD, provided advice and counsel.

References

1. Clemis J, Sarno C: The acoustic reflex latency test: Clinical application. *Laryngoscope* 1980;90:601-611.

2. Clemis J, Sarno C: Acoustic reflex latency test in the evaluation of nontumor patients with abnormal brainstem latencies. *Ann Otol Rhinol Laryngol* 1980;89:296-302.

3. Mangham C, Lindeman R, Dawson W: Stapedius reflex quantification in acoustic tumor patients. *Laryngoscope* 1980;90:242-250.

4. Hung I, Dallos P: Study of the acoustic reflex in human beings: I. Dynamic characteristics. *J Acoust Soc Am* 1972;52:1168-1180.

5. Sundby A, Flottorp G, Djupesland G: *Time Constants of Registrating Equipment in Middle Ear Impedance Investigation: Proceedings of the Second Nordic Meeting on Medical and Biological Engineering.* 1971, pp 207-209.

6. Ruth R, Niswander P: Acoustic reflex latency as a function of frequency and intensity of eliciting stimulus. *J Am Aud Soc* 1976;2:54-60.

7. McPherson D, Thompson D: Quantification of the threshold and latency parameters of the acoustic reflex in humans. *Acta Otolaryngol,* 1978, suppl 353, pp 1-37.

8. Hayes D: Effect of degree of hearing loss on diagnostic audiometric tests. *Am J Otol* 1980;2:91-96.

9. Josey A, Jackson C, Glasscock M: Brainstem evoked response audiometry in confirmed eighth nerve tumors. *Am J Otolaryngol* 1980;1:285-290.

10. Moller AR: Acoustic reflex in man. *J Acoust Soc Am* 1962;34:1524-1534.

11. Borg E: Acoustic middle ear reflexes: A sensory-control system. *Acta Otolaryngol,* 1972, suppl 304, pp 1-34.

12. Jerger J, Hayes D: Diagnostic applications of impedance audiometry: Middle ear disorder, sensori-neural disorder, in Jerger J, Northern J (eds): *Clinical Impedance Audiometry,* ed 2. Acton, Mass, American Electromedics, 1980, pp 109-127.

13. Jerger S: Diagnostic applications of impedance audiometry: Central auditory disorder, in Jerger J, Northern J (eds): *Clinical Impedance Audiometry,* ed 2. Acton, Mass, American Electromedics, 1980, pp 128-140.

SIGNAL-AVERAGING OF THE ACOUSTIC REFLEX: DIAGNOSTIC APPLICATIONS OF AMPLITUDE CHARACTERISTICS

Deborah Hayes, Ph.D. and James Jerger, Ph.D.

Baylor College of Medicine
Houston, Texas

ABSTRACT

We employed simultaneous measurement of the crossed and uncrossed acoustic reflex (AR) and a signal-averaging technique to evaluate supra-threshold amplitude characteristics of the AR. By evaluating AR amplitude relationships in a mathematical model based on known afferent, efferent, and central pathway effects, we are able to compare results from a variety of patients and to make meaningful diagnostic interpretations.

INTRODUCTION

Recently, we developed a technique to evaluate diagnostic significance of supra-threshold acoustic reflex (AR) amplitude characteristics. As noted by previous investigatigators, retrocochlear dysfunction may affect AR amplitude without disturbing the more traditionally evaluated threshold characteristics (Borg, 1973; 1976; Bosatra et al, 1975; Colletti, 1975). By this new approach, we are able to identify and distinguish among the effects of various auditory disorders on AR amplitude characteristics.

METHOD

Procedure

Acoustic reflex activity was recorded using a specially designed system. This system has been described previously (Jerger et al, 1978). Briefly, a reflex eliciting signal is alternated between two commercial probe transducers sealed in the subject's ears. Microphone outputs of the probe transducers are routed through independent lock-in amplifiers to the analog-to-digital input converters of a laboratory minicomputer. Responses to eight consecutive signals are computer-averaged. At the end of each test condition, the four component ARs (right uncrossed, right-to-left crossed, left-to-right crossed, and left uncrossed) are displayed on the same time base. Simultaneous elicitation of the crossed and uncrossed component from each ear permits unequivocal comparisons of uncrossed and crossed reflex characteristics; alternating signal presentation allows unambiguous comparisons of right and left ears.

Reflex activity is measured in 5 dB steps from 110 dB SPL down to apparent threshold (defined as first deviation from pre-stimulus baseline on the signal-averaged display). Amplitude of each of the four component ARs for each signal condition is then measured as dB change in probe tone relative to resting (non-reflex) probe tone level. Resting probe tone SPL is adjusted at the point of maximum immittance to 85 dB SPL in each ear independently before each test condition.

Analysis

Visual examination of signal-averaged AR activity from normal subjects and from subjects with a variety of auditory disorders revealed two important findings. First, there appear to be two general classes of AR amplitude effects, one related to interaural symmetry, and one related to crossed/uncrossed relationships. The first effect (interaural symmetry), can be further subdivided into afferent and efferent effects.

Second, we noted considerable overlap of normal and pathological ranges when the absolute amplitude measures were compared. Therefore, in order to make meaningful diagnostic comparisons, we analyzed the data in two ways. First, we defined a set of three amplitude "indexes" designed to emphasize specific aspects of interaural symmetry and the crossed/uncrossed relationship. One index emphasizes afferent (cochlear and eighth nerve) effects (Afferent Index, or AI); one index emphasizes efferent (seventh nerve and middle ear) effects (Efferent Index, or EI); the third index emphasizes central pathway (brainstem) effects (Central Pathway Index, or CPI). Second, we derived an equation for each index which, in the normal case, would yield a theoretical value of zero (0) for AI and EI, and a theoretical value of two times a constant (2k) for CPI, regardless of absolute AR amplitude. In this manner we attempted to isolate the specific effects influencing AR amplitude relationships and to control for the troublesome overlap of normal and pathological ranges of absolute amplitude measures. The formulae for calculating the three AR amplitude indexes are as follows:

Afferent Index;

$$AI = (Ru + Rc) - (Lu + Lc)$$

Efferent Index;

$$EI = (Ru - Rc) - (Lu - Lc)$$

Central Pathway Index;

$$CPI = (Ru + Lu) - (Rc + Lc)$$

where Ru = absolute amplitude of the right uncrossed AR, Rc = absolute amplitude of the right crossed AR, Lu = absolute amplitude of the left uncrossed AR, and Lc = absolute amplitude of the left crossed AR.

Since it is not altogether clear whether AR amplitude relationships should be examined at equal SPLs or equal SLs, or over a range of reflex-eliciting signal intensities, we calculated each of the three indices at three different points on the amplitude-intensifty function; at a fixed SL relative to each AR threshold (+10 dB), at a fixed SPL (100 dB), and over a range of signal intensities (AR amplitude summed at 90, 100, and 110 dB SPL).

For final data reduction we expressed the three AR indexes in normal deviates (Z scores) based on the distribution of results from a control group of 20 normal hearing, neurologically normal subjects. This reduction aids in immediate identification of "significant" effects; Z scores greater than approximately 2.0 are significant at the 5% confidence level, Z scores greater than approximately 3.0 are significant at the 1% confidence level (two-tailed test).

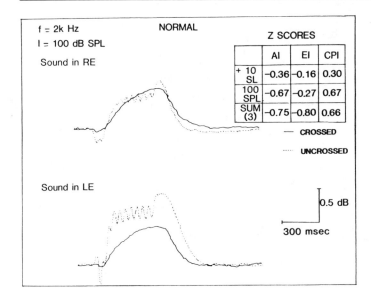

Figure 1.....Signal-averaged acoustic reflexes (AR) from a normal hearing, neurologically normal subject (f=2k Hz; I=100 dB SPL). The reflexes demonstrate two normal relationships; first, the uncrossed AR (dotted traces) is typically larger than the companion crossed AR (solid traces), and second, interaural amplitude relationships are relatively symmetrical. The three AR indexes (afferent, efferent, and central pathway), expressed in Z scores are non-significant.

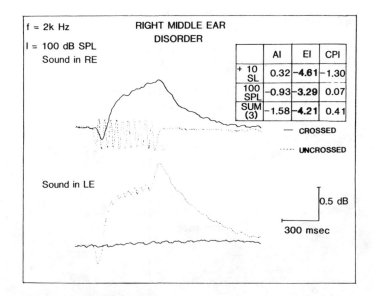

Figure 2.....Signal-averaged ARs from a patient with a right middle ear disorder (f=2k Hz; I=100 dB SPL). Both the right uncrossed and left crossed AR are absent. All three methods of calculating the efferent index (EI) are significant at the 1% level. Note, however, that significant middle ear effects do not contaminate either the afferent (AI) or central pathway (CPI) index.

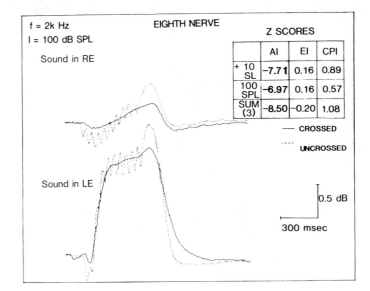

Figure 3.....Signal-averaged ARs from a patient with a right acoustic neuroma (f=2k Hz; I=100 db SPL). Although the crossed/uncrossed AR relationship is normal in both ears, there is considerable interaural amplitude asymmetry. Amplitude of the AR with sound in the affected (right) ear is significantly reduced relative to the unaffected (left) ear. The afferent index (AI) is significant.

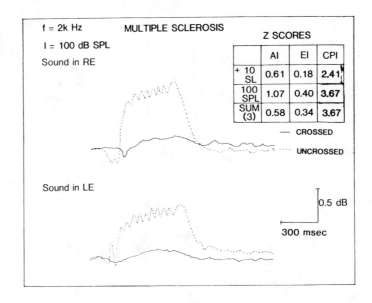

Figure 4.....Signal-averaged ARs from a patient with multiple sclerosis affecting the brainstem pathways (f=2k Hz; I=100 dB SPL). Interaural reflex amplitudes are symmetrical but the crossed/uncrossed AR relationship is abnormal. Crossed ARs are significantly reduced relative to uncrossed ARs. The central pathway index (CPI) is significant.

ILLUSTRATIVE CASES

Figures 1, 2, 3, and 4 show signal-averaged reflex activity from four representative subjects. Z scores for each index and each method of calculation are shown in the upper right corner of each figure.

Figure 1 shows results from a normal subject. Note that uncrossed AR from each ear (dotted traces) is slightly larger than the companion crossed AR (solid traces). In addition, note the relative symmetry of AR amplitude from each ear. Z scores for each of the reflex indices are not significant at either the 5% or 1% level.

Figure 2 shows results from a subject with a minor middle ear disorder on the right resulting in a mild (5 dB air-bone gap) conductive hearing loss. Not unexpectedly, both the left crossed and right uncrossed AR are absent. Note that AR index Z scores are significant for EI only; both AI and CPI Z scores fall within the normal range. The presence of a significant efferent effect does not confound either the afferent index or the central pathway index.

Figure 3 shows results from a subject with an acoustic neuroma on the right. As seen in case 1, the relationship between the uncrossed AR from each ear and its companion crossed AR is normal. In contrast to case 1, however, the relationship of reflex amplitude between the two ears is markedly asymmetrical. Amplitude of both the crossed and uncrossed AR with sound in right ear (ear with acoustic neuroma) is substantially reduced relative to amplitude in the unaffected left ear. In this case, all three methods of calculating the afferent index (AI) are significant.

Finally, figure 4 shows results from a patient with multiple sclerosis affecting the brainstem pathways. The amplitude relationship between the uncrossed and crossed AR components from each ear is quite abnormal. With sound presented to either the right or left ear, amplitude of the crossed AR is markedly reduced relative to the uncrossed companion. Interaural amplitude relationships are symmetrical, however. Not unexpectedly, all three methods of calculating the central pathway index (CPI) are significant.

SUMMARY

This technique of reflex measurement and evaluation yields important diagnostic information. Simultaneous measurement of reflex activity permits unequivocal comparisons of the crossed and uncrossed AR components; alternating signal presentation permits unambiguous comparison of right and left effects.

The index technique of evaluating AR amplitude relationships is especially promising. By applying the index equations to individual subject data, we are able to extract significant retrocochlear effects, (afferent and central pathway) without fear contamination by minor middle ear effects (see case 2). In other words, middle ear dysfuncion, while influencing absolute amplitude of the AR, does not yield a false positive retrocochlear index (AI or CPI).

We believe that diagnostic applications of the acoustic reflex can be significantly expanded by continued evaluation of important supra-threshold characteristics of reflex activity.

ACKNOWLEDGEMENT

This study was supported in part by Public Health Service Research Grants NS-10940 from the National Institute of Neurological and Communicative Disorders and Stroke. Janet Taff assisted in data collection and analysis.

REFERENCES

1. Borg, E. On the neuronal organization of the acoustic middle ear reflex. A physiological and anatomical study. Brain Res. 49:101-123, 1973.
2. Borg, E. Dynamic characteristics of the intra-aural muscle reflex. In Feldman, A., and Wilber, L. (eds) Acoustic Impedance and Admittance. The Measurement of Middle Ear Function. Williams and Wilkins, Balimore, 1976.
3. Bosatra, A., Russola, M. and Poli, P. Modification of the stapedius muscle reflex under spontaneous and experimental brain stem impairment. Acta Otolaryngol., 80: 61-66, 1975.
4. Colletti, V. Stapedius reflex abnormalities in multiple sclerosis. Audiol., 14:63-71, 1975.
5. Jerger, J., Hayes, D., Anthony, L. and Mauldin, L. Factors influencing prediction of hearing level from the acoustic reflex. Monographs in Contemporary Audiol., 1:1-20, 1978.

REPRINTED FROM ANNALS OF OTOLOGY, RHINOLOGY & LARYNGOLOGY, JANUARY-FEBRUARY 1987
Volume 96, Number 1, Part 2   Supplement 128

ELECTRICALLY ELICITED STAPEDIUS REFLEX AND PREFERRED LISTENING LEVEL IN A PATIENT WITH A COCHLEAR IMPLANT

J. F. JERGER, PhD; H. A. JENKINS, MD; R. CHMIEL, MS; T. A. OLIVER, MS

In a patient with a multichannel cochlear implant, it was possible to demonstrate stapedial reflex contraction to intracochlear electrical stimulation. Using a standard immittance measurement technique, characteristics of the electrically evoked reflex were compared to analogous characteristics of the acoustically evoked reflex. Latency-intensity functions were similar for the two modes of excitation, but reflex waveform morphology and amplitude growth functions were different. The effects of electrode position and electrode spacing were of particular interest. In our patient, neither position nor spacing affected onset latency. Both electrode position and electrode spacing did, however, affect reflex amplitude. As position moved from base to apex, reflex amplitude increased systematically and substantially. Although we have reported amplitude results in suprathreshold current level, we also found the same relationship across electrode position for stimulation at constant current level. Reflex amplitude by electrode spacing was also affected. The widest spacing (3 mm) produced the largest reflex amplitude, and the narrowest spacing (1.5 mm) produced the smallest amplitude. The spacing effect, however, showed a strong interaction with electrode position, being greatest at the apical position and least at the basal position.

As cochlear implantation becomes available to younger age groups,[1-3] problems in hardware adjustment inevitably arise. The adult patient is able to provide behavioral estimates of threshold, comfort, and discomfort levels of electrical stimulation on which optimal current level ranges may be confidently based. In the case of very young children, however, especially in the age range below 3 years, such behavioral estimates may lack sufficient reliability and validity. In such cases stapedius muscle contraction in response to electrical stimulation[4,5] may provide an alternative technique for adjusting signal parameters.

In the present paper the relationships between behavioral measures and electrically elicited reflex responses as a function of electrode position are examined in an adult patient with a multichannel cochlear implant. The aim was to determine the extent to which aspects of the reflex would predict the useful dynamic range of electrical stimulation across the electrode array.

METHOD

The single experimental patient was a 59-year-old man who had been implanted with the 22-electrode Nucleus system 3 months previously. The subject was alert and well motivated. Experimental data were gathered over a 3-week period in experimental sessions lasting 60 to 90 minutes each. During each session complete measurements were performed for three to four electrodes.

The apparatus used to measure behavioral responses consisted of the Nucleus speech processor interface unit, coupled to a Sanyo 1000 microcomputer. The special apparatus used to acquire stapedius muscle responses to electrical stimulation has been described in detail in previous publications.[6,7] Briefly, a standard Madsen probe assembly was sealed in the external canal of the contralateral, or unoperated, ear. The probe microphone output was delivered to a lock-in amplifier, phase-coupled to the probe tone source (270 Hz). The rectified output from the lock-in amplifier was digitized and stored in the memory of a microcomputer (Apple II) for subsequent averaging. Responses to ten consecutive signals were acquired and the first two were discarded. The remaining eight were signal averaged. The time constant of the entire reflex recording system was approximately 10 ms.

The same electrical signal, an 800-ms burst of 125/s biphasic electrical pulses, was used to define threshold, preferred loudness level, and maximum comfortable loudness level, as well as to elicit the stapedius muscle reflex. For any given electrode the three behavioral measures were acquired before the reflex measures were obtained. For the latter, current level was increased in 50-μA steps to a level approximately 50 to 100 μA above the previously determined maximum comfortable loudness level.

The three behavioral measures were defined as follows.

1. Behavioral threshold was the lowest level below which the patient could not reliably respond to the presence or absence of the electrical signal.

2. Preferred loudness level was the ideal level at which the patient preferred to listen for long periods of time.

3. Maximum comfortable loudness level was the highest level the patient could comfortably tolerate for long periods, ie, as loud as possible without being actually uncomfortable.

Complete behavioral and reflex data were gathered for 15 electrodes across the 22-electrode array. Electrode spacing was held constant at one (ie, one inactive electrode between each pair of active electrodes).

RESULTS

At each electrode maximum reflex amplitude in decibels was plotted against current level in microamperes to pro-

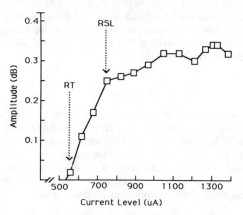

Fig 1. Reflex amplitude as function of current level for electrode 13. RT—reflex threshold, RSL—reflex saturation level.

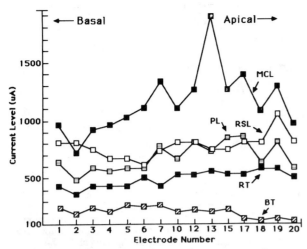

Fig 2. Three behavioral and two reflex measures as functions of electrode position. BT—behavioral threshold, PL—preferred loudness level, MCL—maximum comfortable loudness level.

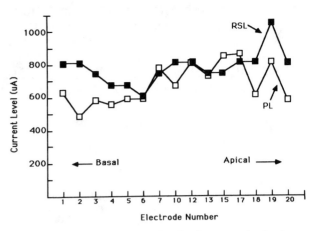

Fig 3. Preferred loudness level and reflex saturation level as functions of electrode position.

duce an amplitude versus current level function. Figure 1 shows an example of one such function for electrode 13. Two measures were extracted for each amplitude versus current level function: 1) reflex threshold, defined as the lowest current level at which a reflex response could be observed; and 2) the reflex saturation level, defined as the current level at which the amplitude versus current level function changed from its initial, rapidly rising phase to its subsequent, slowly rising or completely plateaued level. Figure 2 summarizes all of the data obtained in the study. Included are the behavioral thresholds, the preferred loudness level, the maximum comfortable loudness level, the reflex threshold, and the reflex saturation level, for each of the 15 electrodes tested.

The total dynamic range (behavioral thresholds-maximum comfortable loudness level) widened slightly as electrode position moved from base to apex. Within this range the preferred loudness level was relatively constant at a point in the range approximately 75% above the behavioral threshold. Reflex threshold and reflex saturation level were also relatively constant across electrode position. The reflex threshold tended to bisect the range, being somewhat below 50% in the basal region and somewhat above 50% in the apical region. The reflex saturation level was in remarkably good agreement with the preferred loudness level. This agreement is further illustrated in Fig 3. Here the two measures, preferred loudness level and reflex saturation level, are shown in isolation. Across the entire electrode array reflex saturation level was a relatively good predictor of preferred loudness level.

DISCUSSION

The agreement between preferred loudness level and reflex saturation level in this particular patient may not necessarily hold for other adult patients or for children. Indeed, in an earlier cochlear implant patient on whom we measured electrically elicited reflex responses, reflex saturation level corresponded more closely to maximum comfort loudness level than to preferred loudness level.

Such inconsistency is, perhaps, inevitable when one considers the intersubject variability in comfort settings for acoustic signals and the difficulty in establishing uniform instructions leading to the same internal definitions of subjective comfort and discomfort across individuals.[8] Nevertheless, we are encouraged to believe that the present results could provide the basis for a relatively conservative protocol for setting the dynamic range of individual electrodes without the patient's conscious cooperation.

As a first approximation the reflex saturation level could be used to define the upper boundary of the dynamic range of a given electrode. At the same time reflex threshold could be used to define the lower boundary of the useful range. These settings should place the trial range well within the actual usable range. Then, as the child gains experience with the device, the upper and lower boundaries could be slowly and carefully expanded until the ultimate ideal range had been determined in actual usage over a substantial observational interval.

REFERENCES

1. House WF, Eisenberg LS. The cochlear implant in preschool-aged children. Acta Otolaryngol (Stockh) 1983;95:632-8.

2. Berliner KI, Eisenberg LS. Methods and issues in the cochlear implantation of children; an overview. Ear Hear 1985;6(suppl 3): 65-135.

3. Luxford WM, House WF. Cochlear implants in children: medical and surgical considerations. Ear Hear 1985;6(suppl 3): 205-35.

4. Burnett P. Contralateral intra-aural reflexes elicited by a cochlear prosthesis in non-human primates [Thesis]. Seattle: University of Washington, 1981.

5. Jerger J, Fifer R, Jenkins H, Mecklenburg D. Stapedial reflex to electrical stimulation in a patient with a cochlear implant. Ann Otol Rhinol Laryngol 1986;95:151-7.

6. Hayes D, Jerger J. Signal averaging of the acoustic reflex: diagnostic application of amplitude characteristics. Scand Audiol [Suppl] 1982;17:31-6.

7. Stach B, Jerger J. Acoustic reflex averaging. Ear Hear 1984: 5:289-96.

8. Dirks DD, Kamm C. Psychometric functions for loudness discomfort and most comfortable loudness levels. J Speech Hear Res 1976;19:613-27.

Prediction of Dynamic Range from Stapedius Reflex in Cochlear Implant Patients

James Jerger, Terrey A. Oliver, and Rose A. Chmiel

Department of Otolaryngology and Communicative Sciences, Baylor College of Medicine, Houston, Texas

ABSTRACT

Amplitude growth functions of the electrically elicited stapedius reflex were compared with behavioral estimates of dynamic range in seven patients using multielectrode cochlear implants. The range between threshold and saturation level of the amplitude growth function usually either encompassed or fell between the preferred and uncomfortable listening levels. Implications of these findings for the initial mapping of electrodes in young children are discussed.

The use of cochlear implants, especially multichannel systems, in children raises special problems in setting the dynamic range of the individual electrodes. Adults can identify their own preferred and uncomfortable listening levels, but young children may not be able to provide the audiologist with the same subjective judgments. There is clearly an urgent need to devise procedures for electrode mapping in children that do not depend on subjective patient report. According to Boothroyd (1986) for example:

As cochlear implants become more complex, there is an increase in the range of possible adjustments of the speech processor, and of the number of ways of mapping processor output onto electrode arrays. In the adult population, it is possible to base decisions on patients' reports of sensation. This approach becomes difficult with younger patients, especially if they are prelingually deaf. Objective evaluation methods are clearly required for this aspect of the work (p. 350).

Recent studies of the electrically elicited stapedius reflex in adults (Jerger, Fifer, Jenkins, & Mecklenburg, 1986; Jerger, Jenkins, Chmiel, & Oliver, 1986) suggest a possible approach to the problem. Specifically, the function relating reflex amplitude to stimulating current level, the reflex amplitude growth function, has shown an encouraging relation to the optimal dynamic range as defined by behavioral measures of preferred and uncomfortable listening levels. In a single subject with a 21-channel Nucleus implant the total dynamic range between behavioral threshold and the uncomfortable listening level widened slightly as electrode position moved from base to apex. Within this range the preferred listening level remained relatively constant at a point in the range approximately 75% above the behavioral threshold. Both reflex threshold and reflex saturation level were also relatively constant across electrode position. The reflex threshold tended to bisect the range, somewhat below 50% in the basal region, and somewhat above 50% in the apical region. Reflex saturation level was in good agreement with the preferred listening level.

The purpose of the present study was to examine this relationship in further detail in seven adult cochlear implant patients. We sought to determine whether the amplitude growth function of the electrically elicited stapedius reflex could be used to define an algorithm suitable for adjusting electrode dynamic range in the pediatric population.

METHOD

Subjects

The subjects of this study were seven postlingually deafened adults implanted with the Nucleus 22-electrode, cochlear implant system. Six were male, one was female. Subjects ranged in age from 25 to 60 yr with a mean age of 38.7 yr. The etiologies of hearing loss included meningitis (2), ototoxicity (1), congenital factors (1), and unknown causes (3). The duration of profound hearing loss prior to implant surgery ranged from 8 mo to 4 yr with a mean duration of 2 yr 3 mo.

Subjects utilized from 13 to 20 electrodes, activated in bipolar pairs. There was one inactive band between each pair of active electrodes (BP+1 mode). All subjects had worn the system for at least 3 mo and were considered successful implant users.

Apparatus

The apparatus used to record stapedius muscle activity in response to acoustical or electrical stimulation has been described in previous publications (Hayes & Jerger, 1982; Stach & Jerger, 1984). Briefly, a probe assembly system monitored immittance changes from the contralateral or unoperated ear. The probe tone was a 270 Hz sinusoid whose level was individually adjusted such that the intensity level in the external ear canal was 85 dB SPL, as measured by a microphone calibrated in a 2 cc coupler. The probe tone was amplified and rectified by a lock-in amplifier (Princeton Applied Research, model 129A), then routed to the memory of a microcomputer (Apple II) for averaging. In the present study, this apparatus was interfaced with a microcomputer (Sanyo, MDC-1000) which generated the reflex-eliciting electrical stimulus and provided the syncronized trigger for reflex averaging. The time constant of the reflex- recording apparatus was 10 msec, temporal resolution was 2 msec, and analog-to-digital amplitude resolution was 12 bits.

Procedure

Acoustic Reflex Measures. The patient was seated comfortably and the probe assembly was sealed in the external ear canal. Air pressure was then adjusted to the point of maximum admittance. Next, probe tone intensity was adjusted, to achieve an ear canal SPL of 85 dB.

The same electrical signal was used both to elicit stapedius reflex responses and to define preferred and uncomfortable listening levels behaviorally. Each electrode of the array was tested separately. The eliciting signal was a 800 msec burst of biphasic, charge-balanced, 200 µsec pulses presented at a rate of 125 pulses/sec. The interstimulus interval was held constant at 1000 msec. Current level was varied in approximately 50 µA steps in order to define the amplitude versus current level growth function. From this growth function two measures were extracted; reflex threshold (RT) and reflex saturation level (SAT). RT was defined as the lowest current level at which an averaged stapedius reflex waveform could be visualized oscilloscopically. SAT was defined as the lowest current level at which the largest absolute amplitude of the reflex was observed.

The averaged stapedius reflex waveform was based on the presentation of 16 successive bursts. Reflex thresholds and saturation levels were monitored on-line. In addition, averaged waveforms were stored on floppy disk for subsequent off-line analysis.

Behavioral Measures. All behavioral testing was carried out immediately following stapedius reflex testing. Three behavioral measures were obtained from each patient on each electrode: (1) behavioral threshold (BT), (2) preferred listening level (PL), and (3) uncomfortable listening level (UCL). In each case, the patient adjusted a potentiometer to produce the desired measure. For behavioral threshold the patient was instructed to find a level at which he could just barely hear the pulse train. For preferred listening level the patient was instructed to adjust the potentiometer to a level at which he could easily hear the pulse train and judged it comfortable for prolonged listening, that is neither too faint nor too loud. For the uncomfortable listening level the patient was instructed to adjust the potentiometer to a level which was uncomfortably loud, that is a level at which he would not want to listen for very long. Because all patients had completed at least a 3 month rehabilitation program, they were well practiced at generating stable subjective judgments in an adjustment paradigm before the present study began.

RESULTS

Figure 1 shows illustrative reflex amplitude growth functions for each of the seven patients of the present study. In all cases, the electrode displayed was chosen as representative of the midrange of active electrodes for that subject. In each case, the growth function for a single electrode is displayed along with the current levels corresponding to the three behavioral measures, BT, PL, and UCL.

Reflex amplitude growth functions showed substantial variation among subjects, both in shape and in absolute magnitude. Note, in particular, the considerable variation in range of amplitudes displayed on the ordinates of each of the growth functions of Figure 1. Some functions climbed slowly to a plateau extending over a broad range of current levels. Other functions rose rapidly from minimum to maximum, reflecting a much narrower dynamic range. Still others were extremely limited in absolute magnitude and reflected poorly defined shapes.

In general, despite the variation in shape and height of reflex growth functions, we observed that BT was always well below reflex threshold, that PL was usually in the vicinity of reflex threshold or somewhere on its rising phase, and that UCL was usually in the vicinity of the saturation level of the growth function or well above it. Thus, the range from reflex threshold to reflex saturation level appeared to be well within the subject's behavioral dynamic range for that electrode. In Figure 2, the data of Figure 1 are replotted in order to visualize better the relationships among the behavioral and reflex measures. Note that, in each of the seven subjects, the range between reflex threshold and reflex saturation level either overlaps the preferred listening level or extends between the preferred listening level and the uncomfortable listening level. We were impressed, in particular, with the relatively close correspondence between reflex threshold and the preferred listening level. Table 1 summarizes current levels corresponding to reflex threshold and preferred listening level in each of the seven subjects of Figures 1 and 2. In spite of some variation, especially in subjects 1 and 7, the average current level for RT, 583 µA, was very close to the average current level for PL, 648 µA.

The extent to which these relationships held over different electrodes in the same subject is illustrated in Figure 3. Here the range from reflex threshold to saturation level is compared with the preferred listening level and uncomfortable listening level across each of 15 of the 20 electrodes used by subject 1. Again, we note that the range from reflex threshold to saturation level usually encompasses the preferred listening level.

Figure 4 shows similar results across representative electrodes for each of the seven patients. In general, reflex threshold shows good agreement with preferred listening level, and reflex saturation level is typically close to or below the uncomfortable listening level.

Test-Retest Stability

The stability of the absolute values of the various behavioral and reflex measures is a clinically relevant issue. To this end we examined test-retest data for both reflex and behavioral measures, available for six of the seven patients of the present study. The test-retest interval varied from 3 to 6 mo. Table 2 summarizes test-retest results for reflex threshold, preferred listening level, and uncomfortable listening level on one electrode. For each subject, we show current levels measured on the first date, the second date, and the difference between measures on the two dates.

The mean difference between test and retest was 55 µA for reflex threshold, 97 µA for preferred listening level, and 205 µA for uncomfortable listening level. For all three measures the sign of the mean difference shows that the measure was associated with a higher current level on the retest than on the original test. In the case of the preferred listening level, and especially the uncomfortable listening level, some of the relatively large test-retest differences (+720, in subject 1 and +655 in subject 3) were undoubtedly influenced by practice and/or training effects. It is

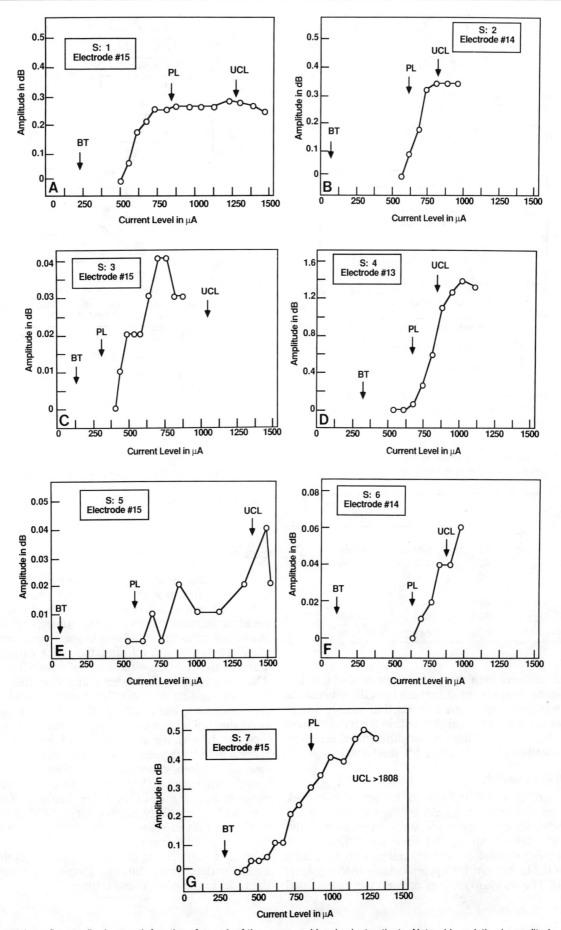

Figure 1. Illustrative reflex amplitude growth functions for each of the seven cochlear-implant patients. Note wide variation in amplitude scales.

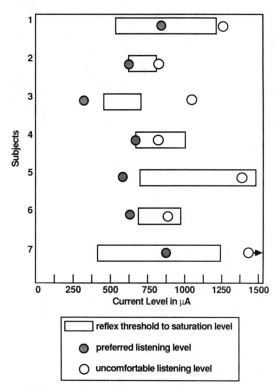

Figure 2. Relations among PL, UCL, and RT and SAT of the reflex amplitude growth function for one electrode in each of the seven cochlear-implant patients.

Table 1. Current levels, in μA, corresponding to stapedius reflex threshold (RT) and preferred listening level (PL) in seven patients with cochlear implant

Subject	RT	PL	Difference (PL-RT)
1	535	848	313
2	620	620	0
3	454	308	−146
4	667	667	0
5	696	584	−112
6	696	638	−58
7	410	870	460
Mean	583	648	65

commonly observed, in the early stages of cochlear implant training, that some patients are initially reluctant to tolerate relatively high current levels, but readily accept them after some weeks or months within the rehabilitative regimen. None of the three mean differences, however, was statistically significant at the 5% level.

Test-Retest Reliability

The extent to which individuals maintain their rank order, from test to retest speaks to the reliability of the various behavioral and reflex measures. Regression analysis showed relatively strong test-retest correlation coefficients for reflex threshold ($r = 0.87$) and preferred listening level ($r = 0.84$), but not for uncomfortable listening level ($r = 0.44$). The standard error of measurement associated

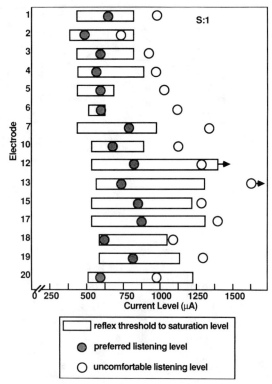

Figure 3. Relations among PL, UCL, and range between threshold and saturation level of the reflex amplitude growth function for 15 electrodes of one cochlear-implant patient.

with each regression equation was 80 μA for reflex threshold, 127 μA for preferred listening level, and 420 μA for uncomfortable listening level.

COMMENT

The present data suggest that the electrically elicited stapedius reflex growth function may provide a basis for the initial estimation of electrode dynamic range in the cochlear implant patient. In the subjects of the present study, the reflex threshold was in good agreement with the preferred listening level, and the reflex saturation level was usually well below the uncomfortable listening level. Thus, if electrodes had been mapped in these seven patients, according to the reflex threshold and saturation level measures, the resulting dynamic range would have been roughly within each subject's range of comfortable listening. Indeed, the upper limit of each subject's dynamic range would have been set relatively conservatively. In the case of children, especially the prelingually deafened, a useful initial approach might be to center the dynamic range of an electrode at the reflex threshold. Then, beginning with a relatively narrow range (200–300 μA), one might carefully increase the range, both upward and downward around this center point, and using the saturation level as a tentative upper limit, until an optimal range could be determined through long-range observation of the child in the educational setting.

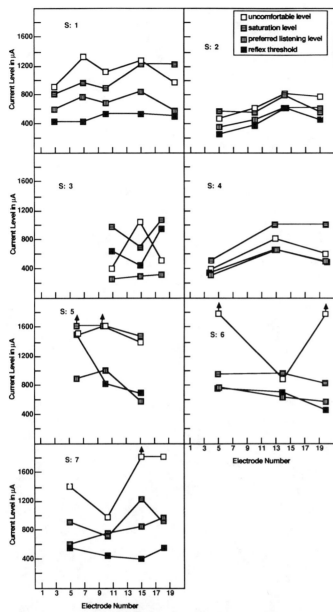

Figure 4. Relations among PL, UCL, RT, and SAT across electrodes in each of the seven cochlear-implant patients.

Table 2. Test-retest differences in current levels (μA) for two behavioral measures (PL and UCL) and one reflex measure (RT) from six patients with cochlear implant.

Measure	Subject	Test		Difference
		1	2	(2-1)
RT	1	535	559	24
	2	564	620	56
	3	498	454	−44
	4	557	667	110
	5	696	882	186
	6	696	696	0
	Mean	591	646	55
PL	1	672	938	266
	2	681	620	−61
	3	308	308	0
	4	557	667	110
	5	584	772	188
	6	559	638	79
	Mean	560	657	97
UCL	1	1114	1834	720
	2	813	828	15
	3	398	1053	655
	4	647	821	174
	5	1390	1485	95
	6	1307	879	−428
	Mean	945	1150	205

References

Boothroyd A. Issues of pre- and postimplant evaluation regarding cochlear implants in children. Semin Hear 1986;7:249–359.

Hayes D, and Jerger J. Signal averaging of the acoustic reflex: diagnostic application of amplitude characteristics. Scand Audiol 1982;Suppl.17:31–36.

Jerger J, Fifer R, Jenkins H, and Mecklenburg D: Stapedius reflex to electrical stimulation in a patient with a cochlear implant. Ann Otol Rhinol Laryngol 1986;95:151–157.

Jerger J, Jenkins HA, Chmiel R, and Oliver TA: Electrically-elicited stapedius reflex and preferred listening level in a patient with cochlear implant. Ann Otol Rhinol Laryngol 1986;95:151–157.

Stach B, and Jerger J: Acoustic reflex averaging. Ear Hear 1984;5:289–296.

Address reprint requests to James Jerger, 11922 Taylorcrest Rd., Houston, TX 77024.

Received March 23, 1987.

VI

Auditory Evoked Potentials

Of the many technological advances over the past three decades, none has had a greater impact on our profession than the averaging computer. It has made possible the recording, not only of the auditory brainstem response (ABR), but of an entire family of electrical potentials evoked by sound. My first contact with averaged evoked potentials came while I was still at Northwestern. In the late 1950s, Dan Geisler, now at Wisconsin, was a graduate student at the University of Chicago. A group of us went down to hear him speak on his recently completed dissertation in which he used, for the first time, an averaging computer to record the brain's response to an acoustic signal. What he was recording, a positivity at about 30 msec, has since come to be called the middle-latency response, or MLR. We were duly impressed, but commercial equipment to make such recording feasible in most laboratories was not yet available. By the time I had moved to Houston in the early 1960s, the first commercial averager, the Computer of Averaged Transients (CAT), could be had for about $10,000. We purchased one and set to work looking, not at the MLR, but at a later response in the 60–180 msec region, which has since come to be called the LVR or late vertex potential. Hallowell Davis, at the Central Institute for the Deaf, was working intensively on this response, hoping to devise an objective test of hearing that could be applied to babies and young children. This was, of course, the principal reason why we were all so interested in evoked potentials. This was the pre-ABR era. Testing the hearing of babies and young children

was not always a happy experience. We had to rely on behavioral techniques, usually involving some sort of conditioning, and results were not always clearcut. (I can see some of my contemporaries rolling their eyes and muttering that this may be the understatement of the month.) So there was very great interest in the development of a hearing test that would not require the child's active cooperation.

One of my less successful ideas during this period was to connect the electrodes on the child's head to a small FM transmitter and telemeter the ongoing EEG to an FM receiver outside the sound room. In this way, I reasoned, the child would be free to move around the test room, unencumbered by restricting wires and be happily at play. But it never seemed to work out that nicely. In fact we, like Davis, soon found that the LVR was too state-dependent to be used as an objective test of anything in young children. But I don't think we wasted all that time, because when ABR came along, a few years later, we were quick to appreciate the value of such a state-independent response.

The first paper in this section, "Prediction of Sensorineural Hearing Level from the Brain Stem Evoked Response" (*Archives of Otolaryngology*, 1978), was one of the earliest attempts to determine what exactly the ABR threshold to clicks was predicting. In light of subsequent findings, our conclusions seem perhaps a bit too simplistic, but we were correct, I think, in concluding that audiometric contour is more important than absolute degree of high-frequency loss in determining wave V latency.

The second paper, "Auditory Brain Stem Evoked Responses to Bone-Conducted Signals" (*Archives of Otolaryngology*, 1979), was one of the earliest attempts to relate the bone-conducted to the the air-conducted ABR. Larry Mauldin and I showed that, because of the differing click spectra transduced by the air- and bone-conduction drivers, the latency of wave V of the bone-conducted ABR is 0.5 msec longer than the latency of wave V of the air-conducted ABR at comparable click sensation levels. But, when correction is made for this difference, the latency-intensity functions of air-conduction and bone-conduction ABRs are similar, making possible precise estimation of air-bone gap from the latency distance between the two functions. This finding has particularly important implications for the evaluation of children with congenital atresia.

The next paper, "Clinical Experience with Auditory Brainstem Response Audiometry in Pediatric Assessment" (*Ear & Hearing*, 1980), is interesting from an historical perspective. In 1980 ABR testing was not yet as widespread as it is today. Many audiologists and centers were standing by, waiting to see whether they should become involved in the new technique. In this paper we were attempting to share our experiences with them, to emphasize both the very important strengths and inherent weaknesses of the technique. As I reread this paper after 13 years, I was struck not only with the accuracy of most of the predictions, but with the historical perspectives the interested reader may gain from the interchange at the end of the paper with Drs. Naunton, Finitzo-Heiber, and Rose.

The last three papers are concerned with the gender difference in ABR latency. Very early on, it became apparent that the latency of wave V of the ABR was, on the average, slightly shorter in females than in males. Three possible mechanisms suggested themselves: distance, temperature, and hormones. The distance hypothesis was based on the fact that the diameter of the average female skull is slightly smaller than the diameter of the average male skull. Hence, there is less distance to travel between auditory nerve and lower brainstem. The temperature hypothesis was based on the fact that the body temperature of the average female is slightly higher than the body temperature of the average male, and nerve conduction time decreases as temperature increases. Finally, the hormone hypothesis was based on the fact of variation in hormonal milieu over the course of the menstrual cycle.

In the first paper, "Effects of Age and Sex on Auditory Brainstem Response" (*Archives of Otolaryngology*, 1980), Jay Hall and I confirmed the significance of the gender difference in both latency and amplitude of wave V of the ABR, not only in subjects with normal hearing but in those with varying degrees of sensorineural hearing loss. In the second paper, "Analysis of Gender Differences in the Auditory Brainstem Response" (*Laryngoscope*, 1990), Chris Dehan and I showed that oral temperature had little effect on ABR latency and amplitude and that head size could explain only part of the gender effect. The remainder of the effect, however, was correlated with hormonal changes as measured from venous blood samples. It was not, however, until we began collaboration with an endocrine specialist, Karen Elkind-Hirsch, that the true picture began to unfold. In the final paper in this section, "Estrogen Influences Auditory Brainstem Responses During the Normal Menstrual Cycle" (*Hearing Research*, 1992), Elkind-Hirsch shows how an increase in ABR latency in mid-cycle is associated with a high estrogen state, and suggests the existence of brainstem auditory neural pathways sensitive to fluctuations in serum estrogen levels during the menstrual cycle.

These six papers sample only some of the many possible applications of auditory evoked potentials. The auditory brainstem response has been successfully brought to center stage and integrated into clinical practice, but other evoked responses, notably the MLR, the LVR, and the various event-related potentials, are still waiting impatiently in the wings.

Prediction
of Sensorineural Hearing Level
From the Brain Stem Evoked Response

James Jerger, PhD, Larry Mauldin

● Correlational analysis was carried out between the auditory brain stem evoked response (BER) threshold, BER latency, and various audiometric indices in 275 ears with varying degrees and configurations of sensorineural hearing loss.

Results confirm the importance of sensitivity in the 1 to 4-kHz region to the brain stem response. Sensitivity over this frequency region is best predicted as 0.6 of the BER threshold. Brain stem evoked response latency in the 70- to 90-dB hearing level range increases about 0.2 ms for each 30-dB increase in the steepness of the audiometric contour between 1 and 4 kHz. Finally, audiometric shape appears to be more important than absolute high-frequency sensitivity in determining BER latency.

(Arch Otolaryngol 104:456-461, 1978)

In 1971, Jewett and Williston[1] first suggested that the auditory brain stem evoked response (BER) might be employed in clinical evaluation. Subse-

quent studies on subjects with normal hearing have shown that the threshold of the BER response is near the behavioral threshold for the same signal. In addition, as signal intensity decreases, latency to the most prominent component wave (wave V) progressively increases.[2-4]

These promising results, coupled with the extraordinary repeatability of the BER, have encouraged clinicians to seek a basis for predicting degree of hearing loss from the BER threshold and latency data. Two recent reports described changes in both measures in patients with sensorineural hearing loss. Both Coats and Martin[5] and Moller and Blegvad[6] reported that the BER threshold correlates best with high-frequency (HF) hearing levels (2 to 4 kHz). In addition, Moller and Blegvad suggested that wave V latency is directly related to audiometric configuration. Latency in flat hearing loss tends to be shorter than latency in HF sloping loss.

Both of these studies were based on a limited number of cases and, as a result, on a restricted selection of both degree of loss and audiometric configuration. Our study extends their preliminary findings by providing correlational analysis on a larger

group of patients with varied losses, rather than on a small number of subjects selected for particular audiometric configurations.

METHOD
Subjects

Threshold and latency measures were obtained from 275 ears of 185 patients with sensorineural hearing loss, who were evaluated by the Audiology Service of the Neurosensory Center of Houston. Of these patients, 106 were male and 79 were female. Average age was 47.2 years, with a range from 7 to 83 years.

The 275 ears that were studied represented only those ears with sensorineural hearing loss on which a BER was observed. No restrictions were imposed on degree of loss or audiometric configuration, with the exception that a response must be present for at least one test level. However, ears with normal hearing, middle ear disorder, or any evidence of retrocochlear disorder were specifically excluded.

Instrumentation

Figure 1 shows a block diagram of the signal and recording instrumentation of our BER system. The acoustic signal used to elicit BER was a half cycle of a 3,000-Hz sinusoid. The half cycle was generated by a function generator (Wavetek, 146) that was triggered by a second function generator (Hewlett-Packard, 3311A) at a rate of 20 cps. The half cycle was amplified (MacIntosh, 250), attenuated (Hewlett-

Accepted for publication March 15, 1978.

From the Department of Otorhinolaryngology and Communicative Sciences, Baylor College of Medicine and the Neurosensory Center, Houston.

Reprint requests to Department of Otorhinolaryngology and Communicative Sciences, Baylor College of Medicine and Neurosensory Center, 1200 Moursund Ave, Houston, TX 77030 (Dr Jerger).

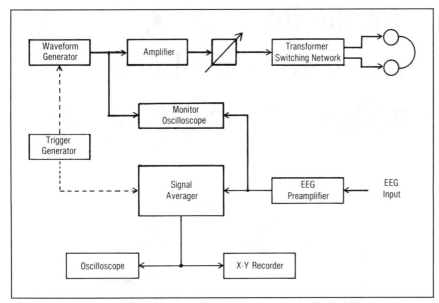

Fig 1.—Simplified block diagram of BER measurement system.

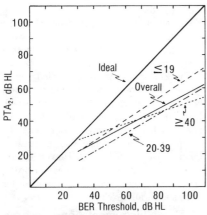

Fig 2.—Linear regression equations for predicting PTA₂ from BER threshold. Functions are shown for total group (overall) and for three subgroups based on 1 vs 4 kHz contour. Also shown is line of ideal (unit) slope.

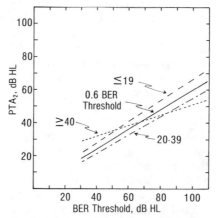

Fig 3.—Linear regression equations for predicting PTA₂ from BER threshold. Functions are shown for three subgroups based on 1 vs 4 kHz contour and for proposed predictive equation (0.6 × BER threshold).

of the sweeps (1,024) were responses to condensation clicks, and half were responses to rarefaction clicks. The two click polarities were employed to facilitate cancellation of signal artifact. Permanent records were obtained by photographing the oscilloscopic display or by plotting the response on an X-Y recorder (Hewlett-Packard, 7035B).

Procedure

The subjects were seated in a double-walled sound room. Each subject was tested at a high intensity (90 or 100 dB HL), and at 10- to 20-dB intensity decrements until the BER was no longer observed. Each signal intensity condition was run twice. The resulting averaged responses were superimposed on the permanent record. The lowest intensity level at which a repeatable response was observed was defined as the BER threshold. The latency of wave V, which is the time from signal onset to the positive peak of wave V, was measured for each response.

In addition to BER threshold and latency measures, a number of pure-tone sensitivity indices were obtained from the patient's clinical audiogram: the pure-tone average of 0.5, 1, and 2 kHz (PTA₁), the pure-tone average of 1, 2, and 4 kHz (PTA₂), the 2-kHz threshold, and the 4-kHz threshold. To provide information relative to audiometric configuration, three contour indicators were calculated: the 0.5- to 4-kHz difference, the 1-to 4-kHz difference, and the 2- to 4-kHz difference. Each contour measure was determined by subtracting the threshold for the lower frequency signal from the threshold at 4-kHz.

Although previous investigators, especially Coats and Martin,[5] have shown that behavioral threshold at 8 kHz relates strongly to the BER, we did not attempt analysis at this frequency because of the relatively large proportion of patients in our sample whose 8-kHz threshold was beyond equipment limits.

Statistical analysis of the various measures was carried out by computer (DEC system 10) that employed the statistical package for the social sciences (University of Pittsburgh, SPSS-10). Standard descriptive statistics were obtained for age, both BER measures, and each pure-tone sensitivity and contour measure. Correlational analysis was carried out between the BER threshold and each behavioral measure, and between the BER latency and each behavioral measure. This correlational analysis supplied scattergrams, coefficient of correlation, standard error (SE) of estimate, and the slope coefficient of the linear regression equation.

Packard, 350D), and routed through an impedance-matching transformer to a switching network before being delivered to standard audiometric earphones (TDH-39) that were mounted in circumaural cushions (CZW-6). The switching network allowed signals of equal voltage to be delivered to either the right or left earphone or to both earphones simultaneously. Click intensities were expressed in hearing level. The behavioral click threshold of ten young adults with normal hearing defined 0 dB HL. At this level, the peak equivalent sound pressure level (peSPL) was 30 dB.

The BER was recorded by a conventional signal-averaging technique. Standard EEG disk electrodes were attached to the vertex (active) and each mastoid. The mastoid of the stimulated ear served as reference, and the opposite mastoid served as a ground. Prior to electrode placement, the three electrode sites were cleaned with an abrasive gel to reduce interelectrode resistance to less than 5K Ω. A standard EEG preamplifier (Grass, P511 H) provided differential amplification of 100,000 to 200,000:1 and band-pass filtering from 0.3 to 3 kHz. The amplified EEG activity was delivered to a signal averager (Nicolet 1010). The ongoing EEG activity was also displayed on an oscilloscope (Hewlett-Packard, 122 AR) to allow continuous on-line monitoring of the EEG.

The signal averager was triggered for a 10-msec sweep at the onset of each signal. A total of 2,048 sweeps was averaged. Half

RESULTS

Table 1 summarizes the statistical description of the study sample. The SDs and ranges show that the 275 ears encompassed virtually every degree and configuration of sensorineural loss. Variation in degree of loss is attested by the range of PTA$_1$, from 0 to 83 dB HL. Similar variation in audiometric configuration is demonstrated by the range of the 0.5 vs 4 kHz contour, from −40 to +90 dB.

Since many losses were so severe that BERs could be observed only at a few very high click levels, complete latency vs intensity functions could not be obtained uniformly. Therefore, for each ear, we chose a single response to represent latency. The level of this response was always in the 70 to 90 dB HL range (100 to 120 dB peSPL). We preferred to measure latency at 70 dB HL whenever possible, to avoid the signal artifacts that are often present in responses at very intense levels, but we used responses at levels as high as 90 dB HL when these were the only data available.

For each behavioral measure, three correlational indices were computed: the coefficient of correlation, the SE of estimate, and the slope coefficient of the linear regression equation. Each index reflects an unique dimension of the overall relationship. The coefficient of correlation (Pearson's r) reflects the proportion of variance in the behavioral measure attributable to its relationship to the BER measure. In effect, it reflects the extent to which an individual's rank order on the BER measure is preserved in the behavioral measure.

The SE of estimate is the SD of the distribution of actual behavioral measures around the result that is predicted by the least-squares linear regression equation. It reflects the precision with which a given behavioral measure can be predicted from the BER measure.

The slope coefficient of the linear regression equation reflects the extent to which the behavioral measure changes as the BER measure changes.

Of the three correlational indices, the most important from the standpoint of the present prediction problem is the SE of estimate. It yields, most directly, the probability of any given degree of error when a BER measure is used to predict a behavioral measure. The slope coefficient of the least-squares linear regression equation is also important to the present prediction problem since it yields an essential component of the predictive rule by which the behavioral measure is predicted from the BER measure. If the slope coefficient is unity, then prediction of the behavioral measure from the BER measure involves only a constant correction. However, for any slope coefficient other than unity, a corresponding multiplier must be involved in the predictive equation.

The coefficient of correlation, itself, is probably of least interest to the present problem, except as a tool by which to survey the various behavioral measures in search of the most promising predictive equations.

Prediction Based on BER Threshold

Table 2 summarizes the overall correlational analysis when the BER threshold is related to seven audiometric indices of sensorineural hearing loss. Review of the coefficients of

Table 1.—Statistical Description of Study Sample*			
Measure†	**Mean**	**SD**	**Range**
BER threshold, dB HL	66.2	16.9	10-100
BER latency,‡ ms	6.0	0.48	4.8-8.1
PTA$_1$, dB HL	31.5	19.2	0-83
PTA$_2$, dB HL	40.3	18.0	5-93
2-kHz threshold, dB HL	36.1	22.1	−5-105
4-kHz threshold, dB HL	54.6	21.5	5-110
0.5 vs 4 kHz contour, dB	26.9	28.0	−40-90
1 vs 4 kHz contour, dB	24.5	25.4	−35-85
2 vs 4 kHz contour, dB	18.5	19.9	−20-97

*Mean, SD, range of various audiometric and BER indices are indicated for 275 ears with sensorineural hearing loss.
†BER indicates brain stem evoked response; PTA$_1$, pure-tone average of 0.5, 1, and 2 kHz; and PTA$_2$, pure-tone average of 1, 2, and 4 kHz.
‡Indicates for signal at 70 to 90 dB HL.

Table 2.—Correlational Analysis of BER Threshold With Selected Behavioral Measures (N = 275)				
Behavioral Measure*	**Coefficient of Correlation (r)**	**Significance Level (P)**	**SE of Estimate, dB**	**Slope of Regression Equation, dB/dB**
PTA$_1$	.34	.00001	18.1	0.38
PTA$_2$	.48	.00001	15.8	0.51
2-kHz threshold	.41	.00001	20.2	0.54
4-kHz threshold	.49	.00001	18.7	0.63
0.5 vs 4 kHz contour	.25	.00001	27.1	0.42
1 vs 4 kHz contour	.17	.002	25.1	0.26
2 vs 4 kHz contour	.07	.11	19.9	0.09

*For explanation of PTA$_1$ and PTA$_2$, see footnote to Table 1.

Table 3.—Correlational Analysis of BER Threshold With PTA$_2$* in Groups With Different Audiometric Contours					
Contour Index (4 kHz − 1 kHz)	**N**	**Coefficient of Correlation (r)**	**Significance Level (P)**	**SE of Estimate, dB**	**Slope of Regression Equation, dB/dB**
≤ 19	107	.55	.00001	16.3	0.64
20-39	83	.53	.00001	15.2	0.56
≥ 40	85	.35	.0006	14.2	0.32
Total group	**275**	**.48**	**.00001**	**15.8**	**0.51**

*For explanation of PTA$_2$, see footnote to Table 1.

correlation shows that, in common with previous investigators, we noted highest correlation in the 2- to 4-kHz threshold region. The highest correlation (0.49) is with the 4-kHz threshold, but the correlation with PTA_2 (0.48) is almost as high. Correlation with the various audiometric contour measures is not strong, and declines as the range of frequencies over which contour is defined decreases from three octaves to one octave.

The SE of estimate is smallest for PTA_2 (15.8 dB) and largest for the 0.5 vs 4 kHz contour (27.1 dB). Herein lies the principal problem in predicting audiometric levels from the BER. The precision with which prediction can be made is limited by a SD of about 15 dB. Thus if, for example, a 50-dB level is predicted, the probability is 0.67 that the actual level is between 35 and 65 dB, and about 0.95 that the actual level is between 20 and 80 dB.

The slope coefficient of the regression equation for the BER threshold with each of the seven behavioral measures varies from 0.09 (2 vs 4 kHz contour) to 0.63 (4-kHz threshold). In the HF region (1 to 4kHz) where the correlation coefficient is highest, the slope coefficient averages about 0.60. The fact that the slope coefficient is not unity (1.00) means that behavioral level cannot be predicted by applying a constant correction to the BER threshold. Instead, the BER threshold must be multiplied by the slope coefficient before a constant (if needed) correction can be applied.

Taken as a whole, the results that are summarized in Table 2 seem to recommend PTA_2 as the behavioral measure best predicted by BER threshold. The correlation coefficient is second highest (0.48), and the SE of

estimate is lowest (15.8 dB). However, we were surprised by the relatively low-slope coefficient (0.51). Clinical experience suggested to us that a low-slope coefficient might be the result of pooling different audiometric configurations. We reasoned that for patients with flat loss, the slope coefficient might be near unity, while for HF sloping losses, the slope coefficient might be much smaller. In other words, the overall slope coefficient might be contaminated by steep HF losses.

To test this assumption, we divided the total group into three subgroups based on audiometric contour. Categorization was based on the 4- to 1-kHz difference. Ranges for the three groups were as follows: (1) 19 dB or less; (2) 20 to 39 dB; and (3) 40 dB or greater.

Table 3 compares the correlational analysis of these three contour subgroups with results for the total group. All correlational indices decrease as audiometric contour increases. The coefficient of correlation decreases from 0.55 to 0.35, the SE of estimate decreases from 16.3 to 14.2, and the slope coefficient of the regression equation decreases from 0.64 to 0.32. This latter change confirms, at least partially, our working hypothesis that the regression slope coefficient is related to audiometric contour.

Contrary to our expectation, however, the regression slope coefficient in the flat or rising audiometric contour group did not approach unity. Figure 2 shows the "ideal" linear equation for a unit slope coefficient and the actual linear equations for the overall group

and for the three contour subgroups.

The implication of departure from unit slope for the regression equation coefficient is that if a unit slope coefficient is assumed, then degree of hearing loss will tend to be overestimated. This arises from the fact that in cochlear hearing loss, the BER threshold elevation occurs much more rapidly than elevation of behavioral threshold. Even the use of a constant correction factor, which is subtracted from the BER threshold, assumes a unit slope coefficient for the regression equation. The technique of employing a constant correction factor will result in an overestimation of hearing loss when the BER threshold is high and an underestimation of hearing loss when the BER threshold is low.

To avoid these problems that plague predictive schema based on unit slope coefficient assumption, one must employ a strategy that takes into account the nonunit slope coefficient. This may be accomplished by multiplying the BER threshold by a slope index. Figure 3 shows the regression lines for the three subgroups with hearing loss and the line for a proposed, clinically applicable equation. The slope coefficient of the proposed line is 0.6. Thus, PTA_2 would be predicted to be 0.6 of the BER threshold ($PTA_2 = 0.6 \times$ BER threshold).

To evaluate the effectiveness of this predictive technique, we computed the difference between actual PTA_2 and predicted PTA_2 (actual $PTA_2 - 0.6 \times$ BER threshold) for the entire group of patients and for the three contour subgroups. Table 4

Table 4.—Error of Estimation of PTA_2 in Groups With Different Audiometric Contours*

Contour Index, dB (4 kHz − 1 kHz)	Mean	SD
≤ 19	4.91	16.2
20-39	−3.63	15.1
≥ 40	−0.84	14.8
Total group	**0.56**	**15.8**

*Mean and SD of difference between actual PTA_2 and PTA_2 was estimated from $0.6 \times$ BER threshold. For explanation of PTA_2, see footnote to Table 1.

Table 5.—Correlational Analysis of BER Latency* With Selected Behavioral Measures (N = 275)

Behavioral Measure	Coefficient of Correlation (r)	Significance Level (P)	SE of Estimate, dB	Slope of Regression Equation, dB/ms
PTA_1	.07	.13	19.2	2.66
PTA_2	.30	.00001	17.2	11.03
2-kHz threshold	.23	.00005	21.6	10.58
4-kHz threshold	.47	.00001	19.0	21.13
0.5 vs 4 kHz contour	.44	.00001	25.2	25.66
1 vs 4 kHz contour	.38	.00001	23.6	19.69
2 vs 4 kHz contour	.25	.00001	19.3	10.41

*Indicates brain stem evoked latency for signal at 70 to 90 dB HL. For explanation of PTA_1 and PTA_2, see footnote to Table 1.

summarizes descriptive statistics for each group. The SD for the overall group is almost identical to the SE of estimate obtained in the correlation analysis (Table 2). We had expected that the SDs shown in Table 4 might show a progressive increase as audiometric contour increased. However, the opposite was true, although the maximum difference between SDs was only 1.38. Although unexpected, this finding is especially encouraging. It suggests that accuracy of prediction is not markedly dependent on audiometric configuration.

In summary, although audiometric contour does systematically affect the slope of the regression equation, prediction of behavioral threshold (PTA_2) can be achieved without substantial constant error if the BER threshold is multiplied by 0.6. Furthermore, predictive precision will not vary substantially with audiometric configuration.

Prediction From BER Latency

Table 5 summarizes the result of correlational analysis by comparing BER latency with the seven behavioral measures. In general, BER latency seems more strongly related to indices of HF contour than to absolute sensitivity level, but both BER threshold and latency correlate best with the threshold at 4 kHz.

In general, the SE of estimate is somewhat larger when threshold prediction is based on BER latency rather than BER threshold, but it is interesting to note that, in the case of PTA_2, the SE based on BER latency (17.2 dB) is not very much larger than the SE based on BER threshold (15.8 dB). Note, also, that BER latency predicts audiometric contour with slightly better precision than does BER threshold.

Effect of HF Loss on Latency

From the standpoint of the clinical application of BER latency, the most important correlational measure is the slope coefficient of the regression equation. This slope coefficient allows us to predict the likelihood that any observed prolongation of latency can be attributed solely to audiometric configuration.

In subjects with normal hearing, the expected BER latency at 70 to 90 dB HL ranges from 4.9 to 6.5 ms. However, it has been well documented that in patients with HF sloping audiograms, latency will be slightly prolonged. When a patient with unilateral sensorineural loss is being evaluated for the possibility of eighth nerve disorder, prolonged latency may be observed in the BER from the suspect ear. Then there is the crucial clinical question: Is the prolonged latency due to eighth nerve disorder, or is it no more than we must expect on the basis of the audiometric configuration? For this analysis, it is necessary to interpose dependent and independent variables to consider the regression of latency on the various behavioral measures.

Figure 4, for example, shows the effect of the 1 vs 4 kHz contour on latency when contour is the independent variable. At a contour index of 0 dB (flat configuration), the expected latency is about 5.8 ms. A contour index of 30 dB can be expected to add about 0.2 ms to this value, and a contour index of 50 dB adds about 0.35 ms. Thus, a delay of 0.5 ms would be within expected limits if the index of the audiometric contour (1 vs 4kHz) were 70 dB, but it would reflect delay that was not explainable by audiomet-

ric configuration if the contour index were only 40 dB. In general, an absolute wave V latency in excess of 7 ms cannot be explained by audiometric contour. In the present series, only 2% of cases had latencies longer than 7 ms no matter how steep the audiometric contour.

Contour vs Absolute Level

In the analysis of audiometric influences on BER latency, it is difficult to separate the effect of audiometric contour from the effect of absolute HF sensitivity, because the two measures are, necessarily, highly

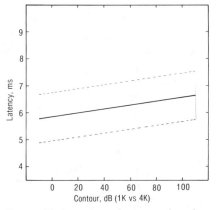

Fig 4.—Linear regression equation for predicting BER latency at 70 to 90 dB HL from audiometric contour (1 vs 4 kHz). Function based on linear regression equation ±2 SE of estimate.

Table 6.—Correlational Analysis of BER Latency* With PTA_2 in Groups With Different Audiometric Contours

Contour Index (4 kHz – 1 kHz)	N	Coefficient of Correlation (r)	Signifcance Level (P)	SE of Estimate, dB	Slope of Regression Equation, dB/ms
≤ 19	107	.24	.006	18.8	11.26
20-39	83	.33	.001	16.9	14.65
≥ 40	85	.40	.00007	13.9	11.38
Total group	**275**	**.30**	**.00001**	**17.2**	**11.03**

*Indicates latency for signal at 70 to 90 dB HL. See footnote to Table 1 for explanation of PTA_2.

Table 7.—Correlational Analysis of BER Latency* With Audiometric Contour (4 kHz – 1 kHz) in Groups With Different PTA_2

PTA_2, dB	N	Coefficient of Correlation (r)	Significance Level (P)	SE of Estimate, dB	Slope of Regression Equation, dB/ms
≤ 29	87	.23	.02	20.0	13.14
30-59	144	.43	.00001	24.8	23.34
≥ 60	44	.54	.00009	23.0	28.87
Total group	**275**	**.38**	**.00001**	**23.6**	**19.69**

*Indicates latency for signal at 70 to 90 dB HL. See footnote to Table 1 for explanation of PTA_2.

correlated. As contour increases, HF threshold level also increases.

In this communication, we have attempted to approach the problem by subdividing the total group in two ways: first, according to contour; second, according to PTA$_2$.

The first categorization holds contour constant while permitting absolute level to vary; the second categorization holds absolute level constant while permitting contour to vary. If contour is, indeed, more important than absolute level, then correlation coefficients and slope coefficients should be higher when contour is permitted to vary than when absolute level is permitted to vary.

Tables 6 and 7 show that this is, indeed, the case. In Table 6, subjects are categorized according to contour (1 vs 4 kHz), and absolute level is permitted to vary. Correlation coefficients range from 0.24 in the subgroup with least contour (≤ 19) to 0.40 in the subgroup with the greatest contour (≥ 40).

In Table 7, subjects are categorized according to PTA$_2$, and contour is permitted to vary. Correlation coefficients range from 0.23 in the subgroup with least loss (≤ 29) to 0.54 in the subgroup with most loss (≥ 60). In Table 7, note also the systematic increase in slope coefficient from

13.14 to 28.87 as degree of loss increases.

Table 6 shows that when contour is held relatively constant there is a definite relation between absolute level of HF sensitivity and BER latency. However, Table 7 shows that when absolute level is held relatively constant there is an even stronger relation between audiometric contour and BER latency.

Therefore, we conclude that although both audiometric shape and level are factors in latency delay, degree of contour in the 1- to 4-kHz region is a more important factor in determining BER latency than absolute level in the same frequency region.

COMMENT

In concert with both Coats and Martin[5] and Moller and Blegvad,[6] we reaffirm the importance of the 1- to 4-kHz frequency region to the BER. In further agreement with both previous investigations, we reaffirm the prolongation of latency in downward sloping audiometric configurations. Finally, the relatively large SEs of estimate associated with the regression equations in the present study reaffirm the admonition of Moller and Blegvad that "attempts to measure hearing capacity exclusively

with the aid of brain stem responses to unfiltered clicks should be regarded as unacceptable."[6]

Our data suggest the following specific conclusions:

1. Threshold of the BER response to clicks best predicts HF sensitivity in the 1- to 4-kHz region.

2. The average pure-tone threshold for 1, 2, and 4 kHz is most accurately predicted by multiplying BER threshold by 0.6.

3. The SE of estimate of such predictions is relatively large (15 to 16 dB), limiting the success with which audiometric level can be predicted from BER alone.

4. Latency of the BER response in the 70 to 90 dB HL region increases about 0.2 ms for a 30-dB increase in the audiometric contour between 1 and 4 kHz.

5. Audiometric contour is more important than absolute sensitivity level in determining BER latency, although both factors are related to latency prolongation.

This study was supported, in part by Public Health Service research grant NS-10940 from the National Institute of Neurological and Communicative Disorders and Stroke, National Institutes of Health.

Lois Anthony, MA, Connie Jordan, MS, Sharron Smith, MS, and Deborah Hayes, MA, assisted in the collection, analysis, and interpretation of data; Alfred C. Coats, MD, provided helpful criticism of the manuscript.

References

1. Jewett D, Williston J: Auditory-evoked far fields averaged from the scalp of humans. *Brain* 94:681-696, 1971.

2. Picton T, Hillyard S, Kransz H, et al: Human auditory evoked potentials: I. Evaluation of components. *Electroencephalogr Clin Neurophysiol* 36:179-190, 1974.

3. Hecox K, Galambos R: Brain stem auditory evoked potentials in human infants and adults. *Arch Otolaryngol* 99:30-33, 1974.

4. Yanada O, Yagi T, Yamane H, et al: Clinical evaluation of the auditory evoked brain stem response. *Auris-Nasus-Larynx* 2:97-105, 1975.

5. Coats AC, Martin JL: Human auditory

nerve action potentials and brain stem evoked responses: Effects of audiogram shape and lesion location. *Arch Otolaryngol* 103:605-622, 1977.

6. Moller K, Blegvad B: Brain stem responses in patients with sensori-neural hearing loss. *Scand Audiol* 5:115-127, 1976.

Auditory Brain Stem Evoked Responses to Bone-Conducted Signals

Larry Mauldin, James Jerger, PhD

● Auditory brain stem evoked responses to air-conducted and bone-conducted signals were recorded in subjects with normal hearing and in subjects with conductive hearing loss. In normal subjects, the latency to wave V for bone-conducted signals was approximately 0.5 ms longer than the latency for air-conducted signals delivered at the same sensation level. In conductive hearing loss, the separation of the latency-intensity functions for air conduction and bone conduction (corrected for the 0.5-ms delay) provided a valid estimate of the behavioral air-bone gap in the 1,000- to 4,000-Hz region.

(Arch Otolaryngol 105:656-661, 1979)

The use of bone-conducted signals in electrocochleography has been reported by Yoshie,[1] who indicated that the separation of the air conduction input-output and latency-intensity functions from the analogous bone conduction functions provides an estimate of the behavioral air-bone gap. In addition, Yoshie described a differ-ence in waveform between the compound action potentials elicited by air-conducted and bone-conducted signals. He also noted that the bone-conduction latency-intensity function was somewhat different than the normal air conduction latency-intensity function. Yoshie suggested that differences in the air conduction and bone conduction click spectra might contribute to these observed dissimilarities in the action potentials recorded with the two signals.

The effects of conductive hearing loss on the auditory brain stem evoked response (ABR) have been reported in a general manner.[2-4] In conductive loss, the ABR to air-conducted clicks has been reported to be affected in three ways: (1) the threshold is elevated; (2) the amplitude is decreased; and (3) the latency to high-intensity clicks is increased (due to a shift in the latency-intensity function). The degree of conductive hearing loss on a given patient has been predicted to be the amount that the patient's air conduction latency-intensity curve is shifted from the "normal" latency-intensity function for air-conducted signals.

If the ABR can be recorded with bone-conducted signals, then the air-bone gap on a patient with conductive hearing loss can be predicted from the separation of the air conduction and bone conduction latency-intensity functions, as in electrocochleography. The goal of the present study was to evaluate the use of bone-conducted click signals in subjects with normal hearing and in subjects with conductive hearing loss. Specific attention was focused on comparison of air conduction and bone conduction latency-intensity functions.

METHOD
Subjects

The ABR latencies to clicks presented by air conduction and by bone conduction were measured on four young adults with normal hearing and 11 patients with conductive hearing loss (12 ears) evaluated at the Neurosensory Center of Houston. On each ear of the patients with conductive hearing loss, ABR latency and threshold measures were obtained for both air-conducted and bone-conducted click signals.

Instrumentation

A detailed description of the signal and recording instrumentation has been reported previously.[5] In brief, the ABR was recorded using a vertex (active) to mastoid (reference and ground) electrode array. The amplified (100,000 to 300,000:1) EEG activity was signal-averaged (Nicolet, 1010). The averaged response was plotted

Accepted for publication Nov 29, 1978.

From the Department of Otorhinolaryngology and Communicative Sciences, Baylor College of Medicine and the Neurosensory Center of Houston.

Reprint requests to 11922 Taylorcrest Rd, Houston, TX 77024 (Dr Jerger).

on an X-Y recorder (Hewlett-Packard, 7035B).

The electrical signal was one-half cycle of a 3,000-Hz sinusoid. This signal was band-pass-filtered (Krohn-Hite, 330 NR), amplified (McIntosh, 250), attenuated (Hewlett-Packard, 350D), and delivered either to standard audiometric earphones (TDH-39) mounted in circumaural cushions (CZW-6) or to a bone conduction vibrator (Radioear, B-70A). Signal polarity was alternated to facilitate cancellation of signal artifact.

Procedure—Subjects With Normal Hearing

Subjects with normal hearing were tested using binaural stimulation for air-conducted signals and without masking noise for bone-conducted signals. Forehead placement was always used for the bone conduction vibrator. Since ABR latency varies as a function of signal intensity, it was necessary to use a constant sensation level (SL) for all the test signals. On each subject, behavioral click threshold was independently determined for the bone-conducted signal and for each of the various air-conducted signals. The ABR was recorded immediately after the threshold determination for a given signal. Click intensity was always adjusted to an SL of 40 dB (40 dB SL).

For testing by bone conduction, the band-pass filter was set for a 40- to 20,000-Hz bandwidth so that the spectrum of the click signal was determined primarily by the frequency response of the bone vibrator. Similarly, a 40- to 20,000-Hz bandwidth was used for air conduction testing. In addition, air conduction responses were obtained using clicks that were low-pass filtered at the following cutoff frequencies: 8,000, 6,000, 4,000, 3,500, 3,000, 2,500, and 2,000 Hz. Thus, nine separate responses at 40 dB SL were recorded on each subject. For each response, the latency of wave V, the time from signal onset to the positive peak of wave V, was measured.

Procedure—Subjects With Conductive Hearing Loss

For evaluation of subjects with conductive hearing loss, click intensities were expressed in hearing level (HL). The behavioral click threshold of ten normal-hearing young adults defined 0 dB HL. Maximum equipment output was 60 dB HL for bone-conducted clicks and 100 dB HL for air-conducted clicks.

Each subject was tested monaurally with unfiltered clicks delivered by both air conduction and bone conduction. In all cases, contralateral masking noise was used as indicated. Responses were recorded

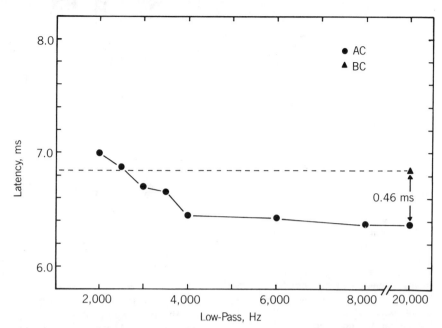

Fig 1.—Average brain stem evoked response wave V latencies to bone-conducted (BC) clicks and low-pass-filtered clicks on four normal subjects at sensation level of 40 dB. For broad-band clicks, BC latency is 0.46 ms longer than air conduction (AC) latency. Latency of AC increases as low-pass-filtering decreases.

Fig 2.—Spectra for broad-band and low-pass-filtered air conduction (AC) click signals. Also shown is spectrum of click signal delivered through bone vibrator (B-70A). Note similar shapes of low-pass AC and bone conduction (BC) curves.

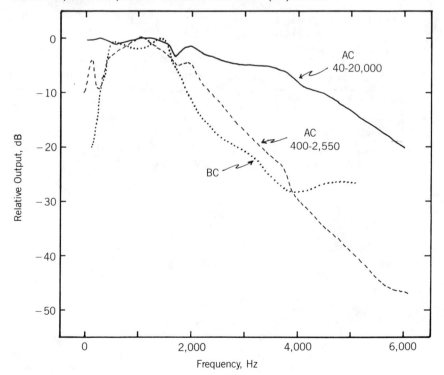

Table 1.—Correlational Analysis of Air Conduction ABR Threshold With Selected Behavioral Air Conduction Threshold Measures*

Behavioral Measure†	Coefficient of Correlation (r)	Standard Error of Estimate, dB	Slope of Regression Equation, dB/dB
500-Hz threshold	.61	19.4	0.74
1,000-Hz threshold	.58	20.0	0.80
2,000-Hz threshold	.71	17.2	0.79
4,000-Hz threshold	.79	15.0	0.63
PTA₁	.68	18.1	0.90
PTA₂	.81	14.3	0.96

*ABR, auditory brain stem evoked response.
†PTA₁, pure tone average of 500, 1,000, and 2,000 Hz; PTA₂, pure tone average of 1,000, 2,000, and 4,000 Hz.

Table 2.—Correlational Analysis of Bone Conduction ABR Threshold With Selected Behavioral Bone Conduction Threshold Measures*

Behavioral Measure†	Coefficient of Correlation (r)	Standard Error of Estimate, dB	Slope of Regression Equation, dB/dB
500-Hz threshold	.53	14.4	0.70
1,000-Hz threshold	.83	9.4	1.14
2,000-Hz threshold	.87	8.2	1.35
4,000-Hz threshold	.84	9.2	0.74
PTA₁	.86	8.7	1.41
PTA₂	.95	5.2	1.28

*ABR, auditory brain stem evoked response.
†PTA₁, pure tone average of 500, 1,000, and 2,000 Hz; PTA₂, pure tone average of 1,000, 2,000, and 4,000 Hz.

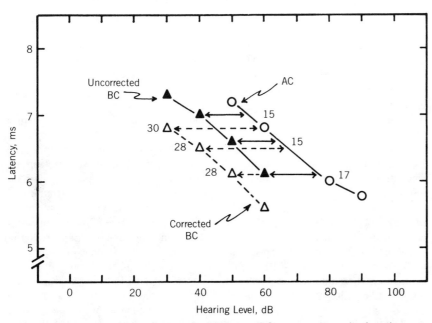

Fig 3.—Air conduction (AC) and bone conduction (BC) latency-intensity functions on subject with conductive hearing loss. Uncorrected BC function represents latencies measured directly from responses. Corrected BC function was generated by subtracting 0.5 ms from each data point along uncorrected BC function. Numbers to right of AC function represent individual estimates of the separation, in decibels, of AC and uncorrected BC functions. Numbers to left of corrected BC function are estimates of separation of AC and corrected BC functions. Average separation of AC and corrected BC functions predicts behavioral air-bone gap for average of 1,000, 2,000, and 4,000 Hz.

at maximum equipment output and at 10- to 20-dB decrements until the response was no longer observed. The lowest intensity level at which a response could be elicited was defined as the ABR threshold. In addition to ABR threshold and latency measures, a number of pure tone sensitivity indexes for air conduction and bone conduction were obtained from the patient's clinical audiogram: thresholds at 500, 1,000, and 2,000 Hz, the pure tone average of 500, 1,000, and 2,000 Hz PTA₁), and the pure tone average of 1,000, 2,000, and 4,000 Hz (PTA₂). The air-bone gap at each of these frequencies was also determined.

Correlational analysis was carried out between ABR air conduction threshold and each behavioral air conduction measure, between ABR bone conduction threshold and each behavioral bone conduction threshold, and between ABR estimates of air-bone gap and each behavioral air-bone gap. The correlational analysis supplied coefficient of correlation, standard error of estimate, and the slope coefficient of the linear regression equation.

RESULTS
Subjects With Normal Hearing

Comparison of wave V latencies for broad-band (40 to 20,000 Hz) clicks delivered by air conduction and by bone conduction showed that the ABR latency to bone-conducted signals averaged 0.46 ms greater than the latency to air-conducted signals at comparable SLs. The frequency response curves for the TDH-39 earphone and the B-70A bone vibrator are quite different. In comparison to the earphone, the bone vibrator responds poorly to high-frequency signals. Thus, when driven by a broad-band signal (such as a click), the vibrator acts as a low-pass filter. To evaluate the effect of low-pass-filtered clicks on the latency of wave V, air-conducted signals of different bandwidths were employed. Mean latencies on the four normal subjects are shown in Fig 1. Low-pass-filtering above 4,000 Hz had only slight effect on the wave V latency. However, low-pass-filtering below 4,000 Hz yielded progressively longer latencies for the successively lower pass-bands. For the four normal subjects represented in Fig 1, low-pass-filtering of the air-conducted signal at 2,550 Hz yields the same latency as the unfiltered bone-conducted click. Air-conducted clicks that are low-pass-filtered below 2,550 Hz give latencies that are greater than the bone conduction latency, whereas the air conduction latency is less than the bone conduction latency when the clicks are low-pass-filtered above 2,550 Hz.

To verify that limited high-pass-filtering had no effect on ABR latency, we tested one subject with clicks that were band-passed from 400 to 3,000 Hz and from 400 to 6,000 Hz. Comparison of the 40- to 3,000-Hz latency with the 400- to 3,000-Hz latency revealed no difference. Similar comparison between the 40- to 6,000-Hz and 400- to 6,000-Hz latencies showed no difference.

To investigate further the hypothesis that spectral differences between air-conducted and bone-conducted signals were responsible for the increased latency by bone conduction, we measured the spectra for the acoustic outputs of the two earphones. Two spectral analyses were performed on each earphone. Spectra were determined for the broad-band (40 to 20,000 Hz) click and for the low-pass band that produced equal air conduction and bone conduction latencies (2,550 Hz). The low-pass-filtered clicks were also high-pass-filtered at 400 Hz since this had no effect on the wave V latency. Figure 2 shows the two spectral curves for the right earphone. The left earphone yielded essentially identical spectra. Also illustrated in Fig 2 is the frequency response curve for our bone-conducted signal as measured on an artificial mastoid. Both curves begin to show a decrease in output in the 1,500- to 2,000-Hz region. Although the output curve for the low-passed air conduction clicks begins to decline at a slightly higher frequency than the bone vibrator curve, the two are sufficiently similar to lend support to our hypothesis. Increased wave V latency to bone-conducted clicks appears to be due to the spectrum of the bone-conducted signal.

Subjects With Conductive Hearing Loss

Table 1 summarizes the correlational analysis when the ABR air conduction threshold is related to six conventional audiometric indexes of air conduction sensitivity. Similar to previous findings in normal-hearing subjects and in patients with sensorineural hearing loss,[5] the highest coefficients of correlation occur with high-frequency threshold measures. The PTA_2 yields the highest coefficient (0.81).

The standard error of estimate systematically declines with increasing frequency. It is smallest for PTA_2 (14.3 dB), although as previously noted,[5] a standard error of estimate of this magnitude limits the precision with which audiometric levels may be predicted from ABR.

The slope coefficient of the regression equation relating ABR air conduction threshold with the various audiometric measures ranges from 0.63 (4,000 Hz threshold) to 0.96 (PTA_2). The nearly unit slope coefficient for PTA_2 suggests that PTA_2 may be directly predicted from the ABR air conduction threshold by applying a suitable correction factor. In addition, since the coefficient of correlation was highest and the standard error of estimate lowest, PTA_2 seems to be the air conduction measure best predicted by the air conduction ABR threshold.

Table 2 summarizes the correlational analysis when the ABR bone conduction threshold is related to six audiometric indexes of bone conduction sensitivity. Again, the highest coefficient of correlation and lowest standard error of estimate are observed when the ABR threshold is related to PTA_2. Inspection of the 1,000-, 2,000-, and 4,000-Hz threshold measures in Table 2 reveals a pattern of results quite different from Table 1. For air conduction threshold estimates (Table 1), the coefficient of correlation increases systematically as the frequency is raised from 1,000 to 4,000 Hz. Over the same frequency range, the standard error of estimate progressively decreases. However, for bone conduction threshold estimates (Table 2), coefficients of correlation and standard errors of estimate are essentially unchanged as the signal frequency increases from 1,000 to 4,000 Hz. These results suggest that frequencies below 4,000 Hz are of greater relative importance for ABR by bone conduction than for ABR by air conduction.

In order to predict air-bone gap from ABR, we compared the air conduction and bone conduction latency-intensity functions. Figure 3 shows such a comparison on one patient with conductive hearing loss. The uncorrected bone conduction function is a plot of the wave V latencies measured directly from the individual responses. The corrected bone conduction function was derived by subtracting the bone conduction response delay observed in normal subjects (rounded to 0.5 ms to facilitate clinical application) from the uncorrected bone conduction function. The air-bone gap prediction was based on the average separation (in decibels) of the latency-intensity functions. In Fig 3, the average separation between the air conduction function and the uncorrected bone conduction function is 16 dB. This value was determined by averaging the separation at three points along the latency-intensity function. The three individual separations are indicated to the right of the air conduction function. Inspection of the air conduc-

Table 3.—Correlational Analysis of 'Corrected' ABR Air-Bone Gap With Selected Behavioral Air-Bone Gaps*			
Behavioral Measure†	Coefficient of Correlation (r)	Standard Error of Estimate, dB	Slope of Regression Equation, dB/dB
500-Hz threshold	.62	11.4	0.84
1,000-Hz threshold	.53	11.4	0.67
2,000-Hz threshold	.65	11.7	0.94
4,000-Hz threshold	.84	9.3	1.35
PTA_1	.48	11.3	0.57
PTA_2	.83	7.4	1.02

*ABR, auditory brain stem evoked response.
†PTA_1, pure tone average of 500, 1,000, and 2,000 Hz; PTA_2, pure tone average of 1,000, 2,000, and 4,000 Hz.

tion and corrected bone conduction functions shows an average separation of 29 dB, with the individual separations shown to the left of the corrected bone conduction function.

Table 3 summarizes the correlational analysis when the ABR air-bone gap prediction (based on the corrected bone conduction latency-intensity function) was related to the various audiometric air-bone gaps. Consideration of coefficient of correlation, standard error of estimate, and slope of regression equation once again point to PTA₂ as the audiometric measure best predicted from ABR. For the patients with conductive hearing loss, the average PTA₂ air-bone gap predicted from ABR is 37.8 dB with a standard deviation of 10.2. The average behavioral PTA₂ air-bone gap is 36.4 dB (SD = 12.6).

COMMENT

In subjects with normal hearing, the latency to wave V was found to be about 0.5 ms longer for responses to bone-conducted clicks than for responses to air-conducted clicks presented at the same SL. When low-pass-filtered clicks were delivered by air conduction, the wave V latency increased as the low-pass cutoff frequency was decreased. The cutoff frequency that yielded the same latency by both air conduction and bone conduction was, averaged across the four normal hearing subjects, 2,550 Hz.

Other investigators have recently reported the effects of different air-conducted signals on the ABR. Don and Eggermont[6] employed high-pass noise bands to derive contributions to the ABR from different regions of the cochlea. Suzuki et al[7] used tone pips at selected frequencies to elicit the ABR. In both studies, regression equations were reported for predicting wave V latency (Suzuki et al) or shift in wave V latency (Don and Eggermont) for different stimulus conditions. The signal predicted to produce a 0.5-ms change in wave V latency is 2,447 Hz if the Don and Eggermont regression equation is used and 2,577 Hz if the Suzuki et al equations are used.

Different experimental procedures were used in the present study, by Don and Eggermont, and by Suzuki et al. However, when each study is focused on the same problem, estimating the frequency that produces a 0.5-ms shift in wave V latency, the results are remarkably similar. Only 130 Hz separates the highest estimate (2,577 Hz) from the lowest estimate (2,447 Hz). Thus, when the spectral content of the stimulus is limited to frequencies below 2,500 Hz, the ABR wave V latency will be approximately 0.5 ms greater than the wave V latency in response to a broad-band signal at the same intensity.

Three separate lines of evidence allow us to draw some conclusions regarding the bone-conducted signal that arrives at the cochlea. First, the spectrum of the bone-conducted click signal is quite similar to the spectrum of the air-conducted signal that resulted in equal air conduction and bone conduction latencies in subjects with normal hearing. Second, in patients with conductive hearing loss, correlational analysis relating ABR air conduction and bone conduction thresholds to their behavioral counterparts suggested that lower frequencies (1,000 and 2,000 Hz) have a greater relative importance for bone-conducted clicks than for air-conducted clicks. Third, three independent estimates of the air conduction signal frequency that results in a wave V delay of 0.5 ms were very close to 2,500 Hz. From these data, we conclude that the effective spectrum of the bone-conducted signal consists primarily of energy below 2,500 Hz.

To allow direct comparison of air conduction latency with bone conduction latency at comparable intensities, one must first correct the bone conduction latency. This is easily accomplished by subtracting 0.5 ms from the measured bone conduction latency. By applying this correction procedure at each intensity tested by bone conduction, one can generate a corrected bone conduction latency-intensity function. The average separation, in decibels, of the air conduction and corrected bone conduction latency-intensity functions then provides a valid estimate of the average air-bone gap at 1,000, 2,000, and 4,000 Hz.

In addition to furnishing an estimate of the air-bone gap in adults with conductive hearing loss, ABR by bone conduction can contribute valuable information in certain difficult to evaluate cases where ABR by air conduction alone is ambiguous. Clemis and Mitchell[8] recently described problems that arise from conductive hearing loss when ABR is used in the diagnosis of acoustic tumors. Latency increases due to conductive losses can be a source of false-positives in this application of ABR. The use of bone-conducted signals offers a solution to this problem. For interaural latency comparisons, the ABR to bone-conducted clicks may be recorded separately for each ear with the use of appropriate masking. The two latency-intensity functions may be directly compared, before or after latency correction. In addition, the corrected bone conduction latency-intensity function on the ear in question may be compared with the latency-intensity function of normal subjects. The use of air conduction alone does not allow these comparisons to be made.

Another area where ABR by bone conduction can be of great value is in the evaluation of infants. It is well established that wave V latency systematically increases as gestational age decreases.[9-11] However, conductive hearing loss also increases wave V latency. In infants with conductive hearing loss, it may be difficult to separate the latency increase due to age from the latency increase due to conductive hearing loss. In such cases, valid estimation of air-bone gap can be accomplished only if bone-conducted signals are used, in addition to air-conducted signals.

Bone-conducted signals may, in some cases, elicit the only observable response. In patients with a mixed hearing loss, the cochlear loss will result in an elevation of the ABR threshold. The conductive loss will elevate the ABR threshold further. The summed threshold elevations may exceed the output capability of the air conduction signal system. Bone-conducted signals are not affected by the conductive loss and need only exceed the cochlear threshold to elicit a response. The bone conduction threshold thus allows a prediction of cochlear sensitivity. This may be important in a young child with congenital atresia, where other techniques for estimating cochlear function cannot be used.

The use of bone-conducted signals, in conjunction with air-conducted signals, increases the diagnostic and predictive capabilities of the ABR. However, ABR by bone conduction is not without limitations. As discussed previously, the wave V latency by bone conduction is about 0.5 ms longer than the air conduction latency at the same intensity. The maximum output intensity for bone conduction is less than that for air conduction. If the maximum air conduction output level is 100 dB HL, the maximum bone conduction output level is about 60 dB HL. This limits the degree of cochlear loss in which a response by bone conduction will be observed to a maximum of 40 to 50 dB. At high-intensity levels by bone conduction (50 to 60 dB HL), electrical artifacts from the signal transducer may present a significant problem. The use of forehead placement of the bone vibrator reduces but does not eliminate this problem. Finally, as with all bone-conducted signals, ABR signals delivered by bone conduction result in binaural stimulation. To record the bone conduction ABR from one ear only, the nontest ear must be appropriately masked.

In subjects with normal hearing, the bone-conducted ABR latency is approximately 0.5 ms greater than the air conduction latency at a comparable intensity level. This increase in bone conduction latency is due to the different spectra of bone-conducted and air-conducted signals. The bone-conducted signal primarily is restricted to energy below 2,500 Hz. When the bone conduction latency-intensity function is corrected for the latency increase, the average separation of the air conduction and bone conduction functions predicts the average behavioral air-bone gap in the 1,000- to 4,000-Hz region. Furthermore, the air conduction and bone conduction ABR thresholds provide valid estimates of the behavioral thresholds in the 1,000- to 4,000-Hz region for air conduction and bone conduction, respectively.

This study was supported in part by Public Health Service research grant NS-10940 from the National Institute of Neurological and Communicative Disorders and Stroke, National Institutes of Health.

References

1. Yoshie N: Diagnostic significance of the electrocochleogram in clinical audiometry. *Audiology* 12:504-539, 1973.

2. Galambos R, Hecox K: Clinical applications of the brain stem auditory evoked potentials, in Desmedt J (ed): *Progress in Clinical Neurophysiology.* New York, S Karger, 1977, vol 2, pp 1-19.

3. Yamada O, Yagi T, Yamane H, et al: Clinical evaluation of the auditory evoked brain stem response. *Auris-Nasus-Larynx* 2:97-105, 1975.

4. Suzuki M, Suzuki J: Clinical application of the auditory-evoked brain stem response in children. *Auris-Nasus-Larynx* 4:19-26, 1977.

5. Jerger J, Mauldin L: Prediction of sensorineural hearing level from the brain stem evoked response. *Arch Otolaryngol* 104:456-461, 1978.

6. Don M, Eggermont J: Analysis of the click-evoked brainstem potentials in man using high-pass noise masking. *J Acoust Soc Am* 63:1084-1092, 1978.

7. Suzuki T, Hirai Y, Horiuchi K: Auditory brain stem responses to pure tone stimuli. *Scand Audiol* 6:51-56, 1977.

8. Clemis J, Mitchell C: Electrocochleography and brain stem responses used in the diagnosis of acoustic tumors. *J Otolaryngol* 6:447-459, 1977.

9. Hecox K, Galambos R: Brainstem auditory evoked responses in human infants and adults. *Arch Otolaryngol* 99:30-33, 1974.

10. Hecox K: Electrophysiological correlates of human auditory development, in Cohen L, Salapatek P (eds): *Infant Perception From Sensation to Cognition.* New York, Academic Press Inc, 1975, pp 152-191.

11. Schulman-Galambos C, Galambos R: Brain stem auditory-evoked responses in premature infants. *J Speech Hearing Res* 18:456-465, 1975.

Effects of Age and Sex on Auditory Brainstem Response

James Jerger, PhD, James Hall, PhD

We examined amplitude and latency of the auditory brainstem response (ABR) waveform as functions of chronological age in 182 male and 137 female subjects. Hearing sensitivity was within normal limits in 98 subjects. The remaining 221 subjects had varying degrees of sensorineural hearing loss. Age had a slight effect on both latency and amplitude of wave V. In subjects with normal hearing, latency increased about 0.2 ms over the age range from 25 to 55 years. In the same group, wave V amplitude decreased about 10%. In subjects with sensorineural hearing loss, the latency increase was smaller, but the amplitude decrease was equivalent. Sex also affected the ABR. In both normal and hearing-impaired subjects, female subjects showed consistently shorter latency and larger amplitude at all age levels. Wave V latency was about 0.2 ms shorter and wave V amplitude was about 25% larger in female subjects.

(Arch Otolaryngol 106:387-391, 1980)

In less than a decade, auditory brainstem response (ABR) audiometry has assumed a prominent role in clinical audiology. Following the Jewett and Williston[1] report in 1971, numerous investigators have studied the ABR in subjects with normal hearing[2-11] and a range of otologic and neurologic disorders.[12-30] The developmental aspects of the ABR in neonates, infants, and young children are also well established.[3,10,31-35] From birth to approximately 18 months, latency of the ABR, in particular the wave V component, systematically decreases, while amplitude increases.

In contrast to the interest in the developmental changes in the ABR, the potential influence of aging in adults has received remarkably little attention. Age is an important factor in behavioral audiometry. The age-related decrease in pure-tone sensitivity for higher frequencies[36,37] and, in some patients, lower frequencies,[38-40] is well documented. Depressed performance in speech understanding for both single words[37,41-43] and, especially, sentences in competition[40,43] is associated with aging. Age is also a factor in impedance audiometry. Static compliance decreases as a function of age.[44,45] With increasing age, acoustic reflex thresholds usually improve slightly for pure-tone signals, and are elevated for noise signals, even in subjects with normal hearing.[46] Consequently, the noise-tone difference (NTD) is decreased as a function of age.[46,47] Recently, Gersdorff[48] reported decreased amplitudes for crossed (contralateral) and uncrossed (ipsilateral) acoustic reflexes, again, in subjects with normal hearing sensitivity. In view of these documented age effects in other aspects of auditory function, it seems reasonable to suspect an age factor in the ABR.

There is mounting evidence that sex is a factor in both behavioral and impedance audiometry. In older adults, pure-tone sensitivity for high-frequency, pure-tone signals is usually better in women than in men, while sensitivity for low-frequency pure-tone signals is usually better in men than women.[40,49,50] Sex differences in performance on diagnostic speech audiometric procedures have also been reported.[40] Sex is a factor in some impedance audiometry measures. Static compliance tends to be greater in male than in female subjects.[44,45,51] However, a sex effect is not apparently reflected in acoustic reflex thresholds.[44]

Recent evidence suggests that both age[9,52-55] and sex[52,53,55] affect the ABR. We report the effects of age and sex for ABR wave V latency and amplitude.

METHOD
Subjects

The subjects were 319 patients, aged 20 to 79 years, whose clinical records were studied retrospectively. All subjects had received a routine audiologic evaluation at the Methodist Hospital/Neurosensory Center, Houston. There were 182 male and 137 female subjects. In 98 subjects, hearing sensitivity was within normal limits; that is, equal to or better than 20 dB hearing level (HL) for octave frequencies from 250 through 4,000 Hz. The remaining 221 subjects had varying degrees of sensorineural hearing loss. All subjects had normal middle ear function, as defined by impedance audiometry, and no audiometric evidence

Accepted for publication July 5, 1979.

From the Department of Otorhinolaryngology and Communicative Sciences, Baylor College of Medicine, Houston. Dr Hall is now with the Department of Hearing and Speech Sciences, University of Maryland, College Park.

Reprint requests to 11922 Taylorcrest Rd, Houston, TX 77024 (Dr Jerger).

of retrocochlear disorder. In the sensorineural group, ABR latency and amplitude are always reported for the ear with better hearing sensitivity.

Instrumentation and Procedure

The instrumentation and procedure used in this study have been described previously.[28](pp 456-457) In brief, the acoustic signal used to elicit the ABR was a half-cycle of a 3,000-Hz sinusoid. Signal intensity is expressed in HL (ie, decibels above average normal hearing for the click). The ABR was recorded by conventional signal-averaging technique. Standard EEG disk electrodes were attached to the vertex (active) and to each mastoid. The mastoid of the stimulated ear served as reference, and the opposite mastoid served as ground. Prior to electrode placement, the three electrode sites were cleaned with an abrasive gel to reduce interelectrode resistance to less than 4,000 ohms. The EEG signal was preamplified (Grass P511) with a voltage gain of 200,000 and band-pass filtered from 300 to 3,000 Hz (6 dB/octave skirt). The signal averager (Nicolet, 1010) was triggered for a 10-ms sweep at the onset of each signal. A total of 2,048 sweeps was averaged. Half of the signals (1,024) were condensation clicks, and half were rarefaction clicks.

Subjects were seated in a double-walled sound-treated room. Each subject was tested at a high intensity (90 or 100 dB HL) and at 10- to 20-dB intensity decrements until the ABR was no longer observed. However, for this study, only ABRs for signal intensities of 70 to 90 dB HL were analyzed. The latency of wave V (the time, in milliseconds, from signal onset to the positive peak of wave V) and the amplitude of wave V (in microvolts) measured from the peak of wave V to the following trough were determined for each response.

RESULTS

Figure 1 shows mean ABR latency (wave V) as a function of age in both the normal and sensorineural groups. Results for male and female subjects are plotted separately. The average signal intensity was comparable (83 to 85 dB HL) for all groups of subjects. In the normal group, latency increased as a function of age for both sexes. For both male and female subjects, the average latency in the oldest group was 0.20 ms longer than the average latency in the youngest group. However, while the relative age effect was comparable for male and female subjects, there was a dis-

tinct difference in the absolute latencies between sexes. In each age group, the average latency of the ABR was longer for male than for female subjects. In male subjects, the latency ranged from 5.70 ms in the youngest group to 5.89 ms in the oldest group. For female subjects, the latency ranged from 5.57 ms for the youngest group to 5.76 ms for the oldest group. Combining all age groups, the average latency for male subjects was 0.14 ms greater than the latency for female subjects.

In the sensorineural group, latency showed little change as a function of age. For male subjects, the average latency in the oldest group was only 0.10 ms longer than the average latency in the youngest group. For female subjects, there was no consistent change in latency as a function of age. In contrast to the small age effect, the difference in absolute latencies between male and female subjects was substantial, ranging from 0.19 ms in the youngest age group to 0.35 ms in the oldest age group. Collapsed across age, the average sex difference was 0.25 ms.

Figure 2 shows mean ABR amplitude (wave V) as a function of age in both groups. Results for male and female subjects are plotted separately. Again, the average signal intensity was comparable (83 to 85 dB HL) for all groups of subjects. In the normal group, wave V amplitude for female subjects showed a very slight decrease (0.025 μV) from the youngest to oldest age groups. For male subjects, the amplitude decrease was twice as great (0.050 μV) from the youngest to the oldest age groups. Compared with the weak age effect on normal ABR amplitude, the sex difference was robust. Female amplitude consistently exceeded male amplitude by amounts ranging from 0.080 μV in the youngest group to 0.120 μV in the oldest group.

In the sensorineural group, there was a slightly greater age effect on wave V amplitude. For female subjects, amplitude decreased by about 0.050 μV. For male subjects, amplitude decreased by about 0.020 μV. Again, a sex difference in wave V amplitude is clearly evident. The amplitude for

female subjects exceeded the amplitude for male subjects by up to 0.150 μV (in the 50 to 59 year age group).

In view of the dependence of both amplitude and latency of the ABR on auditory sensitivity in the high-frequency (1,000 to 8,000 Hz) region,[19] it is possible that the sex differences observed in Fig 1 and 2 could be due to subtle differences in high-frequency hearing sensitivity, differences favoring the female group. To investigate this possibility, we calculated the mean and standard deviation of the threshold HL at each test frequency from 250 through 8,000 Hz for each sex. Table 1 summarizes these data for the normal group (40 female and 58 male subjects).

Average HLs between sexes differed in excess of 2 dB at only one test frequency; at 250 Hz, the average threshold level was 2.17 dB better for male subjects. At 8,000 Hz, the average level for female subjects was 1.29 dB poorer than the average level for male subjects. It is unlikely that these differences in sensitivity level could produce significant effects on either ABR amplitude or latency. However, if they did, the effects would be in the direction of decreasing amplitude and increasing latency in the group with greater loss, the female group. However, in fact, actual results were reversed. In spite of poorer sensitivity, female subjects showed larger amplitude and shorter latency. Therefore, we conclude that the sex differences in ABR amplitude and latency cannot be accounted for by subtle differences in high-frequency hearing sensitivity in the normal group.

Table 2 summarizes means and standard deviations for wave V latency and amplitude collapsed across age subgroups, along with the probability of α error derived from tests of statistical significance of mean differences in latency and amplitude. For latency, the mean sex difference, collapsed across age, was 0.14 ms. For amplitude, the mean sex difference was 0.088 μV.

In the total sensorineural group (N = 221), there was an inevitable interaction among age, sex, audiometric contour, and the amplitude and latency of ABR. Not unexpectedly,

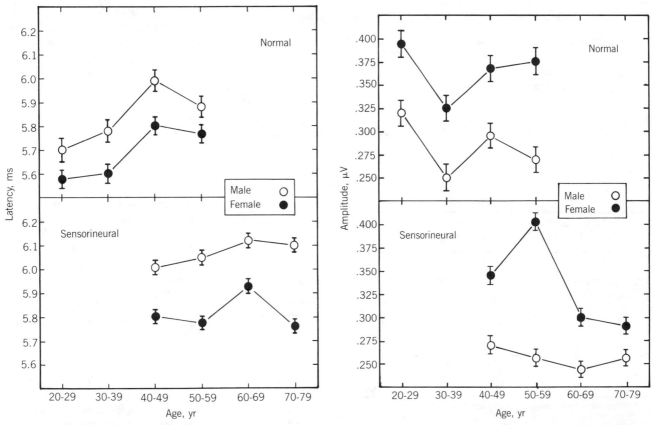

Fig 1.—Mean latency of wave V of auditory brainstem response as function of age for male and female subjects with both normal hearing (N = 98) and sensorineural hearing loss (N = 221). Brackets indicate SEM.

Fig 2.—Mean amplitude of wave V of auditory brainstem response as function of age for male and female subjects with both normal hearing (N = 98) and sensorineural hearing loss (N = 221). Brackets indicate SEM.

male subjects, especially in the older age groups, had more high-frequency sensitivity loss than female subjects. To control for this factor, we formed two matched subgroups of 35 male and 35 female subjects from the total sensorineural pool. The subgroups were selected in such a way that average age and average audiometric contour were matched as closely as possible. Table 3 summarizes average audiometric threshold HLs for these male and female subgroups. At all test frequencies, average threshold levels for the two sexes were within 3 dB, except at 8,000 Hz, where female subjects were actually 12 dB poorer than male subjects. Again, if this difference at 8,000 Hz had an effect on the ABR, it would be in the direction of penalizing female subjects. Thus, shorter latency and larger amplitude in the female subgroup cannot be attributed to audiometric contour.

Table 4 summarizes mean latency and amplitude measures for these two matched sensorineural subgroups. Wave V latency was an average of 0.250 ms shorter in the female group, and wave V amplitude was an average of 0.069 μV larger.

COMMENT

Two conclusions seem warranted. First, there is a slight age effect on the ABR. In subjects with normal hearing, latency increased about 0.20 ms over the age range from 25 to 55 years, and amplitude decreased about 0.050 μV. Beagley and Sheldrake[53] noted a similar but smaller effect in 70 normal subjects. In the sensorineural group, age had relatively little effect on latency, but amplitude showed the same 0.050-μV decrease. The age effect, albeit relatively modest, should be taken into account in ABR audiometry. Slightly delayed wave V latency, and smaller wave V amplitude, must be expected in older patients.

Second, there is a pronounced sex effect in the ABR. In subjects with normal hearing, female subjects showed consistently shorter latency and larger amplitude at all age levels. Beagley and Sheldrake[53] noted a similar effect on latency in their 70 normal subjects. In contrast to the influence of age, the differential effect of sex on the ABR seems to be slightly enhanced by sensorineural loss.

The clinical implications of the age and sex effects in the ABR are important. For example, the proportion of male to female subjects in normative data groups is a prime consideration. Many audiology facilities, especially in university settings, find it convenient to test young, normal-hearing female subjects during the standardization process.

Values derived from such groups must be regarded as highly suspect when used as a normal standard for evaluation of the clinical population. In fact, in evaluating the ABR in older, adult male subjects, the use of such normal values could easily con-

Table 1.—Means and Standard Deviations of Threshold Hearing Levels in Normal Group*

Sex	No.	Measure	Frequency, Hz					
			250	500	1,000	2,000	4,000	8,000
M	40	Mean	8.54	8.23	5.23	3.45	10.30	11.50
		SD	7.81	6.12	5.55	6.13	7.04	15.88
F	58	Mean	10.71	7.43	5.80	3.91	9.18	12.79
		SD	10.60	9.71	6.18	6.63	7.6	15.05

*N = 98.

Table 2.—Sex Differences in Wave V Latency and Amplitude for 98 Subjects With Normal Hearing

Measure	Index	Sex		Sex Difference	P*
		M	F		
Sample size	No.	40	58	...	...
Age, yr	Mean	39.0	40.0	...	...
Wave V latency, ms	Mean	5.83	5.69	0.14	.020
	SD	0.34	0.30	...	...
	SEM	0.05	0.04	...	...
Wave V amplitude, μV	Mean	0.284	0.372	0.088	< .003
	SD	0.081	0.124	...	...
	SEM	0.013	0.016	...	...

*Probability of incorrectly rejecting null hypothesis (α error).

Table 3.—Means and Standard Deviations of Threshold Hearing Levels in Matched Sensorineural Loss Subgroups

Sex	No.	Measure	Test Frequency, Hz					
			250	500	1,000	2,000	4,000	8,000
M	35	Mean	17.50	16.70	19.00	23.77	46.87	39.59
		SD	10.69	11.23	14.09	17.68	12.47	20.93
F	35	Mean	19.80	19.00	17.97	28.13	45.67	51.93
		SD	12.82	10.18	9.08	13.84	14.47	18.51

Table 4.—Sex Differences in Wave V Latency and Amplitude for 70 Selected Subjects With Sensorineural Hearing Loss

Measure	Index	Sex		Sex Difference	P*
		M	F		
Sample size	No.	35	35	...	...
Age, yr	Mean	55.0	55.5	...	...
Wave V latency, ms	Mean	5.99	5.74	0.25	< .002
	SD	0.31	0.34	...	...
	SEM	0.05	0.06	...	...
Wave V amplitude, μV	Mean	0.268	0.328	0.069	.026
	SD	0.088	0.136	...	...
	SEM	0.015	0.023	...	...

*Probability of incorrectly rejecting null hypothesis (α error).

tribute to inaccurate clinical interpretation. For example, at a signal intensity of 85 dB HL, the average wave V latency in our young female subjects was less than 5.6 ms. At the same signal intensity, the average wave V latency in our male subjects of 40 to 49 years was greater than 6.0 ms. Since the standard deviation for the wave V latency in the young female group was about 0.20 ms, the latency of the older male subjects would, in comparison, appear abnormally delayed.

We have stressed that both age and sex must be routinely considered in the generation of normal values for the ABR. Since the Jewett and Williston[1] 1971 report, abundant data on the normal ABR have been reported in the literature. We hypothesized that by compiling these normal data, and examining them for age and sex effects, we might augment the present findings. With this objective in mind, we surveyed 37 studies reporting ABR data for 617 normal adults, published from 1971 to 1978. In general, information on subject age and sex was rarely reported. Only 6% of the studies reported ABR data as a function of age. Of the remaining studies, 56% reported only the age range of subjects; 36% provide no age data. Subject sex was noted in 67% of the studies. The ABR data were reported as a function of subject sex in only two studies (6% of the total). Thus, although normal data for the ABR have been reported for at least 617 subjects, the effects of age and sex are accounted for in only 120 or 19%. Clearly, the potential influences of age and sex on the ABR have been grossly unappreciated.

The age effect on the ABR was not unexpected. Anatomic and physiologic changes in the peripheral and central auditory system have long been associated with aging.[56-59] It is not unreasonable to expect that the ABR would reflect such changes. What, then, is the basis of the sex difference in the ABR? We can only speculate with Stockard et al[55] that, due to the relatively smaller dimensions of the female CNS, neural transmission time of the ABR is reduced. The actual basis for the conspicuous sex difference deserves further investigation.

References

1. Jewett DL, Williston JS: Auditory-evoked far fields averaged from the scalp of humans. *Brain* 94:681-696, 1971.

2. Terkildsen K, Osterhammel P, Hius in't Veld F: Electrocochleography with a far-field technique. *Scand Audiol* 2:141-148, 1973.

3. Hecox K, Galambos R: Brainstem auditory evoked responses in human infants and adults. *Arch Otolaryngol* 99:30-33, 1974.

4. Picton TW, Hillyard SA, Krausz HI, et al: Human auditory evoked potentials: I. Evaluation of components. *Electroencephalogr Clin Neurophysiol* 36:179-190, 1974.

5. Yamada O, Yagi T, Yamane H, et al: Clinical evaluation of the auditory evoked brain stem response. *Auris Nasus Larynx* 2:97-105, 1975.

6. Hyde ML, Stephens SDG, Thornton ARD: Stimulus repetition rate and the early brainstem responses. *Br J Audiol* 10:41-50, 1976.

7. Don M, Allen AR, Starr A: Effect of click rate on the latency of auditory brainstem responses in humans. *Ann Otol* 86:186-195, 1977.

8. Goff WR, Allison T, Lyons W, et al: Origins of short latency auditory evoked potentials in man. *Prog Clin Neurophysiol* 2:30-44, 1977.

9. Rowe MJ III: Normal variability of the brainstem auditory evoked response in young and old adult subjects. *Electroencephalogr Clin Neurophysiol* 44:459-470, 1978.

10. Salamy A, McKean CM, Pettett G, et al: Auditory brainstem recovery processes from birth to adulthood. *Psychophysiology* 15:214-220, 1978.

11. Chiappa KH, Gladstone KJ, Young RR: Brainstem auditory evoked responses: Studies of waveform variations in 50 normal human subjects. *Arch Neurol* 36:81-87, 1979.

12. Robinson K, Rudge P: Auditory evoked responses in multiple sclerosis. *Lancet* 1:1164-1166, 1975.

13. Robinson K, Rudge P: Abnormalities of the auditory evoked potentials in patients with multiple sclerosis. *Brain* 100:19-40, 1977.

14. Starr A, Achor LJ: Auditory brainstem responses in neurological disease. *Arch Neurol* 32:761-768, 1975.

15. Stockard JJ, Rossiter VS, Wiederholt WL, et al: Brainstem auditory evoked responses in suspected central pontine myelinolysis. *Arch Neurol* 33:726-728, 1976.

16. Chiappa KH, Norwood AE: A comparison of the clinical utility of pattern-shift visual evoked responses and brainstem auditory evoked responses in multiple sclerosis. *Neurology* 27:397, 1977.

17. Chiappa KH, Norwood AE: Brainstem auditory evoked responses in clinical neurology: Utility and neuropathological correlates. *Electroencephalogr Clin Neurophysiol* 43:518, 1977.

18. Clemis JD, Mitchell C: Electrocochelography and brainstem responses used in the diagnosis of acoustic tumors. *J Otolaryngol* 6:447-459, 1977.

19. Coats AC, Martin JL: Human auditory nerve action potentials and brainstem evoked responses: Effects of audiogram shape and lesion location. *Arch Otolaryngol* 103:605-622, 1977.

20. Daly DM, Roeser RJ, Aung MH, et al: Early evoked potentials in patients with acoustic neuroma. *Electroencephalogr Clin Neurophysiol* 43:151-159, 1977.

21. Gilroy J, Lynn GE, Riston GE, et al: Auditory evoked brainstem potentials in a case of "locked-in" syndrome. *Arch Neurol* 34:492-495, 1977.

22. Rosenhamer HJ: Observations on electric brainstem responses in retrocochlear hearing loss. *Scand Audiol* 6:179-196, 1977.

23. Selters WA, Brackman DE: Acoustic tumor detection with brainstem electric response audiometry. *Arch Otolaryngol* 103:181-187, 1977.

24. Selters WA, Brackmann DE: Brainstem electric response audiometry in acoustic tumor detection, in House WF, Leutje CM (eds): *Acoustic Tumors*. Baltimore, University Park Press, 1979, vol 1, pp 225-235.

25. Stockard JJ, Rossiter VS: Clinical and pathologic correlates of brainstem auditory response abnormalities. *Neurology* 27:316-325, 1977.

26. Stockard JJ, Stockard JE, Sharbrough FW: Detection and localization of occult lesions with brainstem auditory responses. *Mayo Clin Proc* 52:761-769, 1977.

27. Terkildsen K, Hius in't Veld F, Osterhammel P: Auditory brainstem responses in the diagnosis of cerebellopontine angle tumors. *Scand Audiol* 6:43-47, 1977.

28. Jerger J, Mauldin L: Prediction of sensorineural hearing level from the brainstem evoked response. *Arch Otolaryngol* 104:456-461, 1978.

29. Jerger J, Mauldin L, Anthony L: Brainstem evoked response audiometry. *Audiol Hear Ed*, June/July 1978, pp 17-19.

30. Thomsen J, Terkildsen K, Osterhammel P: Auditory brainstem responses in patients with acoustic neuromas. *Scand Audiol* 7:179-183, 1978.

31. Lieberman A, Sohmer H, Szabo G: Cochlear audiometry (electrocochleography) during the neonatal period. *Dev Med Child Neurol* 15:8-13, 1973.

32. Salamy A, McKean CM, Borda FB: Maturational changes in auditory transmission as reflected in human brainstem potentials. *Brain Res* 96:361-366, 1975.

33. Schulman-Galambos C, Galambos R: Brainstem auditory-evoked responses in premature infants. *J Speech Hear Res* 18:456-465, 1975.

34. Salamy A, McKean CM: Postnatal development of human brainstem potentials during the first year of life. *Electroencephalogr Clin Neurophysiol* 40:418-426, 1976.

35. Mokotoff B, Schulman-Galambos C, Galambos R: Brainstem auditory evoked responses in children. *Arch Otolaryngol* 103:38-43, 1977.

36. Bunch CC: Age variations in auditory acuity. *Arch Otolaryngol* 9:625-636, 1929.

37. Goetzinger CP, Proud GO, Dirks D, et al: Study of hearing in advanced age. *Arch Otolaryngol* 73:662-674, 1961.

38. Saxén A: Inner ear in presbycusis. *Acta Otolaryngol* 41:213-227, 1952.

39. König E: Pitch discrimination and age. *Acta Otolaryngol* 48:473-489, 1957.

40. Hayes D, Jerger J: Aging and hearing aid use. *Scand Audiol* 8:33-40, 1979.

41. Gaeth JH: *A Study of Phonemic Regression in Relation to Hearing Loss*, thesis. Northwestern University, Evanston, Ill, 1948.

42. Pestalozza G, Shore I: Clinical evaluation of presbycusis on the basis of different tests of auditory function. *Laryngoscope* 65:1136-1163, 1955.

43. Jerger J: Audiologic findings in aging. *Adv Otorhinolaryngol* 20:115-124, 1973.

44. Jerger J, Jerger S, Mauldin L: Studies in impedance audiometry: I. Normal and sensorineural ears. *Arch Otolaryngol* 96:513-523, 1972.

45. Hall JW: Effects of age and sex on static compliance. *Arch Otolaryngol* 105:153-156, 1979.

46. Jerger J, Hayes D, Anthony L, et al: Factors influencing prediction of hearing level from the acoustic reflex. *Contemp Monogr Audiol* 1:1-20, 1978.

47. Hall JW: Predicting hearing level from the acoustic reflex: A comparison of three methods. *Arch Otolaryngol* 104:601-605, 1978.

48. Gersdorff MC: Modifications du reflexe acoustico-facial chez l'homme en fonction de l'age, par etude impedancemetrique. *Audiology* 17:260-270, 1978.

49. Bunch CC, Raiford TS: Race and sex variations in auditory acuity. *Arch Otolaryngol* 13:423-434, 1931.

50. Corso JF: Aging and auditory thresholds in men and women. *Arch Environ Health* 6:350-356, 1963.

51. Hall JW: Impedance audiometry in a young population: Effects of age, sex, and minor tympanogram abnormality. *J Otolaryngology*, to be published.

52. Thomsen J, Terkildsen K, Osterhammel P: Auditory brainstem responses in persons with acoustic neuromas. *Scand Audiol* 7:179-183, 1979.

53. Beagley HA, Sheldrake JB: Differences on brainstem response latency with age and sex. *Br J Audiol* 12:69-77, 1978.

54. Fujikawa SM, Weber BA: Effects of increased stimulus rate on brainstem electric response (BER) audiometry as a function of age. *J Am Audiol Soc* 3:147-150, 1977.

55. Stockard JJ, Stockard JE, Sharbrough FW: Nonpathologic factors influencing brainstem auditory evoked potentials. *Am J EEG Technol* 18:177-209, 1978.

56. Schuknecht HF: Presbycusis. *Laryngoscope* 65:402-419, 1955.

57. Kirikae I, Sato T, Shitara T: A study of hearing in advanced age. *Laryngoscope* 74:205-220, 1964.

58. Kirikae I: Auditory function in advanced age with reference to histological changes in the central auditory system. *Int Audiol* 8:221-230, 1969.

59. Hanson CC, Reske-Nielsen E: Pathological studies in presbycusis. *Arch Otolaryngol* 82:115-132, 1965.

Invited Paper

Clinical Experience with Auditory Brainstem Response Audiometry in Pediatric Assessment

James Jerger, Deborah Hayes, and Connie Jordan

ABSTRACT

We discuss our experience with evaluation of 167 children by auditory brainstem response audiometry in 1978. We summarize experience with referral sources, medication for sedation, and interpretation of test outcome. Medication for sedation was required for 136 children. Concommitant central nervous system involvement rendered auditory brainstem response ambiquous in some children; however, the technique still provide useful information about status of peripheral auditory sensitivity obtainable in no other way. Finally, agreement among auditory brainstem response, behavioral, and impedance audiometry predictions was usually quite good.

INTRODUCTION

During the past 5 years, auditory brainstem response (ABR) audiometry has come to play an increasingly important role in pediatric audiological assessment (1–7, 9, 12). In children who can be tested by conventional behavioral and/or impedance techniques, ABR audiometry provides an invaluable cross-check on the behavioral and/or impedance prediction (3, 4). In children who cannot be successfully tested by conventional techniques, ABR audiometry may provide the only basis for prediction of auditory status. It is an especially powerful technique for the evaluation of very young infants and multiply handicapped children (2, 5, 9). For these reasons, an increasing number of audiologists and audiology centers have added ABR audiometry to their pediatric test battery, and still other audiologists are contemplating such action.

We address this brief report to the latter group in the hope that our clinical experience with ABR audiometry at the Neurosensory Center of Houston will assist them in evaluating the advantages, disadvantages, and problems associated with the technique.

In this report, we summarize our experience with the evaluation of children by ABR audiometry during a 1-year period, 1978. We present results for only 1 year because our medication for sedation procedure underwent several modifications, until its present form was finally established in late 1977. We present results of 1978 then as illustrative of our experience during a period when our procedure for sedation was standardized. We specifically discuss experience with referral sources, medication for sedation, and interpretation of test outcome.

CLINICAL EXPERIENCE

In the 1-year period, January through December, 1978, we evaluated 665 children by various audiometric techniques. Of these, 167 children, or 25%, of all children tested, were evaluated by ABR audiometry. Age ranged from 4 days to 83 months. The decision to carry out ABR audiometry in these children was made either to confirm behavioral and/or impedance test results or to define sensitivity level in high-risk infants or multiply involved children whose evaluation by more conventional test procedures yielded only limited information.

Referral Sources

Children were referred for ABR audiometry by a variety of sources. Table 1 summarizes the distribution of referral sources of the 167 children tested in 1978. Otolaryngologists referred more children for ABR audiometry than did any other source. They accounted for 75 referrals (45%). Audiologists referred another 47 children (28%). Pediatricians accounted for 21 referrals (13%), and neurologists accounted for 15 referrals (9%). Finally, 9 children (5%) were referred from other sources. These included school districts, centers for the multiply handicapped, and university speech and hearing programs.

It is not surprising that otolaryngologists and other audiologists accounted for the majority (73%) of referrals. Still, 1 in 5 children was referred by either a pediatrician or a neurolgist. In essence, the addition of ABR audiometry to our clinical services has had the effect of broadening our referral basis.

Medication for ABR Audiometry

To ensure adequate technical quality for recording auditory brainstem responses, the child must be either resting quietly or asleep. Most children, therefore, must be medicated with a mild sedative.

Our sedation procedure is as follows. At the time an appointment for ABR audiometry is scheduled, the referral source is asked to provide an order for sedation. All orders are written on a 3-part standard form. The physician completes part A, which specifies the type and amount of medication ordered. The parent or guardian completes part B, which authorizes administration of the medication. Finally, the recovery room nurse, who administers the medication, completes part C. This section records the time of drug administration. A permanent copy of the 3-part sedation form is kept both in the recovery room files and in the Audiology Service's patient record.

On the day of testing, the child is taken to the postoperative recovery room of the neurosensory center. The parent or guardian signs part B of the sedation form, and a recovery room nurse administers the medication. The child is then returned to the Audiology Service and placed with his parents in a quiet, darkened room. If the medication fails to take effect in approximately 30 to 45 min and the child remains awake and active, he is returned to the recovery room for remedication, if authorized.

Once the child is asleep, he is placed in a standard hospital crib in the ABR test suite. Electrodes are attached, and testing begins. Upon completion of testing, the child is released from the Audiology Service. If he is awake, he is released to go home. If, however, the child is still asleep, he is returned to the recovery room. The recovery room medical staff monitors the child until sedation has effectively worn off. The child is then released to go home.

In our experience, chloral hydrate in rectal suppository form provides a safe, effective sedation for ABR audiometry. A dose of 40 to 50 mg/kg of body weight usually induces sleep of sufficient duration to permit complete evaluation by ABR

audiometry (25 to 35 min). In those cases where chloral hydrate is not effective, some combination of demerol (meperidine), phenergran (promethazine), and thorazine (chlorpromazine) is usually recommended. In a few instances (4 in 1978), children are sedated with nembutal (pentobarbital). In general, the nature of the medication inducing the level of sleep necessary for ABR audiometry is not critical (8).

Table 2 summarizes our experience with medication for sedation of the 167 children evaluated by ABR audiometry in 1978. Not all children required sedation. Thirty-one (18%) could be tested without medication. These children were either (1) in natural sleep, or (2) sitting quietly. One child was tested while comatose. Age was bimodally distributed within this group. Sixteen of 31 children were age 12 months or younger; 9 were age 60 months or older.

Eighty-four children (50%) were sedated effectively with a single administration of chloral hydrate; five (3%) were sedated effectively with a single administration of another medication. These included medication with nembutal (3 children) and medication with demerol, phenergran, and thorazine (2 children). Average age of children sedated with chloral hydrate was 23 months. Average age of children sedated with other medications was 31 months.

Thirty-six children could be tested only after 2 administrations of medication. Twenty children (12%) were both medicated and remedicated with chloral hydrate. Sixteen children (10%) were either medicated initially with chloral hydrate and remedicated with another drug or both medicated and remedicated with a drug other than chloral hydrate. Some combination of demerol, phenergran, and thorazine was the most usual medication (10 children). Average age of children sedated with chloral hydrate was 30 months; average age of children sedated with other drugs was 28 months.

In 10 children (6%), medication was not effective. These children could not be evaluated by ABR audiometry because medication failed to induce the necessary sedated state. Chloral hydrate (6 children) and demerol, phenergran, and thorazine (4 children) were the medications administered. Average age of these children was 40 months.

Finally, one child, age 41 months, was tested under general anesthesia. This child was hospitalized for middle ear surgery. ABR audiometry was carried out in the operating room immediately before surgery.

When we first initiated ABR audiometry in our pediatric service, we had hoped that medication for sedation would be unnecessary. From our experience both with and without

Table 1. Distribution of referral source of 167 children (age 4 days to 83 months) evaluated by ABR audiometry in 1978

Referral Source	N	%
Otolaryngologist	75	45
Audiologist	47	28
Pediatrician	21	13
Neurologist	15	9
Other	9	5

Table 2. Experience with medication of 167 children for ABR audiometry in 1978.

	N	%	Average Age (mos.)	Range (mos.)
Medication not necessary	31	18	[a]	1–83
Medicated once- chloral hydrate	84	50	23	1–83
Medicated once- other	5	3	31	12–54
Medicated twice- chloral hydrate	20	12	30	6–72
Medicated twice- other	16	10	28	11–51
Medication not effective	10	6	40	26–67
Tested under general anesthesia	1	<1	41	

[a] Bimodal age distribution. Sixteen children age 12 months and younger; 6 children age 13 to 59 months; 9 children age 60 months and older.

medication, however, we came to the reluctant conclusion that medication for sedation was usually necessary with children tested. It is a fact of life to which the audiologist who contemplates pediatric assessment must resign himself. In addition, in our experience, this has been the single most frustrating aspect of the activity. Unless medication is effective on first application, successful testing may be a time-consuming, difficult process requiring considerable professional dedication to the task at hand. On the positive side, however, we have been encouraged by the fact that with a vigorous commitment to medication almost all children referred to us (94% in 1978) could be successfully tested.

Effect of CNS Involvement on Test Interpretation

Interpreting the outcome of ABR audiometry in children is not always straightforward. When responses to click signals at 80 to 90 dB HL are absent and the child has no obvious central nervous system (CNS) involvement, we may predict with reasonable certainty the presence of at least a severe hearing loss. However, when the ABR response is absent, but the child has concomitant CNS involvement, the test result may be ambiguous. In this case, absence of the response may be due to profound peripheral sensitivity loss or to central auditory pathway disorder at the brainstem level (9–11). In this situation, absence of the response as an indication of severe hearing loss must be interpreted cautiously.

To examine our ability to interpret unambiguously ABR results, the 157 children successfully evaluated in 1978 (10 of the original total of 167 could not be effectively sedated) were classified by CNS integrity. Children with no known history, diagnosis, or behavior consistent with CNS involvement were classified as "uninvolved." Children with previous diagnosis of CNS disorder were classified as "involved." Included in this category were children with cerebal palsy, mental retardation, cerebral atrophy, Down's syndrome, hydrocephalus, microcephaly, and seizure disorders. One hundred twenty-six children (80%) were classified as uninvolved; 31 children (20%) were classified as involved.

Table 3 shows 3 levels of sensitivity predicted by ABR audiometry for both uninvolved and involved children. An ABR in either or both ears at 40 dB HL or less was considered consistent with a prediction of "normal sensitivity or mild sensitivity loss." An ABR in either ear to click signals of 50 to 90 dB HL was considered consistent with a prediction of "moderate to severe sensitivity loss." Finally, absence of an ABR in both ears to click signals of 90 dB HL was regarded as consistent with a prediction of "profound sensitivity loss."

Results of ABR audiometry in 72 uninvolved children (46% of the total group) were consistent with normal sensitivity or mild sensitivity loss. Results in 24 uninvolved children (15% of the total group) were consistent with a moderate-to-severe sensitivity loss. Finally, results of ABR audiometry in 30 uninvolved children (19% of the total group were consistent with a profound sensitivity loss.

Fourteen involved children (9% of the total group) exhibited responses consistent with normal sensitivity or a mild sensitivity loss; 8 involved children (5% of the total group) demonstrated responses consistent with a moderate-to-severe sensitivity loss. Finally, in 9 involved children (6% of the total group), no ABR was observed at 90 dB HL.

Table 3. Summary of degree of sensitivity loss predicted by ABR audiometry in 157 children evaluated in 1978. Children are categorized by CNS integrity.

	Uninvolved		Involved	
	N	% of total	N	% of total
Normal-to-mild sensitivity loss (ABR threshold from 0–40 dBHL)	72	46	14	9
Moderate-to-severe sensitivity loss (ABR threshold from 50–90 dBHL)	24	15	8	5
Profound sensitivity loss (no ABR at 90 dBHL)	30	19	9	6

In the 14 involved children with normal-to-mild sensitivity loss, results were useful and unambiguous in showing that at least peripheral auditory sensitivity was quite good. In the 8 children with moderate-to-severe prediction, we can only say that peripheral sensitivity can be no worse than the prediction, but might be better than predicted. We cannot exclude the possibility that the CNS involvement has compromised ABR amplitude. In the 9 children with absent ABR at 90 dB HL, the situation is quite ambiguous. We cannot tell whether the ABR is absent due to severe hearing loss or simply to the CNS involvement.

Thus, of the total of 31 CNS-involved children tested, results could be considered unambiguous in only 14. In the remaining 17 children, results were either relatively (8 children) or totally (9 children) ambiguous in the sense that the effects of peripheral hearing disorder could not be differentiated from the effects of generalized CNS involvement.

Thus, in children with concomitant CNS involvement, the information obtained from ABR audiometry is, in a certain sense, nontransitive. That is, when responses are relatively normal they contribute valuable information about peripheral sensitivity. But when responses are abnormal or absent, the information contributed by ABR is to a greater or lesser extent ambiguous.

Agreement with Cross-checks

In general, our approach to pediatric audiometry uses the "cross-check principle." That is, the results of a single test are cross-checked by an independent test measure. Whenever possible, therefore, results of ABR audiometry are cross-checked by impedance audiometry and/or behavioral audiometry. Behavioral audiometry is usually attempted before the child is medicated for ABR audiometry; impedance audiometry is usually attempted after ABR audiometry while the child is still sedated.

Of the 157 children successfully evaluated by ABR audiometry in 1978, results were cross-checked in 141. No cross-check was available for 16 children. Either (1) the child slept through the evaluation, and behavioral testing could not be carried out; (2) impedance audiometry was noncontributory in quantifying sensorineural level due to middle ear disorder; or (3) the child awoke before impedance audiometry could be attempted.

Table 4 summarizes agreement among ABR audiometry and its cross-checks in the 141 children who were additionally evaluated with impedance and/or behavioral audiometry.

Table 4. Agreement among ABR audiometry, impedance audiometry, and behavioral audiometry in 2 groups of children categorized by CNS integrity and ABR sensitivity prediction

Number in each group reflects number of children in whom cross-checks were available. Some groups, therefore, may be smaller than original number tested (see Table 3).

| | Agreement among Tests | | | |
| | Uninvolved Child | | Involved Child | |
	Con-sistent	Incon-sistent	Con-sistent	Incon-sistent
ABR prediction				
Normal-to-mild loss	60	3	10	4
Moderate-to-severe loss	19	2	6	0
Profound loss	29	0	8	0
Total	108	5	24	4

Children are categorized by both CNS involvement (uninvolved versus involved) and by ABR prediction of hearing sensitivity.

Table 4 shows that for both groups of children results of ABR audiometry were usually consistent with results of impedance audiometry and/or behavioral audiometry. Of the 63 uninvolved children with a normal or mild loss prediction whose results could be cross-checked, results of ABR audiometry were consistent with impedance and/or behavioral audiometry in 60 children and inconsistent in only 3 children.[1] Of the 21 uninvolved children with a moderate-to-severe prediction, results of ABR audiometry were consistent with results of impedance and/or behavioral audiometry in 19 children and inconsistent in only 2 children. Finally, of the 29 uninvolved children with a profound prediction, results of ABR audiometry were consistent with results of impedance audiometry and/or behavioral audiometry in all 29 children. In this group, there were no inconsistencies among test results.

Agreement among test results of involved children with normal-to-mild sensitivity loss prediction was somewhat poorer than agreement among test results of uninvolved children with similar sensitivity prediction. In the involved group, test results were consistent in 10 children but inconsistent in 4 children. In both the moderate-to-severe and the profound prediction categories of involved children, however, there were no inconsistencies among test results. Results of ABR audiometry were consistent with results of impedance and/or behavioral audiometry in all children tested.

Although there were no inconsistencies among test results in the group of involved children with absent ABR (profound sensitivity loss prediction), the interpretation of a peripheral sensitivity loss in this group must necessarily remain uncertain. Results of both behavioral and impedance audiometry may be compromised by a brainstem auditory pathway disorder in a fashion similar to the auditory brainstem response. Thus, site

[1] Results were considered inconsistent when ABR audiometry predicted normal sensitivity to mild sensitivity loss and either behavioral and/or impedance audiometry predicted severe or profound sensitivity loss. Most inconsistencies arose between ABR audiometry and behavioral audiometry. In agreement with Mokotoff et al. (4) we found that ABR Audiometry and results of impedance audiometry agreed in a vast majority of cases.

Table 5. Role of ABR audiometry in the audiometric evaluation of 157 children, age 4 days to 83 months

	N	%
Only test available	16	10
Confirm conventional test results (impedance and/or behavioral audiometry)	132	84
Fails to confirm conventional test results	9	6

of auditory disorder (peripheral vesus central) in these involved children remains relatively ambiguous.

Table 5 summarizes the contribution of ABR audiometry to the audiometric assessment of all 157 children tested in 1978. In 16 children (10%), ABR audiometry was the only test result available. Prediction of hearing sensitivity, then, was dependent solely on these results. In 132 children (84%), ABR audiometry provided confirmatory information. In these children, results of ABR audiometry agreed with results of more conventional test procedures. Finally, in 9 children (6%) ABR audiometry failed to confirm results of more conventional test procedures; results of ABR audiometry did not agree with results of either behavioral or impedance audiometry.

SUMMARY

Audiologists and audiology centers contemplating the addition of ABR audiometry to their pediatric test battery should consider the following important factors.

First, medication for sedation is the single most challenging aspect of the technique. In our experience, almost every child in the age range 0 to 6 years requires some form of medication to induce sleep of sufficient depth and duration to carry out the test. With a vigorous commitment to medication and the cooperation of the medical staff at the Neurosensory Center, we have arrived at what we consider to be a safe, effective procedure for medication. In fact, we were able to to complete ABR audiometry successfully in 94% of all children scheduled for this technique in 1978. In only 6% of cases did ineffective sedation preclude evaluation. We recommend that audiologists contemplating ABR audiometry for children work out a procedure for medication with the medical staff at their facility prior to initiating the service.

Second, the presence of concommitant CNS involvement may render ABR results ambiguous. In our 1978 series, results in 17 of 31 children with CNS involvement were to some extent ambiguous due to CNS disorder. In spite of this problem, however, ABR results in this group of children often provided useful data about status of the peripheral auditory system obtainable in no other way.

Finally, in our experience, agreements among ABR, behavioral, and impedance audiometry predictions is typically quite good. In our 1978 series of children, the 3 techniques showed good agreement in 132 children, and poor agreement in only 9 children.

Our experience with ABR audiometry in pediatric, audiometric assessment has been positive. We have found that the results of ABR audiometry provide an invaluable cross-check on behavioral and impedance audiometry and often provide the only available information on auditory status in difficult-to-test infants and children. Nonetheless, ABR audiometry for children may not be useful or even desirable in all settings. Specifically, in audiology centers where medical facilities and personnel are not available to administer and monitor sedation, ABR audiometry may not be a feasible procedure. Similarly, in centers with a limited pediatric case load, ABR audiometry may not be cost effective.

References

1. Davis, H., and S. Hirsh. 1976. The audiometric utility of brain stem responses to low-frequency sounds. Audiology (Basel) **15**, 181–195.
2. Hecox, K., and R. Galambos. 1974. Brain stem auditory evoked responses in human infants and adults. Arch. Otolaryngol. **99**, 30–33.
3. Jerger, J., and D. Hayes. 1976. The cross-check principle in pediatric audiometry. Arch. Otolaryngol. **102**, 614–620.
4. Mokotoff, B., C. Schulman-Galambos, and R. Galambos. 1977. Brain stem auditory responses in children. Arch. Otolaryngol. **103**, 38–43.
5. Schulman-Galambos, C., and R. Galambos. 1979. Brain stem evoked response audiometry in newborn hearing screening. Arch. Otolaryngol. **105**, 86–90.
6. Sohmer, H., and M. Feinmesser. 1973. Routine use of electrocochleography (cochlear audiometry) on human subjects. Audiology (Basel) **12**, 167–173.
7. Sohmer, H., and M. Feinmesser. 1974. Electrocochleography in clinical audiological diagnosis. Arch. Oto-Rhino-Laryngol. **206**, 91–102.
8. Sohmer, H., M. Gafni, and R. Chisin. 1978. Auditory nerve and brain stem responses: comparison in awake and unconscious subjects. Arch. Neurol. **35**, 228–230.
9. Sohmer, H., and M. Student. 1978. Auditory nerve and brain-stem evoked responses in normal, autistic, minimal brain dysfunction and psychomotor retarded children. Electroencephalogr. Clin. Neurophysiol. **44**, 380–388.
10. Starr, A., and J. Achor. 1975. Auditory brain stem responses in neurological disease. Arch. Neurol. **32**, 761–768.
11. Stockard, J., and V. Rossiter. 1977. Clinical and pathologic correlates of brain stem auditory response abnormalities. Neurology **27**, 316–325.
12. Suzuki, M., and J. Suzuki. 1977. Clinical application of the auditory evoked brain stem response in children. Auris-Nasus-Larynx (Tokyo) **4**, 19–26.

From the Division of Audiology and Speech Pathology. Department of Otorhinolaryngology and Communicative Sciences, Baylor College of Medicine and The Methodist Hospital, Houston, Texas 77030.

Acknowledgments: Lorraine Gipe and Jay Hall assisted in data analysis.

Send reprint requests to: Dr. James Jerger, Audiology, Neurosensory Center of Houston, 6501 Fannin Street, NA200, Houston, Texas 77030

Comments of Ralph Naunton, M. D., National Institutes of Health

In describing their impressive experience with ABR audiometry, the authors have provided a valuable practical guide for those entering or already in this field of study. It is refreshing to see a discussion of the vexing problem of the time (and hence cost) commonly involved in working with an unsedated or inadequately sedated child, but this section of the manuscript would be improved were it to include a discussion of the question of responsibility for the care of a sedated child and for the decision that sedation has effectively worn off and the child may go home. In my experience, some children recover more slowly than others, and the slow ones are always those who live 100 miles away; this may require an overnight bed in the hospital or a motel room.

The authors' comments on the ambiguity of results obtained in children with recognized CNS involvement are critical. Just as the neurologist using the test method to assess CNS activity must be cautious lest his results be confounded by a hearing deficit, so the audiologist must recognize that response abnormalities he sees may be wholly or partially the result of recognized or unrecognized CNS disorder. The manuscript would be strengthened by more detailed reference to this important problem.

REPLY TO DR. NAUNTON

Dr. Naunton highlights the importance of safety in medication for sedation of children for ABR audiometry. Care of the sedated child and responsibility for medical release are certianly of paramount importance. We appreciate Dr. Naunton's reemphasis of this point. We have not elaborated on our own procedure in greater detail, however, because the procedure established by any facility must necessarily depend on available staff and resources. A procedure which is acceptable in a medical/surgical hospital may differ substantially from one which is feasible in a private practice office. It is the responsibility of each clinical setting to establish a suitable sedation procedure.

Dr. Naunton also emphasizes the important problem of test result ambiguity in evaluating children with CNS involvement. We refer the interested reader to the important work of Sohmer et al. for further discussion of this problem. Dr. Heiber, in her review of this article, offers some specific suggestions for recognizing and minimizing test result ambiguity.

Comments of Terese Finitzo-Hieber, Callier Center/University of Texas at Dallas

The addition of the ABR assessment to our pediatric test battery has as Jerger et al. point out, proven invaluable in the identification of hearing impairment. I agree, that the ABR procedure is not useful in all audiology setting, but belongs rather in the large referral centers for the reasons mentioned by the authors. Because results are not always unambiguous, accurate interpretation is most likely in centers with large caseloads and more extensive experience with the procedure.

The paper is an excellent introduction for the audiologist about the benefits and pitfalls of the ABR procedure. However, I would like to comment on the routine need for sedation and the large number of patients with ambiguous ABR results.

First, although it has not been our experience that sedation be required on almost every child, I agree that a crying, awake infant is the most frustrating part of the assessment. We seldom sedate the infant (to date over 200 infants) under 12 months. I suspect that because of the "wait it out" attitude of our staff, testing, or more precisely our "waiting time," is slightly longer than that in Houston. However, with luck, we have tested 5 and 6 infants a day without sedation.

Secondly, the authors state that the presence of concomitant CNS involvement rendered ABR results ambiguous in 20% of their cases. This percentage is higher than we have found. Because we use ABR primarily with our intensive care unit infants and multihandicapped children, differentiating peripheral from brainstem involvement has been vital. To facilitate such interpretation, we evaluate multiple parameters of the response beyond the presence or absence of wave V. The ABR threshold and the way wave V latency changes with intensity (the latency-intensity function) provide precise audiological information. However, these 2 parameters cannot be used in isolation. The wave I latency is also important. Neurological information is defined by the conduction time through the brainstem, that is, the wave I to V interval and the relative amplitudes of the various components. In addition, we also compare the changes in latency that occur as the repetition rate of the stimulus is increased.

Thus, in the author's 8 "involved" babies with moderate-to-severe losses, if the I-V interval was normal, but thresholds were elevated and Wave V was prolonged, the diagnosis would be primarily peripheral disease. If the latency of Wave I was WNL but the amplitudes of the components were abnormal, the diagnosis would be primarily neurological. In the absence of an ABR, despite signal presentations of up to 90 or 100 dB, we would state that these infants had a peripheral impairment and that the severity of the loss precluded assessment of the brainstem pathways. If Wave I appeared without additional components, the impairment would again be neurological. Of course, many youngsters often exhibit both brainstem and peripheral impairment.

Certainly, such an approach will not eliminate 100% of the ambiguous ABR results. It has, however, greatly decreased the questionable cases we see. It is our hope that the audiologist will approach the ABR assessment the way audiologists approach impedance audiometry or special testing, by considering and evaluating multiple components of the response. As Dr. Jerger has pointed out, our diagnostic capabilities with impedance audiometry are strengthened with the complete test battery, so too will our ability to differentiate peripheral from brainstem disease be strengthened if the latency of Waves I and V, the interwave interval, and the amplitude ratio are assessed along with the presence or absence of a response.

REPLY TO DR. HEIBER

We agree with Dr. Heiber that sedation of very young children (i.e., 12 months and younger) for ABR audiometry is not always necessary. Of the 31 children we evaluated without sedation in 1978, one one-half (16) were age 12 months and younger. For children between the ages 12 months and 5 years, however, we continue to observe that medication for sedation is almost always necessary.

We have recently introduced the use of videotaped cartoons to amuse unsedated children. The silent cartoons are presented during the entire ABR evaluation. The results have exceeded our initial expectations. Children willingly sit quietly for up to 1 hr of test time while watching cartoons. This technique does not replace sedation, of course, because the children tested while watching cartoons would not have been sedated anyway. It has had the positive result of extending available test time with these children, however.

Dr Heiber's specific suggestions for minimizing test result ambiguity are certainly valuable. We, too, scrutinize multiple parameters of the auditory brainstem response: the absolute wave V latency, the interwave latency of waves I and V, the effect of stimulus repetition rate on response latency, and the monaural/binaural response amplitude ratio. For pediatric applications, many of these components need further experimental investigation to differentiate the effects of maturation and sensorineural hearing loss from the effects of CNS involvement.

REPLY TO DR. HEIBER

We agree that the wave I to V interwave latency is an especially promising technique for differentiating peripheral from central auditory involvement. By conventional vertex to mastoid ABR recording techniques, however, wave I may be observed only to relatively high-intensity (80 dB HL and greater) click stimuli. Unfortunately, stimulus artifact at high-click levels often precludes recording a wave I response, especially in young children. Thus, although we, too, find the wave I to V interwave latency helpful in cases of potentially ambiguous test results, it does not eliminate the problem entirely. In those cases where we are unable to record a wave I and its presence would unequivocally define hearing sensitivity, we refer the child for electrocochleography which is available at another laboratory in The Neurosensory Center.

Comments of Darrell E. Rose, Mayo Clinic

(1) Dr. Jerger et al. make a statement in the introduction section which is somewhat confusing. They state, "In children who can be tested by conventional behavioral and/or impedance techniques, ABR audiometry provides an invaluable cross-check of the behavioral and/or impedance predictions (3, 4)."

Is it possible that for the child who can be tested by conventional behavioral techniques "ABR audiometry" is a gross waste of professional time and money? Is not this a very costly procedure?

(2) Why have the authors failed to define their stimuli? Is it not possible to know what they are comparing (click stimuli (rep rate) from the ABR audiometry with pure tones from behavior? click ABR audiometry with noise from the impedance technique?)

(3) Is it possible to use pure tone pips and obtain information which is more meaningful than with a click?

(4) Why have the authors used the terminology "ABR audiometry" instead of the more widely used "BSER audiometry?"

(5) In the summary, the authors mention 2 rather profound concepts: (*a*) sedation should be used only where a medical staff is present. One is hard pressed to make a case for the use of sedation without medical staff in attendance. Speech and hearing clinics should be made aware of this; (*b*) the authors tie the need for such a procedure with a large pediatric population. In a speech and hearing facility, one might be inclined to justify it on the basis of neurological involvement in adults. However, this type of rationale is equally tough to justify because although the procedure is easier to do with adults and easier to pay for, unjustifiable testing is usually the result.

REPLY TO DR. ROSE

Dr. Rose raises a number of important points that warrant comment. We would reply to each of his 4 questions as follows.

(1) It is certainly possible that ABR audiometry is a waste of time and money for some children who can be tested successfully by behavioral techniques. This could almost be regarded as self-evident. The point we want to stress, however, is that you can never be absolutely sure of the validity of behavioral estimates of sensitivity in all children. Therefore, independent cross-checks are vitally important. Even though you are relatively confident of your behavioral results, you will increase the objectivity of your work by demanding an independent cross-check. This is one of the most important contributions that ABR audiometry makes to modern pediatric assessment. In our experience, the increased cost is more than justified by the increased diagnostic accuracy.

(2) We should have mentioned that our click stimulus is the haversine transformation of a single cycle of a 7500 Hz sinusoid. In previous publications, we have noted that the ABR to this stimulus is dominated by sensitivity in the 1000 to 4000 Hz region, a finding noted by a number of other investigators using similar broad-spectrum, brief-duration impulses.

Dr. Rose is quite right in drawing us out on this point. Clinicians should be aware that, whereas behavioral results may be frequency specific, predictions based on the ABR to clicks and predictions based on relations among acoustic reflex thresholds, are dominated by sensitivity in the 1000 to 4000 Hz range.

(3) In our view, the final answer is not yet in on the value of tone pips for frequency specificity. Based on our own experience to date, we feel (with modestly flagging enthusiasm), that we must continue to regard this as an experimental area worthy of continuing research. We do not feel that the clinical efficacy of tone pips has as yet been adequately documented.

(4) Our use of the "ABR" terminology is based on the unanimous recommendation of the joint *USA-Japan Seminar on Auditory Responses from the Brain Stem* held in Honolulu, Hawaii January 5 to 7, 1979 (see Davis, H. Laryngoscope, **89**, 1336–1339, 1979).

Analysis of Gender Differences in the Auditory Brainstem Response

Christopher P. Dehan, MD; James Jerger, PhD

This study examined the effects of hormones, head size, and oral temperatures on latencies and amplitudes of the auditory brainstem response in 10 young women, 10 young men, and 5 postmenopausal women. Significant gender differences between men's and women's auditory brainstem responses were confirmed. Men showed longer latencies and smaller amplitudes than women. Results showed that oral temperature has little effect on auditory brainstem response latencies and amplitudes. Head size affects waves III, V, and the amplitude of wave V, but is not entirely responsible for the gender latency difference. By examining young women with normal monthly hormonal cycles, significant changes in the absolute latencies of wave V were observed. These changes were correlated with hormonal changes as measured from venous blood samples. It was concluded that the etiology of the gender difference is a combination of hormonal and head-size differences.

INTRODUCTION

Auditory brainstem response (ABR) audiometry has achieved a prominent role in both audiology and otolaryngology since its description by Jewett and Williston in 1971.[1] It has become an important objective measure of hearing. Its many clinical applications include evaluation of newborns with suspected hearing loss and patients with suspected retrocochlear lesions.[2]

Numerous studies of both normal and hearing-impaired subjects have documented significant gender differences in both ABR latencies and amplitudes. Investigators have shown that both absolute and interwave latencies are shorter in women than in men.[3–15] In Kjaer's studies,[6] the average wave V latency of men was .20 millisecond longer than the average women's latency. The latency gender difference in-

creased as the impulse traversed the brainstem: .025 millisecond for wave I, and .087 millisecond for wave III. In addition, women tended to have greater wave I through V amplitudes than men. Because of these gender differences, separate norms have been established for ABR latencies and amplitudes.

The etiology of these gender differences is not clear from the literature. The ABR latency gender differences do not occur in normal young children, and there is not agreement in the literature as to precisely when the adult differences begin. McClelland and McCrea[8] did not find a gender latency difference until age 14, which suggests a relationship to the physical changes of puberty. O'Donovan[16] noted in his studies, however, that gender latency differences were present at age 8.

Most investigators have speculated that the shorter latencies in women were due to the smaller dimension of the brainstem, resulting in reduced neural transmission times. Until recently, studies demonstrating head size as a cause of the gender difference were lacking. Trune, et al.[14] looked at the relative importance of head size, gender, and age on the ABR and demonstrated that the ABRs of men and women were sensitive to head-size changes. However, when they compared men and women with similar head sizes, the women still had shorter latencies. Trune, et al. concluded that head size explained only part of the gender difference. Another study by Antonelli, et al.[17] showed that brainstem length, as measured by magnetic resonance imaging (MRI), correlated with wave V latency and I to V interpeak latency.

Jerger and Johnson[18] studied the interrelationship of age, gender, and sensorineural hearing loss (SNHL) on ABR latencies and found that younger women (less than 50 years) with SNHL had shorter ABR wave V latencies as compared to older women (greater than 50 years) with a similar SNHL. When ABR wave V latencies in younger men and older men with similar SNHL were compared, there was no statistical difference. Jerger and Johnson concluded that factors other than head size must distinguish the younger women

Presented at the Meeting of the Southern Section of the American Laryngological, Rhinological and Otological Society, Inc., Naples, Fla., January 14, 1989.

From the Department of Otorhinolaryngology and Communicative Sciences, Baylor College of Medicine, Houston.

Send Reprint Requests to James Jerger, PhD, Department of Otorhinolaryngology and Communicative Sciences, Baylor College of Medicine, One Baylor Plaza, Houston, TX 77030.

from the older women to account for the latency difference and suggested the possibility of a hormonal effect.

The effect of body temperature is also related to ABR latencies and amplitudes. Numerous investigators have shown that a decrease in body temperature can increase the latencies of ABR waves I to V in both experimental animals and humans.[19–21] In addition, Marshall and Donchin[22] have shown that variations in ABR waves I, III, and V occurred in relation to circadian variations in body temperature in the three men studied, demonstrating that a 1°C decrease in body temperature was associated with a 0.2 millisecond increase in the latency of wave V. This variation of ABR with circadian temperature changes was also observed by Picton, et al.,[23] who suggested that an increase in body temperature may cause action potentials and postsynaptic potentials to have a more rapid onset and shorter duration, which would increase neuronal conduction velocity and decrease synaptic transmission time.

Another frequently postulated etiology of the ABR gender difference is the hormonal milieu of young women. The only study of this variable was done by Picton, et al.,[23] who reported slight interpeak latency changes during the menstrual cycle. They related these differences to the temperature changes during menses. No examination of the effects of menstrual cycle hormonal changes on ABR has been reported.

MATERIALS AND METHODS

Participants

Twenty-nine paid white volunteers participated in the study, including 14 women ranging in age from 23 to 36 years (4 women from this group were excluded from data analysis because of irregular menses and incomplete data), 10 young men ranging in age from 22 to 27 years, and 5 postmenopausal women ranging in age from 48 to 73 years. Oral contraceptive use, pregnancy, hearing disorders, and menstrual irregularities excluded young women from participation in the study. Any hearing loss or medical disorders excluded young men from participation. Estrogen therapy, hearing loss, or any significant medical problem excluded postmenopausal women from participation. Each participant had normal hearing with pure tone average (1, 2, 4 kHz average) less than or equal to 20 dB. The age, gender, menstrual histories, and head diameter of each participant were recorded. The intertemporal diameter of the head was measured from the root of the helix, using the base of the nose as a reference. The average difference on repeated measures was .12 cm.

Audiometric Testing

Subjective pure-tone thresholds were established at 250, 500, 1000, 2000, and 4000 Hz by standard audiometric testing (American National Standards Institute, 1969). The acoustic signal, a 100-microsecond click, was presented at the rate of 21.1/s. Clicks were delivered monaurally via insert tubephones with foam eartips. One ear in each participant was tested at 80 dB above the average normal hearing level for the click. The right ear was tested in half of the participants, and the left ear was tested in the other half. The ABR was recorded by conventional signal averaging technique. Standard EEG disk electrodes (impedance less than 5 kΩ) were attached to the vertex (active) and to each earlobe, with the fore-

TABLE I.
Average ABR Latencies (milliseconds) and Wave V Amplitudes (μV) in Three Groups of Subjects.

	Waveform Measure			
	Latency Wave I	Latency Wave III	Latency Wave V	Amplitude Wave V
Young male	1.69	4.03	5.95	0.54
Young female	1.63	3.91	5.72	0.74
Postmenopausal female	1.78	4.10	6.10	0.68

head serving as the reference electrode. The EEG signal was preamplified, with a voltage gain of 200,000 and band pass filtered from 30 to 3000 Hz. The signal averager was triggered for a 10-millisecond sweep at the onset of each signal. A total of 4096 sweeps were averaged. Half of the signals were condensation clicks, and half were rarefaction clicks. Both ipsilateral and contralateral recordings were made. The ABR peak latency (I, III, V), the last positive value before the sharp decline from positive to negative, was measured using visual overlay cursors. Wave V amplitudes were measured from the peak of the wave IV to V complex to the valley prior to wave VI. The recordings from the contralateral ear verified wave V latencies. Contralateral recordings were not significantly different from the ipsilateral recordings in the participants studied. Waves II and IV were not evaluated.

Experimental Protocol

Each participant was tested three afternoons a week for 4 consecutive weeks (12 ABRs). Two of the young women had two additional sessions because their menstrual cycles were longer than 28 days. Participants were seated in a reclining chair in a double-walled, sound-treated room. After the ABR was performed, the participants took their own digital oral temperatures (participants had been instructed not to smoke or drink hot or cold beverages before each session). In addition, blood was drawn from the antecubital fossa of each young woman after each session. Hormonal assays of follicle stimulating hormone (FSH), luteinizing hormone (LH), estradiol (E2), and progesterone (P) were performed. The basic statistical methods used were linear regression analysis and one-factor analysis of variance.

RESULTS

The results of this study will be presented in two main sections: first, the effects of temperature and head size on ABR latencies and wave V amplitudes are discussed; second, the influence of hormones on the wave V latency will be examined. Before proceeding to these sections, the average latencies and amplitudes recorded in the 25 participants must be examined.

The waves I, III, and V latencies and the wave V amplitudes were averaged in each subject over 12 sessions. Table I summarizes the averages for each group.

The wave I latency difference between the young men and the young women was .06 millisecond, showing little gender effect. The wave III latency difference was .12 millisecond, which is consistent with the latency difference of .15 millisecond reported by Picton, et al.[23]

The largest difference, .23 millisecond, occurred at wave V. This value is consistent with previously published studies, which have shown a wave V latency gender difference ranging from .12 to .30 milliseconds[8,15] and averaging .22 milliseconds, according to Picton, et al.[23]

The wave V amplitude difference is usually reported in the literature as the percent difference between the women's amplitude and the men's amplitude (this value is approximately 30%[7,9,23]). This means that the women's wave V amplitude is, on average, 30% larger than the men's amplitude average. We found in our series of participants an average young man-young woman amplitude difference of .20 mV, which is a 27% amplitude difference.

The data from the five postmenopausal women are also presented in Table I. Their data was excluded from analysis in the next section, in which the effects of temperature and head size are discussed, because the effects of aging on their latencies would skew the results. The importance of their data comes later when the hormonal influences on ABR are examined.

SECTION I

Temperature differences. Large temperature changes can significantly affect ABR latencies[19–22] in two ways. First, the overall temperature difference between women and men could contribute to the overall gender difference. Second, the variation of the young women's temperatures over their menstrual cycles could affect the overall gender difference. In this section, we will discuss the possibility of an overall gender effect.

In the young men, temperature varied slightly in each participant and averaged 36.5°C (SD = 0.27). In the young women, there were minimal daily variations in temperatures, with an average temperature of 36.6°C (SD = 0.28).

The effect of temperature on wave V latency was analyzed by plotting the wave V latency versus the temperature at each ABR session. In the young men, the linear regression line ($y = -.025x + 6.84$) shows that minimal fluctuations in temperature did not significantly affect wave V latency.

The same analysis was done in the young women. The temperature versus wave V latency plot showed a minimal effect of temperature, with a linear regression line of $y = -.10x + 9.53$.

Since the overall effect of temperature was greater in the young women, the slope of their wave V latency-temperature linear regression line ($-.10$) was used to calculate the overall contribution of temperature on the gender difference. The average woman-man temperature difference was .1°C which, according to the slope of the aforementioned regression line, would correspond to a .01 millisecond latency difference. From Table I, the actual wave V latency difference is .23 millisecond. Thus, temperature could account for less than the 5% overall gender difference and is,

TABLE II.
Average ABR Latencies (milliseconds) and Wave V Amplitudes (μV) Adjusted to 14-cm Head Size in Three Groups of Subjects.

	Waveform Measure			
	Latency Wave I	Latency Wave III	Latency Wave V	Amplitude Wave V
Young male	1.66	4.01	5.90	0.60
Young female	1.66	3.94	5.80	0.65
Postmenopausal female	1.77	4.09	6.08	0.70

therefore, inconsequential in explaining the wave V latency difference between young men and young women. How menstrual-cycle temperature changes could affect ABR wave V latency will be examined later.

Head size. After overall temperature difference is ruled out as a significant variable, the effect of head size on ABR latencies and wave V amplitudes must be considered. The young men had an average head size of 14.3 cm. The young women averaged 13.4 cm, while the postmenopausal women averaged 14.1 cm.

The young men and young women average wave I latencies were plotted against their head sizes, and a linear regression line was recorded ($y = 0.78 + .063x$). Using the slope of this line, each participant's average wave I latency was adjusted to a head size of 14 cm. These adjusted values are presented in Table II. Note that head size has little effect on wave I.

Next, wave III latencies were adjusted to 14 cm using the slope of the wave III latency-head size regression line ($y = 3.08 + .064x$) plotted from the young man-young woman data. After correcting for head size, the young women still had shorter wave III latencies (Table II).

The wave V latencies were corrected for head size using the slope of the regression line ($y = 3.85 + 0.14x$) from the wave V latency-head size plot. These corrected values show a .10 millisecond latency difference between the young men and young women. The slope of our wave V latency-head size regression line (.14), although based on a limited sample, closely approximates the slope of the wave V latency-head size regression line from the data of Trune, et al. (.13).[14]

Finally, wave V amplitudes were adjusted for head size using the regression equation $y = 3.05 - 0.17x$. This adjustment resulted in a reduction of the young woman-young man amplitude difference from 27% to 8% (Table II). Thus, the majority of the gender amplitude difference can be explained by head size.

SECTION II

Endocrine background. The menstrual cycle is divided into a preovulatory phase and a postovulatory phase. The length of the preovulatory phase varies from individual to individual, whereas the postovulatory phase lasts approximately 14 days. During the preovulatory phase, FSH and E2 gradually rise until

WAVE V

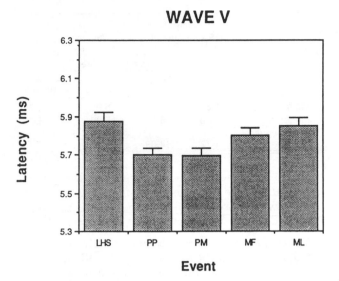

Fig. 1. Average wave V latency (corrected to head size of 14 cm) and its standard error from ten young women recorded during five key events in the menstrual cycle.

WAVE I

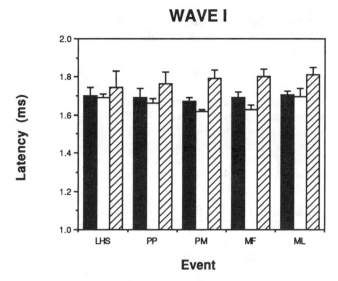

Fig. 2. Average wave I latency (corrected to head size of 14 cm) and its standard error from 10 young men, 5 postmenopausal women, and 10 young women recorded during 5 key events in the menstrual cycle. ■ = Young men; □ = Young women; ▨ = Postmenopausal women.

there is an LH surge (LHS), which results in ovulation from one of the ovaries being stimulated by FSH, E2, and LH. The basal body temperature begins to rise gradually from the LHS to the middle of the post-ovulatory phase. After ovulation, the follicle which extruded the oocyte becomes the corpus luteum and begins to produce P and E2. Progesterone has many effects, including preparing the uterine endometrium for implantation and directly affecting the hypothalamus and causing a rise in the basal body temperature. Although varying from woman to woman, the P level peaks between 4 to 10 days after ovulation. The corpus luteum involutes if there is no pregnancy, and both P and E2 levels sharply drop. This fall in P and E2 is the hallmark of the premenstrual (PM) phase and the proposed cause of PM tension. Shortly thereafter, menses occur and a new cycle begins.[24]

Hormonal influences on ABR. In reviewing the ABR wave V latency data from the ten young women studied, there appeared to be a significant trend in the majority of these women. Five key events in the menstrual cycle seemed to affect wave V latencies. At LHS, there was a lengthening of the wave V latency. At the progesterone peak (PP), the wave V latency shortened significantly. In addition, there was a shortening of the wave V latency in the PM phase when the P and E2 levels dropped. During the first day of menses (MF) studied, the wave V latency began to lengthen until the last day of menses (ML) studied, when it nearly returned to LHS level. These changes are illustrated in Figure 1.

To rule out the possibility that these findings were random phenomena, the young men and post-menopausal women (who do not have fluctuating hormone levels) were used as controls. Five ABR sessions (of the 12 performed) for each young man and post-menopausal woman were randomly chosen to provide

control data for the five events in the young women's menstrual cycles.

Figure 2 shows that the latencies of wave I vary little with the monthly cycle in all three groups. Figure 3 shows that wave III latencies vary little during the time of the month in the young men's control group, but the young women begin to show a trend toward shortened latencies during PP and PM. The postmenopausal women show some random variation at wave III. None of these changes was statistically significant. The main difference occurs in the wave V latencies (Fig. 4). At LHS, the latency of wave V

WAVE III

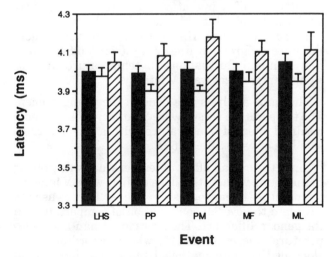

Fig. 3. Average wave III latency (corrected to head size of 14 cm) and its standard error from 10 young men, 5 postmenopausal women, and 10 young women recorded during 5 key events in the menstrual cycle. ■ = Young men; □ = Young women; ▨ = Postmenopausal women.

WAVE V

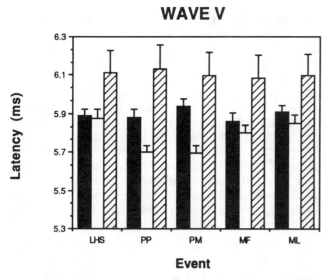

Fig. 4. Average wave V latency (corrected to head size of 14 cm) and its standard error from 10 young men, 5 postmenopausal women, and 10 young women recorded during 5 key events in the menstrual cycle. ■ = Young men; □ = Young women; ▨ = Postmenopausal women.

for the young men is nearly identical to the young women. At PP and PM, the wave V latency drops in the young women and varies little in the young men and postmenopausal women. At MF, a gradual trend to the LHS latency begins; at the ML, the wave V latency approaches LHS level. The difference between LHS and PP and PM was statistically significant by one-factor analysis of variance. In the two control groups, no statistically significant variation was present.

Figure 5 shows that changing hormone levels have little effect on the amplitude of wave V in the young women. There were some random variations in the

WAVE V AMPLITUDE

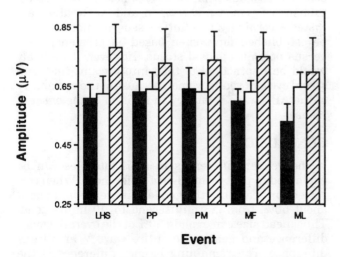

Fig. 5. Average wave V amplitude (corrected to head size of 14 cm) and its standard error from 10 young men, 5 postmenopausal women, and 10 young women recorded during 5 key events in the menstrual cycle. ■ = Young men; □ = Young women; ▨ = Postmenopausal women.

LATENCY DIFFERENCE

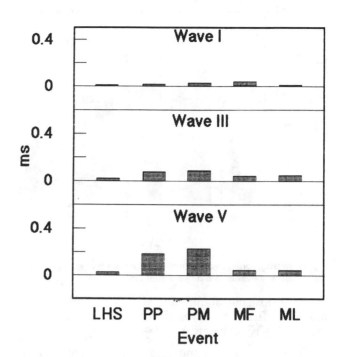

Fig. 6. The latency difference between young men and young women (corrected to head size of 14 cm) for waves I, III, and V during five key events in the menstrual cycle.

wave V amplitudes in the two control groups, but these were not statistically significant.

Thus, the hormonal effect on ABR wave V latency is the difference between the LHS and the PP and PM (approximately .20 milliseconds). Figure 6 compares the young man-young woman latency difference, and thus summarizes the hormone effect in all latencies.

Progesterone affects the hypothalamus and causes a temperature elevation in young women. Figure 7 shows how the temperature changed during the menstrual cycle. Note that an average .45°C difference exists between LHS and PP. Marshall and Donchin[22] noted in their studies on three men that a 1°C change in oral temperature corresponded to a .2 millisecond difference in wave V latency. Our previous temperature-wave V latency regression equation would predict that a 1°C change in temperature would cause a .07 millisecond change in latency. Marshall and Donchin's data, which show a more robust temperature effect, do not explain the .2 millisecond difference between LHS and PP with a .45°C temperature difference. Therefore, it seems that the temperature differences during menses are not the cause of the gender difference, but rather a result of the P effect on the hypothalamic temperature control center.

DISCUSSION

The present data confirm previous studies in which conspicuous sex differences were found in ABR latencies and amplitudes. The differences between ABR

YOUNG FEMALES

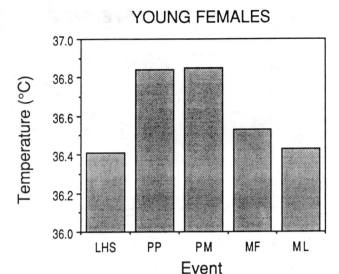

Fig. 7. Average oral temperatures recorded for ten young women during five key events in the menstrual cycle.

latencies are not significant at wave I and become more significant as waves III and V are encountered, confirming Kjaer's data.[7]

When the latencies and amplitudes are adjusted to 14 cm, the extent of the head size effect can be seen. The head size measurement we used is similar to that used by Trune, *et al.*[14] In this study, head size correlates with ABR latencies and amplitudes. Wave I is not really affected by head size, indicating that head size affects central conduction time through the brain stem. Although brainstem size was not directly measured in this study, it is likely that part of the gender difference at wave V is due to gender brainstem size differences. This was seen by Antonelli, *et al.*,[17] when they noted a correlation between brainstem length (as measured by MRI) and wave V latency.

When corrected for head size, the amplitudes of wave V are not significantly different when the young men are compared with young women (Table II). It does not appear that hormones have an effect on wave V amplitude differences (Fig. 5).

After correcting for head size, there is still a significant gender difference. This was seen by Trune, *et al.*,[14] also. The gender difference that remains (after head-size adjustments are made) is related to the hormonal differences between young women and young men. At LHS, the young men's wave V latency is nearly identical to the young women's. At PP and PM, these latencies drop in the young women, whereas the young men remain nearly the same. The difference between LHS and PP and PM is the hormonal effect on wave V latency.

The exact mechanism of this effect is not clear. Since E2 is elevated at both LHS and PP, it would seem unlikely that E2 is the main factor. Progesterone, however, may be the main factor. Studies on brainstem thresholds in cats by Kawakami and Saw-

yer[25] demonstrated that at PP there was a lowering of the brainstem arousal threshold for a few hours, followed by an elevation of the thresholds. When P levels dropped, there was a rebound phenomenon, and the thresholds were lowered once again. This observation is similar to the wave V latencies in the young women. When PP occurred, there was a shortening of the wave V latency, perhaps due to a lowering of the thresholds of the neurons in the auditory pathways. After PP, many of the young women showed a lengthening of the latencies until PM, when P dropped sharply. At this point, a rebound phenomenon similar to that seen by Kawakami and Sawyer[25] may have occurred, causing another lowering of the thresholds of the brainstem auditory pathways.

How P levels affect brainstem thresholds is unknown. One possibility is that P has an effect on the ionic channels at the neuronal level, causing the neuron to be more sensitive to electrical stimulation and causing more rapid depolarizing of the neuron. Another possible effect of P is at the neurotransmitter level, where it possibly causes the proteins to bind more efficiently to their respective binding sites.

It is interesting that other studies have shown gender differences in other evoked potentials. Allison, *et al.*[26] showed gender differences in visual-evoked potentials and short-latency, somatosensory-evoked potentials in addition to ABR. These differences could not be explained on the basis of size differences alone. Perhaps the gender differences in these systems are the effects of the women's hormones, as in ABR latencies. Further studies in these evoked potentials would help to confirm the hormonal effects seen in this study.

The clinical significance of the head size differences and the hormonal effects are yet to be studied. It seems reasonable that head-size norms could be established for men and women and ABR values adjusted accordingly. In addition, separate norms would be established for women based on premenopausal versus postmenopausal status. However, it probably would be impractical to take into account the menstrual cycle in young women because of the variability of the ABR wave V latency in relation to the onset of menses.

CONCLUSION

The gender differences in ABR latencies can be explained in part by head-size differences. When corrected for head size, the gender difference is reduced about 50%, from .23 millisecond to .10 millisecond. Thus, head size can explain 50% of the overall gender difference and nearly the entire wave V amplitude difference. The remaining latency difference is the average hormone effect. The ABR wave V latencies vary significantly during the changing hormonal environment of the young woman. The average effect of the hormones is .10 millisecond, with the maximum effect of the hormones seen at PP and PM. Thus, nearly half of the ABR wave V latency difference can be explained by hormonal differences. Temperature differences do not seem to have a significant effect on ABR wave V latencies or amplitudes. Further studies in other evoked potentials would help to confirm the conclusions of this study. In addition, the exact mechanism of the hormonal effect needs further investigation.

BIBLIOGRAPHY

1. Jewett, D.L. and Williston, J.L.: Auditory Evoked Far Fields Averaged From the Scalp of Humans. *Brain,* 94:681–696, 1971.
2. Hall, J.W.: Auditory Brainstem Response Audiometry. In: *Hearing Disorders in Adults: Current Trends.* J. Jerger, Ed. College Hill Press, San Diego, 1983.
3. Beagley, H.A. and Sheldrake, J.B.: Differences in Brainstem Response Latency With Age and Sex. *Br. J. Audiol.,* 12:69–77, 1978.
4. Eberling, C. and Parbo, J.: Reference Data for ABRs in Retrocochlear Diagnosis. *Scand. Audiol.,* 16:49–55, 1987.
5. Jerger, J. and Hall, J.: Effects of Age and Sex on Auditory Brainstem Response. *Arch. Otolaryngol.,* 106:387–391, 1980.
6. Kjaer, M.: Recognizability of Brainstem Auditory Evoked Potential Components. *Acta Neurol. Scand.,* 62:20–33, 1980.
7. Kjaer, M.: Differences in Latencies and Amplitudes of Brain Stem Evoked Potentials in Subgroups of a Normal Material. *Acta Neurol. Scand.,* 59:72–79, 1979.
8. McClelland, R.J. and McCrea, R.S.: Intersubject Variability of the Auditory Evoked Brain Stem Potentials. *Audiologie,* 18:462–471, 1979.
9. Michalewski, H.J., *et al.*: Sex Differences in the Amplitude and Latencies of the Human Auditory Brain Stem Potential. *Electroencephalogr. Clin. Neurophysiol.,* 48:351–356, 1980.
10. Patterson, J.V., *et al.*: Age and Sex Differences in the Human Auditory Brainstem Response. *J. Gerontol.,* 36:455–462, 1981.
11. Stockard, J.J., *et al.*: Brainstem Auditory Evoked Responses: Normal Variation as a Function of Stimulus and Subject Characteristics. *Arch. Neurol.,* 36:823–831, 1978.
12. Stockard, J.J., *et al.*: Nonpathologic Factors Influencing Brainstem Auditory Evoked Potentials. *Am. J. EEG Technol.,* 18:177–209, 1978.
13. Rosenhall, U., *et al.*: Brainstem Auditory Evoked Potentials in Different Age Groups. *Electroencephalogr. Clin. Neurophysiol.,* 62:426–430, 1985.
14. Trune, D.R., *et al.*: The Relative Importance of Head Size, Gender and Age on the Auditory Brainstem Response. *Hear. Res.* 32:165–174, 1988.
15. Sturzebecher, E. and Werbs, M.: Effects of Age and Sex on Auditory Brainstem Response. *Scand. Audiol.* 16:153–157, 1987.
16. O'Donovan, C.A.: Latency of Brainstem Response in Children. *Br. J. Audiol.,* 14:23–24, 1980.
17. Antonelli, R.A., *et al.*: The Relationship of Head and Brainstem Size to Main Parameters of ABR in the Developmental Age and in Adults. *Acta Otolaryngol.,* 105:587–590, 1988.
18. Jerger, J. and Johnson, K.: Interaction of Age, Gender and Sensorineural Hearing Loss on ABR Latency. In press.
19. Jones, T.A., *et al.*: The Effects of Temperature and Acute Alcohol Intoxication on Brainstem Auditory Evoked Potential in the Cat. *Electroencephalogr. Clin. Neurophysiol.,* 49:23–30, 1980.
20. Kaga, K., *et al.*: Effects of Deep Hypothermia and Circulatory Arrest on the Auditory Brainstem Responses. *Arch. Otolaryngol.,* 225:199–205, 1979.
21. Stockard, J.J., *et al.*: Effects of Hypothermia on the Human Brainstem Response. *Ann. Neurol.,* 3:363–370, 1978.
22. Marshall, N.K. and Donchin, E.: Circadian Variations in the Latency of Brainstem Responses: Its Relation to Body Temperature. *Science,* 212:356–358, 1981.
23. Picton, T.W., *et al.*: Auditory Evoked Potentials. *J. Otolaryngol.,* 14:1–41, 1981.
24. Tepperman, J.: *Metabolic and Endocrine Physiology.* Year Book Medical Publishers, Chicago, pp. 118–143, 1980.
25. Kawakami, M. and Sawyer, C.H.: Neuroendocrine Correlates of Changes in Brain Activity Thresholds by Sex Steroids and Pituitary Hormones. *Endocrinology,* 65:652–668, 1969.
26. Allison, T., *et al.*: Brainstem Auditory, Pattern-Reversal Visual, and Short Latency Somatosensory Evoked Potentials: Latencies in Relation to Age, Sex, and Grain and Body Size. *Electroencephalogr. Clin. Neurophysiol.,* 55:619–636, 1983.

Estrogen influences auditory brainstem responses during the normal menstrual cycle

K.E. Elkind-Hirsch [a], W.R. Stoner, B.A. Stach and J.F. Jerger

Departments of Otorhinolaryngology, Communicative Sciences and [a] Medicine, The Methodist Hospital, Baylor College of Medicine, Houston, Texas, USA

(Received 7 October 1991; Revision received 13 February 1992; Accepted 18 February 1992)

We evaluated the impact of the menstrual cycle on auditory brainstem response (ABR) latency in nine normally cycling women. Subjects (age 23–40 years) using no hormonal therapy were recruited and underwent ABR testing during four different phases of the same menstrual cycle: early follicular (cycle days 1 to 3); mid-cycle (cycle days 12 to 15); mid-luteal (cycle days 17 to 22), and premenstrual (cycle days 25–27). Cycles were verified by basal body temperature, and serum estrogen (E_2), progesterone (P), and gonadotropin levels. A control group of nine women (age 23–40 years) on oral contraceptives (Nordette-28) was also studied four times during a pill cycle. Results show a significant increase in the latency of wave III and wave V peak latencies and in the I-V interpeak interval associated with a high estrogen state at the mid-cycle phase. No statistically significant variations in latency were found in the birth control pill group. These data suggest the existence of brainstem auditory neural pathways that are sensitive to fluctuations in E_2 levels during the menstrual cycle.

Auditory brainstem response; Menstrual cycle; Estrogen effect; Oral contraceptives

Introduction

The speed with which sound-elicited nerve impulses travel through the structures of the auditory brainstem is faster in women than in men. Numerous studies have shown that latencies of the waveform components of the auditory brainstem response (ABR), particularly component wave V, are consistently shorter in women (Beagley and Sheldrake, 1978; Stockard et al., 1978; Trune et al., 1978; McClelland and McCrea, 1979; Jerger and Hall 1980; Jerger and Johnson, 1988). Although the cause of this gender difference remains unclear, several clinical studies suggest that female sex hormones may contribute to these functional differences (Fagan and Church, 1986; Dehan and Jerger, 1990). More specifically, some investigators have implicated sex steroids as a contributing factor by suggesting that ABR latencies change during the menstrual cycle.

Two ovarian steroids have been proposed to be responsible for the change in latency seen in regularly cycling women: estrogen or progesterone. During the first half (follicular phase) of the the 28 day cycle, the follicle grows and matures under the dominant influence of follicle stimulating hormone (FSH) and some luteinizing hormone (LH). Early in this phase, follicular estradiol (E_2) secretion is low, but toward the middle of the cycle there is a burst of E_2 from the dominant follicle. If estrogen contributes to the change in ABR latency, then the effect would occur during this phase of the menstrual cycle. Following the rise in E_2 production, a surge of LH secretion occurs, which causes ovulation. After ovulation, marking the second phase of the cycle (luteal phase), the follicle undergoes luteinization and is converted to a progesterone-secreting structure, the corpus luteum. Progesterone (P) acts to stimulate both endometrial gland and stroma maturation. If P leads to the change in ABR latency, then it is during this luteal phase that the effect would be seen. The corpus luteum involutes after about 12 days of secretion. With involution of the corpus luteum, the fall in plasma E_2 and P leads to withdrawal menstrual bleeding. Both estrogen and progesterone drop to their lowest level around the time of menses, and the cycle begins again. Menstruation marks the end of the luteal phase and the beginning of the next follicular phase.

Contradictory findings concerning the impact of the menstrual cycle on ABR have left this issue unresolved. Studies of the auditory brainstem response report variable alterations in latency during the menstrual cycle. A shortening of wave V latency was found during the luteal phase in one study (Dehan and Jerger, 1990), while, in another, no latency change as a function of the phase of the menstrual cycle was identified (Fagan and Church, 1986). These inconsistent findings are difficult to evaluate for two reasons: 1) studies

Correspondence to: K. Elkind-Hirsch, Department of Medicine, The Methodist Hospital, 6565 Fannin Street, B 200 Houston, TX 77030, USA.

were performed without hormonal verification of the actual cycle phase; and 2) the effect of individual hormones is difficult to factor out when the actual measurement of those hormones has not been performed. Previous studies have failed to document ovulation, which is a requirement for the production of progesterone. The purpose of this study was to evaluate ABR latency in females to determine if it varies with measured fluctuations in circulating hormone levels during the menstrual cycle.

Materials and Methods

Subjects

Eleven normally cycling women (cycle length 27–30 days), who were within 10% of ideal body weight, were recruited as experimental subjects. None of the women had taken any medications, including hormonal contraception, for the previous six months. The age, menstrual histories, and head diameter of each participant were recorded. The head diameter was measured from tragus to tragus using a specially-built, calibrated caliper. The subjects' mean age was 29.5 years and ranged from 23 to 40 years. One month prior to the study, all patients' cycles were documented as ovulatory by biphasic basal body temperature charts and a serum P of greater than 31.8 nmol/l within five to seven days following the temperature rise. Baseline levels of E_2, testosterone (T), dehydroepiandrosterone sulfate (DHEAS), and prolactin (Prl) were also determined prior to the start of any studies. One patient was excluded from the study because of an elevated basal T level (> 50 ng/dl). All subjects had behavioral hearing threshold levels of 20 dB HL or better at octave interval frequencies from 250 to 8000 Hz. Nine subjects had normal middle ear function as determined by conventional immittance audiometry. One patient was excluded from the data analysis due to abnormal middle ear function.

Normally cycling women subjects were studied four times during a single cycle. A group of ten women (age 23–40 years) who were currently and voluntarily using the same oral contraceptives (Nordette-28; Wyeth Laboratories, Philadelphia, PA) served as a control group and were tested four times, at one-week intervals, during their pill-regulated cycles. One participant on oral contraceptives was excluded from the study due to abnormal middle ear function. Thus the final study (cycling and pill) groups each contained nine subjects.

Clinical Protocol

Hormone Measurements
A butterfly catheter was placed in the forearm for blood sampling. Estradiol, LH, FSH and P levels were drawn after intravenous placement before each auditory test. Each normal cycling study patient underwent four ABR tests during a single menstrual cycle. The early follicular phase study (cycle day 2–3) was performed within 1 to 3 days of the onset of menstrual bleeding. The mid-cycle study (cycle day 12–15) was performed on the day after an increase in E_2 to at least 551 pmol/l, as determined by drawing E_2 levels daily. The mid-luteal phase study (cycle day 17–22) was performed 7 to 9 days after the mid-cycle study, and premenstrual phase studies were performed on cycle days 25 to 27. Cycles were followed by measurement of basal body temperature, serum E_2 levels and serum P levels. The oral contraceptive subjects were required to have been using Nordette oral contraceptive pills for at least 1 month prior to being studied. Women who were using Nordette-28 oral contraceptive pills were on a 28-day cycle during which they took chemically inert pills and menstruated during the first 7 days. For the remaining 21 days, subjects were taking a combination oral contraceptive containing 30 mcg of ethinyl estradiol (synthetic estrogen) and 0.15 mg levonorgestrel (synthetic progestin). They were tested on day 2 or 3, day 9, 10 or 11, day 16, 17, or 18, and on day 23 or 24 of their pill-regulated cycle.

ABR Measurements

Subjects reclined on a comfortable bed in a darkened room with their eyes closed. Click stimuli of alternating polarity and 100 ms duration were presented independently to each ear through insert earphones (Etymotic ER-3A) with foam eartips at a level of 70 dB nHL and a rate of 21.1/s. Two-channel recordings were obtained from scalp electrodes placed on the vertex (active), each earlobe (reference), and the forehead (ground). EEG activity was preamplified at a voltage gain of 200,000:1 and bandpass filtered from 150 to 3000 Hz. The amplified EEG was signal averaged over a time base of 10 ms using the Nicolet CA-1000 Averager. A total of 1,200 sweeps was averaged. ABR waveforms were analyzed separately for each ear. Absolute peak latencies of component waves I, III, and V were measured, and interwave intervals were calculated. To avoid measurement bias, the examiner was unaware of both group placement and phase of the cycle of individual subjects.

Analytical Techniques and Calculations

Serum E_2, LH, FSH, Prl, DHEAS, T, and P concentrations were measured, in duplicate, with commercial assay kits (Diagnostic Products; Los Angeles, CA) in the General Clinical Research Center Radioimmunoassay (RIA) core laboratory. The interassay coefficients of variation of all hormone assays were less than 12%.

Comparisons of baseline measurements between groups were performed using one way analyses of variance (ANOVAs). Statistical analyses of serum steroid and ABR measurement values in the cycling and pill groups were performed using subjects-by-treatments repeated-measures ANOVAs with the between-subjects variable being either cycle or birth-control-pill group and the within-subjects variable being either hormone (E_2, LH, FSH, and P) levels or ABR measurements for the four tests. Since the observations were made repetitively on the same subject, these observations are correlated. This violates the validity of the probability (P) values for the univariate repeated measures hypothesis tests (F tests). Therefore, all the F tests were corrected using the Greenhouse-Geisser estimate of epsilon, which is the most conservative adjustment of the F-test. The amount of adjustment is determined by the factor epsilon. The reported P values reflect this correction.

Results

Hormone Measurements

No significant differences in baseline concentrations of Prl, DHEAS, or T were found in either the cycling or pill groups ($P > 0.05$). At the time of menses (first study in each group), levels of E_2 and P were equivalent in cycling and pill patients. E_2 levels in cycling patients increased significantly from the early follicular phase to mid-cycle and remained elevated during the luteal phase, as compared with follicular, premenstrual, and all four studies of the pill group ($P < 0.0001$), as shown in Fig. 1A and B. P levels in normal cycling females were significantly elevated during the luteal phase ($P < 0.0001$), as compared to all other phases in the cycling group and all four studies in the control group (Table I). The rise in P observed for each cycling woman confirmed that ovulation had occurred. No statistically significant differences between the groups were found in LH and FSH concentrations during the cycle ($P > 0.05$).

ABR Measurements

When the ABR latency data from the nine cycling women were compared to those of the nine women on oral contraceptives, there was a significant trend in the cycling females. The main difference occurred in wave V latencies and was associated with a rise in estrogen secretion. A significant lengthening of wave V peak latency was observed during the mid-cycle estrogen peak ($P < 0.007$) as illustrated in Fig. 2A. In addition, the wave I-V interpeak intervals were also increased in the cycling group at mid-cycle ($P < 0.04$) (Table II). No

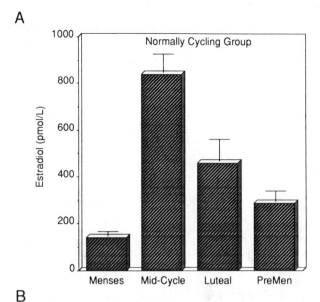

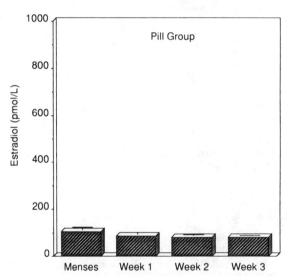

Fig. 1. Mean endogenous estradiol concentrations, measured on four occasions in (A) nine normal cycling women and (B) nine women taking Nordette-28 oral contraceptive pills. Error bars represent one standard error of the mean.

significant differences were found in ABR wave V latency (Fig. 2B) or wave I-V interpeak interval (Table II) in the oral contraceptive pill group. As shown in Table II, wave III peak latency increased slightly at mid-cycle and decreased during the premenstrual period ($P < 0.007$). A significant, gradual increase in wave III peak latency was observed in oral contraceptive users during the period in which pills were being ingested, days 8–28, which included all phases of the cycle other than menstruation. The latencies of wave I varied little with the monthly cycle in both groups.

The changing hormone levels had no apparent effect on the amplitude of wave V (as measured from positive peak to following negative peak) in cycling women. Similarly, no significant differences were found

TABLE I

Mean estradiol and progesterone concentrations in cycling and pill patients

Evaluation	Estradiol (pmol/l)	Progesterone (pmol/l)
Cycling		
Follicular	141 (18)	1.2 (0.16)
Mid-cycle	839 (81) **	2.2 (0.60)
Luteal	461 (92) *	39 (5.4) **
Premenstrual	285 (47)	12 (2.0)
Pill		
1- no hormone	105 (11)	0.91 (0.13)
2- week 1 replacement	88 (6)	0.84 (0.13)
3- week 2	81 (5)	0.77 (0.10)
4- week 3	82 (5)	0.83 (0.13)

** $P < 0.001$ compared to other groups; * $P < 0.01$ compared to other groups. Data are expressed as mean ($+/-$S.E.M).

in wave V amplitude in patients taking oral contraceptive pills ($P > 0.05$).

Basal Body Temperature

All normal cycling female subjects demonstrated ovulatory biphasic basal body temperature (BBT) changes. Cycling women displayed a rise in temperature in response to the secretion of progesterone during the luteal phase. Patients on oral contraceptives had nonovulatory monophasic BBT charts with no observable changes in temperature during the pill cycle.

Discussion

We found an increase in wave III and V peak latencies and I-V interpeak interval associated with a high estrogen state at mid-cycle. This suggests the existence of brainstem auditory neural pathways sensitive to the surge in E_2 during the menstrual cycle.

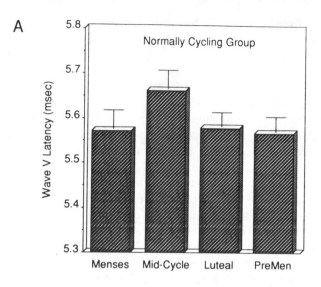

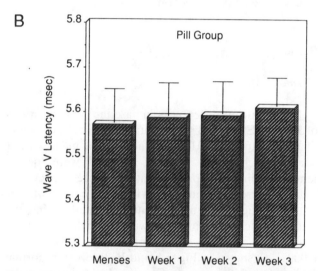

Fig. 2. Average wave V latency recorded on four occasions in (A) nine normal cycling women and (B) nine women taking Nordette-28 oral contraceptive pills. Error bars represent one standard error of the mean.

TABLE II

Mean ABR latency in cycling and pill patients

Evaluation	Wave I (ms)	Wave III (ms)	Wave V (ms)	Wave I–V (ms)
Cycling				
Follicular	1.56 (0.03)	3.66 (0.04)	5.57 (0.04)	4.01 (0.04)
Mid-cycle	1.56 (0.03)	3.70 (0.04) **	5.70 (0.04) **	4.10 (0.05) *
Luteal	1.57 (0.04)	3.66 (0.04)	5.58 (0.03)	4.00 (0.04)
Premenstrual	1.56 (0.04)	3.60 (0.04)	5.57 (0.03)	4.00 (0.04)
Pill				
1- no hormone	1.57 (0.04)	3.68 (0.07)	5.57 (0.08)	4.00 (0.05)
2- week 1	1.57 (0.5)	3.70 (0.06)	5.60 (0.07)	4.02 (0.05)
3- week 2	1.57 (0.05)	3.70 (0.07)	5.60 (0.07)	4.02 (0.05)
4- week 3	1.61 (0.04)	3.70 (0.07)	5.61 (0.06)	4.00 (0.05)

** $P < 0.01$ compared to other groups, * $P < 0.05$ compared to other groups. Data are expressed as mean($+/-$S.E.M.).

These findings are in contrast to previous studies which reported either a decreased wave V latency in the luteal phase (Dehan and Jerger, 1990) or no changes in wave V latency during the menstrual cycle (Fagan and Church, 1986).

The source of the latency change appears to be in the central auditory neural pathways rather than in the auditory periphery. Wave I latency, which reflects peripheral conduction time, does not change. However, waves III and V, which reflect central conduction time, are increased at mid-cycle. If the changes in latency were peripheral in nature, then the latencies of all component waves should be increased by the same amount. In addition, the fact that the latency increase is greater for the wave III-V interpeak interval than for the wave I-III interpeak interval suggests that the effect is more pronounced at increasingly rostral brain sites.

Our findings also showed that wave III and wave V peak latency gradually increased in oral contraceptive users during the period in which pills were being ingested. However, wave III and wave V peak latencies appeared equivalent among the two groups during menses, when no differences in hormone levels were evident. While the endogenous levels of gonadal steroids of patients on oral contraceptive therapy were suppressed, exogenous supplied hormones result in constant hormone levels in the pill group of 30 mcg of synthetic estrogen and 0.15 mg of synthetic progesterone daily. This gradual increase in latency in the oral contraceptive group may result from the presence of the exogenous hormone replacement.

Our findings suggest that an elevation in estrogen alters the speed with which sensory information travels through the auditory brainstem nuclei. One explanation as to how a rise in the circulating levels of E_2 could modify auditory conduction time is by the E_2 effect on neurotransmitter synthesis. Gamma-aminobutyric acid (GABA) is one such neurotransmitter. GABA has been reported to play a role as an inhibitory neurotransmitter in the efferent fibers of the cochlea (Altschuler and Fex, 1986; Eybalin and Pujol, 1986; Schwartz and Ryan, 1986). Far-field auditory evoked potentials are altered by systemic application of the GABA analog- (-) baclofen {p-chlorophenyl GABA) (-) baclofen}. Auditory evoked potential (AEP) response studies in cats suggest that an excitatory amino acid is the transmitter at the auditory nerve-cochlear nucleus synapse which is blocked by baclofen. Martin (1982) found that the AEP latencies of peaks I and II did not change after injection of baclofen, whereas there was a tendency for the latencies of peaks IV and V to increase. Iontophoretic application of baclofen greatly reduces tone-evoked activity of cochlear nucleus (CN) neurons. Baclofen typically causes a parallel shift to the right of the rate-intensity function. Dose-

response curves obtained from neuron recordings from the anteroventral cochlear nucleus display dose-dependent decreases in discharge rates with increasing iontophoretic doses of GABA (Caspary, 1986). Collectively, studies suggest that GABA may be partially responsible for acoustically evoked inhibition seen in the response patterns of certain CN neurons.

There appears to be an intricate interaction among sex steroids in regulating GABA-mediated signals. When steroid levels are high in the bloodstream, they will be high in the cerebrospinal fluid (CSF) that bathes the brain. Steroids are very soluble in cell membranes and would be expected to cross the blood-brain barrier and enter the CSF. Levels of ovarian hormones, estrogen in particular, could affect ABR latencies by modulating GABA action. Physiological fluctuations in ovarian hormones have been shown to modify GABA/benzodiazepine (BZD) receptor sites in the cerebral cortex and hypothalamus of female mice. In both brain areas, BZD receptor binding was significantly higher in the estrus phase, when estrogen concentrations were elevated, as compared to other phases of the cycle (Martin et al, 1991). Estrogen has been shown to have a dual effect on release rates of GABA in the female primate. Roosen-Runge et al (1984) demonstrated the pulsatile release of hypothalamic GABA in female monkeys was significantly increased during the time of estrogen surge and abolished during the negative feedback phase. Fluctuations in circulating E_2 levels during the menstrual cycle could influence availability of GABA at the synapse and, in turn, influence conduction time. The biphasic response of GABA to estrogen action helps to further explain the increase in latency in the cycle group. At mid-cycle, estrogen has a positive feedback action which most likely results in enhanced GABA secretion in the brain, whereas estrogen has a negative feedback action during the early follicular phase and late luteal phase.

One factor which has been implicated as affecting ABR latency changes during the normal cycle is alterations in basal body temperature. All female subjects plotted changes in their basal body temperature (BBT) occurring over the menstrual cycle. The shift in BBT did not appear to alter ABR latencies in our subjects. Characteristically, the basal body temperature prior to ovulation is in the 36.1 to 36.3°C range, and after ovulation the basal temperature is over 36.7°C. The change in plateaus is caused by progesterone, which has a slight heat-producing effect. Wave III and V peak latencies did not change as a function of biphasic variations in basal body temperature records observed in all normally cycling patients. The increase in latency of wave III and V during the mid-cycle estrogen surge (study 2) was not related to a drop in body temperature. Nor was an elevation in body temperature during the mid-luteal phase (study 3) associated with shortening in wave III and V peak latencies. However, BBTs are measured in the 'basal' or resting state, i.e.; immediately upon awakening and before any activity. Any activity or even lack of sleep will raise the temperature. Since the ABR testing was performed after the patients had been active, these slight temperature fluctuations were probably eliminated.

Head size has also been implicated as a possible source of ABR variation. Variation in head size as an explanation for ABR latency changes was not applicable to this study for two reasons. Head size variation attributed to gender differences is due to the presence of a longer auditory pathway in males as compared with females (Trune et al., 1978; Jerger and Johnson, 1988; Dehan and Jerger, 1990). As this study was an intra-sex study, head size differences which exist between the two groups would not alter the results. The effect that was studied was a within-subjects effect, not a between-groups effect. Given that head size did not vary over the four trials, head size could not affect our analysis of latency change.

Acknowledgements

We express our thanks to all personnel in the Methodist Hospital General Clinical Research Center for their unselfish co-operation and to Wyeth Laboratories in Philadelphia, PA for the generous gift of Nordette-28 oral contraceptive pills.

This work was funded in part by the Division of Research Resources of the National Institutes of Health under grant MO1RR00350.

References

Altschuler, R.A. and Fex, J. (1986) Efferent neurotransmitters. In: R.A. Altschuler, D.W. Hoffman and R.P. Bobbin (Eds.) Neurobiology of hearing: The cochlea, Raven Press, New York, NY, pp. 383–396.

Beagley, H.A. and Sheldrake, J.B. (1978) Differences in brainstem response latency with age and sex. Br. J. Audiol. 12, 69–77.

Caspary, D.M. (1986) Cochlear nuclei: functional neuropharmacology of the principal cell types. In: R.A. Altschuler, D.W. Hoffman and R.P. Bobbin (Eds.), op cit pp. 303–3332.

Dehan, C.P. and Jerger, J. (1990) Analysis of gender differences in the auditory brainstem response. Laryngoscope 100, 18–24

Eybalin, M; and Pujol, R (1986) Cochlear neuroactive substances. Arch. Otorhinolaryngol. 246, 228–234.

Fagan, P.L. and Church, G.T. (1986) Effect of the menstrual cycle on the auditory brainstem response. Audiology 25, 321–8.

Jerger, J. and Hall, J. (1980) Effects of age and sex on auditory brainstem response. Arch. Otolaryngol. 106, 387–391.

Jerger, J. and Johnson, K. (1988) Interactions of age, gender, and sensorineural hearing loss on ABR latency. Ear Hear. 9, 168–175.

Martin, J.V., Agrawal, N. and Lee, H. (1991) Effect of ovariectomy or stage of estrous cycle on benzodiazepine binding in female mouse brain. Soc. Neurosci. Abstr. 17, 264.

Martin, M.R. (1982) Baclofen and the brainstem auditory evoked potential. Exp. Neurology 76, 675–680.

McClelland, R.J. and McCrea, R.S. (1979) Intersubject variability of the auditory-evoked brain stem potentials. Audiologie 18, 462–471.

Roosen-Runge, G., Epler, M., Duker, E., Fuchs, E., Siegel, R.A., Demling, J. and Wuttke, W/ (1984) In vivo release of neurotransmitters in the medial basal hypothalamus of the monkey. Exp. Brain Res. 54, 575–578.

Schwartz, I.R. and Ryan, A.F. (1986) Uptake of amino acids in the gerbil cochlea. In: R.A. Altschuler, D.W. Hoffman and R.P. Bobbin (Eds.) Neurobiology of hearing: The cochlea, Raven Press, New York, NY, pp. 173–190.

Stockard, J.E., Stockard, J.J., and Sharborough, F.W. (1978) Non-pathologic factors influencing brainstem auditory evoked potentials. Am. J. Electroencephalogr. Technol 18, 177–193.

Trune, D.R., Mitchell, C. and Phillips, D.S. (1978) The relative importance of head size, gender and age on the auditory brainstem response. Hear. Res 32, 165–174.

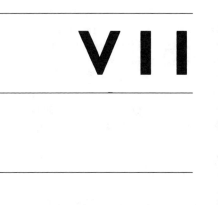

Aging

Aging produces unique auditory dysfunction. We are used to thinking about hearing problems resulting from changes in the auditory periphery, the middle and inner ears, and we are just getting used to thinking about hearing problems resulting from changes in the central auditory pathways. In aging, however, we have to think about hearing problems due to changes throughout the auditory system, involving both peripheral and central mechanisms. And central changes may refect both specifically auditory and more generalized, age-related cognitive disorders.

The first article in this section, "Audiological Findings in Aging" (*Advances in Otorhinolaryngology*, 1973), was a paper presented at an aging conference organized by Merle Lawrence at the University of Michigan in 1972. I took the opportunity to ask whether, in a very large sample, one could derive support for John Gaeth's idea of a disproportionate loss in monosyllabic word recognition scores in the elderly. The answer was quite positive. When results for 4,095 ears were grouped according to pure tone average (PTA), for every category of degree of loss, ranging from 0–69 dB, there was a systematic decline in the PB_{max} score with advancing chronological age. Then, in subgroups matched on various dimensions, I showed that the phenomenon was related to the difficulty of the speech recognition task, and could be dramatically enhanced by stress in the time domain. All of this suggested a primarily central rather than peripheral interpretation of the effect.

Virtually everything that we have learned in our laboratory in the 20 years since the publication of this paper has tended to support these early conclusions. One of the most convincing lines of evidence was the series of events leading up to the case presentation, "Central Presbyacusis: A Longitudinal Case Study" (*Ear & Hearing*, 1985). A dynamic businessman, the CEO of one of the major oil companies headquartered in Houston, originally came to us at age 70. Five years later, we fitted him with a hearing aid. From the very beginning, he complained of difficulty in noisy situations, but seemed to fare pretty well in quiet places. Over the next four years, his complaints increased. Even in quiet situations, he was forced to rely more and more on lip reading to understand what was being said. Then, one day he brought the aid in for repair, convinced that it was not working properly. He said that he could hear better without it. When we checked the aid, we found it to be in good working order. What had changed was not the hearing aid but his auditory processing ability. Because we had tested him thoroughly on four different occasions over a 9-year period, we were able to document the change in central auditory function and to differentiate the auditory from the cognitive changes. The pure-tone audiogram and the PB_{max} scores had changed very little over the 9-year period, but SSI scores had declined dramatically, demonstrating a waxing and waning "rollover" effect in the process. Occasionally a single case study like this one can give you as much insight as a formal investigation of hundreds of subjects.

The paper entitled, "Effect of Response Criterion on Measures of Speech Understanding in the Elderly" (*Ear & Hearing*, 1988), is a favorite because it shows the versatility of the "signal-detection" paradigm. Here, we were concerned with the question: "Is the poorer performance of elderly persons on speech recognition tests due to a shift in criterion with age?" In other words, do elderly persons perform less well simply because they become more conservative and rigid in their attitudes and are less willing to guess when they are not sure of an answer?

Previous investigators of this problem generally had used a design in which an elderly group was compared with a young group matched for degree of hearing loss. The rationale would be that if the elderly subjects perform less well on the speech recognition task, and were also shown to be more conservative listeners, then the point was made that change in response criterion is the explanation for the poorer speech recognition scores in the elderly.

But this is a very weak approach, beset by many problems in controlling all possible relevant variables, and based on the assumption that all elderly people change criterion in the same direction. It seemed to us that a better design would be to divide elderly people into different groups according to whether they were strict, intermediate, or lax listeners and then see whether there was, in fact, any difference in speech recognition performance scores across the groups. When we did this, we found, not unexpectedly, that the dominating influence on PB, SSI, DSI, and SPIN scores was degree of hearing loss. When this factor was taken into account, listener strategy had no significant differential effect on the speech recognition scores.

Two papers, "Speech Understanding in the Elderly" (*Ear & Hearing*, 1989) and "Correlational Analysis of Speech Audiometric Scores, Hearing Loss, Age, and Cognitive Abilities in the Elderly" (*Ear & Hearing*, 1991), summarize our 5-year study, supported by the National Institute on Aging, of the relative influence of a number of variables on speech recognition in the elderly. The research was motivated by the important question: "Can the decline in speech understanding in the elderly be explained as a consequence of cognitive decline?" In other words, it is well established that a number of cognitive abilities, especially memory and speed of mental processing, decline with age. Are these changes sufficient to explain the progressive decline in speech understanding with age? To approach this question, we enlisted the aid of a Baylor neuropsychologist, Francis Pirozzolo. Together we planned a test battery that included tests of both auditory and cognitive function, then administered the battery to 130 elderly persons. We categorized results as normal or abnormal according to the auditory test results, and Pirozzolo categorized results as normal or abnormal according to the tests of cognitive function. Each of us was blind to the interpretation of the other. Not unexpectedly, we found a good deal of abnormality in both dimensions. Indeed, 27% of the total group was abnormal in both the auditory and cognitive areas. In 37% of cases, however, there was an important lack of congruence between the two sets of results. In 23%, or almost one

in four elderly persons, auditory status was abnormal but cognitive status was normal, whereas in 14% cognitive status was abnormal but there was no auditory abnormality.

In a later correlational study of 200 elderly persons we asked how much of the variability in performance on tests of speech understanding can be predicted from knowledge of hearing loss, age, and cognitive function. Results were consistent with our previous findings. Degree of hearing loss accounted for the lion's share of the variance. Cognitive status accounted for very little. Interestingly, however, speed of mental processing, as measured by the Digit-Symbol subtest of the Wechsler Adult Intelligence Scale-Revised (WAIS-R), accounted for significant variance in the DSI score, and age accounted for significant variance in the SSI score.

An interesting variant on the general theme of dichotic listening is the "cued-listening" task, which Craig Jordan and I developed in an attempt to simulate the listening situation so frequently complained about by elderly hearing-aid users, difficulty in attending to a target talker while there is competing speech coming from other directions. We set up a listening task in which the subject is "cued," by a signal light, to attend to what is coming from a loudspeaker either to his right or to this left, in the presence of voice babble from a loudspeaker directly above the subject's chair. The two loudspeakers, to right and left, are playing the same recording of continuous discourse, a detective story written in the first person, but the recording is delayed 60 seconds from one loudspeaker relative to the other. The speech target is the personal pronoun "I." During the entire test run, the "I" target is presented 50 times from the right side and 50 times from the left side. A computer keeps track of correct identification (hits) and laterality errors (false alarms). Our original idea in creating this task was to have a method for comparing monaural and binaural hearing aid performance. But in the process of running elderly persons in the unaided condition, we noticed an unexpected laterality effect. In young adult listeners, we observed the expected right-ear advantage to be expected in any dichotic or, in this case, quasi-dichotic paradigm. The effect, however, was small, less than 4%. But in elderly listeners the right-ear advantage was substantially larger, averaging almost 16%. Various lines of evidence suggest that this may represent an age-related compromise of the auditory pathways in the corpus callosum. In any event, the data provided by the cued-listening task highlight, anew, the value of the dichotic paradigm in the study of central auditory processing.

Finally, I have chosen for this section two papers concerned with the low-frequency region of the audiogram in the elderly population. Both were motivated by persistent clinical observations. "Low-Frequency Hearing Loss in Presbycusis" (*Archives of Otolaryngology*, 1979) documented our clinical impression that elderly persons with central auditory signs had flatter audiograms than elderly persons without such signs. We showed that this was, indeed, the case and that the effect could not be explained by either age or audiometric contour. At this point, however, we were not clever enough to factor in a possible gender difference as an explanatory factor.

Another persistent clinical observation was that, whenever we compared average audiograms of elderly males and elderly females, it seemed that the males always showed more high-frequency loss, but the females always showed more low-frequency loss. We have documented this observation in the paper entitled, "Gender Affects Audiometric Shape in Presbyacusis." Here we show, from surveys large and small, and from many different countries, that males lose more high-frequency sensitivity than females, but that the reverse is true in the frequency region below 1000 Hz. In this region, females lose more sensitivity with age than males.

Is it possible that these two sets of observations can be related? Is it the case that females experience more central auditory changes with age than males? Clearly we need to pay more attention to possible gender differences in the way aging affects auditory processing ability.

Adv. Oto-Rhino-Laryng., vol. 20, pp. 115–124 (Karger, Basel 1973)

Audiological Findings in Aging[1]

J. Jerger

Department of Otolaryngology, Baylor College of Medicine, Houston, Texas

Introduction

The aging process produces systematic changes in each of the two critical dimensions of hearing impairment – loss in threshold sensitivity and loss in the ability to understand suprathreshold speech.

The pattern of loss in threshold sensitivity is well documented. Since Zwaardemaker's pioneering report [17] several investigators [1, 4–6] have quantified the progressive loss in pure-tone sensitivity as a function of frequency, culminating in the mathematical expression of a general exponential law governing the relation [8].

Concomitant changes in the second critical dimension, the ability to understand speech, are less well understood. Gaeth [3] was one of the earliest investigators to describe a disproportionate loss in single-syllable word intelligibility in the aged patient. He coined the expression 'phonemic regression' to describe the phenomenon. In retrospect, this highlights the hazard inherent in ascribing descriptive terms to phenomena before they are well understood. In the light of present knowledge it seems doubtful that the effect involves either 'phonemes' or 'regressive' tendencies. Nevertheless, the observation that elderly patients have more difficulty in word intelligibility tests than one would expect from younger subjects with comparable sensitivity loss was a pioneering contribution to the audiologic study of aging.

The present paper summarizes the results of a series of experiments designed to further our understanding of the effects of aging on suprathreshold speech intelligibility.

1   This research was supported by US Public Health Service grants NS08542 and NS08810 from the National Institute of Neurological Diseases and Stroke.

Reality of the Aging Effect

The concept of disproportionately poor speech understanding in the aged has been widely accepted in spite of the fact that the effect has not been documented with anything like the depth of study accorded changes in threshold sensitivity

As a first step, therefore, in an analysis of the phenomenon, we analyzed the PB scores of virtually all patients with sensorineural hearing loss who were tested in the Audiology Service of the Methodist Hospital during the past four years. The analysis was based on 4,095 ears of 2,162 patients ranging in age from 6 to 89 years. The number of ears in each age decade ranged from a maximum of 740 in the 60th to 69th year to a minimum of 109 in the 80th to 89th year. The speech audiometric evaluation of each ear involved the generation of a complete performance vs. intensity (PI) function for monosyllabic, phonetically-balanced (PB) words. Lists of 25 words each were presented at 4–6 suprathreshold levels in order to define the shape of the function relating intelligibility to speech intensity. A true maximum PB score (PB_{max}) could, therefore, be determined for each ear of each patient.

For all patients PB test materials were NDRC lists 1–6 recorded on magnetic tape in our laboratory by a male speaker with general American dialect.

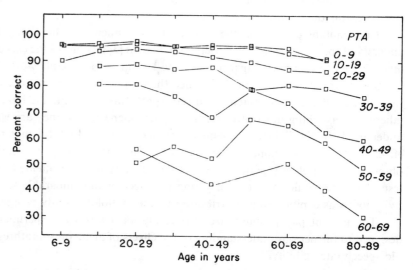

Fig. 1. Average PB_{max} as a function of age with hearing loss (PTA) held constant. Note systematic decline in PB_{max} with advancing age. 2,162 patients, 4,095 ears.

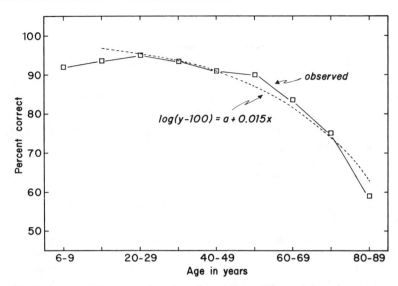

Fig. 2. Average PB$_{max}$ as a function of age. Data of figure 1 have been averaged across PTA. Note exponential shape of decline. 2,162 patients, 4,095 ears. PTA=0–69.

Figure 1 shows the average PB$_{max}$ as a function of age with the average pure-tone threshold (500–2,000 Hz) loss (PTA) held constant.

Here we see, with dramatic immediacy, the reality of the aging effect on speech intelligibility. At virtually any level of PTA there is a systematic decrement in performance with advancing age. The effect is slight for the PTA category 0–9 dB but increases substantially with greater hearing loss. In the PTA category 40–49 dB, for example, the average PB$_{max}$ declines from 80%, in the 10 to 19-year age group, to 60% in the 80 to 89-year age group, a result in very close agreement with the earlier work of PESTALOZZA and SHORE [13].

Figure 2 is a single curve obtained by averaging the data of figure 1 across PTA in order to illustrate the general shape of the functional relationship between PB score and age. The expected exponential form is evident.

The equation:

$$\log (y - 100) = a + 0.015 \, x$$

where y is the PB$_{max}$ score and x is age in years fits the observed trend reasonably well, and may be compared with HINCHCLIFFE's [8] general equation for pure-tone sensitivity changes with age:

$$\log (\varnothing - \varnothing_k) = 0.032 \, x - a$$

where $\varnothing$ is threshold sensitivity expressed in dyn/cm², $\varnothing_k$ is a reference intensity unique to frequency, and x is age.

Possible Relation to Loudness Recruitment

In view of a steady accumulation of evidence (1) that speech intelligibility loss tends to be unusually severe in patients with acoustic tumors and other lesions affecting the first order neuron, and (2) that speech understanding may be dramatically altered in patients with lesions of the central auditory system, it is compelling to speculate that the phenomenon of 'phonemic regression' is the result of aging in the central rather than in the peripheral auditory system. For example, HINCHCLIFFE [7, p. 307] concludes:

'This implies that temporal lobe deficit is a component of presbycusis. Decrease in the intelligibility of distorted speech with age must, therefore, be correlated with a decrease in cell count of the temporal lobe with age.'

On the other hand, SCHUKNECHT implicates the VIIIth nerve itself [14, p. 418]:

'The second type, termed "neural atrophy", is characterized by degeneration of spiral ganglion cells beginning at the basal end of the cochlea as well as neurons of the higher auditory pathways and is superimposed upon varying degrees of epithelial atrophy. Its onset is late in life, it progresses slowly for years, and is characterized clinically by high tone deafness with disproportionately severe loss in auditory discrimination.'

In a pioneering survey of the audiologic manifestations of aging, PESTALOZZA and SHORE [13] studied the relation between PB score and the recruitment phenomenon in a subset of 24 elderly patients. In effect, they found that discrimination might be good or bad when recruitment was absent, but tended to be bad only when recruitment was present, a finding in seeming contradiction to the notion that 'phonemic regression' is the result of retrocochlear rather than cochlear aging.

The purpose of the present study was to extend the exploration of the relation between loudness recruitment and loss in speech understanding through the use of a more satisfactory method for the detection of loudness recruitment than was available to PESTALOZZA and SHORE [13]. These investigators employed a monaural loudness balance procedure which required that the elderly patient equate the loudnesses of two relatively dissimilar frequencies on the same ear. We felt that a more objective procedure based on the sensation level required to elicit the acoustic reflex [2] would provide a more satisfactory index of loudness recruitment in the elderly patient. Accordingly, we compared PB scores in two groups of presbycusics, one with and one without recruitment (as defined by the sensation level of the acoustic reflex).

Subjects were 36 patients chosen from our audiological files. They were subdivided into 3 groups of 12 each: old persons without recruitment, old persons with recruitment, and young persons with recruitment.

Table I. Median age, air conduction hearing levels (ACHL), and acoustic reflex sensation levels (SL), in 3 groups of 12 patients each

Group	Age, years		ACHL				Reflex SL			
	median	range	500 Hz	1 kHz	2 kHz	4 kHz	500 Hz	1 kHz	2 kHz	4 kHz
Old with recruitment	67	60–78	25	35	50	53	58	53	45	40
Old without recruitment	67	60–80	15	23	30	40	75	>75	>70	>70
Young with recruitment	37	8–54	35	40	60	50	43	48	40	>40

Three measures were abstracted from the clinical data on each patient: (1) the pure-tone audiogram, (2) the PB_{max} score, and (3) the sensation level of the acoustic reflex.

Presence or absence of loudness recruitment was defined by the sensation level at which the acoustic reflex was elicited. Reflex sensation levels were measured by means of an electroacoustic impedance bridge (Madsen ZO-70). Patients were considered to have recruitment when the sensation

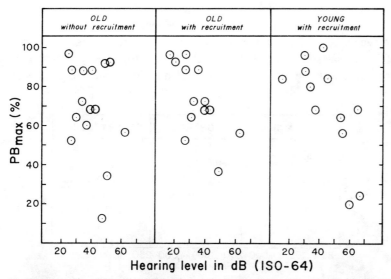

Fig. 3. PB_{max} as a function of PTA in 3 groups of patients: (1) old without recruitment, (2) old with recruitment, and (3) young with recruitment.

level of the acoustic reflex was less than 60 dB at 2 or more of the 4 frequencies: 0.5, 1, 2 and 4 kHz.

Table I describes salient features of the three experimental groups. It summarizes the median and range of ages for each of the three groups, the median air conduction hearing loss for each group, and the median reflex sensation level for each group.

Figure 3 plots, for each of the three groups separately, the PB_{max} score of each patient as a function of the average audiometric hearing loss (PTA). Careful analysis of these plots fails to reflect substantial differences among the three groups. We note that the relationship between PB_{max} and PTA seems equivalent whether we are dealing with young people with recruitment, old people with recruitment, or old people without recruitment. The *disproportionate loss in speech understanding* in aging patients is apparently not strongly related to the loudness recruitment phenomenon.

Relation to Difficulty of Speech Intelligibility Task

In a search for aspects of speech intelligibility loss unique to the aging process, we next compared the behavior of elderly patients with the behavior of younger patients showing the same degree and configuration of sensorineural loss on a variety of suprathreshold tasks involving speech understanding under difficult listening conditions.

After generating complete performance-intensity functions for PB words we generated analogous functions for sentence identification in the presence of ipsilateral speech competition (SSI-ICM) [10], then repeated the same procedure with the test sentences subjected to 50% time compression.

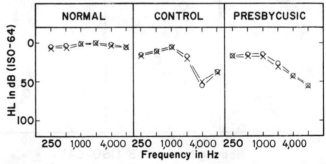

Fig. 4. Average pure-tone audiograms for 18 presbycusics, 5 young adults with similar audiometric loss, and 5 normals.

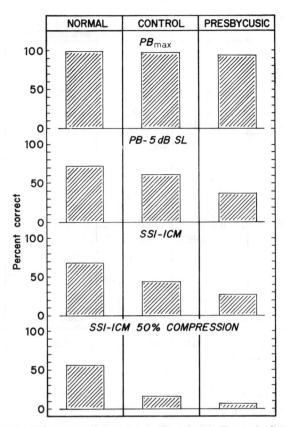

Fig. 5. Average scores on 4 speech understanding tasks for the three patient groups.

18 presbycusics were compared with 5 young adult patients matched for average hearing level (control group), and with 5 subjects with normal hearing. Figure 4 shows the average audiogram for each group. Figure 5 shows the average score for each group for PB_{max}, PB score at 5 dB sensation level, sentences in competition, and sentences time-compressed.

We see that, for the relatively easy task of repeating back PB words at a level well above threshold (PB_{max}) there is little difference among the three groups. When the task is made somewhat more difficult, however, by simply presenting the words at a very faint level (5 dB SL) the presbycusic group has more difficulty than either the normal or the control groups. Sentence identification in the presence of ipsilateral competing message (SSI-ICM) shows

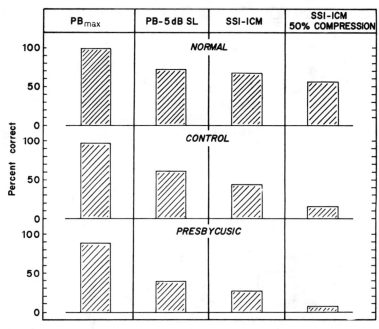

Fig. 6. Same data as figure 5 but recast in order to highlight effect of increasing difficulty of listening task on each group.

an even more pronounced effect. Controls break down relative to normals, but presbycusics show an even greater loss.

Finally, subjecting the SSI sentences to time compression accentuates the effect even more. Both the control and presbycusic groups show a severe breakdown in comparison with the normal group.

Figure 6 recasts these same data in a manner which emphasizes how both the control and presbycusic groups decline to a greater degree than the normal group as the nature of the speech intelligibility task becomes more difficult.

Presbycusics show a slightly greater effect than the younger controls.

Discussion

If we make the not unreasonable assumption that cochlear disorders account for the bulk of sensorineural hearing loss in young adults, then it seems clear from figure 1 that we must look beyond the cochlea to explain the loss in speech understanding unique to the elderly.

A number of previous investigators [7, 11, 12], especially HINCHCLIFFE [7], have hypothesized that central rather than peripheral changes are responsible for the speech intelligibility loss in the aged. The present results certainly concur with this conceptualization. In particular we are in accord with those investigators [9, 11, 16], notably KIRIKAE [11], who have stressed the importance of temporal factors in aging. Our own results with time-compressed English sentences are in close agreement with analogous data obtained by KIRIKAE [11] using Japanese monosyllables.

Taken as a whole, the present results support the following conclusions:

(1) There is, indeed, in the elderly, disproportionate loss in speech understanding, over and above what can be accounted for by the loss in threshold sensitivity. When hearing loss is held constant across age, the progressive effect of aging on speech intelligibility loss is easily documented.

(2) The phenomenon is not strongly related to the presence or absence of loudness recruitment.

(3) The phenomenon is related to the difficulty of the listening task. In particular, it can be dramatically enhanced by stress in the time domain.

(4) Available evidence supports a central rather than peripheral interpretation of the phenomenon.

Summary

The aging process produces systemic changes in both threshold sensitivity and suprathreshold speech intelligibility. The latter phenomenon is demonstrated as a progressive decline in PB_{max} with increasing age when degree of hearing loss is held constant.

Various characteristics of the phenomenon implicate a central rather than peripheral locus of the disorder.

References

1 BUNCH, C.C.: Age variations in auditory acuity. Arch. Otolaryng. *9:* 625–636 (1929).

2 EWERTSEN, H.; FILLING, S.; TERKILDSEN, K., and THOMSEN, K.A.: Comparative recruitment testing. Acta oto-laryng., Stockh. suppl. *140:* 116–122 (1958).

3 GAETH, J.H.: A study of phonemic regression in relation to hearing loss; Diss. Northwestern Univ. Chicago (1948).

4 GLORIG, A. and NIXON, J.: Hearing loss as a function of age. Laryngoscope *72:* 1596–1610 (1962).

5 GUILD, S.R.: The ear; in COWDRY Problems of aging, biological and medical aspects, 2nd ed., pp. 556–566 (Williams & Wilkins, Baltimore 1942).

6   HINCHCLIFFE, R.: Correction of pure tone audiograms for advancing age. J. Laryng. *73:* 830–832 (1959).

7   HINCHCLIFFE, R.: The anatomical locus of presbycusis. J. Speech Dis. *27:* 301–310 (1962).

8   HINCHCLIFFE, R.: Aging and sensory thresholds. J. Geront. *17:* 45–50 (1962).

9   HOLMGREN, L.: Psychology of deafness in the aged. Int. Audiol. *8:* 281–289 (1969).

10 JERGER, J.; SPEAKS, C., and TRAMMELL, J.L.: A new approach to speech audiometry. J. Speech Dis. *33:* 318–328 (1968).

11 KIRIKAE, I.: Auditory function in advanced age with reference to histological changes in the central auditory system. Int. Audiol. *8:* 221–230 (1969).

12 KÖNIG, E.: Audiological tests in presbycusis. Int. Audiol. *8:* 240–259 (1969).

13 PESTALOZZA, G. and SHORE, I.: Clinical evaluation of presbycusis on the basis of different tests of auditory function. Laryngoscope *65:* 1136–1163 (1955).

14 SCHUKNECHT, H.F.: Presbycusis. Laryngoscope *65:* 402–419 (1955).

15 SCHUKNECHT, H.F. and WOELLNER, R.C.: An experimental and clinical study of deafness from lesions of the cochlear nerve. J. Laryng. *69:* 75–97 (1955).

16 STICHT, T.G. and GRAY, B.B.: The intelligibility of time compressed words as a function of age and hearing loss. J. Speech Res. *12:* 443–448 (1969).

17 ZWAARDEMAKER, H.: Der Verlust an hohen Tönen mit zunehmendem Alter, ein neues Gesetz. Arch. Ohr. Nas.-KehlkHeilk. *47:* (1899).

Author's address: J.F. JERGER, Ph D, 11922 Taylorcrest, *Houston, TX 77024* (USA)

Low-Frequency Hearing Loss in Presbycusis

A Central Interpretation

Deborah Hayes, MA, James Jerger, PhD

● **Elderly subjects with a central phonemically balanced (PB) and synthetic sentence identification (SSI) pattern show greater low-frequency (LF) sensitivity loss than elderly subjects with a peripheral PB-SSI pattern. This LF hearing loss is not the simple consequence of age, nor does the LF hearing loss account for depressed SSI performance. We conclude that LF sensitivity loss and a central PB-SSI pattern are both components of central aging. We discuss the implications for auditory rehabilitation of elderly subjects.**

(Arch Otolaryngol 105:9-12, 1979)

The aging process affects both the peripheral and central auditory systems. Histopathologic studies[1-3] have shown age-related changes in the cochlea, major brain stem nuclei, and auditory cortex. Behaviorally, these changes are reflected in decreased pure-tone sensitivity and depressed suprathreshold speech intelligibility.[4,5]

The change in pure-tone sensitivity in aging is typically represented as a progressive loss in sensitivity as a function of frequency. High-frequency sensitivity is more affected than low, which gives the audiometric contour a gently sloping configuration.

The change in speech intelligibility is generally considered to be a slight but consistent decrease in speech-understanding ability with increasing age, as measured by the monosyllabic, phonemically balanced (PB) word score.[6] This decrease in speech intelligibility is thought to reflect the contribution of central auditory involvement in presbycusis. Consequently, several investigators have studied this phenomenon with various altered or degraded speech materials that were originally designed for the evaluation of central auditory disorders.[7] Popular procedures include filtered, distorted, or time-compressed PB words.[8,9] The results of these experiments typically show decreasing performance with increasing age, even in the presence of normal hearing.

In a recent report,[10] we proposed an alternative speech test that promised to be useful in the determination of the central-aging component in speech processing, the synthetic sentence identification (SSI) test at a 0-dB message-to-competition ratio. The results of this procedure, when compared with the results of the conventional PB word test, demonstrate several useful diagnostic patterns. One of these patterns is a "central effect" in which the performance-intensity (PI) function for sentences (PI-SSI) falls well below the PI function for PB words (PI-PB). The effect of age on these speech functions is considered a special case of the central effect. Many elderly patients perform substantially poorer on the SSI test than on the PB test. This central-aging effect begins at about the age of 60 years and increases substantially thereafter.

We have been performing complete PB and SSI speech audiometric functions on adult patients at the Audiology Service, The Methodist Hospital, Houston, since 1974. About a year ago, we began a systematic review of the pure-tone and speech audiometric findings in these subjects. As we reviewed the audiograms of elderly subjects, we noticed an interesting pattern. The audiometric configurations of elderly subjects with a central PB-SSI effect seemed to show more low-frequency (LF) sensitivity loss than the audiometric configuration of elderly subjects without the central PB-SSI effect. This suggested to us that evidence of "central aging" might appear not only in speech audiometry, but in the pure-tone audiogram as well. The purpose of the present study was to explore this possibility in presbycusis by comparing the audiometric findings in subjects with the clearly peripheral PB-SSI pattern to the audiometric find-

Accepted for publication Nov 24, 1977.

From the Department of Otorhinolaryngology and Communicative Sciences, Baylor College of Medicine, Houston.

Reprints not available.

ings in subjects with the clearly central PB-SSI pattern.

METHOD
Subjects

The subjects of this study were drawn retrospectively from the clinical files of the Audiology Service, The Methodist Hospital, Houston. All experimental subjects were aged 60 years or older. They had received a complete audiometric evaluation, including impedance audiometry, pure-tone audiometry, and diagnostic speech audiometry (complete PI-PB and PI-SSI functions).

All patients had either normal hearing or a sensorineural hearing loss; subjects with conductive losses were excluded from the study. Speech thresholds for spondees, PB words,[11] or sentences were at a 59-dB hearing level or less, and the difference in speech thresholds between the two ears was 19 dB or less. The resulting 197 subjects (100 female and 97 male) were divided into three groups on the basis of their PB-SSI performance.

The first experimental group consisted of 70 subjects who exhibited the peripheral PB-SSI pattern, ie, the SSI maximum (SSI_M) was either equal to $\pm 4\%$ or better than the PB maximum (PB_M) in both ears. This group was called experimental-peripheral (EP). The second experimental group consisted of 90 subjects who exhibited neither a purely peripheral nor a purely central PB-SSI pattern. Patients in this group showed an SSI_M poorer than the PB_M by 4% to 19% in both ears. We called this group experimental-intermediate (EI). The third experimental group consisted of 37 patients whose SSI_M was poorer than the PB_M by 20% or more bilaterally. This, of course, is the central PB-SSI pattern. This group was called experimental-central (EC).

In addition to these three experimental groups, we also analyzed audiometric findings in two control groups. These two groups were formed during the course of this investigation, as needed to control for certain experimental variables.

The first control group provided a control for age. This age-control group (CA) consisted of 16 subjects who were more than the age of 70 years; these subjects were drawn from the original pool of group EP. Their PB-SSI pattern, then, was purely peripheral.

The second control group provided a control for audiometric configuration. This slope-control group (CS) consisted of 35 subjects with LF, rising audiometric configurations. All subjects in this group were under the age of 60 years (average age, 40.2 years) to remove the possibility of aging effects on the speech scores.

Analysis

Results were analyzed separately for each ear of each group. Since there was a larger number of subjects who were under the age of 70 years, a strong right-left ear difference[10] did not emerge. Therefore, we have chosen to present data from the right ear only.

RESULTS

Not unexpectedly, subjects in group EC were somewhat older than subjects in groups EP and EI. The average age in each group was as follows: EP, 66.4 years; EI, 67.0 years; EC, 74.1 years. In other words, the group with the central pattern was, on the average, almost eight years older than the group with no central effect.

Speech audiometric results are shown in Fig 1. The average PB_M and SSI_M scores are shown for each group. Although the average PB_M for group EC is slightly poorer than for either groups EP or EI, all three PB_M scores are quite similar (EP = 83.1%; EI = 88.5%; EC = 77.7%). The fact that the PB_M should be only mildly depressed for group EC suggests that central aging has only a slight effect on undistorted, monosyllabic word understanding, which is a fact well documented by previous investigators.[6,9] The fact that the average SSI_M scores are dissimilar (EP = 90.4%; EI = 78.8%; EC = 33.5%) is, of course, due to the fact that the three groups were originally formed on the basis of this score.

The average audiograms and average acoustic reflex thresholds for the right ear of each group are seen in Fig 2. Acoustic reflex thresholds are virtually identical for all three groups. Pure-tone sensitivity above 2,000 Hz is also similar for the three experimental groups. However, below 2,000 Hz, an interesting trend emerges. Group EC shows poorer LF sensitivity than either group EP or EI. The difference between groups EP and EC is a substantial 16.9 dB at 250 Hz and diminishes to less than 1.0 dB at 4,000 Hz.

It is possible that the LF sensitivity loss of group EC is merely an expression of its greater average age (EP = 66.4 years; EC = 74.1 years). To control for this possibility, we compared the pure-tone audiometric findings from group EC with an age-matched control group CA. Its average age (74.4 years) was matched to group EC, but its PB SSI pattern was peripheral.

Figure 3 compares the average audiogram of group CA with the average audiogram of the original group EC. In spite of the age-matching procedure, group EC continues to show more LF sensitivity loss than group CA. The difference at 250 Hz is 12.8 dB, diminishes to 5.6 dB at 1,000 Hz, and disappears altogether above 1,000 Hz. In other words, the LF sensitivity loss of group EC cannot be attributed to chronological age, per se.

It is possible that the poor average SSI_M score of group EC is the simple consequence of its greater average LF sensitivity loss, rather than a more complex central-aging effect. To control for this possibility, we compared the pure-tone and speech audiometric findings for group EC with these same findings for a group of young subjects with rising audiometric configurations (group CS). The purpose of group CS was to match the LF sensitivity loss of group EC, but to remove the aging effect.

Figure 4 compares the average audiogram of group CS with the average audiogram of group EC. We see that the control group shows even greater LF sensitivity loss than group EC. Nonetheless, its average SSI_M score is considerably better (CS = 78.6%; EC = 33.5%). In other words, young subjects with LF sensitivity loss performed more than 40% better on the SSI task than did elderly subjects with similar audiometric configurations. Thus, the substantially depressed sentence identification performance of group EC cannot be attributed to LF sensitivity loss, per se.

The Table summarizes the average audiometric test results for the three experimental groups (EP, EI, EC) and the two control groups (CA, CS). The pure-tone averages for 500, 1,000, and 2,000 Hz and the speech thresholds for

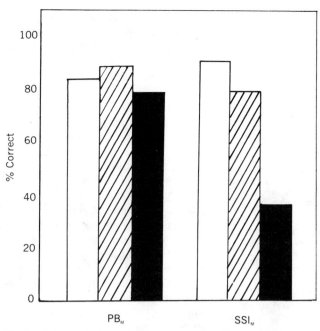

Fig 1.—Average PB$_M$ and SSI$_M$ scores for three experimental groups of elderly subjects. Average PB scores are similar, but average SSI$_M$ scores are dissimilar. Open bar indicates experimental-peripheral group; shaded bar, experimental-intermediate group; closed bar, experimental-central group.

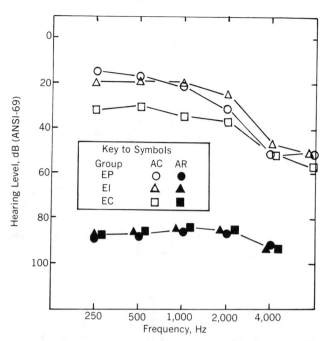

Fig 2.—Average pure-tone audiograms and average acoustic reflex thresholds for three experimental groups. Acoustic reflex thresholds and pure-tone sensitivity above 2,000 Hz are similar for all three groups. However, below 2,000 Hz, group EC shows greater sensitivity loss. AC indicates air conduction; AR, acoustic reflex.

Fig 3.—Average pure-tone audiograms for group EC and for age-matched control group CA. Group EC shows greater LF sensitivity loss. AC indicates air conduction.

Fig 4.—Average pure-tone audiograms for group EC and for slope-control group CS. Group CS shows greater LF sensitivity loss. AC indicates air conduction.

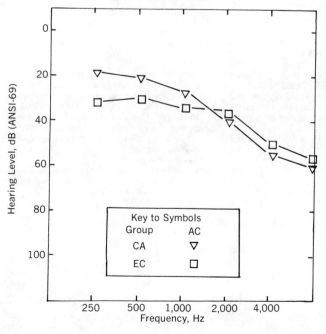

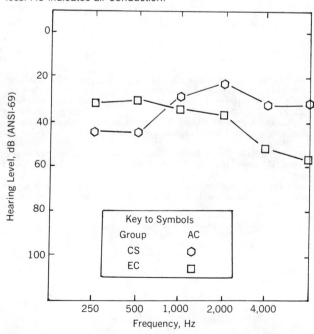

Average Audiometric Test Results for Three Experimental Groups and Two Control Groups*					
	Experimental Group			**Control Group**	
Measure	EP	EI	EC	CA	CS
Age, yr	66.4	67.0	74.1	74.4	40.2
PTA, dB HL	23.7	20.8	32.6	29.8	29.0
ST, dB HL	22.4	22.6	31.0	28.3	30.2
PB_M, %	83.1	88.5	77.7	78.2	83.8
SSI_M, %	90.4	78.8	33.5	86.2	78.6
PB_M-SSI_M, %	−7.3	+ 9.7	+ 44.2	−8.0	+ 5.2

*EP indicates experimental-peripheral; EI, experimental-intermediate; EC, experimental central; CA, age-control; CS, slope-control; PTA, pure-tone average; HL, hearing level; ST, speech threshold; PB_M, phonemically balanced maximum; SSI_M, synthetic sentence identification maximum.

all five groups indicate mild hearing loss. The average PB_M scores indicate relatively good, undistorted word understanding for all five groups. The average SSI_M scores for the two control groups (CA and CS) and two of the experimental groups (EP and EI) show good to excellent sentence identification. Only group EC shows depressed sentence identification performance. The difference between the average PB_M and SSI_M scores of group EC is a substantial + 44.2%. Group CA indicates that this PB-SSI discrepancy is not a purely age-related phenomenon because its average PB_M-SSI_M difference score is only −8.0%. Similarly, group CS indicates that this discrepancy is not the simple consequence of LF hearing loss because its average PB_M-SSI_M difference score is only + 5.2%. We conclude that neither age nor audiometric configuration can account for the substantial PB-SSI discrepancy that was observed in group EC.

COMMENT

The results of this investigation confirm our impression that elderly subjects who demonstrate the central PB-SSI effect also show LF sensitivity loss. We have seen that this loss is not the simple consequence of age. Furthermore, the LF sensitivity loss, itself, does not account for the depressed sentence identification performance in elderly subjects. Thus, although the LF sensitivity loss is often present in elderly subjects with a PB-SSI discrepancy, it does not account for this discrepancy.

To what can we attribute this unique constellation of results? Several factors must be considered. The possibility that the LF sensitivity loss is due to a middle ear disorder can be ruled out by the acoustic reflex findings. All three experimental groups had virtually identical acoustic reflex threshold levels. Furthermore, we would not expect a middle ear disorder to alter speech intelligibility scores substantially.

Similarly, the possibility that the depressed sentence identification is due to a purely cochlear phenomenon can be ruled out by the pattern of speech test results that were obtained from the young subjects in group CS. These young subjects with LF, rising audiometric contours showed, on the average, good sentence identification scores. Low-frequency cochlear loss did not substantially alter SSI performance.

We believe that the two phenomena, summarized in the Table and in Fig 2, the LF sensitivity loss and the PB-SSI discrepancy of group EC, are best explained as concomitant components of the central-aging effect.

In any event, the effect of the LF sensitivity loss is to give these elderly subjects a relatively flat audiometric contour. Classically, it is thought that subjects with such a configuration are the best candidates for hearing aid use.[12] However, central auditory effects decrease the likelihood of successful auditory rehabilitation. Possibly then, in elderly subjects, a sloping audiometric configuration is a better prognosis for successful hearing aid use than a more relatively flat audiometric contour.

References

1. Hansen C, Reske-Neilsen E: Pathological studies in presbycusis: Cochlear and central findings in 12 aged patients. *Arch Otolaryngol* 82:115-132, 1965.

2. Kirikae I, Sato T, Shitara T: A study of hearing in advanced age. *Laryngoscope* 74:205-220, 1964.

3. Hinchcliffe R: The anatomical locus of presbycusis. *J Speech Hearing Disord* 27:301-310, 1962.

4. Jerger J: Audiological findings in aging. *Adv Otorhinolaryngol* 20:115-124, 1973.

5. Palva A, Jokinen K: Presbycusis: V. Filtered speech test. *Acta Otolaryngol* 70:232-241, 1970.

6. Committee on Hearing, Bioacoustics, and Biomechanics: *Speech Understanding and Aging.* Washington, DC, National Academy of Science, 1977.

7. Bocca E, Calearo C: Central hearing processes, in Jerger J (ed): *Modern Developments in Audiology.* New York, Academic Press Inc, 1963.

8. Antonelli A: Sensitized speech tests in aged people, Rojskjaer C (ed): *Speech Audiometry.* Second Danavox Symposium, 1970, pp 66-79.

9. Konkle D, Beasley D, Bess F: Intelligibility of time-altered speech in relation to chronological aging. *J Speech Hearing Res* 20:108-115, 1977.

10. Jerger J, Hayes D: Diagnostic speech audiometry. *Arch Otolaryngol* 103:216-222, 1977.

11. Jerger S, Jerger J: Estimating speech threshold from the PI-PB function. *Arch Otolaryngol* 102:487-496, 1976.

12. Berger K, Millin J: Hearing aids, in Rose D (ed): *Audiological Assessment.* Englewood Cliffs, NJ, Prentice-Hall Inc, 1971.

Central Presbyacusis: A Longitudinal Case Study

Brad A. Stach, James F. Jerger, and Katherine A. Fleming

The Methodist Hospital and Baylor College of Medicine, Houston, Texas

ABSTRACT

An elderly patient with presbyacusis was tested on four occasions over a 9-year interval. Although there was little change in peripheral hearing sensitivity, central auditory function declined substantially. Diminished success as a hearing aid user seemed to parallel the change in central function. Results suggest that the central changes were auditory-specific rather than generalized cognitive in origin.

Many cross-sectional studies have documented progressive decline in auditory function with age, but few longitudinal studies have revealed the fine grain of this decline in the individual aging patient. During the past 9 yr, we have had a unique opportunity to follow senescent changes in auditory function in the same individual. Results, over this 9-yr period, suggest a substantial decline in central auditory function but little change in peripheral sensitivity.

The patient, a 79-yr-old man, was first evaluated by the Audiology Service, The Methodist Hospital, at the age of 70. He has since been evaluated on three occasions, at ages 75, 76, and 79 yr. Figure 1 shows the results of audiometric evaluation on the initial visit at age 70 (*left panel*) and the final visit at age 79 (*right panel*). The initial audiometric results revealed a typical presbyacusic profile. The pure-tone audiogram showed a mild, gradually falling contour from low to high frequencies, and speech understanding was only mildly impaired. Maximum phonemically balanced (PB) word scores were 96% for the right ear and 88% for the left ear. Maximum synthetic sentence identification (SSI) scores were slightly depressed; 80% on the right ear, and 80% on the left ear, suggesting a mild central component. On the whole, however, results were consistent with a mild, primarily peripheral, presbyacusic profile.

On the final visit, at age 79 (*right panel*), neither the pure-tone audiogram nor the maximum PB scores had changed appreciably, but the maximum SSI score had declined substantially on both ears. The latter profile suggested that the principal change, over the 9-yr period, had been a marked change in central function in spite of a relatively stable peripheral loss.

Figure 2 shows the actual progression of decline in pure-tone sensitivity (PTA2; average of HTLs at 1000, 2000, and 4000 Hz), the PB maximum score, and the SSI maximum score. The PTA2 declined only about 10 dB over the 9-yr period and the PB maximum score declined about 20%. Over this same period, however, the SSI maximum score declined by about 80% on the right ear and 60% on the left ear.

Figure 3 shows this decline in SSI performance in greater detail. For each ear, the performance versus intensity (PI) function is shown for each test date. These PI functions show an interesting progression, especially on the right ear. Initially, the maximum right ear SSI score did not change, but the degree of rollover (i.e., decrease in performance at intensities above the point of maximum performance) increased from 20% in 1975 to 50% in 1980. Then, the maximum, itself, dropped from 70% in 1980 to only 10% in 1984. A similar, but less dramatic, progression characterized the left ear as well.

This patient's experience as a hearing aid user is noteworthy, especially in view of the progression illustrated in Figure 2. He was fitted with an aid on the right ear in 1980. During the next 4 yr, he consistently complained of difficulty understanding speech in noisy situations, but used the aid successfully in quiet situations. Finally, in 1984, he asserted that the aid no longer worked, that while it still seemed to be amplifying, clarity was very poor. He suspected that the battery was weak. He thought his hearing must have decreased, since the aid was issued, because he could no longer understand any better with it than without it. While he had always had trouble in crowds, he now found increasing difficulty in one-on-one situations. He felt that he now had to "read lips" more as the benefit derived from the aid gradually decreased.

In short, he felt that amplification no longer gave him sufficient benefit to warrant its use. He strongly suspected that there was something very wrong with the hearing aid.

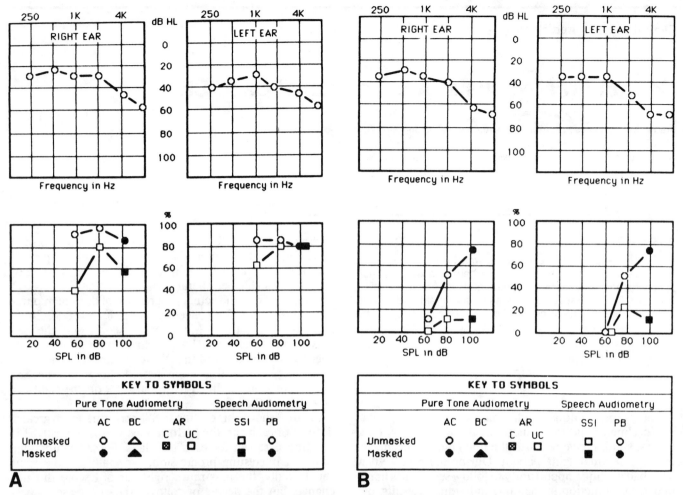

Figure 1. Pure tone and speech audiometric results in a patient with presbyacusis: A, at age 70; B, 9 yr later at age 79.

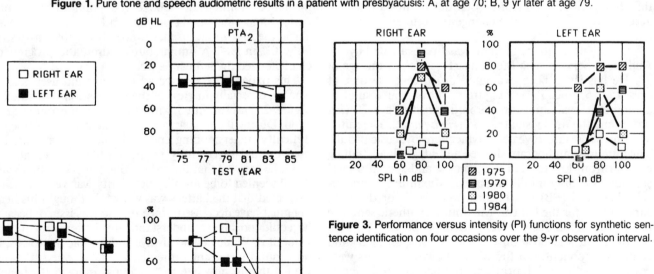

Figure 2. Changes in pure tone and speech audiometric scores over the 9-yr period: PTA2, average of HTLs at 1000, 2000, and 4000 Hz; PB Max, maximum of PI function for phonemically balanced (PB) words; SSI Max, maximum of PI function for synthetic sentences.

Figure 3. Performance versus intensity (PI) functions for synthetic sentence identification on four occasions over the 9-yr observation interval.

An electroacoustic analysis of the aid showed it to be in good working order and to be performing according to specifications.

COMMENT

This patient's experience illustrates the impact of central auditory function on successful hearing aid use.[1-5] As central function declined (apparently independently of peripheral status), the benefit derived from amplification diminished concomitantly.

It is appropriate to ask whether the progressive decline in SSI scores, over the 9-yr period, was due to specifically auditory changes or to more generalized cognitive decline. Two sets of data, in the present case, argue for specifically auditory changes. First, when the message-to-competition ratio (MCR) was changed 10 dB, from 0 to +10, SSI scores increased to 100%, indicating that the patient could perform the task satisfactorily when the signal-to-noise ratio was made more favorable. Second, the progressive change in shape of the performance versus intensity (PI) functions for SSI at 0 dB MCR illustrated in Figure 3, are difficult to reconcile with a generalized decline in cognitive function. The fact that changes were level-specific, leading to progressively greater "rollover" at high intensities, argues for an auditory rather than a general cognitive interpretation.

By conventional criteria (i.e., audiometric contour and PB score), this patient could be considered an ideal candidate for hearing aid use. On the initial visit, at age 70, the audiogram showed a mild, gradually sloping, symmetric contour with maximum PB scores in the range from 88 to 96%. On the final visit, at age 79, this overall picture had not changed appreciably. Conventional criteria still suggested an ideal candidate for amplification, yet actual benefit from hearing aid use had declined substantially.

It is noteworthy that neither the audiogram nor the PB scores, nor real-ear gain measures revealed this dramatic change. Only a test sensitive to central auditory disorder reflected the systematic decline, presumably underlying diminished benefit from amplification.

References

1. Hayes, D., and J. Jerger. 1979a. Low-frequency hearing loss in presbyacusis. A central interpretation. Arch. Otolaryngol. **105**, 9–12.
2. Hayes, D., and J. Jerger. 1979b. Aging and the use of hearing aids. Scand. Audiol. **8**, 33–40.
3. Hayes, D., J. Jerger, J. Taff, and B. Barber. 1983. Relation between aided synthetic sentence identification scores and hearing aid user satisfaction. Ear Hear. **4**, 158–161.
4. Jerger, J., and D. Hayes. 1977. Hearing and aging. pp. 109–118. *in* S. S. Han, and D. H. Coons, eds. *Special Senses in Aging.* University of Michigan Press, Ann Arbor.
5. Otto, W. C., and G. A. McCandless. 1982. Aging and auditory site of lesion. Ear Hear. **3**, 110–117.

Address reprint requests to Brad A. Stach, Audiology Service, Neurosensory Center, 6501 Fannin, NA200, Houston, TX 77030.

Received April 12, 1985; accepted May 19, 1985.

Effect of Response Criterion on Measures of Speech Understanding in the Elderly*

James Jerger, Karen Johnson, and Susan Jerger

Division of Audiology and Speech Pathology, Baylor College of Medicine, Houston, Texas

ABSTRACT

Twenty-four elderly subjects were divided into three groups on the basis of response criterion in a signal-detection task. The groups, representing strict, lax, and intermediate listeners, were then compared on the basis of performance on several conventional speech audiometric measures. When the data were corrected for degree of hearing loss, group differences were not significant. Thus, conventional speech audiometric results did not appear to be significantly influenced by response criterion.

A recurring theme, in the literature on aging, is that, in perceptual tasks requiring decisions, older adults tend to be more conservative than younger adults (Botwinick, Brinley, & Robbin, 1958; Clark & Mehl, 1971; Danzinger & Botwinick, 1980; Harkins & Chapman, 1976, 1977). In other words, older individuals seem to require a more complete sensory target than younger individuals before they are willing to make a decision about the target and they are less willing to make such a decision when the target is degraded or incomplete. It is interesting to ask, therefore, whether the well-documented decline in speech understanding with age may be related to a tendency toward the use of strict response criteria by the elderly. If audiological test results are significantly influenced by a conservative response bias in the elderly, then as Marshall (1981, p. 227) suggests, ". . . . . a whole body of literature, including aging norms, is in error."

Response criteria in perceptual tasks may be defined within the context of the theory of signal-detectability (see Clarke & Bilger, 1973, for a detailed discussion of signal-detection theory and its applications in the measurement of hearing). In the theory-of-signal detectability (TSD) paradigm a trial consists of an observation interval during which a target signal may, or may not, be presented against a background of noise or other competition. At the conclusion of each observation interval the subject's task is to indicate whether or not the target signal was presented during the interval. After a sufficient number of such trials one may compute the dual metric of the TSD paradigm, the "hit rate" and the "false alarm rate." Hit rate is the percentage of times that the subject voted "yes" when the target signal was, in fact, presented. False alarm rate is the percentage of times that the subject voted "yes" when the target signal was, in fact, not presented. The exact values that these measures will take depend upon the inherent detectability (d') of the target signal, the a priori probability that the signal will occur in a given trial, and the observer's unique response strategy.

Central to the theory underlying the description of an observer's behavior, in this paradigm, is the axiom that hit rate and false alarm rate are not free to vary independently. In fact, they are closely linked by a trade-off principle. To maximize hit rate one must accept an inevitably high false alarm rate. In order to be sure that he has identified every target signal that was, in fact, presented, the observer must, necessarily, be willing to adopt a relatively "lax" attitude toward guessing affirmitavely about those trials where he is not sure about the target. Thus, hit rate and false alarm rate must necessarily rise together. Conversely, to minimize false alarm rate one must accept an inevitably low hit rate. In order to be sure that he does not incorrectly identify the presence of a signal when, in fact, it was not presented, the observer must adopt a relatively cautious, or "strict" attitude toward voting yes in those trials where he is not sure about the target. Thus, to keep false alarm rate low one must accept that the hit rate will suffer.

The exact manner in which hit rate and false alarm rate covary is defined by three factors: (1) the inherent detectability of the target signal (d'), (2) the a priori probability that a signal will occur during an observation interval, and (3) the unique response strategy that the observer employs.

If the inherent detectability (d'), and the a priori probability are held constant, then the exact combination of hit rate and false alarm may be used to reveal the nature of the observer's response strategy. Some observers may employ a relatively lax strategy in the sense that they are willing to accept a high false alarm rate in order to achieve

* This research was supported by NIA grant AG-05680 and NINCDS grant NS-10940 from the National Institutes of Health, U.S. Public Health Service.

a high hit rate. Other observers may employ a relatively strict strategy in the sense that they are willing to sacrifice a high hit rate in order to preserve a low false alarm rate. Still others may employ an intermediate strategy in which neither the hit rate nor the false alarm rate is differentially emphasized. The exact listening strategy employed by an observer is called his "response criterion."

The relations among detectability, a priori probability, and response criterion are illustrated in Figure 1. This figure shows a family of iso-detectability (d') curves and iso-criterial curves. An observer's actual performance may be varied over the entire range of possible combinations of hit rate and false alarm rate in one of two ways: either (1) by manipulating the listener's response criterion while holding the d' and a priori probability constant, or (2) by manipulating the a priori probability while permitting the response criterion to vary freely.

The iso-detectability curves of Figure 1 are generated by option one. At each value of d' the a priori probability is held constant (usually at 0.5) while the observer's response criterion is manipulated, usually by a "payoff matrix," or system of rewards and punishments (frequently monetary) designed to encourage a particular response criterion.

Similarly, the iso-criterial curves of Figure 1 are generated by option two. For a given a priori probability the d' is varied to generate a curve reflecting the way in which hit rate and false alarm rate change with d' at that probability. For low a priori probabilities the observer's response criterion is forced into the strict zone by the fact that so few trials contain a target signal. Similarly, when the a priori probability is relatively high, the the observer's response criterion is forced into the lax zone by the fact that so many trials contain a target signal. The functions generated in this fashion are called "iso-criterial" curves, since the a priori probability determines the constant criterion across various levels of d'.

Finally, it may be noted that, if the a priori probability is set at 0.50, and the payoff matrix is not defined, then actual performance, under varying conditions of inherent signal detectability defines a particular observer's iso-criterial curve (i.e., his inherent response criterion). The rationale for subject categorization in the present paper is based on this observation.

The extent to which response criterion does, in fact, affect conventional audiologic measures of speech understanding is not clear. A number of investigators have shown that, for tonal detection in noise, elderly listeners tend to use a more conservative response criterion than young listeners (Craik, 1969, Potash & Jones, 1977; Rees & Botwinick). Citing such evidence, Marshall (1981) suggested that older listeners might also refuse to respond to words that were not clear. Yantz and Anderson (1984), however, comparing young and elderly listeners on an open-set word recognition task, found no difference between groups in either performance or response criterion. In a follow-up to the study by Yantz and Anderson, Gordon-Salant (1986) compared the response criteria of young and elderly listeners, matched for degree of hearing loss, on both open- and closed-set speech recognition tasks. In contrast to previous studies, Gordon-Salant found that,

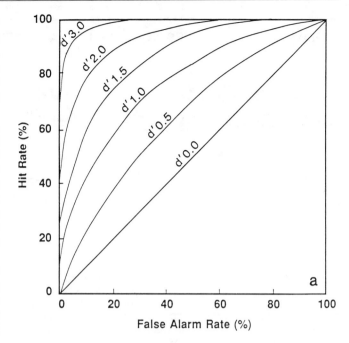

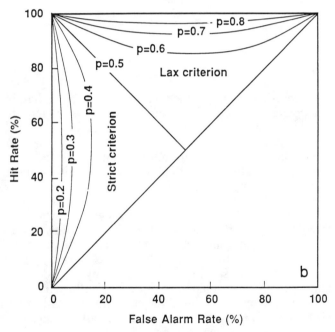

Figure 1. Iso-detectability curves (*panel a*), and iso-criterial curves (*panel b*), defining performance in the TSD paradigm.

in her sample, elderly listeners showed less conservative response criteria than young listeners.

The literature summarized above may be criticized on at least three grounds. First, virtually every study has employed a research design in which a single elderly (experimental) group is compared with a single young (control) group. The weakness of this design, especially in studies involving the elderly, is the danger that a spurious group difference may arise due to the influence of a relevant, but uncontrolled, variable. Investigators have generally recognized, for example, the importance of controlling for degree of hearing loss when comparing speech recognition scores of the young and the elderly. Matching on other potentially relevant variables, however, has been less common. Little attention, for example, has been directed toward matching on variables of cognitive function, although cognitive status must certainly impact response criterion. Nor have such potentially relevant variables as socioeconomic level or educational level been considered. Group comparisons, in general, are hazardous because of the possibility that not every relevant variable has been controlled. They are especially hazardous, however, when one group passed through the educational system, formulated its standards and values, and entered society 40 or more years before the other.

A second problem with previous studies is the assumption of homogeneity of change. Inherent in the group comparison design is the tacit assumption that aging will modify the response criteria of elderly subjects in an essentially homogenous fashion. Either all become more conservative, all become less conservative, or all stay the same. But such an assumption runs counter to much that we know of the effects of aging. In general, one may safely predict that, on virtually any dimension one may study, the inexorable effect of aging will be to increase variability relative to the distribution of that dimension in young people. The pure-tone audiogram, itself, is a prime example. At any test frequency the distribution of threshold sensitivity in an elderly group will be modified, relative to the analogous distribution in a young group, in two ways: (1) an increase in the central tendency, and (2) an increase in variability around the central tendency (Corso, 1963). It is not unreasonable to suppose, therefore, that aging may increase the dispersion of response criteria in the elderly. Some may become more conservative, but others may become less conservative. Still others may not change at all. Indeed, such an hypothesis, coupled with the ever-present possibility of sampling error, might explain the conflicting results of Yanz and Anderson, on the one hand, and Gordon-Salant, on the other.

A third potential flaw in previous studies has been the use of a criterial measure based on performance at a single level of difficulty of the speech recognition task. The hazard here is that, if the level of difficulty is not sufficient to force performance below a relatively high d′ level, then true differences in listening strategy may not be adequately reflected in the criterial measures. Because the iso-criterial contours converge toward the upper left hand corner of the response space (Fig. 1b), small variation in the hit rate and/or the false alarm rate can substantially affect the apparent response criterion.

In the present study we attempted to address each of these three methodological issues. In order to avoid the problem of matching young and elderly subjects on all variables thought to be relevant to such a comparison, and in order to avoid the assumption that the elderly share a common change in response criterion, we used a design in which elderly subjects were divided into three groups according to response criterion. Comparison of performance on conventional measures of speech understanding was then made across the three criterial groups. In order

to avoid the problem of criterial definition at a single performance level, we varied task difficulty, in a signal detection paradigm, until a relatively complete criterial function had been defined. We then classified elderly subjects as lax, intermediate, or strict listeners according to the shape of this criterial function.

The goal of the present study was to determine whether the elderly subjects' listening strategies, as defined by their criterial categorization, influenced performance on certain audiologic tests of speech understanding. The measures examined were phonemically balanced monosyllabic words (PB; Egan, 1948), Synthetic Sentence Identification (SSI; Jerger, Speaks, & Trammel, 1968), the Revised Speech Perception in Noise Test (SPIN; Bilger, Nuetzel, Rabinowitz, & Rzeczkowski, 1984), and a test of dichotic sentence identification (DSI; Fifer, Jerger, Berlin, Tobey, & Campbell, 1983).

METHOD

Subjects

Twenty-four adults, ranging in age from 53 to 83 yr, served as subjects in the present experiment. Ten were male, 14 were female. All were paid volunteers. Each subject was screened by a physician to rule out the presence of obvious otologic disease, neurologic disease, or other significant health problem that might compromise performance in the experiment.

Degree of peripheral hearing loss and interaural asymmetry were limited in order to exclude severe hearing loss and markedly asymmetric loss. The PTA_1 (average of hearing threshold levels at 500, 1000, and 2000 Hz) did not exceed 55 dB in either ear, and the PTA_2 (average of hearing threshold levels at 1000, 2000, and 4000 Hz) could not exceed 65 dB. For either PTA_1 or PTA_2 no interaural difference exceeded 20 dB. To rule out significant conductive hearing loss, we required normal (type A) tympanograms, with a peak air pressure not in excess of -100 daPa.

Apparatus and Procedure

For the criterial phase of the experiment, 20 synthetic sentences (Speaks & Jerger, 1965) were digitized and stored on the hard disk of a microcomputer (Compaq 286). Sampling rate was 20 kHz and amplitude resolution was 12 bits. A computer program selected one of the sentences, at random, and presented it to the listener against a background of speech competition provided by an endless-loop cassette tape. Sampling at random, but without replacement, the program presented the 20 sentences successively. Arrayed before the subject, on a response panel, was a bank of 11 response buttons. Ten buttons corresponded to a list of 10 sentences on the target list; the 11th was labeled "none of these." After each sentence had been presented, the subject scanned the list to determine whether it was one of the 10 target sentences, or whether it was one of the 10 sentences not on the list. If he found the sentence on the list, he responded by pushing the appropriate button. If not, he responded by pushing the 11th (none of these) button. The subject initiated the presentation of each sentence by pushing a "ready" button. Thus, no time limit was placed on his deliberation. In this sense, the experimental procedure was self-paced. All scoring was computer automated. Hit rate was defined as the percentage of times that 1 of the 10 target sentences was correctly identified as being on the list (buttons 1 through 10). Whether the identification of the exact sentence presented was correct or incorrect was disregarded. A response was scored as a hit if 1 of the 10 target sentences was presented and the subject responded by pressing one of the buttons 1 to 10. False alarm rate was defined as the percentage of times that one of the buttons 1 to 10 was pressed in response to the presentation of a nontarget sentence. No attempt was made to manipulate the subject's listening strategy. He was instructed only that the a priori probability of a target sentence was 0.50.

In order to generate criterial functions, it was necessary to vary task difficulty (i.e., detectability or d'). To this end the 20-item procedure was repeated at three to five different sentence or message-to-competition ratios, representing different degrees of difficulty of the listening task. The choice of exact message-to-competition ratios (MCRs) varied from subject to subject. Choices were made adaptively, on-line, in order to define a relatively complete iso-criterial function for each subject across the receiver-operating characteristic (ROC) space.

For conventional speech measures, stimuli were presented via cassette tape recorder feeding a two-channel diagnostic audiometer. All materials were presented under earphones in standard clinical fashion using commercially available taped materials. Following routine immittance and pure-tone audiometry, each subject's threshold for 12-talker tape-recorded babble (Kalikow, Stevens, & Elliot, 1977) was obtained. The SPIN (both high and low-probability items), SSI, and PB tests were then administered at 50 dB SL relative to the babble threshold in each ear. The DSI was administered at 70 to 100 SPL, depending on the degree of loss. For the SPIN test, both speech signal and babble were routed through a mixer to achieve the recommended +8 dB signal-to-noise ratio. For the remaining measures, the mixer was not used.

With the exception of the DSI, all speech materials, whether criterial or conventional, were carried out monaurally. In the case of the DSI, however, the dichotic paradigm required that both ears be tested. The DSI is a dichotic test of central auditory function which is only minimally affected by peripheral hearing loss when PTA_1 does not exceed 49 dB HL (Fifer et al, 1983). The test consists of 90 pairs of third-order synthetic sentences randomly chosen from a six-sentence subset of the SSI. The sentence pairs, which have been temporally aligned in onset and offset to within 100 μsec, are presented simultaneously to the two ears. Following each pair, the subject scans the list of six sentences and reports the numbers of the sentences heard.

RESULTS

Criterial Groups

Figure 2 shows the criterial functions generated by each of the 24 elderly subjects. Each subject is represented by a unique series of symbols. In general, message-to-competition (MCR) ratios varied from +10 to −10 dB. In the lax criterion group, all criterial functions moved toward the upper right sector of the response space as the level of

difficulty of the listening task increased. In the case of the intermediate criterion group, all criterial functions tended to follow the diagonal representing the behavior of the ideal listener. Finally, in the case of the strict criterion group, all criterial functions moved toward the lower left sector of the response space as the MCR became more difficult. Statistical analysis revealed no significant difference among the three groups with respect to chronological age, years of education completed, or verbal and full scale IQ (Wechsler Adult Intelligence Scale).

Conventional Speech Audiometry

Initial inspection of the data indicated that the DSI test result showed no trend across criterial group. Average DSI scores for right and left ears are shown in Figure 3. Performance was uniformly high across all three groups. Criterial group difference was statistically significant for neither the right ($F = 0.124$, $p = 0.884$) nor the left ($F = 0.579$, $p = 0.569$) ear. In the case of the other four measures (PB, SSI, SPIN-low probability, and SPIN-high probability), however, we observed a consistent trend across criterial group. Each measure showed best performance in the lax group and poorest performance in the strict group. A two-way analysis of variance, with criterial group as a between-group factor and speech measure as a within-group factor, yielded significant F ratios for criterial group ($F = 4.406$, $p = 0.025$) and speech measure ($F = 39.44$, $p = 0.0001$), but not for the interaction between group and

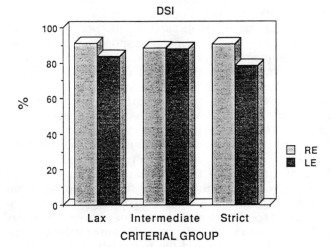

Figure 3. Average DSI Scores for right and left ears as a function of criterial group. (□), Right ear; (■), left ear.

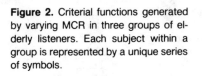

Figure 2. Criterial functions generated by varying MCR in three groups of elderly listeners. Each subject within a group is represented by a unique series of symbols.

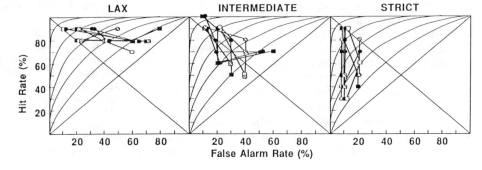

measure ($F = 1.355$, $p = 0.247$). However, a comparison of the average audiograms of the three groups showed that the change in speech scores across criterial group was paralleled by a change in high-frequency sensitivity loss. Figure 4 shows the average audiogram for each of the three criterial groups. The lax group shows best hearing, whereas the strict group shows poorest hearing, in the 1000 to 4000 Hz region. Thus, the change in speech measures across criterial groups could be due simply to greater hearing loss in the intermediate and strict criterial groups.

To evaluate this possibility, we carried out multiple regression analysis separately on each of the four remaining speech measures. For this purpose we quantified degree of sensitivity loss as the average of the hearing threshold levels at 1000, 2000, and 4000 Hz. Throughout the remainder of this paper we label this average as PTA_2, to distinguish it from the more familiar PTA_1, or average of the pure-tone threshold hearing levels at 500, 1000, and

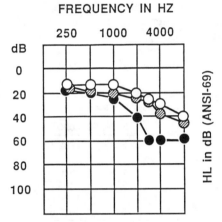

Figure 4. Average audiograms of the three criterial groups. (O), Lax; (◉), intermediate; (●), strict.

2000 Hz. We chose PTA_2 as the measure of hearing loss because of its well known influence on conventional speech audiometric measures, especially monosyllabic word intelligibility.

PB Score Figure 5 shows the PB scores of each of the 24 subjects, plotted against PTA_2. There is a clear trend toward poorer PB performance as PTA_2 increases. Across this trend, however, there appears to be little systematic effect of criterial group. Table 1 summarizes the multiple regression analysis. We first asked whether variance in PB scores could be accounted for by knowledge of degree of hearing loss (PTA_2), criterial group, or interaction between PTA_2 and group. The overall regression effect was significant ($F = 7.68$, $p < 0.001$). We next asked which factor contributed significantly to the variance accounted for in each measure after controlling for the contributions of the other two factors. This analysis revealed that hearing loss (PTA_2) was the only significant predictor of PB score ($F = 18.04$, $p < 0.001$). Neither regression due to group nor regression due to interaction between group and PTA_2 yielded a significant F ratio.

All three factors together accounted for 68% of the variance in PB scores. Knowledge of PTA_2 alone, however, accounted for 58% of the total variance. The addition of knowledge of criterial group contributed only 2% to the prediction of performance on the PB task. Thus, knowledge of degree of high-frequency hearing loss was the most important predictor of PB score. Additional knowledge of criterial group was essentially superfluous.

SSI Score Figure 6 shows the SSI scores of each of the 24 subjects, plotted against PTA_2. Again there is a clear trend toward poorer speech performance as PTA_2 increases, but little systematic effect of criterial group. Table 2 summarizes the multiple regression analysis for SSI scores. The overall regression effect was significant ($F = 6.53$, $p < 0.01$), and again, hearing loss (PTA_2) was the only significant predictor of the speech score ($F = 12.81$,

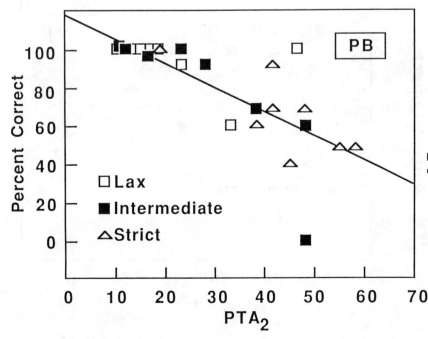

Figure 5. PB scores of individual subjects as a function of degree of high-frequency hearing loss (PTA_2).

$p < 0.01$). Neither regression due to group nor regression due to interaction between group and PTA$_2$ yielded a significant F ratio.

All three factors together accounted for 65% of the variance in SSI scores. Knowledge of PTA$_2$ alone, however, accounted for 51% of the total variance. The addition of criterial group contributed only 3% to the prediction of performance on the SSI task. Thus, like the PB score, knowledge of degree of high-frequency hearing loss was the most important predictor of the SSI score. Additional knowledge of criterial group contributed little toward SSI score prediction.

Spin-Low Figure 7 plots the Spin-Low scores of each of the 24 subjects, against PTA$_2$. Again, speech performance decreases systematically as PTA$_2$ increases. Across this trend, however, there appears to be little systematic effect of criterial group. Table 3 summarizes the multiple regression analysis for Spin-Low scores. The overall regression effect was significant ($F = 7.77$, $p < 0.001$), and, as in the case of both PB and SSI, hearing loss (PTA$_2$) was the only significant predictor of the speech score ($F = 20.10$, $p < 0.001$). Neither regression due to group nor regression due to interaction between group and PTA$_2$ yielded a significant F ratio.

All three factors together accounted for 68% of the variance in Spin-Low scores. Knowledge of PTA$_2$ alone, however, accounted for 62% of the total variance. The addition of criterial group contributed only 1% to the prediction of performance on the Spin-Low task. Thus, like the PB and SSI scores, knowledge of degree of high-frequency hearing loss was the most important predictor of the Spin-Low score. Additional knowledge of criterial group contributed little toward Spin-Low score prediction.

Spin-High Figure 8 shows the Spin-High scores of each of the 24 subjects, plotted against PTA$_2$. Again there is a clear trend toward poorer performance as PTA$_2$ increases, but little systematic effect of criterial group. Table 4 summarizes the multiple regression analysis for Spin-High scores. We first asked whether variance in scores could be accounted for by knowledge of degree of hearing loss (PTA$_2$), criterial group, or interaction between PTA$_2$ and group. The overall regression effect was significant ($F = 16.58$, $p < 0.001$), but, for the Spin-High measure, regression due to interaction between group and PTA$_2$ was also significant ($F = 6.37$, $p < 0.01$), indicating that the slopes of the regression lines relating Spin-High scores to PTA$_2$ differed among criterial groups. Such an effect must be interpreted cautiously, however, in view of the limited range of scores on the Spin-High measure. In any event, Figure 7 shows that criterial group did not order Spin-

Table 1. Regression analysis of PB scores

Source	df	Sum of Squares	F-ratio
Overall regression	5	11,015.58	7.68**
Regression unique to			
PTA$_2$	1	5174.65	18.04**
Group	2	5676.13	0.99
PTA$_2$ × group	2	1288.50	2.25
Residual	18	5163.03	

** $p < 0.001$.

Table 2. Regression analysis of SSI scores

Source	df	Sum of Squares	F-ratio
Overall regression	5	7282.18	6.53*
Regression unique to			
PTA$_2$	1	2856.60	12.81*
Group	2	495.76	1.11
PTA$_2$ × group	2	1188.60	2.67
Residual	18	4013.65	

* $p < 0.01$.

Figure 6. SSI scores of individual subjects as a function of degree of high-frequency hearing loss (PTA$_2$).

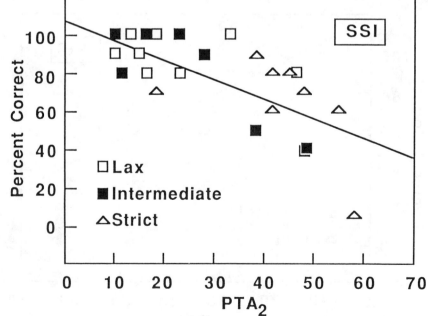

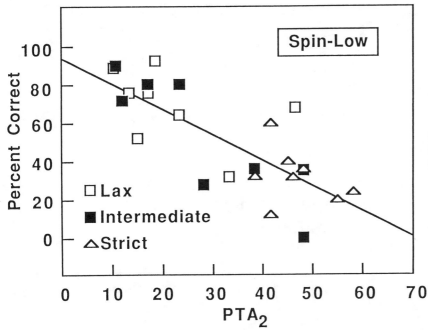

Figure 7. Spin-Low scores of individual subjects as a function of degree of high-frequency hearing loss (PTA_2).

Table 3. Regression analysis of Spin-Low scores

Source	df	Sum of Squares	F-ratio
Overall regression	5	11,241.57	7.77**
Regression unique to			
PTA_2	1	5817.20	20.10**
Group	2	347.43	0.60
$PTA_2 \times$ group	2	808.46	1.40
Residual	18	5209.38	

** $p < 0.001$.

High scores in the direction predicted by the hypothesis that strict listeners will have the poorest scores. If there is any group effect on Spin-High scores it is in the direction of poorest performance by the intermediate listeners, with essentially equivalent results for the lax and strict groups when PTA_2 is taken into account.

In general, then, it seems safe to conclude that, when elderly subjects are appropriately matched for degree of high-frequency sensitivity loss, listening strategy, as defined by the iso-criterial function, does not significantly bias conventional speech audiometric measures.

DISCUSSION

The present results suggest that whether an elderly listener uses a relatively strict or a relatively lax listening strategy has little impact on the results of conventional speech audiometric measures. We conclude, therefore, that in studies of speech understanding in the elderly, rigid control of response criterion is not essential. Nor are present age norms in serious jeopardy.

Still unresolved, however, is the interesting question of whether aging does, in fact, change response criterion. The present experiment was not designed to address this issue directly. It is interesting to observe, however, that we had

little difficulty in finding elderly listeners demonstrating a relatively lax response criterion. Indeed, we had the impression that the distribution of response criteria in our elderly subjects was not unlike the distribution to be anticipated in listeners of any age. Once the a priori probability of 0.50 had been defined, our subjects seemed about equally divided among strict, intermediate, and lax listeners. In further study of this issue, the assumption that aging exerts a fixed, unidirectional effect on listening strategy should be avoided. More attention should, perhaps, be focused on the manner in which the distribution of response criterion differs between young and elderly listeners.

An important methodological issue concerns the d' level at which the response criterion is measured. Reference to Figure 2 will show that, if the inherent difficulty of the listening task was associated with a d' level in excess of 1.5, criterial measures based on the hit and false alarm rates would not have differentiated among the three groups of listeners. Differences in response criteria were not revealed until the d' level associated with the listening task fell well below 1.5.

A second methodological issue concerns the use of the same speech materials both to define criterion and as conventional measures of speech understanding. Both Yantz and Anderson and Gordon-Salant employed a technique in which the subject responds to a target word, then rates his confidence in the correctness of his answer. The response to the word represents the conventional measure of speech understanding, and the subject's criterion is computed from the confidence rating. In the present experiment, synthetic sentences were used in the TSD paradigm to define the iso-criterial functions. The same synthetic sentences were used to define two of the five conventional measures of speech understanding (SSI and DSI). If we had observed a systematic trend, in either of

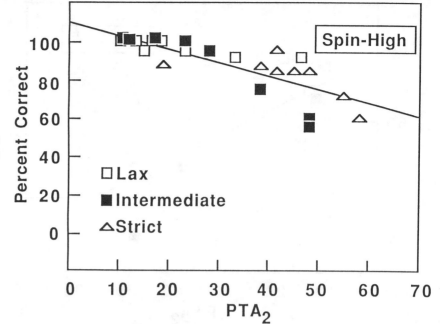

Figure 8. Spin-High scores of individual subjects as a function of degree of high-frequency hearing loss (PTA$_2$).

Table 4. Regression analysis of Spin-High scores

Source	df	Sum of Squares	F-ratio
Overall regression	5	3678.67	16.58**
Regression unique to			
PTA$_2$	1	1633.65	36.82**
Group	2	221.27	2.49
PTA$_2$ × group	2	564.85	6.37*
Residual	18	798.66	

* $p < 0.01$.
** $p < 0.001$.

these two conventional speech audiometric measures across criterial groups, it could be argued that the result was forced by the use of the same materials both to define group membership and to define performance as a function of group. But, such trends were not observed. No differences in performance were observed as a function of group membership, whether the performance measures were based on the synthetic sentences, the PB words, or the SPIN materials.

It may be of more than passing interest that the only systematic trend we did observe, as a function of response criterion, was degree of high-frequency sensorineural hearing loss. Whether the fact of hearing loss, per se, renders the elderly subject a more conservative listener might profitably be the subject of further study.

In any event, the present results highlight, once again, the critical importance of controlling for degree of hearing sensitivity loss with some precision, when studying variables associated with, or assumed to be associated with, speech understanding in the elderly.

References

Bilger RC, Nuetzel JM, Rabinowitz WM, and Rzeczkowski C. Standardization of a test of speech perception in noise. J Speech Hear Res 1984;27:32–48.
Botwinick J, Brinley JF, and Robbin JS. The interaction effects of perceptual difficulty and stimulus exposure time on age differences in speech and accuracy of response. Gerontologia 1958;2:1–10.
Clark WC, and Mehl L. Thermal pain: A sensory decision theory analysis of the effect of age and sex on d', various response criteria, and 50% pain threshold. J Abnorm Psychol 1971;78:202–212.
Clarke FR, and Bilger RC. The theory of signal detectability and the measurement of hearing. In Jerger JF, ed, Modern Developments in Audiology, 2nd ed. New York: Academic Press, 1973.
Craik FM. Applications of signal detection theory to studies of aging. Interdisciplinary Topics Gerontol 1969;4:147–157.
Corso J. Age and sex differences in pure-tone thresholds—survey of hearing levels from 18 to 65 years. Arch Otolaryngol 1963;8:33–40.
Danzinger WL, and Botwinick J. Age and sex differences in sensitivity and response bias in a weight discrimination task. J Gerontol 1980;35:388–394.
Egan J. Articulation testing methods. Laryngoscope 1948;58:955–991.
Fifer R, Jerger J, Berlin C, Tobey E, and Campbell J. Development of a dichotic sentence identification test for hearing-impaired adults. Ear Hear 1983;4:300–305.
Gordon-Salant S. Effects of aging on response criteria in speech recognition tasks. J Speech Hear Res 1986;29:155–162.
Harkins SW, and Chapman CR. Detection and decision factors in pain perception in young and elderly men. Pain 1976;2:253–264.
Harkins SW, and Chapman CR. The perception of induced dental pain in young and elderly women. J Gerontol 1977;32:428–435.
Jerger J, Speaks C, and Trammel J. A new approach to speech audiometry. J Speech Hear Disord 1968;33:318–328.
Kalikow DN, Stevens KN, and Elliot LL. Development of a test of speech intelligibility in noise using sentence materials with controlled word predictability. J Acoust Soc Am 1977;61:1337–1351.
Marshall L. Auditory processing in aging listeners. J Speech Hear Disord 1981;46:226–240.
Potash M, and Jones B. Aging and decision criteria for the detection of tones in noise. J Gerontol 1977;32:436–440.
Rees JN, and Botwinick J. Detection and decision factors in auditory behavior of the elderly. J Gerontol 1971;26:133–136.
Speaks C, and Jerger J. Method for measurement of speech identification. J Speech Hear Res 1965;8:185–194.
Yantz JL, and Anderson SM. Comparison of speech perception skills in young and old listeners. Ear Hear 1984;5:134–137.

Acknowledgments: We are indebted to Danny Holden and Tina Holden for assistance in computer programming.

Address reprint requests to James F. Jerger, Ph.D., 11922 Taylorcrest, Houston, TX 77024.

Received June 22, 1987; accepted September 14, 1987.

Speech Understanding in the Elderly*

James Jerger, Susan Jerger, Terrey Oliver, and Francis Pirozzolo

Division of Audiology, Department of Otolaryngology & Communicative Sciences [J. J., S. J., T. O.] and Neuropsychology Service, Department of Neurology [F. P.], Baylor College of Medicine, Houston, Texas

ABSTRACT

Both auditory and cognitive status were determined in 130 elderly persons, in the age range from 51 to 91 years. Data were analyzed from the standpoint of the congruence of auditory and cognitive deficits. The prevalence of central auditory processing disorder was 50%, and the prevalence of cognitive deficit was 41%. Findings in the two areas were congruent, however, in only 63% of the total sample. Central auditory status was abnormal in the presence of normal cognitive function in 23% of subjects. Central auditory status was normal in the presence of cognitive deficit in 14% of subjects. In general, results did not support the hypothesis that decline in speech understanding in the elderly can be explained as the consequence of concomitant cognitive decline.

Speech understanding declines progressively with age. Traditionally it has been assumed that this decline could be explained by the well documented concomitant progressive decline in auditory sensitivity with age. In recent years, however, some investigators have suggested that at least a part of this decline may be the result of age-related changes in the central auditory system rather than in the auditory periphery. Gaeth (1948) was among the first to observe that some elderly individuals show poorer performance on tests of monosyllabic word intelligibility than would be expected on the basis of the degree and configuration of the audiometric loss. Subsequent investigations have revealed a similar picture of disproportionately poor performance among the elderly on measures of speech understanding involving time-altered speech (Bergman, Blumenfeld, Cascardo, Dash, Levitt, & Margulies, 1976; Konkle, Beasley, & Bess, 1977; McCroskey & Kasten, 1982; Schmitt & Carroll, 1985; Sticht & Gray, 1969), interrupted speech (Bergman, 1971; Bergman et al, 1976; Kirikae, Sato, & Shitara, 1964; Marston & Goetzinger, 1972), and sentences against a background of speech com-

* This research was supported by research grant AG-05680 from the National Institute of Aging.

petition (Dubno, Dirks, & Morgan, 1984; Jerger, 1973; Jerger & Hayes, 1977a; Orchik & Burgess, 1977; Otto & McCandless, 1982; Shirinian & Arnst, 1982).

Such deficits in speech understanding are not confined, however, to the elderly. Similar findings have been described in patients with focal brain lesions affecting the auditory pathways in the central nervous system. Indeed, it has become axiomatic that the fundamental nature of central auditory processing disorder (CAPD) in such patients is a deficit in speech understanding that cannot be explained on the basis of the peripheral sensitivity deficit (Jerger & Jerger, 1974; Jerger & Hayes, 1977b; Noffsinger & Kurdziel, 1979).

The similarity in the pattern of results between brain-lesioned and elderly individuals has led to the hypothesis that age-related changes in the central auditory pathways produce CAPD in the same manner as known lesions of the central auditory system (Hayes & Jerger, 1979; Jerger & Hayes, 1977b; Stach, Jerger, & Fleming, 1985). Support for this hypothesis derives from the considerable evidence of progressive structural changes in central auditory system with increasing age. Histopathologic and morphologic studies have demonstrated age-related alterations in the auditory nerve (Fisch, 1972; Krmpotic-Nemanic, 1971; Schuknecht, 1974) and the central auditory pathways at both the brain stem and temporal lobe levels (Corso, 1977; Hansen & Reske-Nielsen, 1965; Hinchcliffe, 1962; Kirikae et al, 1964).

It is the case, however, that senescent changes are not confined to the auditory system. There is considerable evidence, for example, that certain cognitive abilities decline progressively with age as well (e.g., Salthouse, 1985). Age-related declines have been observed in working memory, episodic memory, and speed of information processing (for a review of age-related cognitive changes, and their possible effects on speech understanding, see "Speech understanding and aging," the report of the CHABA working group on speech understanding and aging, 1988).

It can be hypothesized that the age-related deficits in cognitive abilities might explain much, if not all, of the age-related decline in speech understanding. To the extent that performance on speech audiometric measures depends on such factors as memory, semantic knowledge, perceptual organization and attention, deficits in these areas might be sufficient to explain the depressed speech audiometric scores on an entirely extra-auditory basis. It is relevant to ask, therefore, whether elderly patients with deficits in speech understanding do, in fact, show related cognitive deficits that might explain poor performance on tests of speech understanding. A related question is whether elderly patients with documented cognitive decline will necessarily show related decline in speech understanding.

In summary, there are at least three possible explanations for the decline in speech understanding with age. First, it is possible that age-related changes in the auditory periphery (Igarashi, 1968; Johnsson & Hawkins, 1972; Jorgensen, 1961; Nadol, 1979, 1981) could account for changes in speech understanding. To the extent, for example, that speech understanding depends upon the audibility of the spectral information identifying consonant sounds, speech understanding for tasks heavily dependent upon consonant identification (e.g., PB lists) must necessarily be compromised.

Second, it is possible that aging in the central auditory pathways leads to a specific central auditory processing deficit whose impact on speech understanding adds to the problem produced by peripheral sensitivity loss.

Still a third possibility is that deficits in speech understanding not explicable by peripheral sensitivity loss might be explained by concomitant changes in those cognitive abilities important to the tasks involved in measures of speech understanding.

The purpose of the present study was to assess the relative contributions of peripheral, central, and cognitive factors to senescent speech understanding problems by investigating the relation between auditory and cognitive changes in a sample of elderly subjects with varying degrees of peripheral sensitivity loss. We sought answers to the following specific questions: (1) What deficits in speech understanding are observed in the elderly? (2) To what extent can these deficits in speech understanding be explained by the degree and configuration of the audiometric loss? (3) To what extent can the deficits in speech understanding be explained by concomitant changes in cognitive function?

METHOD

Subjects

We tested a total of 130 elderly subjects (51 males, 79 females), ranging in age from 51 to 91 years. The average age was 69.9 years with a standard deviation of 7.7 years. All subjects were volunteers who responded to advertisements soliciting participation in a study on auditory aging. Each subject was paid for his participation. All subjects were ambulatory and in good general health. The Minnesota Multiphasic Personality Inventory (MMPI) and a clinical interview were used to screen subjects for evidence of mental disorders. Subjects who had two significant elevations (T scores greater than 80) or one subscale eleva-

tion over 90 on the MMPI were excluded. Most subjects had no serious auditory complaints and had not previously sought help for a hearing problem. All were Caucasians who spoke English as their first language.

The hearing sensitivity loss in all subjects was primarily sensorineural. Results of immittance audiometry were within normal limits in 125 subjects, but suggested middle ear abnormality in 5 subjects. Pure-tone audiometry failed, however, to demonstrate a significant air-bone gap in any subject.

Subjects were rejected for participation in the study if the hearing loss exceeded either of two predetermined criteria of severity: (1) if the average pure-tone hearing threshold level (HL) over the frequency range from 500 to 2000 Hz (PTA_1) exceeded 50 dB in either ear, or (2) if interaural asymmetry (difference between PTA_1 on left and right ears) exceeded 19 dB. The purpose of the audiometric severity criterion was to ensure that all speech materials could be presented to the subject at a suprathreshold sensation level of 50 dB (Gang, 1976; Kasden, 1970).

In general audiometric contours were mild-to-moderate, sloping curves, consistent with the classic presbyacusic configuration. The sensitivity loss (PTA_1) ranged from 2 to 48 dB HL for the right ear and from 0 to 47 dB HL for the left ear. The average PTA_1 was 23 dB HL for the right ear and 21 dB HL for the left ear. Sensitivity loss averaged across the frequency range from 1000 to 4000 Hz (PTA_2) ranged from 5 to 70 dB HL in the right ear and from 5 to 65 dB HL in the left ear. The average PTA_2 was 31 dB HL for the right ear and 30 dB HL for the left ear.

Apparatus and Materials

Pure-tone and speech audiometric measures were carried out on a two-channel diagnostic audiometric system comprised of two single-channel audiometers (Rion, BA-75) and a two-channel cassette tape recorder (Sansui, SC-3110). Four speech audiometric measures—the phonemically balanced (PB) word test, the synthetic sentence identification (SSI) test, the speech perception in noise (SPIN) test, and the dichotic sentence identification (DSI) test—were used. All were administered using magnetically recorded materials. For the PB word lists and SSI test, we used tapes previously recorded in this laboratory by a male speaker with General American Dialect. PB lists were the PAL PB-50 word lists developed by Egan (1948). SSI lists were the third-order sentences developed by Speaks and Jerger (1965). For the SPIN test we used tapes supplied to us by Dr. Robert Bilger of the University of Illinois. These tapes were based on the developmental work of Kalikow, Stevens, and Elliott (1977), and of Bilger, Nuetzel, Rabinowitz, and Rzeczkowski (1984). For the DSI test we used a taped version recorded by Dr. Charles Berlin at the Kresge Hearing Research Laboratory of the South, based on the developmental work of Fifer, Jerger, Berlin, Tobey, and Campbell (1983).

Conventional immittance audiometry was carried out on a standard clinical impedance bridge (Amplaid, model 720). All pure-tone and speech signals were delivered to the subject via a single pair of matched earphones (Telephonic TDH-50P) mounted in circumaural cushions (Zwislocki CZW-6). All instrumentation was calibrated to the ANSI-69 standard for diagnostic audiometric equipment.

Simple auditory and visual reaction times and four-choice visual reaction times were obtained by means of a commercially available Visual Choice Reaction Time Apparatus (Lafayette Instrument Co., model 63035) and Digital Display Stop Clock (model 54030). The reaction time apparatus consisted of a panel with four stimulus lamps (red, white, blue, and green), an audio speaker, and five circular (20.5 mm diameter) response buttons. The response buttons were situated 28.5 mm apart in a horizontal row below their respective stimuli with the auditory response button in the middle. Stop clock timing was activated by the stimulus onset and terminated by a button press.

Procedure

Each subject was tested on two consecutive days. One day of testing was devoted to various auditory measures including the pure-tone and speech audiometric data reported in the present paper, and to the measurement of a series of auditory evoked potentials and cognitive potentials not herein reported. The second day of testing was devoted to the administration of a neuropsychological test battery.

We first obtained the conventional pure-tone audiogram by air conduction at octave frequencies from 250 to 8000 Hz on each ear. We then administered a conventional immittance battery including tympanograms at 220 Hz, measurement of static compliance in cm^2 and determination of crossed and uncrossed acoustic reflex thresholds (ARTs). For crossed ARTs test frequencies were 500, 1000, 2000, and 4000 Hz. For uncrossed ARTs test frequencies were 1000 and 2000 Hz. In addition, if immittance audiometry indicated the possibility of middle ear disorder, then conventional bone-conduction audiometry was carried out at frequencies of 500, 1000, 2000, and 4000 Hz.

In order to equate test presentation levels for the battery of speech audiometric tests, we first determined, on each ear separately, the subject's threshold for the multitalker babble of the SPIN test. The presentation level for PB, SSI, and SPIN testing was set at 50 dB above the babble threshold of each ear. Thus, test sensation level was held constant at 50 dB for all monaural test conditions. In the case of PB testing, there was no competing signal. In the case of SSI testing, a competing signal of continuous speech discourse was set to a message-to-competition ratio (MCR) of 0 dB. That is, the intensities of the target sentence and of the competing discourse were identical. For the SPIN test, the intensity level of the competing multitalker babble was held constant at a sentence-to-babble ratio of +8 dB. In the case of the DSI, a dichotic paradigm test, the intensity level to each ear was 50 dB HL unless the patient complained of difficulty in hearing the items or did not achieve 100% correct performance monaurally. In either event, the test level was increased to 60 or 70 dB HL. PB testing was carried out in an open set mode. Words were presented at 4 sec intervals. After the presentation of each target word, the subject repeated back to the examiner, through a high-fidelity talk-back system, what he heard. Each response was scored either correct or incorrect. The PB score for each ear was based on a 25 word list.

SSI sentences were presented in a closed set mode. Sentences were presented at 10 sec intervals. Each of the 10 possible sentences appeared on a numbered, printed list. After each sentence had been presented, the subject scanned the list and reported the number of the sentence that he believed had been presented. The SSI score was based on the presentation of 10 sentences.

The SPIN test sentences were presented in an open-set mode. A total of 50 sentences was presented; 25 high-context and 25 low-context items. Sentences were presented at 10 sec intervals. After the presentation of each sentence, the subject reported back the last word of the sentence he heard. Scores were tabulated separately for the high and low-context sentence items on each ear.

The DSI test sentences were presented in a closed-set mode at 10 sec intervals. Six sentences of the original 10 sentence third-order approximation list were used to generate 30 sentence pairs. These 6 sentences appeared on a numbered, printed list. After each pair had been presented (one sentence to the right ear, the other sentence simultaneously to the left ear), the subject responded by indicating the numbers of the 2 sentences he had heard from the 6-sentence list. He was simply instructed to report both sentences. No further instructions were given relative to order of ear report. DSI scores were calculated separately for the right and left ears.

All subjects underwent a neuropsychologic evaluation. The neuropsychological tests selected for use in this study are among the most commonly used measures of cognitive function in neuropsychological research. The various standardized tests were administered by an experienced neuropsychologist (FP) according to established procedures. The complete neuropsychologic test battery included:

1. Minnesota Multiphasic Personality Inventory The MMPI is a 556 item questionnaire containing 14 scales, such as depression, hypochondriasis, mania, etc.

2. Wechsler Adult Intelligence Scale—Revised The WAIS-R is the the most popular battery of cognitive tests in clinical neuropsychological practice. It contains 11 subtests of such cognitive skills as arithmetic, vocabulary, picture arrangement, etc.

3. Wechsler Memory Scale This is a battery of seven subjects of memory skills. The subtests include measures of paragraph memory, mental tracking, digit span, paired associate learning, etc.

4. Boston Naming Test This is a 60 item test of visual confrontation naming that has recently been studied extensively in elderly subjects.

5. Spatial Orientation Memory Test The SOMT is a 20 item memory-for-geometric-designs test commonly used in geriatric settings.

6. Buschke Selective Reminding Test The selective reminding procedure is a clinical test of memory commonly employed in geriatric settings. The subject is read a list of words and asked to recall the list. He/she is reminded of the words omitted from recall and asked to repeat the list until it has been learned completely.

7. Simple Auditory Research Time Test

8. Simple Visual Reaction Time Test

9. Four-Choice Visual Reaction Time Test

The testing protocol for the various reaction time measures was as follows:

In the simple auditory RT task, the subject rested his index finger on the button below the audio speaker. Upon hearing the tone, the subject pressed the button as quickly as possible to extinguish the tone. In the simple visual RT task, the subject rested his index finger on the button below the white light before each trial. Subjects pressed the button as quickly as possible after seeing the light in order to extinguish it. Eight trials were recorded with each hand on the simple RT tasks.

In the four-choice visual RT task, the subject rested his index finger on a button, located in the center of the display, before each RT trial. Subjects were instructed to lift off this "home" button and press the response button corresponding to the trial-determined illuminated lamp as quickly as possible. As in the simple visual RT task, the stimulus lamp illumination continued until the subject made a correct response. A total of 16 responses were required from each hand with each light position represented randomly four times.

A minimum of five practice trials were administered for each hand on all RT tasks. The starting hand was alternated on each successive task, with starting hand on the first task counterbalanced between right and left across subjects. A variable intertrial interval (ITI) was used with mean ITI of 10 sec. Trials in which the response time exceeded 20 sec without a correct response were not included in the analysis.

Scoring and Categorization

Speech audiometric results were categorized as either "normal" or "consistent with CAPD," according to the following criteria:

1. The SSI test was scored as abnormal if the difference between the PB score and the SSI score (PB minus SSI) exceeded 20% on either ear (Jerger & Hayes, 1977b).

2. The SPIN test was scored according to the nomograph supplied with the manual of the revised SPIN test materials. This nomograph defines a region of normalcy based on the joint outcome of the high- and low-context subtests. The SPIN test was categorized as abnormal if the subject's position on the nomograph, on either ear, fell two steps below the normal acceptance region. In general this occurred when the high-context score was reduced to a relatively greater extent than the low-context score. The exact cutoff score varied according to basic performance on the low-context items.

3. The DSI test (Fifer et al, 1983) was scored as abnormal if the difference between individual ear scores exceeded 16%, provided that the PTA_1 was less than 40 dB HL in both ears. If, however, PTA_1 exceeded 40 dB HL in at least one ear, then the criterion of abnormality was a difference greater than 37%. A third criterion of abnormality was invoked if the best absolute ear score fell below the criterion of individual ear score abnormality specified in Figure 3 of Fifer et al.

In the subsequent "Results" section, subjects were categorized as CAPD if performance on any one of the three speech measures was abnormal.

The neuropsychologic examination was interpreted by a neuropsychologist (F. J. P.) who had no knowledge of either the audiologic or medical data. On the basis of the neuropsychologic evaluation, subjects were placed into one of the following categories:

(1) Normal; (2) evidence of cerebral dysfunction limited to the right hemisphere—degree of impairment ranged from mild to moderate; (3) evidence of cerebral dysfunction limited to the left hemisphere—degree of impairment ranged from mild to moderate; (4) evidence of bilateral cerebral dysfunction—degree of impairment ranged from mild to moderate. In the subsequent "Results" section, subjects were categorized as cognitively abnormal if there was evidence of cerebral dysfunction, either mild or moderate, in one or both hemispheres.

RESULTS

How Does Aging Affect Speech Understanding?

The prevalence of CAPD in our sample, as defined by abnormality on one or more of the three speech measures, was 50%. The prevalence of cognitive deficit in this same sample was 41%. To what extent were deficits congruent on these two aspects of aging? Figure 1 presents the matrix of outcomes. Of the entire group of 130 subjects, 47 (36% of total group) were within normal limits on both dimensions, central auditory processing, and cognitive status. Thirty-five subjects (27% of total group) were abnormal

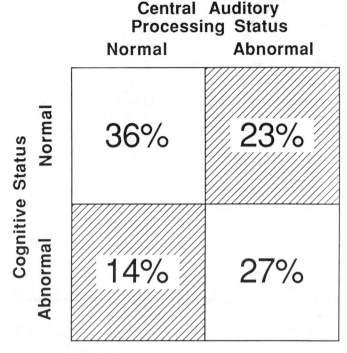

Figure 1. Prevalence of CAPD in subjects with normal and abnormal cognitive findings. Matrix of possible combinations of auditory and cognitive status.

on both aspects. In the remaining 48 subjects, however, we observed abnormality of only one of the two dimensions. In 30 of these 48 subjects (23% of total group), cognitive status was normal but CAP status was abnormal. In 18 subjects (14% of total group) cognitive status was abnormal but CAP status was normal. Thus, cognitive status and central auditory status were congruent (both normal or both abnormal) in 63% of the total group. In the remaining 37%, however, abnormality in one aspect was not matched by an associated abnormality in the other aspect. In these 48 subjects central auditory status, whether normal or abnormal, was not congruent with cognitive status.

The four outcomes shown in the matrix of Figure 1 may be illustrated by individual case reports. Figure 2 presents the audiometric and cognitive results of four subjects illustrating each of the four combinations of CAP and cognitive status. Figure 2A summarizes the pure-tone, speech audiometric, and neuropsychological test results in a 78-year-old female who had normal auditory status and normal cognitive status. The audiogram showed a mild, relatively flat audiometric contour through a 3 kHz and a relatively sharp drop in the higher frequency region. Speech audiometric results were within normal limits. The neuropsychologic examination was also normal. General intellectual ability was approximately 1 SD above age norms. Other cognitive areas tested, such as language, memory, visuospatial, executive, and speed of information processing functions were all within normal limits. There was no selective loss of "fluid intellectual" abilities.

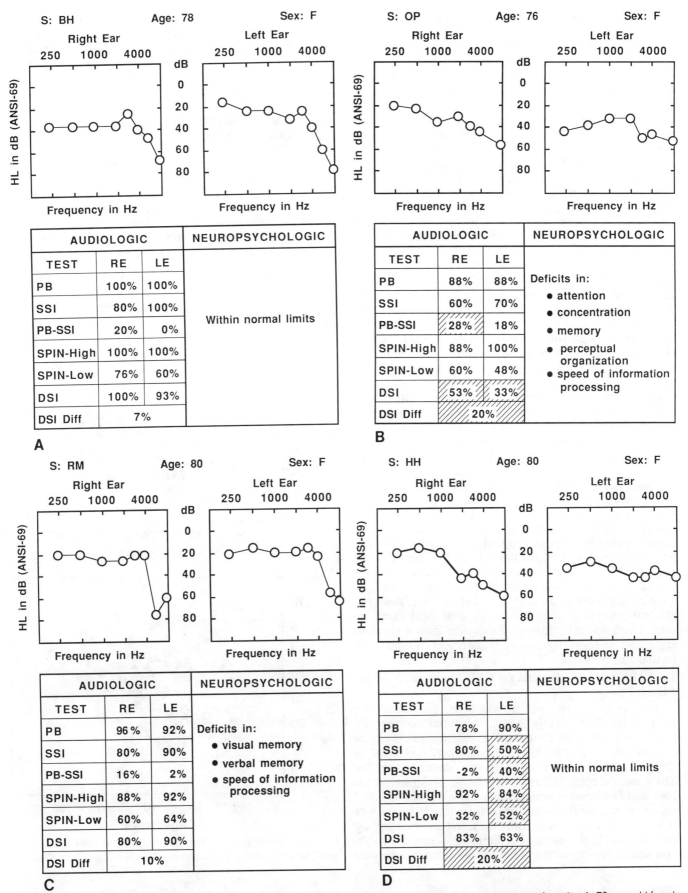

Figure 2. Audiologic and neuropsychologic data in four elderly subjects illustrating the four possible combinations of results: A, 78-year-old female, illustrating combination of normal audiologic and normal neuropsychologic results; b, 76-year-old female, illustrating combination of abnormal audiologic and abnormal neuropsychologic results; C, 80-year-old female, illustrating combination of normal audiologic and abnormal neuropsychologic results; d, 80-year-old female, illustrating combination of abnormal audiologic and normal neuropsychologic results.

Figure 2B summarizes audiometric and neuropsychological data in a 76-year-old female, illustrating the combination of abnormal CAP status and abnormal neuropsychologic status. The audiogram showed a moderate, gradually sloping loss in the right ear and a somewhat flatter configuration in the left ear. Speech audiometric scores were consistent with an abnormality of CAP. The PB-SSI difference was 28% on the right ear and the DSI scores were 53% on the right ear and 33% on the left ear. On the neuropsychological examination this subject showed evidence of a decline from a previously higher level of cognitive functioning. With 14 years of education, her vocabulary, information, and comprehension scaled scores averaged above the means for her age, but she showed deficits in attention, concentration, memory, perceptual organizational ability, and some slowing in speed of information processing.

Figure 2C summarizes audiometric and neuropsychologic data in an 80-year-old female, illustrating the combination of CAP normality in combination with cognitive deficits. The audiogram showed a mild, relatively flat, audiometric contour through 4 kHz. All speech audiometric results were within normal limits but the neuropsychological examination showed evidence of deficits in several areas of cognitive function. In spite of normal general intellectual and verbal abilities, she showed a marked deficit in performance I.Q.-type functioning. There was evidence of a speed of information processing deficit, with most timed tests (e.g., WAIS-R Performance) and reaction time tests showed slower than normal execution. In addition, she showed poor visual and verbal memory.

Figure 2D summarizes audiometric data in an 80 year old female illustrating the combination of CAP abnormality and normal cognitive ability. The audiogram showed a moderate sensitivity loss in both ears. Speech audiometric results indicate a CAP abnormality. The PB-SSI difference was 40% on the left ear, the high and low context SPIN scores were outside the normal range on the left ear, and the DSI test was abnormal on the left ear. Despite some scatter in cognitive performance, however, this subject had a normal neuropsychological examination. There was no evidence of a decline from a previous state, and no focal or selective impairment of fluid intellectual ability.

Does Hearing Loss Account for CAP Abnormality in the Elderly?

Because of the manner in which the present speech audiometric data have been scored, central auditory abnormality is, virtually by definition, independent of degree of peripheral sensitivity loss. The SSI criterion is based on the difference in word and sentence identification, the SPIN test outcome is based on relative performance for high and low context sentences, and the DSI test is based on either interaural or absolute performance in such a way that both degree of loss and interaural asymmetry are incorporated in the norms. Furthermore, degree of peripheral sensitivity loss in the present study group was limited

to less than 50 dB HL (PTA$_1$) on both ears. It is unlikely, therefore, that variation in peripheral sensitivity loss could explain the present central auditory results. Nevertheless, we examined the question by comparing the relation between audiometric level and age, separately for the central auditory processing disorder (CAPD) and non-CAPD groups. If degree of hearing loss is an important factor in the genesis of CAPD, then the functional relation between age and degree of hearing loss should be different for CAPD and non-CAPD groups. Specifically, as age increases we should expect to see relatively more loss in the CAPD group than in the non-CAPD group. At any given age CAPD subjects should show, on the average, more loss than non-CAPD subjects. Figure 3 shows the actual scatterplots of age versus pure-tone average (PTA) for both groups, Figure 3A shows data for PTA$_1$ and Figure 3B for PTA$_2$. Inspection of the individual points in each scatterplot suggests substantial overlap among the CAPD and non-CAPD subjects. Although the CAPD subjects are

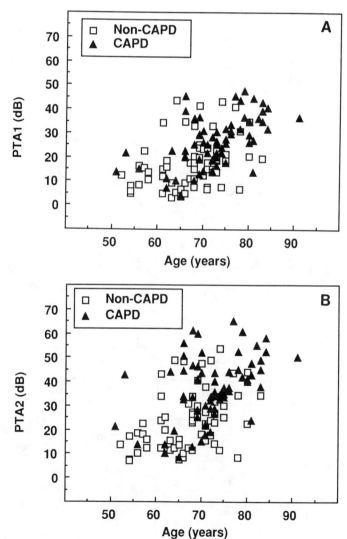

Figure 3. Scatterplot of auditory sensitivity versus age for CAPD and non-CAPD subjects; A, scatterplot for PTA$_1$; B, scatterplot for PTA$_2$.

somewhat older than the non-CAPD subjects, all data points seem to be following the same trend lines. It seems difficult to reconcile these negative findings with the hypothesis that central auditory processing disorders in the elderly can be successfully explained by degree of peripheral sensitivity loss.

Does Cognitive Deficit Account for CAP Abnormality in the Elderly?

The matrix of Figure 1 shows that cognitive status could not explain CAP abnormality in at least 30 of the 65 subjects with CAPD, since cognitive status was judged to be unimpaired in each of these subjects. Thus, the hypothesis that CAP abnormality in the elderly can be explained by cognitive deficit is difficult to justify. Nevertheless, we entertained the possibility that subtle deficits in specific areas of cognitive function, especially those relating to memory and speed of information processing, might explain some of the CAP abnormalities observed.

To investigate this possibility we examined the relation between speech audiometric scores and specific cognitive measures in greater detail. On the dimension of central auditory processing status, 65 subjects were normal and 65 subjects were abnormal. We categorized the 65 subjects of the latter group into five experimental subgroups on the basis of speech audiometric scores. In experimental subgroup E_1, the only CAP abnormality was a significant PB-SSI difference on one or both ears. In experimental subgroup E_2, the only CAP abnormality was an abnormal SPIN test result on one or both ears. In experimental subgroup E_3, only the DSI test result was abnormal. In experimental subgroup E_4, both SPIN and PB-SSI difference were abnormal. Finally, in experiment subgroup E_5, there was abnormality in DSI and SPIN and/or PB-SSI difference.

For each for the five experimental subgroups, we formed a separate control group, matched on the variables of age, hearing loss, and intellectual ability. The subjects for each control group were drawn from the pool of 65 subjects with normal CAP status. For each pair of experimental and control groups mean age was matched to within less than 2 years, for subgroups E_1 through E_4, through to within 8 years for subgroup E_5. Mean hearing loss was matched to within 6 dB for PTA_1 and to within 10 dB for PTA_2. In order to control for premorbid intellectual ability, the averages of the WAIS-R "hold" subtests (i.e., those subtests that are thought to be preserved with age and not selectively vulnerable to age-associated diffuse cerebral dysfunction) were calculated. These subtests, the WAIS-R Vocabulary, Information, and Comprehensive tests, are measures of crystallized intellectual abilities and are used clinically to contrast with fluid intellectual measures (e.g., Block Design, Digit Symbol, and Arithmetic) in order to assess evidence for cognitive impairment. A total hold item score was computed by averaging the three individual subtest scores. The mean hold item score of the WAIS-R (Information, Vocabulary, Comprehension) was matched to within 0.60.

Table 1 summarizes the results of this matching procedure for each for each of the five pairs of experimental and control groups. Included are the number of subjects in each group, means and SDs for chronological age, means and SDs for PTA_1 (average of both ears), means and SDs for PTA_2 (average of both ears), and means and SDs for hold item scores of the WAIS-R.

It is important to note that, whereas the five experimental groups represent five different groups of subjects, the five control groups represent varying subgroups of the same basic pool of non-CAPD subjects. The exact composition of the five control subgroups varied depending

Table 1. Means and standard deviations for age (years), hearing loss (dBHL), and hold items (average) of the WAIS-R in the experimental and control groups.

Group	N	Age Mean	Age (SD)	PTA_1 Mean	PTA_1 (SD)	PTA_2 Mean	PTA_2 (SD)	WAIS Hold Items Mean	WAIS Hold Items (SD)
E_1	16	73.1	(7.0)	27.1	(12.3)	35.4	(16.9)	13.1	(1.5)
C_1	21	72.8	(4.3)	22.1	(10.8)	27.8	(11.4)	13.2	(2.4)
E_2	5	68.0	(6.9)	23.8	(6.8)	35.8	(14.8)	14.4	(1.8)
C_2	40	68.9	(6.5)	22.2	(9.8)	30.0	(10.6)	13.8	(2.0)
E_3	12	67.5	(6.7)	18.2	(8.6)	27.8	(12.5)	12.1	(1.6)
C_3	44	66.5	(7.2)	17.0	(9.8)	23.8	(12.0)	12.1	(1.8)
E_4	6	82.3	(5.4)	36.0	(8.1)	45.0	(7.6)	12.1	(2.0)
C_4	10	74.5	(4.2)	30.8	(11.1)	35.7	(12.6)	12.6	(2.6)
E_5	26	73.1	(6.4)	28.5	(8.1)	41.2	(10.0)	11.6	(2.4)
C_5	22	70.3	(7.1)	26.5	(11.0)	34.4	(12.5)	12.2	(2.1)

Table 2. Mean performance of experimental group E_1 (only PB-SSI difference abnormal, $N = 16$) and control group C_1 ($N = 21$) on 10 cognitive measures.[a] Two-factor, repeated measures ANOVA based on standard scores.

Cognitive Measure	Group E_1	C_1	t
WAIS-R: digit span-forward[b]	7.88	8.20	−0.40
WAIS-R: digit span-backward[b]	7.38	7.15	0.28
WAIS-R: performance IQ[c]	110.31	109.55	0.17
WAIS-R: "don't-hold" items[c]	11.67	11.57	0.16
WMS: associate learning[c]	15.09	14.19	0.77
WMS: passages[c]	10.56	9.71	0.89
BSR: long-term storage[b]	29.88	28.24	0.34
BSR: recall[b]	42.25	40.10	0.57
Spatial orientation memory[b]	15.50	14.33	1.18
Boston Naming Test[b]	55.00	53.52	0.76

Analysis of Variance					
Source	df	SS	MS	F	p
Group	1	2.183	2.183	0.669	0.419
Ss within groups	35	114.276	3.265		
Cognitive measures	9				
Group × measures interaction	9	1.849	0.205	0.277	0.981
Measures × Ss within groups	315	233.692	0.742		

[a] WAIS-R, Wechsler Adult Intelligence Scale-Revised; WMS, Wechsler Memory Scale; BSR, Buschke Selective Reminding Test.
[b] Raw score.
[c] Age-corrected score.

on requirements to achieve the desired degree of match for age, degree of hearing loss, and WAIS-R hold items.

The cognitive measures used to compare the control and experimental groups included the performance I.Q. score from the WAIS-R (age-corrected); the Boston Naming Test (raw score); the Spatial Orientation Memory Test (raw score); the associate learning and passages scores from the Wechsler Memory Scale (age-corrected); long-term storage and recall scores from the Buschke Selective Reminding test (raw scores); forward and backward scores from the digit span subtest of the WAIS-R (raw scores), and the "don't hold" items (block design, digit symbol, and arithmetic) of the WAIS-R (age-corrected). Tables 2 to 5 summarize mean scores on these cognitive measures and the result of statistical analysis with a two-factor, split-plot analysis of variance (ANOVA). For each of the five ANOVAs, the between-subjects factor consisted of the experimental and control groups. The within-subjects factor consisted of the various cognitive measures. All raw and age-corrected scores were converted to standard scores for the analysis. Also included in each table are the Student's t scores associated with each pairwise comparison. The interested reader may derive the standard deviations and standard errors of the means associated with each group on each measure from these t scores.

Table 2 compares group E_1 (PB-SSI diff only) with its control group (C_1). There was no significant group difference ($p = 0.419$) and no significant interaction between group and cognitive measures ($p = 0.981$).

Table 3 compares group E_2 (SPIN only) with its control group (C_2). Again there was no significant difference between groups ($p = 0.498$) and no significant group-by-measures interaction ($p = 0.411$).

Table 4 compares group E_3 (DSI only) with its control group (C_3). In this comparison the difference between groups was significant ($p = 0.007$), but the interaction between group and cognitive measures was not significant ($p = 0.523$). The largest differences between groups were observed on digit span forward ($t = 2.69$), long-term storage ($t = 3.04$), recall ($t = 2.77$), and associate learning ($t = 2.05$).

Table 5 compares group E_4 (SPIN and PB-SSI difference abnormal) with its control group (C_4). In this comparison there was no significant difference between groups ($p = 0.374$) and no significant interaction between group and cognitive measures ($p = 0.720$).

Table 6 compares group E_5 (DSI and SPIN and/or PB-SSI difference) with its control group (C_5). Like group E_3, group E_5 included subjects with DSI abnormalities. In this comparison the group difference approached significance at the 5% level ($p = 0.058$) but no significant interaction between group and cognitive measure was observed ($p = 0.448$). The largest difference between group means was observed for Associate Learning ($t = 3.55$), but the other three measures showing large differences between groups E_3 and C_3, (digit span forward, long-term storage, and recall), were not remarkable in this experimental group.

An aspect of cognitive function of particular relevance to measures of speed understanding is speed of information processing, as measured by simple and choice reaction times. Table 7 summarizes mean performance of groups E_1 and C_1 on measures of simple auditory, simple visual,

Table 3. Mean performance of experimental group E_2 (only SPIN abnormal, $N = 5$) and control group C_2 ($N = 40$) on 10 cognitive measures.[a] Two-factor, repeated measures ANOVA based on standard scores.

	Group		
Cognitive Measure	E_2	C_2	t
WAIS-R: digit span-forward[b]	8.80	8.80	0
WAIS-R: digit span-backward[b]	9.20	7.78	1.21
WAIS-R: performance I.Q.[c]	106.80	114.45	−1.12
WAIS-R: "don't-hold" items[c]	12.60	12.23	0.40
WMS: associate learning[c]	15.90	14.75	0.78
WMS: passages[c]	12.75	10.69	1.54
BSR: long-term storage[b]	34.20	28.92	0.78
BSR: recall[b]	48.20	42.64	1.13
Spatial orientation memory[b]	15.40	15.12	0.19
Boston Naming Test[b]	52.80	55.10	0.76

		Analysis of Variance			
Source	df	SS	MS	F	p
Group	1	1.685	1.685	0.466	0.498
Ss within groups	43	155.433	3.615		
Cognitive measures	9				
Group × measures interaction	9	6.560	0.729	1.036	0.411
Measures × Ss within groups	387	272.322	0.704		

[a] WAIS-R, Wechsler Adult Intelligence Scale-Revised; WMS, Wechsler Memory Scale; BSR, Buschke Selective Reminding Test.
[b] Raw score.
[c] Age-corrected score.

Table 4. Mean performance of experimental group E_3 (only DSI abnormal, $N = 12$) and control group C_3 ($N = 44$) on 10 cognitive measures.[a] Two-factor, repeated measures ANOVA based on standard scores.

	Group		
Cognitive Measure	E_3	C_3	t
WAIS-R: digit span-forward[b]	6.33	8.34	−2.69
WAIS-R: digit span-backward[b]	6.25	6.95	−1.04
WAIS-R: performance I.Q.[c]	104.08	108.42	−0.93
WAIS-R: "don't-hold" items[c]	10.81	11.25	−0.73
WMS: associate learning[c]	11.88	14.02	−2.05
WMS: passages[c]	9.92	10.62	−0.86
BSR: long-term storage[b]	18.00	30.70	−3.04
BSR: recall[b]	35.73	43.48	−2.77
Spatial orientation memory[b]	14.50	15.77	−1.42
Boston Naming Test[b]	51.08	54.50	−1.60

		Analysis of Variance			
Source	df	SS	MS	F	p
Group	1	26.975	26.975	7.936	0.007
Ss within groups	54	183.551	3.399		
Cognitive measures	9				
Group × measures interaction	9	5.479	0.609	0.902	0.523
Measures × Ss within groups	486	327.995	0.675		

[a] WAIS-R, Wechsler Adult Intelligence Scale-Revised; WMS, Wechsler Memory Scale; BSR, Buschke Selective Reminding Test.
[b] Raw score.
[c] Age-corrected score.

Table 5. Mean performance of experimental group E$_4$ (SPIN and PB-SSI difference abnormal, N = 6) and control group C$_4$ (N = 10) on 10 cognitive measures.[a] Two-factor, repeated measures ANOVA based on standard scores.

	Group		
Cognitive Measure	E$_4$	C$_4$	t
WAIS-R: digit span-forward[b]	8.17	7.80	0.29
WAIS-R: digit span-backward[b]	5.83	6.50	−0.77
WAIS-R: performance I.Q.[c]	99.33	106.60	−1.14
WAIS-R: "don't-hold" items[c]	10.00	10.63	−0.67
WMS: associate learning[c]	11.83	15.10	−1.63
WMS: passages[c]	10.00	9.10	0.94
BSR: long-term storage[b]	21.17	27.80	−0.76
BSR: recall[b]	34.17	36.44	−0.40
Spatial Orientation Memory[b]	12.50	12.60	−0.06
Boston Naming Test[b]	46.83	51.30	−1.00

Analysis of Variance

Source	df	SS	MS	F	p
Group	1	2.672	2.672	0.845	0.374
Ss within groups	14	44.281	3.163		
Cognitive measures	9				
Group × measures interaction	9	4.819	0.535	0.687	0.720
Measures × Ss within groups	126	98.228	0.780		

[a] WAIS-R, Wechsler Adult Intelligence Scale-Revised; WMS, Wechsler Memory Scale; BSR, Buschke Selective Reminding Test.
[b] Raw score.
[c] Age-corrected score.

Table 6. Mean performance of experimental group E$_5$ (DSI and SPIN and/or PB-SSI difference abnormal, N = 26) and control group C$_5$ (N = 22) on 10 cognitive measures.[a] Two-factor, repeated measures ANOVA based on standard scores.

	Group		
Cognitive Measure	E$_5$	C$_5$	t
WAIS-R: digit span-forward[b]	7.23	7.59	−0.53
WAIS-R: digit span-backward[b]	5.58	6.46	−1.64
WAIS-R: performance I.Q.[c]	102.88	107.86	−1.40
WAIS-R: "don't-hold" items[c]	10.29	11.15	−1.45
WMS: associate learning[c]	11.67	14.75	−3.55
WMS: passages[c]	9.27	9.91	−0.79
BSR: long-term storage[b]	23.80	24.87	−0.29
BSR: recall[b]	36.48	37.95	−0.51
Spatial Orientation Memory[b]	13.54	14.27	−0.78
Boston Naming Test[b]	51.04	53.50	−1.06

Analysis of Variance

Source	df	SS	MS	F	p
Group	1	13.500	13.500	3.77	0.058
Ss within groups	46	164.418	3.574		
Cognitive measures	9				
Group × measures interaction	9	6.151	0.683	0.989	0.448
Measures × Ss within groups	414	285.931	0.691		

[a] WAIS-R, Wechsler Adult Intelligence Scale-Revised; WMS, Wechsler Memory Scale; BSR, Buschke Selective Reminding Test.
[b] Raw score.
[c] Age-corrected score.

Table 7. Mean performance of experimental group E$_1$ (only PB-SSI difference abnormal, N = 16) and control group C$_1$ (N = 21) on three measures of reaction time (msec).

	Group		
Reaction Time Measure	E$_1$	C$_1$	t
Simple auditory	314.8	304.4	0.42
Simple visual	324.9	340.6	−0.62
4-Choice visual	668.9	713.8	−0.93

Analysis of Variance

Source	df	SS	MS	F	p
Group	1	7580.6	7580.6	0.450	0.507
Ss within groups	35	589878.8	16853.7		
Reaction time measures	2				
Group × measures interaction	2	13897.4	6948.7	1.499	0.230
Measures × Ss within groups	70	324594.4	4637.1		

Table 8. Mean performance of experimental group E$_2$ (only SPIN abnormal, N = 5) and control group C$_2$ (N = 40) on three measures of reaction time (msec).

	Group		
Reaction Time Measure	E$_2$	C$_2$	t
Simple auditory	322.1	293.0	0.91
Simple visual	311.9	316.7	−0.12
4-Choice visual	613.0	645.4	−0.55

Analysis of Variance

Source	df	SS	MS	F	p
Group	1	96.3	96.3	0.006	0.941
Ss within groups	43	745597.9	17339.5		
Reaction time measures	2				
Group × measures interaction	2	8431.3	4215.7	1.094	0.339
Measures × Ss within groups	86	331358.0	3853.0		

Table 9. Mean average performance of experimental group E$_3$ (only DSI abnormal, N = 12) and control group C$_3$ (N = 44) on three measures of reaction time (msec).

	Group		
Reaction Time Measure	E$_3$	C$_3$	t
Simple auditory	283.6	296.9	−0.64
Simple visual	312.5	328.3	−0.68
4-Choice visual	663.4	637.8	0.66

Analysis of Variance

Source	df	SS	MS	F	p
Group	1	39.6	39.6	0.003	0.958
Ss within groups	54	762393.8	14118.4		
Reaction time measures	2				
Group × measures interaction	2	10126.7	5063.3	1.445	0.240
Measures × Ss within groups	108	378451.4	3504.2		

and 4-choice visual reaction time. Included also is a summary of the ANOVA, as well as the Student's t scores associated with each pairwise comparison. The ANOVA failed to demonstrate either a significant group effect (p = 0.507) or a significant group-by-measures interaction (p

= 0.230). Tables 8, 9, 10, and 11 summarize analogous findings for the other four experimental groups and their associated control groups. In no case was there evidence of a significant group difference or group-by-measure interaction.

DISCUSSION

Is the high prevalence of abnormality in speech understanding in the elderly (50% in the present sample) explainable by peripheral hearing loss? Three lines of evidence argue against this possibility. First, the various CAPD measures were all designed to be relatively free of dependence on audiometric level. The PB-SSI criterion is based on the difference between word recognition in quiet and sentence identification in the presence of background speech competition; the SPIN criterion is based on the relation between performance for low context and high context sentences; and the DSI criteria are based on interaural differences in performance and on absolute norms based on findings in patients with various degrees of cochlear sensitivity loss. Second, the scatterplots of Figure 3 provide little support for the hypothesis that peripheral hearing loss is greater in subjects with CAPD than in their non-CAPD counterparts at comparable ages. It is the case, however, that subjects with CAPD are, on the average, older than non-CAPD subjects. Thus, failure to control for the age factor could lead to the erroneous conclusion that CAPD subjects have greater loss than their non-CAPD counterparts. Third, it is not difficult to match CAPD and non-CAPD subjects on degree of peripheral loss. In the present group E_1 (only PB-SSI difference abnormal) and C_1, for example, the mean PTA_1 differed, between the two groups, by only 5.0 dB. The mean PTA_2 differed, in these two groups, by only 7.6 dB. Yet the PB-SSI difference was substantially greater in the experimental group than in the control group. Furthermore, the direction of the difference, SSI score less than PB score, cannot be explained by high-frequency hearing loss. The effect of such peripheral loss should be to reduce the PB score more than the SSI score, because of the greater dependence of

Table 10. Mean performance of experimental group E_4 (SPIN and PB-SSI difference abnormal, $N = 6$) and control group C_4 ($N = 10$) on three measures of reaction time (msec).

Reaction Time Measure	Group		
	E_4	C_4	t
Simple auditory	301.3	332.4	−0.72
Simple visual	313.5	355.6	−0.85
4-Choice visual	660.3	723.6	−0.80
Analysis of Variance					
Source	df	SS	MS	F	p
Group	1	23267.6	23267.6	0.873	0.366
Ss within groups	14	372990.6	26642.2		
Reaction time measures	2				
Group × measures interaction	2	2008.3	1004.1	0.234	0.793
Measures × Ss within groups	28	120254.3	4294.8		

Table 11. Mean performance of experimental group E_5 (DSI and SPIN and/or PB-SSI difference abnormal, $N = 26$) and control group C_5 ($N = 22$) on three measures of reaction time (msec).

Reaction Time Measure	Group		
	E_5	C_5	t
Simple auditory	322.7	307.9	0.61
Simple visual	329.1	326.4	0.11
4-Choice visual	686.9	675.3	0.30
Analysis of Variance					
Source	df	SS	MS	F	p
Group	1	3380.6	3380.6	0.206	0.652
Ss within groups	46	756005.3	16434.9		
Reaction time measures	2				
Group × measures interaction	2	950.0	475.0	0.077	0.926
Measures × Ss within groups	92	566114.9	6153.4		

monosyllabic word intelligibility than sentence identification on high-frequency sensitivity. Groups E_2 (only SPIN abnormal) and C_2 are also enlightening in this regard. Here the task was specifically designed to eliminate the possibility of contamination by high-frequency sensitivity loss. The physical stimuli are all single syllable words embedded in sentences in which the context influences the predictability of the word to be recognized. The central sign is the difference between scores for words embedded in low-predictability versus high-predictability sentences. Additionally, the mean PTA_1 differed by only 1.6 dB, and the mean PTA_2 by only 5.8 dB, between groups E_2 and C_2. Yet performance on this test of speech understanding differentiated the two groups.

It could be argued that we have not ruled out the possibility that changes in the auditory periphery not revealed by the pure-tone audiometric level were responsible for the deficits in speech understanding. Is it possible, for example, that age-related changes in the sensory structures of the inner ear could affect measures of speech understanding without at the same time affecting the pure-tone audiogram? Although the present design did not address this question directly, the fundamental problems underlying relative changes in word and sentence recognition, word recognition in a low- versus a high-context sentence environment, or difficulty in the dichotic paradigm seem to implicate processing disorders well above the sensory structures in the auditory periphery, especially if these peripheral changes are so subtle that auditory sensitivity is unimpaired.

Another possible explanation for the decline in speech understanding in the elderly is the hypothesis that poor performance on the various speech measures can be explained by concomitant cognitive decline. The present data, however, provide only limited support for this hypothesis. The processing problems revealed by the PB-SSI and SPIN measures could not be explained by concomitant cognitive decline. When CAPD and non-CAPD subjects were matched on the relevant variables of age, hearing loss, and intellectual ability, there were no significant group differences on the cognitive measures. It is difficult to reconcile the data of Tables 2, 3, 5 and 6 with the hypothesis that problems in speech understanding are the consequence of cognitive decline. It is noteworthy, moreover, that performance on both SPIN and PB-SSI difference was unimpaired in the one group that did show clear evidence of concomitant cognitive deficits (E_3, only DSI abnormal).

In the case of the DSI test, we did observe significant differences in cognitive function between CAPD and non-CAPD subjects. In retrospect, the DSI procedure certainly seems to place greater cognitive demands on the subject. Two different sentences are presented simultaneously to the two ears. The subject's task is to report, from a closed response set of six possibilities, the two numbers corresponding to the two sentences heard. Although all cognitive measures were relatively poorer in group E_3, the largest differences were observed on memory tests (digit span, long-term storage, recall, associate learning).

One important clinical implication of this finding is that, if an elderly subject shows an isolated deficit on DSI, as herein scored, such a result is ambiguous. One cannot be sure whether the deficit represents a specific auditory problem, a generalized cognitive decline, or a combination of the two. Further information might be obtained, however, by changing the procedure such that the subject reports only the sentence heard from a single ear. A single response procedure should have the effect of diminishing the cognitive demands on the listener. If, therefore, performance improves in this procedural mode, then the possibility of a cognitive component to the problem must be entertained.

SUMMARY

In summary, the speech understanding problems of the elderly cannot be explained as simple functions of either degree of peripheral hearing loss or degree of cognitive decline. The present results show that elderly subjects with CAPD have no more sensitivity loss than elderly subjects without CAPD. In addition, the present results suggest that CAPD and cognitive decline are relatively independent in the elderly population. CAPD can exist in the absence of cognitive decline, and cognitive decline can exist in the absence of CAPD.

References

Bergman M, Blumenfeld VG, Cascardo D, Dash B, Levitt H, and Margulies MK. Age-related decrement in hearing in speech: Sampling and longitudinal studies. J Gerontol 1976;31:533–538.

Bergman M. Hearing and aging. Audiology 1971;10:164–171.

Bilger RC, Nuetzel J, Rabnowitz WM, and Rzeczkowski C. Standardization of a test of speech perception in noise. J Speech Hearing Res 1984;27:32–48.

Committee on Hearing, Bioacoustics, and Biomechanics (CHABA). Speech understanding and aging. J Acoust Soc Am 1988;83:859–893.

Corso J. Auditory perception and communication. In Birren JE, Schaie KW, Eds. Handbook of the Psychology of Aging. 1st ed. New York: Van Nostrand Reinhold, 1977:535–553.

Dubno JR, Dirks DD, Morgan DE. Effects of age and mild hearing loss on speech recognition in noise. J Acoust Soc Am 1984;76:87–96.

Egan JP. Articulation testing methods. Laryngoscope 1948;58:955–991.

Fifer RC, Jerger JF, Berlin CI, Tobey EA, and Campbell JC. Development of a dichotic sentence identification test for hearing-impaired adults. Ear Hear 1983;4:300–305.

Fisch U. Degenerative changes of the arterial vessels of the internal auditory meatus during the process of aging. Acta Otolaryngol 1972;73:259–266.

Gaeth JH. A study of phonemic regression in relation to hearing loss. Northwestern University, 1948. Unpublished doctoral dissertation.

Gang RP. The effects of age on the diagnostic utility of the rollover phenomenon. J Speech Hear Disord 1976;41:63–69.

Hansen C, Reske-Nielsen E. Pathological studies in presbycusis: Cochlear and central findings in 12 aged patients. Arch Otolaryngol 1965;82:115–132.

Hayes D, Jerger J. Low-frequency hearing loss in presbycusis. A central interpretation. Arch Ontolaryngol 1979;105:9–12.

Hinchcliffe R. The anatomical locus of presbyacusis. J Speech Hearing Disord 1962;27:301–310.

Igarashi M. Pathology of inner ear endorgans. In Minckler J, Ed. Pathology of the Nervous System, Vol. 3. New York: McGraw Hill, 1968:2856–2879.

Jerger J. Audiological findings in aging. Adv Otorhinolaryngol 1973;20:115–124.

Jerger J, Hayes D. Hearing and aging. In Han SS, Coons DH, Eds. Special Senses in Aging. Ann Arbor: University of Michigan Press, 1977a:109–118.

Jerger J, Hayes D. Diagnostic speech audiometry. Arch Otolaryngol 1977b;103:216–222.

Jerger J, Jerger S. Auditory findings in brain stem disorders. Arch Otolaryngol 1974;99:342–350.

Johnsson L, Hawkins J. Vascular changes in the human inner ear associated with aging. Ann Otolaryngol 1972;81:364–376.

Jorgensen MB. Changes of aging in the inner ear: Histological studies. Arch Otolaryngol 1961;74:164–170.

Kalikow DN, Stevens KN, and Elliott L. Development of a test of speech intelligibility in noise using sentence materials with controlled word predictability. J Acoust Soc Am 1977;61:1337–1351.

Kasden SD. Speech discrimination in two age groups matched for hearing loss. J Aud Res 1970;10:210–212.

Kirikae I, Sato T, and Shitara T. A study of hearing in advanced age. Laryngoscope 1964;74:205–220.

Konkle DF, Beasley DS, and Bess FH. Intelligibility of time-altered speech in relation to chronological aging. J Speech Hear Res 1977;20:108–115.

Krmpotic-Nemanic J. A new concept of the pathogenesis of presbycusis. Arch Otolaryngol 1971;93:161–166.

Marston LE, Goetzinger CP. A comparison of sensitized words and sentences for distinguishing nonperipheral auditory changes as a function of aging. Cortex 1972;8:213–223.

McCroskey RL and Kasten RN. Temporal factors and the aging auditory system. Ear Hear 1982;3:124–127.

Nadol JB. Electron microscopic findings in presbycusic degeneration of the basal turn of the human cochlea. Otolaryngol Head Neck Surg 1979;87:818–836.

Nadol JB. The aging peripheral hearing mechanism. In Beasley DS, Davis GA, Eds. Aging: Communication Processes and Disorders. New York: Grune & Stratton, 1981:63–85.

Noffsinger PD and Kurdziel SA. Assessment of central auditory lesions. In Rintelmann WF, Ed. Hearing Assessment. Baltimore: University Park Press, 1979: 351–377.

Orchik DJ and Burgess J. Synthetic sentence identification as a function of the age of the listener. J Am Audiol Soc 1977;3:42–46.

Otto WC and McCandless GA. Aging and auditory site of lesion. Ear Hear 1982;3:110–117.

Salthouse TA. Speed of behavior and its implications for cognition. In Burrow JE, Schaie KW, Eds. Handbook of the Psychology of Age, 2nd ed. New York: Van Nostrand Reinhold, 1985: 400–426.

Schmitt JF and Carroll MR. Older listeners' ability to comprehend speaker-generated rate alteration of passages. J Speech Hear Res 1985;28:309–312.

Schuknecht HF. Pathology of the Ear. Cambridge: Harvard University Press, 1974.

Shirinian MJ and Arnst DJ. Patterns in the performance-intensity functions for phonetically balanced word lists and synthetic sentences in aged listeners. Arch Otolaryngol 1982;108:15–20.

Speaks C and Jerger J. Method for measurement of speech identification. J Speech Hear Res 1965;8:185–194.

Stach BA, Jerger JF, and Fleming KA. Central presbyacusis: a longitudinal case study. Ear Hear 1985;6:304–306.

Sticht TG and Gray BB. The intelligibility of time compressed words as a function of age and hearing loss. J Speech Hear Res 1969;12:443–448.

Acknowledgments: We are grateful to Rose Chmiel, Roderick Mahurin, Norma Cooke, and Richard Jones for assistance in data acquisition and analysis.

Address reprint requests to Dr. James Jerger, Division of Audiology, Department of Otolaryngology and Communications Sciences, Baylor College of Medicine, Houston, TX 77030.

Received September 10, 1988; accepted November 10, 1988.

Correlational Analysis of Speech Audiometric Scores, Hearing Loss, Age, and Cognitive Abilities in the Elderly

James Jerger, PhD; Susan Jerger, PhD; Francis Pirozzolo, PhD

Department of Otorhinolaryngology & Communicative Sciences [J. J., S. J.] and Department of Neurology [F. P.], Baylor College of Medicine, Houston, Texas

ABSTRACT

A battery of speech audiometric measures and a battery of neuropsychological measures were administered to 200 elderly individuals with varying degrees of pure-tone sensitivity loss. Results were analyzed from the standpoint of the extent to which variation in speech audiometric scores could be predicted by knowledge of pure-tone hearing level, age, and cognitive status. For the four monotic test procedures (PB, SPIN-Low, SPIN-High, and SSI) degree of hearing loss bore the strongest relation to speech recognition score. Cognitive status accounted for little of the variance in any of these four speech audiometric scores. In the case of the single dichotic test procedure (DSI), both degree of hearing loss and speed of mental processing, as measured by the Digit Symbol subtest of the WAIS-R, accounted for significant variance. Finally, age accounted for significant unique variance only in the SSI score. (Ear Hear 12 2:103–109)

IT HAS BEEN repeatedly observed that average performance on speech audiometric tests declines with age. Disproportionately poor performance in the elderly has been observed on measures of speech understanding involving words (Jerger, 1973), sentences (Orchik & Burgess, 1977; Plomp & Mimpen, 1979), time-altered speech (Bergman et al, 1976; Konkle, Beasley, & Bess, 1977; Marston & Goetzinger, 1972; Schmitt & Carrol, 1985) and sentences against a background of speech competition (Dubno, Dirks, & Morgan, 1984; Jerger & Hayes, 1977; Otto & McCandless, 1982; Shiranian & Arnst, 1982).

Both auditory and cognitive factors have been proposed to account for these age-related effects. For comprehensive reviews of the extensive literature in these areas, see Olsho, Harkins, and Lenhardt (1985) and CHABA Working Group on Speech Understanding & Aging (1988).

The purpose of the present study was to explore the extent to which speech recognition could be predicted from a set of both auditory and extra-auditory variables. We sought to explore, in elderly listeners, the relations among (1) performance on a battery of speech audiometric tests, (2) pure-tone hearing levels, (3) age, and (4) performance on a battery of neuropsychological measures. To this end we carried out canonical and multiple regression analysis on a sample of elderly subjects ($N = 200$), representing a large range of performance on both audiologic and neuropsychologic measures. The present study asks, "In a sample of elderly individuals, how much of the variability in performance on tests of speech understanding can be predicted from knowledge of hearing loss, age, and cognitive function?"

METHOD

Subjects

We tested 200 elderly subjects (79 males and 121 females) in the age range from 50 to 91 years. The average age was 69.7 years with a standard deviation of 7.7 years. Details of subject recruitment and selection criteria are given in a previous publication (Jerger, Jerger, Oliver, & Pirozzolo, 1989). Briefly, all subjects were ambulatory volunteers in good general health who were paid for their participation in the study. Data on this subject sample have not been previously reported.

In general, audiometric contours were mild to moderate, sloping curves, consistent with the classic presbyacusic configuration. Sensitivity losses (PTA_1) ranged from 0 to 55 dB HL for the right ear and from 0 to 63 dB HL for the left ear. The average PTA_1 was 23 dB HL for the right ear and 22 dB HL for the left ear. Sensitivity loss averaged across the frequency range from 1000 to 4000 Hz (PTA_2) ranged from 3 to 73 dB HL in the right ear and from 0 to 78 dB HL in the left ear. The average PTA_2 was 32 dB HL for the right ear and 31 dB HL for the left ear. Finally, the interaural difference in PTA_1 never exceeded 19 dB.

Speech Audiometric Measures

All speech audiometric measures were carried out on a two-channel diagnostic audiometric system comprised of two

0196/0202/91/1202-0103$03.00/0 · EAR AND HEARING

Copyright © 1991 by The Williams & Wilkins Co. · Printed in U.S.A.

single-channel audiometers (Rion, BA-75) and a two-channel cassette tape recorder (Sansui, SC-3110). Four speech audiometric measures—the phonemically balanced (PB) word test, the synthetic sentence identification (SSI) test, the speech perception in noise (SPIN) test, and the dichotic sentence identification (DSI) test—were used. All were administered using magnetically recorded materials. For the PB word lists and SSI test, we used tapes previously recorded in this laboratory by a male speaker with General American Dialect. PB lists were the PAL PB-50 word lists. SSI lists were the third-order sentences developed by Speaks and Jerger (1965). For the SPIN test we used tapes supplied to us by Dr. Robert Bilger of the University of Illinois. These tapes were based on the developmental work of Kalikow, Stevens, and Elliott (1977), and of Bilger, Nuetzel, Rabinowitz, and Rzeczkowski (1984). For the DSI test we used a taped version recorded by Dr. Charles Berlin at the Kresge Hearing Research Laboratory of the South, based on the developmental work of Fifer, Jerger, Berlin, Tobey, and Campbell (1983).

In order to equate test presentation levels for the battery of speech audiometric tests, we first determined, on each ear separately, the subject's threshold for the multitalker babble of the SPIN test. The presentation level for PB, SSI, and SPIN testing was set to 50 dB above the babble threshold of each ear. Thus, test sensation level was held constant at 50 dB for all monaural test conditions. In the case of PB testing, there was no competing signal. In the case of SSI testing, a competing signal of continuous speech discourse was set to a message to competition ratio (MCR) of 0 dB. That is, the intensities of the target sentence and of the competing discourse were identical. For the SPIN test, the intensity level of the competing multitalker babble was held constant at a sentence to babble ratio of +8 dB. In the case of the DSI, a dichotic paradigm test, the intensity level to each ear was 50 dB HL unless the patient complained of difficulty in hearing the items or did not achieve 100% correct performance monaurally. In either event, the test level was increased to 60 dB or to 70 dB HL. Previous research has demonstrated that DSI scores do not change significantly over this range of intensities (Fifer et al, 1983).

PB testing was carried out in an open set mode. Words were presented at 4 sec intervals. After the presentation of each target word, the subject repeated back to the examiner, through a high-fidelity, talk-back system, what he heard. Each response was scored either correct or incorrect. The PB score for each ear was based on a 25 word list.

SSI sentences were presented in a closed-set mode. Sentences were presented at 10 sec intervals. Each of the 10 possible sentences appeared on a numbered, printed list. After each sentence had been presented, the subject scanned the list and reported the number of the sentence that he believed had been presented. The SSI score was based on the presentation of 10 sentences.

The SPIN test sentences were presented in an open-set mode. A total of 50 sentences was presented; 25 high-context and 25 low-context items. Sentences were presented at 10 sec intervals. After the presentation of each sentence, the subject reported back the last word of the sentence he heard. Scores were tabulated separately for the high and low-context sentence items on each ear.

The DSI test sentences were presented in a closed-set mode at 10 sec intervals. Six sentences of the original 10-sentence, third-order approximation list were used to generate 30 sentence pairs. These 6 sentences appeared on a numbered, printed list. After each pair had been presented (one sentence to the right ear, the other sentence simultaneously to the left ear), the subject responded by indicating the numbers of the 2 sentences he had heard from the 6-sentence list. He was instructed to report both sentences. No further instructions were given relative to order of ear report. DSI scores were calculated separately for the right and left ears.

For each of these five speech tests (PB, SSI, SPIN-high context, SPIN-low context, DSI) we derived a single score for each subject by averaging the individual ear scores.

Neuropsychologic Measures

The neuropsychologic tests selected for use in this study are commonly used measures of cognitive function in neuropsychological assessment. The various standardized tests were administered by an experienced neuropsychologist (FP) according to established procedures. The neuropsychologic test battery included:

Wechsler Adult Intelligence Scale—Revised (WAIS-R) The WAIS-R contains 11 subtests of intellectual function: arithmetic, vocabulary, picture arrangement, picture completion, information, digit span, similarities, comprehension, block design, object assembly, and digit symbol.

Wechsler Memory Scale (WMS) We administered three of the seven subtests of the WMS: passages, visual reproduction, and paired associate learning.

Boston Naming Test (BNT) This is a test of visual confrontation naming.

Spatial Orientation Memory Test (SOM) This is a test of memory-for-geometric designs.

Buschke Selective Reminding Test (BSRT) This is a clinical test of long-term memory commonly used in geriatric settings. The subject is read a list of words and asked to recall the list. He/she is reminded of the words omitted from recall and asked to repeat the list until it has been learned completely.

Four-Choice Visual Reaction Time Test Reaction times were obtained by means of a commercially available Visual Choice Reaction Time Apparatus (Lafayette Instrument Company, model 63035) and Digital Display Stop Clock (model 54030). The reaction-time apparatus consisted of a panel with four stimulus lamps (red, white, blue, and green), an audio speaker, and five circular (20.5 mm diameter) response buttons. The response buttons were situated 28.5 mm apart in a horizontal row below their respective stimuli with the auditory response button in the middle. Stop clock timing was activated by the stimulus onset and terminated by a button press. In the four-choice visual RT task, the subject rested his index finger on a button, located in the center of the display, before each RT trial. Subjects were instructed to lift off this "home" button and press the response button corresponding to the trial-determined illuminated lamp as quickly as possible. The stimulus lamp illumination continued until the subject made a correct response. A total of 16 responses were required from each hand with each light position represented randomly four times.

A minimum of five practice trials was administered for each hand on the RT task. The starting hand was alternated on each successive task, with starting hand on the first task counterbalanced between right and left across subjects. A variable intertrial interval (ITI) was used with mean ITI of 10 sec. Trials in which the response time exceeded 20 sec without a correct response were not included in the analysis. For purposes of the present statistical analysis we computed a single reaction time score for each subject as the average of the separate scores for the two hands.

Data Analysis

Tests of statistical significance may be adversely affected by high intercorrelations, or high multicollinearity, among predictor variables (Pedhazur, 1982). To address the potential problem of high multicollinearity among cognitive predictor variables, a preliminary principal component analysis was carried out to study the nature of the dependencies among the battery of neuropsychological measures (Harris, 1975). From these data, the original set of 20 cognitive variables was reduced to 14 variables by deriving six "combination" variables that were linear combinations of two "component" or associated variables. The six derived variables were based on the following combinations: (1) Digit Span-forward and Digit Span-backward (WAIS-R), (2) Associate Learning (WMS) and Long Term Memory (BSRT), (3) Picture Arrangement and Similarities (WAIS-R), (4) Spatial Orientation Memory (SOM) and Arithmetic (WAIS-R), (5) Picture Completion and Object Assembly (WAIS-R), and (6) Visual Reproduction (WMS) and Block Design (WAIS-R). This approach allowed us to construct a smaller set of cognitive predictor variables without significant multicollinearity and with as little loss of information as possible (Tabachnick & Fidell, 1983).

Table 1 details the specific set of cognitive predictor variables submitted to statistical analyses, along with a brief description of the cognitive dimension assumed to be measured by each. To complete the full array of predictor variables we added degree of hearing loss, as quantified by PTA_2 (average of hearing threshold levels at 1000, 2000, and 4000 Hz, averaged across both ears) and chronological age, in years. Condition Indices for the entire set of predictor variables indicated with multicollinearity was not a significant problem (Wilkinson, 1989). Pearson product-moment significant problem (Wilkinson, 1989). Pearson product-moment correlation coefficients between all variable-pairs ranged from 0.002 (between Passages and Digit Span) to 0.382 (between age and hearing loss) with an average coefficient, independent of sign, of 0.098.

Statistical analyses were carried out with both canonical and multiple regression approaches. Canonical analysis examines the relation between the set of criterial variables (speech audiometric measures) and the set of predictor variables simultaneously. The analysis yields a weight for each criterial and predictor variable that maximizes the correlation between the two sets of variables. The correlation between the sets of variables is called the canonical correlation (R_c). Canonical analysis calculates several R_cs based on variable-sets with different weights.

The significance of the overall canonical analysis is determined by Wilks' lambda. If the overall test is significant, then the first R_c is removed from the analysis and lambda is recomputed. The procedure continues, with successive removal of lower-order R_cs, until lambda is not significant. At this point, it is concluded that the R_cs preceding this step are statistically significant and the remaining ones are not. For the significant R_cs, it is of interest to study the weights, or structure coefficients, of the variables as an indication of the relative importance of the individual variables. If the canonical analysis is significant, then a series of multiple regression analyses is carried out to determine the extent to which each of the individual speech understanding measures can be predicted by the set of predictor measures.

All statistical analyses were carried out on arcsin transformations of the speech audiometric scores and on normalized, or standard, scores of the cognitive predictor measures. Statistical significance was evaluated at the 0.01 level of confidence.

RESULTS

Canonical analysis indicated a significant overall relation between the sets of criterial and predictor variables (Wilks' Lambda = 0.121, df = 70,727, $p < 0.01$). Both the first ($\chi^2 = 337.747$, df = 70, $p < 0.001$) and the second ($\chi^2 = 103.988$, df = 52, $p < 0.001$) canonical correlations were significant, indicating that the senescent changes in speech recognition were significantly affected by two independent dimensions. Table 2 presents the correlation coefficients (R_c), the squares of the correlation coefficients (R_c^2) and the associated structure coefficients for these two canonical correlations. The same data are illustrated graphically in Figure 1.

The first pair of canonical variates suggests that the most powerful contributor to speech recognition performance in the elderly is degree of hearing loss. Hearing loss was a significant dimension affecting performance on all of the five speech tests, particularly the four monotic procedures. Along with hearing loss, age and the Digit Symbol test also appeared to contribute to senescent changes in speech recognition. The proportion of variance shared between the variable-sets for the first pair of canonical variates was large, about 75%.

The second pair of canonical variates suggests that overall cognitive status is also a significant independent dimension affecting performance on two of the speech recognition measures, the SSI and DSI measures. The structure coefficients for the cognitive variables as a group appear to be relatively uniform. The relation between the second pair of canonical variates was noticeably weaker, however, than the first, with only about 30% of shared variance.

Table 1. The 12 neuropsychological predictor variables and the cognitive dimensions assumed to be measured by each.

Variable	Cognitive Dimension
1. Vocabulary	Fund of information and knowledge
2. Comprehension	Fund of information and knowledge
3. Digit symbol	Speed of mental processing
4. Passages	Short-term verbal memory
5. Boston naming	Lexical access; speed of mental processing
6. Choice reaction time	Speed of mental processing
7. Digit span	Memory
8. Associate learning and long-term storage	Verbal learning and memory
9. Picture arrangement and similarities	Higher level conceptual reasoning
10. Spatial orientation memory and arithmetic	Cognitive fluidity
11. Picture completion and object assembly	Gestalt perception
12. Visual reproduction and block design	Visuo-spatial learning and constructional ability

Table 2. Summary of the canonical analysis between the set of criterial variables (speech audiometric measures) and the set of predictor variables (hearing loss, age, and neuropsychological measures).

	Canonical Correlation	
	$R_c = 0.876$ $R_c^2 = 0.767$	$R_c = 0.544$ $R_c^2 = 0.296$
Variables	Structure Coefficients	
Criterial		
DSI	0.727	−0.493
SSI	0.848	−0.420
SPIN-High	0.865	0.137
SPIN-Low	0.898	0.253
PB	0.923	0.234
Predictor		
Hearing loss	−0.947	0.200
Age	−0.606	−0.44
Visual reproduction and block design	0.308	0.532
Picture completion and object assembly	0.349	0.514
Spatial orientation memory and arithmetic	0.171	0.704
Picture arrangement and similarities	0.410	0.411
Associate learning and long-term storage	0.317	0.303
Digit span	0.141	0.625
Choice reaction time	−0.196	−0.596
Boston naming	0.186	0.544
Passages	0.180	0.437
Digit symbol	0.545	0.433
Comprehension	0.208	0.418
Vocabulary	0.137	0.299

The significant overall relation between the variable-sets was investigated in greater detail by means of multiple regression analysis. We asked to what extent performance on the individual speech audiometric tests could be predicted from knowledge of hearing loss, age, and the cognitive measures. Table 3 and Figure 2 summarize the multiple regression analyses for the two single-word tests, PB and SPIN-Low. Overall, the predictor variables were significantly associated with both PB (F = 21.57, $p < 0.001$) and SPIN-Low (F = 20.18, $p < 0.001$) performance. Overall knowledge of the variables predicted about 64% of the performance variability in both PB (R = 0.797, $R^2 = 0.636$) and SPIN-Low (R = 0.802, $R^2 = 0.643$) measures. When the effects of the other predictor variables were controlled, only hearing loss made a significant, unique contribution to the prediction of single-word performance, as indicated by the beta coefficients. In a stepwise regression approach with hearing loss entered first, knowledge of hearing loss alone predicted 58% of the variance in PB word scores and 61% of the variance in SPIN-Low scores. In other words, for PB and SPIN-Low measures, the variance accounted for was incremented by only 3 to 6% by adding all of the other measures to hearing loss.

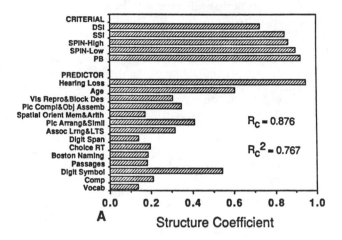

First Canonical Correlation

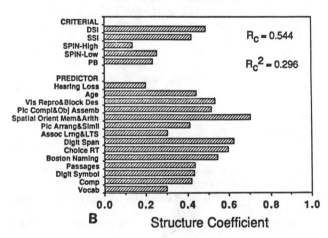

Second Canonical Correlation

Figure 1. Canonical correlation analysis. A, Structure coefficients of criterial and predictor variables from first canonical correlation; B, structure coefficients from second canonical correlation.

Table 4 and Figure 3 summarize the multiple regression analyses for the two monotic, word-in-context measures, SSI and SPIN-High scores. The overall set of predictor measures was significantly associated with both SSI (F = 18.75, $p < 0.001$) and SPIN-High (F = 16.46, $p < 0.001$) performance. Overall knowledge of cognitive abilities, hearing loss, and age again predicted about 60% of the variance in both tests (SSI: R = 0.776, $R^2 = 0.603$; SPIN-High: R = 0.771, $R^2 = 0.595$). As with the single-word test analyses, degree of hearing loss showed a unique, significant contribution to the prediction of performance on both of the word-in-context procedures. However, age was also uniquely related to SSI performance, although not to SPIN-High performance. Again, with a stepwise approach, with hearing loss entered first, knowledge of only degree of hearing loss predicted 42% of the variance in SSI performance and 54% of the variance in SPIN-High performance. Knowledge of both the degree of hearing loss and age, but nothing else, predicted 54% of the varia-

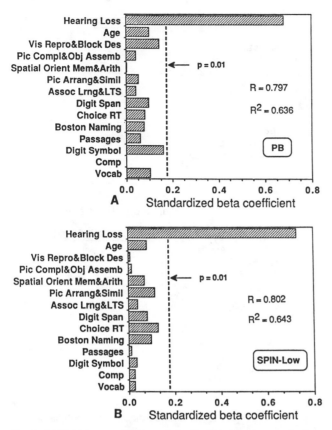

Figure 2. Multiple regression analysis of single-word tests. A, Correlation coefficient and standardized beta coefficients (sign disregarded) for PB scores; B, correlation coefficient and standardized beta coefficients (sign disregarded) for SPIN-Low scores.

Table 3. Multiple correlation and beta coefficients for the prediction of the two single-word criterial variables (PB and SPIN-Low) from the set of predictor variables (hearing loss, age, and neuropsychological measures).

| Predictor | Multiple Correlation | |
| | PB | SPIN-Low |
	$R = 0.797$ $R^2 = 0.636$	$R = 0.802$ $R^2 = 0.643$
	beta	beta
Hearing loss	−0.681*	−0.727*
Age	−0.099	−0.081
Visual reproduction and block design	−0.146	−0.009
Picture completion and object assembly	0.043	0.013
Spatial orientation memory and arithmetic	−0.004	0.069
Picture arrangement and similarities	0.053	0.113
Associate learning and long-term storage	0.043	0.038
Digit span—forward and backward	−0.098	−0.081
Choice reaction time	0.081	0.129
Boston naming	0.078	−0.098
Passages	−0.062	0.012
Digit symbol	0.161	0.033
Comprehension	0.000	0.026
Vocabulary	0.103	0.025

*$p < 0.01$.

bility in SSI scores. The total variance accounted for (60%) was incremented only 6% by the addition of all other variables.

Table 5 and Figure 4 summarize the multiple regression analysis for the dichotic speech test, DSI. Overall, the predictor variables (cognitive, hearing loss, age) were significantly associated with DSI performance (F = 12.82, $p < 0.001$). Knowledge of all the predictor variables accounted for 51% of the variance in dichotic performance. Both hearing loss and speed of mental processing, the cognitive skill measured by the Digit Symbol subtest of the WAIS-R, made significant, unique contributions to the prediction of DSI performance. In the stepwise analysis, knowledge of hearing loss alone accounted for 30% of the variability in DSI scores. Knowledge of both degree of hearing loss and the Digit Symbol score, but nothing else, accounted for 43% of the variability in DSI scores. The total variance accounted for (51%) was incremented only 8% by the addition of all other variables.

DISCUSSION

Canonical analysis suggested that two independent dimensions, degree of hearing loss and cognitive status,

significantly affect speech recognition in the elderly. Hearing loss was the most important dimension. It affected performance on all five speech audiometric measures. General cognitive status affected performance on two of the five speech measures, the SSI and DSI tests. This set of results is certainly not surprising. It would be remarkable, indeed, if degree of hearing loss did not have a substantial impact on speech audiometric scores. Nor is the apparent association between cognitive status and SSI and DSI scores entirely unexpected. The behavioral test paradigms of speech audiometry necessarily invoke a variety of cognitive dimensions for their successful execution. The present analysis sought to assess the relative importance of such cognitive dimensions by asking how much of the variance in speech recognition scores could be explained by knowledge of cognitive abilities.

Multiple regression analyses revealed that the influence of cognitive status varied considerably across the various individual speech measures. In the case of the PB score, knowledge of hearing loss alone predicted 58% of the total variance. The addition of age and all cognitive measures increased prediction by only 6%, suggesting that cognitive status has relatively little unique impact on this speech measure. A similar situation held for both SPIN-Low and SPIN-High scores. Knowledge of hearing loss alone predicted 61% of the

Table 4. Multiple correlation and beta coefficients for the prediction of the two word-in-context criterial variables (SSI and SPIN-High) from the set of predictor variables (hearing loss, age, and neuropsychological measures).

Predictor	Multiple correlation	
	SSI	SPIN-High
	R = 0.776 R² = 0.603	R = 0.771 R² = 0.595
	beta	beta
Hearing loss	−0.484*	−0.702*
Age	−0.259*	−0.051
Visual reproduction and block design	−0.127	−0.086
Picture completion and object assembly	0.108	0.100
Spatial orientation memory and arithmetic	0.104	0.126
Picture arrangement and similarities	0.108	0.056
Associate learning and long-term storage	−0.006	0.034
Digit span—forward and backward	0.016	−0.057
Choice reaction time	0.004	0.170
Boston naming	0.114	0.019
Passages	−0.039	−0.031
Digit symbol	0.058	0.041
Comprehension	0.091	0.074
Vocabulary	−0.048	0.010

*p < 0.01.

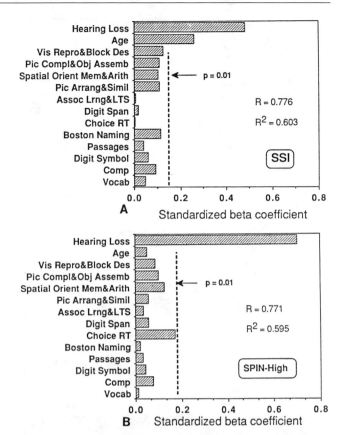

Figure 3. Multiple regression analysis of word-in-context tests. A, Correlation coefficient and standardized beta coefficients (sign disregarded) for SSI scores; B, correlation coefficient and standardized beta coefficients (sign disregarded) for SPIN-High scores.

total variance of SPIN-Low performance; age and cognitive measures increased prediction by only 3%. Knowledge of hearing loss alone predicted 54% of the total variance in SPIN-High performance; age and cognitive measures increased prediction by only 6%.

In the case of SSI, age also contributed significant unique information to the prediction of performance. Knowledge of degree of hearing loss alone predicted 42% of the total variance in SSI performance. But the addition of age to degree of loss predicted 54% of the variance, an increase of 12% attributable to knowledge of age. The addition of all cognitive variables further increased prediction by only an additional 6%.

In the case of the dichotic test, DSI, degree of hearing loss was less strongly related to the speech recognition score. Knowledge of degree of hearing loss accounted for only 30% of the total variance in DSI scores. A cognitive measure, speed of mental processing, as measured by the Digit Symbol subtest of the WAIS-R, contributed significant, unique information to DSI performance. Knowledge of both degree of hearing loss and the Digit Symbol score predicted 43% of the total variance. The addition of age and all other cognitive variables further increased prediction by only 8%.

The Digit Symbol subtest is a complex measure of information processing and speed of manual response. A horizontal visual array displays nine digits, under

Table 5. Multiple correlation and beta coefficients for the prediction of the dichotic criterial variable (DSI) from the set of predictor variables (hearing loss, age, and neuropsychological measures).

Predictor	DSI Multiple Correlation
	R = 0.715 R² = 0.511
	beta
Hearing loss	−0.436*
Age	−0.092
Visual reproduction and block design	−0.072
Picture completion and object assembly	0.013
Spatial orientation memory and arithmetic	0.163
Picture arrangement and similarities	0.012
Associate learning and long-term storage	0.118
Digit span—forward and backward	0.138
Choice reaction time	−0.014
Boston naming	0.050
Passages	−0.069
Digit symbol	0.189*
Comprehension	−0.051
Vocabulary	0.098

*p < 0.01.

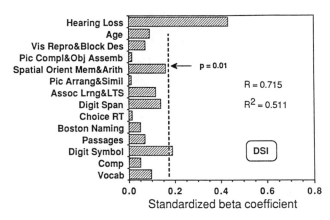

Figure 4. Multiple regression analysis of DSI test. Coefficient of correlation and standardized beta coefficients (sign disregarded).

each of which is a different abstract symbol. With this array as reference, the subject is presented with a 90-item random sequence of digits and asked to enter the corresponding abstract symbol under each digit. The score is based on the number of symbols correctly recording during a timed interval. The relevance of the Digit Symbol test for speech audiometric procedures, especially DSI, resides in the fact that it is a sensitive measure of speed of mental processing. The speed with which an elderly subject can process mental events is undoubtedly relevant to the success with which that subject can process an incoming speech target and execute an appropriate response. It is not surprising that this cognitive dimension should affect performance on DSI, which requires the subject to identify two sentences presented simultaneously, one in each ear, from a closed set of alternatives. Successful performance on this task would undoubtedly be facilitated by an ability to process mental events efficiently.

In summary, degree of hearing loss bore the strongest relation to the four monotic speech recognition scores. This single measure predicted 58 to 61% of the total variance in the two single-word tests, PB and SPIN-Low, and 42 to 54% of the variance in the two word-in-context measures, SSI and SPIN-High. The total variance accounted for, in this group of four monotic tests, was incremented only 3 to 6% by knowledge of all cognitive variables. Age emerged as a significant unique predictor of performance only for the SSI score. In the case of the dichotic test (DSI), degree of hearing loss accounted for less of the total variance, and speed of mental processing, as measured by the Digit Symbol test, emerged as a significant cognitive measure. Degree of hearing loss alone predicted 30% of the total variance. The Digit Symbol score predicted an additional 13%. The addition of age and all other cognitive variables further incremented prediction by only 8%.

REFERENCES

Bergman M, Blumenfeld V, Cascardo D, Dash B, Levitt H, and Margulies M. Age-related decrement in hearing for speech. J Gerontol 1976;31:533–538.

Bilger R, Nuetzel J, Rabinowitz W, and Rzeczkowski C. Standardization of a test of speech perception in noise. J Speech Hear Res 1984;27:32–48.

Dubno JR, Dirks DD, and Morgan DE. Effects of age and mild hearing loss on speech recognition in noise. J Acoust Soc Am 1984;76:87–96.

Fifer R, Jerger J, Berlin C, Tobey E, and Campbell J. Development of a dichotic sentence identification test for hearing-impaired adults. Ear Hear 1983;4:300–305.

Harris R. A Primer of Multivariate Statistics. New York: Academic Press, 1975.

Jerger J. Audiological findings in aging. Adv Otorhinolaryngol 1973;20:115–124.

Jerger J and Hayes D. Diagnostic speech audiometry. Arch Otolaryngol 1977;103:216–222.

Jerger J, Jerger S, Oliver T, and Pirozzolo F. Speech understanding in the elderly. Ear Hear 1989;10:79–89.

Kalikow D, Stevens K, and Elliot L. Development of a test of speech intelligibility in noise using sentence materials with controlled word predictability. J Acoust Soc Am 1977;61:1337–1351.

Konkle D, Beasley D, and Bess F. Intelligibility of time altered speech in relation to chronological aging. J Speech Hear Res 1977;20:108–115.

Marston LE and Goetzinger CP. A comparison of sensitized words and sentences for distinguishing nonperipheral auditory changes as a function of aging. Cortex 1972;8:213–223.

Olsho LW, Harkins SW, and Lenhardt ML. Aging and the auditory system. In Birren J, Schaie K W, Eds, Handbook of the Psychology of Aging, 2nd Ed. New York: Van Nordstrand, Reinhold, 1985: 332–377.

Orchik D, and Burgess J. Synthetic sentence identification as a function of age of the listener. J Am Audiol Soc 1977;3:42–46.

Otto WC and McCandless GA. Aging and auditory site of lesion. Ear Hear 1982;3:110–117.

Pedhazur E. Multiple Regression in Behavioral Research. Explanation and Prediction. New York: Holt, Rinehart & Winston, 1982.

Plomp R and Mimpen AM. Speech-reception threshold for sentences as a function of age and noise level. J Acoust Soc Am 1979;66:1333–1342.

Schmitt JF and Carroll MR. Older listeners' ability to comprehend speaker-generated rate alteration of passages. J Speech Hear Res 1985;28:309–312.

Shirinian M and Arnst D. Patterns in performance intensity functions for phonetically balanced word lists and synthetic sentences in aged listeners. Arch Otolaryngol 1982;108:15–20.

Tabachnick B and Fidell L. Using Multivariate Statistics. New York: Harper & Rose, 1983.

Wilkinson L. SYSTAT: The System For Statistics. Evanston, IL: SYSTAT, Inc., 1989.

Working Group on Speech Understanding and Aging. Speech understanding and aging. J Acoust Soc Am 1988;83:859–893.

This research was supported by grant AG-05680 from the National Institute of Aging.

Acknowledgment: We are grateful to Terrey Oliver Penn, Norma Cooke, and Renae Stoner for assistance in data acquisition and analysis.

Address reprint requests to Dr. James Jerger, Division of Audiology, Department of Otolaryngology & Communicative Sciences, Baylor College of Medicine, Houston, TX 77030.

Received August 27, 1990; accepted December 17, 1990.

Age-Related Asymmetry on a Cued-Listening Task

James Jerger, PhD; Craig Jordan, MS

Division of Audiology, Department of Otolaryngology and Communicative Sciences, Baylor College of Medicine, Houston, Texas

ABSTRACT

We report results on a cued-listening task designed to simulate the listening problems commonly described by individuals with sensorineural hearing loss, especially those experienced by elderly persons. Against a background of multitalker babble, the subject detected targets embedded in continuous discourse. Noncoherent segments of this discourse were presented simultaneously from loudspeakers on the right and left sides. A signal light cued the side to be monitored during a listening trial. The overall difficulty of the task was manipulated by variation of the message to competition intensity ratio. A sequence of listening trials, half-cued to the right side, half cued to the left side, was executed at each of four message to competition intensity ratios. Nineteen young adults with normal hearing and 28 elderly persons with presbyacusic hearing loss were evaluated. All subjects, young and elderly, were able to complete the cued-listening task successfully. Results showed a small but significant right-side advantage in the young group and a substantial right-side advantage in the elderly group. The application of the testing technique to the evaluation of hearing aid performance is illustrated in two elderly persons. (Ear Hear 13 4:272–277)

ONE OF THE MOST COMMON complaints of individuals with sensorineural hearing loss, especially among the elderly, is difficulty in understanding speech against a background of noise or other speech competition. The problem is typically described as a unique problem in following what one person is saying when other individuals are talking simultaneously, or when there is other noise in the background.

Audiologists have long sought to measure this effect clinically. More than 40 yr ago, Carhart (1946) suggested that the familiar PB list should be administered not only in quiet, but also in the presence of a competing, steady state noise. Two decades later, Jerger, Speaks, and Trammel (1968) incorporated the continuous discourse of a single talker as background competition in the Synthetic Sentence Identification (SSI) Test. More recently, the developers of the Speech Perception in Noise (SPIN) Test (Bilger, Nuetzel, Rabinowitz, & Rzeczkowski, 1984; Kalikow, Stevens, & Elliot, 1977) included multitalker babble as competition for their target sentences.

Typically these test procedures are carried out monotically under earphones, but they are often used in the sound field as well. Here the target word or sentence is presented from one loudspeaker, and the background noise or competition is presented from another loudspeaker. Whether delivered by loudspeaker or by earphone, these procedures may be criticized on the ground that they lack validity as predictors of how well a hearing-impaired individual will actually be able to understand ongoing speech in a realistic environment, because of inappropriateness of the targets (e.g., single syllable words), competition (e.g., noise of invariant level), and/or physical arrangements under which the tests are administered (e.g., target at 0° azimuth, competition at 180° azimuth).

The purpose of the present study was to develop and evaluate a new procedure for the measurement of hearing ability in the presence of competing background speech. We sought to construct a more realistic test paradigm in terms of its simulation of everyday listening. At the same time, we sought to retain as much as possible laboratory control over the test environment. A related purpose was to evaluate the extent to which the right ear advantage, already well documented in the dichotic listening paradigm under earphones (cf., Berlin & McNeil, 1976), is retained in the sound field.

METHOD

Subjects

We tested a total of 47 subjects: 19 young adults with normal hearing and 28 elderly persons with varying degrees of sensorineural hearing loss. Young adults with normal hearing were in the age range from 21 to 30 yr. Seventeen were female, two were male. None had any hearing complaint and each passed an audiometric screen at 15 dB HTL across the frequency range from 250 to 8000 Hz for both ears.

In the elderly group, age ranged from 52 to 84 yr. The average age was 71.9 yr. Elderly subjects all had some degree of sensorineural hearing loss. In general, audiometric contours

0196/0202/92/1304-272$03.00/0 · EAR AND HEARING

were mild to moderate, sloping curves, consistent with the classic presbyacusic configuration. The pure-tone HTL averaged over the three frequencies of 500, 1000, and 2000 Hz (PTA$_1$) extended for individual subjects from 8 to 45 dB for the right ear and from 5 to 45 dB for the left ear. The average PTA$_1$ was 22.5 dB HL for the right ear and 21.6 dB HL for the left ear. Hearing sensitivity, averaged over the three frequencies of 1000, 2000, and 4000 Hz (PTA$_2$), ranged from 8 to 62 dB HL in the right ear and from 12 to 55 dB HL in the left ear. The average PTA$_2$ was 30.9 dB HL for the right ear and 30.5 dB HL for the left ear. There was little interaural asymmetry in the mean sensitivity loss. The difference between the two ears in any subject never exceeded 11 dB for PTA$_1$ or 14 dB for PTA$_2$.

All elderly subjects were ambulatory volunteers in good general health who were paid for their participation in the study. Exclusion criteria included evidence of pathological aging, neurological or systemic disease, or dementia. Twenty elderly subjects were tested in the unaided condition only. The remaining eight were tested in both unaided and aided conditions.

Apparatus and Procedure

Figure 1 shows the experimental arrangement. The subject was seated in a sound-treated room equidistant between, and 1.6 m from, two loudspeakers. A third loudspeaker was mounted on a floor stand and positioned 0.5 m above and slightly behind the subject's head. A pair of signal lights, labeled "right" and "left," were mounted directly in front of the subject at eye level. A two-channel system played speech messages to the right and left loudspeakers. One channel contained 20 min of continuous discourse: a male talker with general American dialect reading an adventure story written in the first person. The second channel contained the same

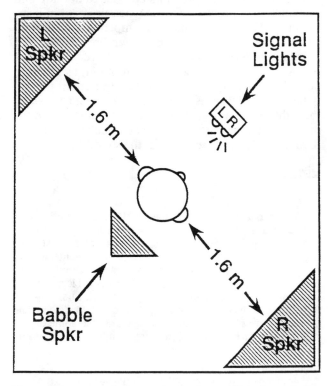

Figure 1. Arrangement of apparatus for the cued-listening task. Signal light cues side to be attended.

recording, but offset by about 1 min relative to the first channel. Thus, the identical discourse was presented on both channels, but, at any moment in time, different parts of the story appeared on the two channels. When both loudspeakers were activated, therefore, the continuous discourse was "noncoherent" in the sense that different speech messages were directed to each ear.

The presentation level of the continuous discourse containing the "I" targets was adjusted separately to each subject's comfortable listening level for continuous discourse. The intensity level of the multitalker babble was varied to produce message to competition ratios (MCRs) of 0, −5, −10, and −15 dB.

A trial, or cued-listening interval, was defined by one of the two lights directly in front of the subject. The subject was directed to attend to the discourse from the side indicated by the signal light, and to attend as long as it was illuminated. The subject's task, during this cued interval, was to press a response button each time she/he heard the personal pronoun "I" from the cued direction. An error was scored if the subject failed to respond within 1.5 sec after an "I" had been presented. In order to manipulate the difficulty of the task, continuous multitalker babble was played via a magnetic tape playback system through the loudspeaker mounted above the subject's head.

Data were gathered on two different sets of apparatus and with two slightly different procedures. In the first, or pilot, version, the continuous speech messages were transduced via magnetic tape recordings and scoring was executed manually. There were four cued intervals at each MCR. Each cued interval contained eight target "I"s. The order of the four cued intervals was always right-left-right-left. Initial results obtained with this pilot version were sufficiently interesting that we upgraded both the apparatus and the procedure. In the second, or final, version, the continuous speech messages were stored on the hard disk of a microcomputer (22 K sampling rate, 16 bit amplitude resolution) and routed directly from the digital to analog converter to the two audio channels feeding the target-right and target-left loudspeakers. Also, in the final version, the number of cued intervals at each MCR was increased from 4 to 10 and the number of target "I"s in each cued interval was increased from 8 to 10. The order of presentation over the 10 cued intervals was quasi-random, with the constraints that the target-right and target-left speakers were each cued on five intervals, and that no target speaker was cued on more than two successive cued intervals. In both the pilot and final versions, the order in which MCR conditions were tested was always from easiest (0 dB) to most difficult (−15 dB).

The results obtained with the pilot and final versions of the apparatus and procedure were equivalent. In all subsequent analyses, therefore, subjects have been collapsed into a single young adult group and a single elderly group.

Sound Field Calibration

In order to ensure that the continuous speech targets from the two loudspeakers were equally intense at the two ears, the two-channel amplifier gains were adjusted such that a broadband noise from either loudspeaker produced the same SPL at the position of the subject's head in the sound field. The subject was absent when these measurements were taken. The continuous speech targets in the two channels were then adjusted such that a 1000 Hz calibration tone, recorded at the average level of frequent peaks of the continuous speech, registered on the channel VU meter at the same point that the broadband noise had been metered.

RESULTS

Figure 2 shows average performance, as a function of MCR, for targets delivered from both right and left loudspeakers to the 19 young adults from normal hearing. In subsequent analysis and discussion, we shall use the term "ear" to refer to these target lateralities, despite the fact that both ears could receive stimulation from either of the loudspeakers. We use the term here in the sense of the ear receiving maximal stimulation from a particular loudspeaker rather than in the traditional sense of an ear being stimulated monaurally via earphone. In the case of the young adults, there was a slight overall advantage for the right ear. A two-factor, within-subjects ANOVA (MCR and Ear as repeated measures) showed a significant effect for Ear ($F = 7.93$; df = 1,18; $p = 0.011$) and a significant effect for MCR ($F = 198.68$; df = 3,54; $p = 0.0001$), but no significant interaction between ear and MCR ($F = 0.97$; df = 3,54, $p = 0.413$).

Because of floor effects, not all elderly subjects could be tested at all MCRs. We have chosen, therefore, to present individual results from the 28 elderly subjects in the form of a scatterplot (Fig. 3) of the right-left (R-L) difference scores at the various MCRs. In general, performance in the elderly subjects was substantially better when the target came from the right side than when it came from the left side. The average R-L difference, collapsed across MCR, averaged 15.97%. Evaluation of this average difference by paired t-test revealed a significant ear effect ($t = 7.38$; df = 27; $p = 0.0001$). This apparent right ear advantage was, on the average, larger in the elderly subjects with presbyacusis than in the young subjects with normal hearing. When the right-left difference was collapsed across MCRs in the young group, the average difference was 3.35%.

Comparison of the overall mean R-L difference between the young and elderly groups (3.35 versus 15.97%) by unpaired t-test was also significant ($t = 4.49$; df = 45; $p = 0.0001$). It is often recommended that the right ear advantage be expressed by the quantity $[(R - L)/(R + L)]$ in order to control for overall performance differences across groups. When the present data are recast in this form, the right ear advantage for the young group was 2.37%. The corresponding right ear advantage for the elderly group was 15.78%.

It is appropriate to ask whether audiometric asymmetries may have accounted for the substantial right ear advantages observed in the elderly group. Perhaps hearing sensitivity was slightly better on the right ear than on the left ear in this group of presbyacusic subjects. Figure 4 shows the average audiogram for separate ears of the elderly group. In fact, average sensitivity was slightly better for the left ear. Thus, the observed differences between ears on the cued-listening task cannot

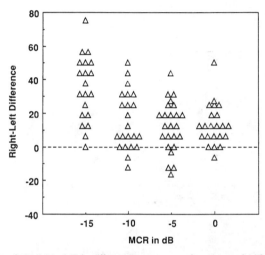

Figure 3. Individual R-L difference scores as functions of MCR on the cued-listening task in 28 elderly subjects with presbyacusis.

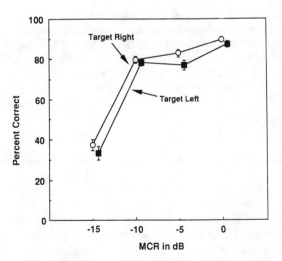

Figure 2. Mean performance of 19 young adults with normal hearing as a function of MCR on the cued-listening task. Error bar denotes SEM.

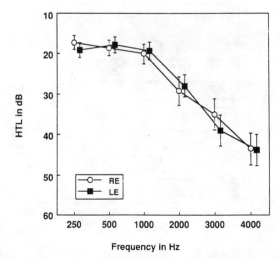

Figure 4. Mean pure-tone, air conduction audiograms of the 28 elderly subjects with presbyacusis. Note slightly better audiometric sensitivity for the left ear.

be explained by better average hearing sensitivity of elderly subjects' right ears. Nor were there significant interaural differences in speech understanding. Average PB scores for the elderly subjects were 84.7% for the right ear and 84.3% for the left ear. Similarly, average SSI scores were 80.0% for the right ear and 81.1% for the left ear. Interear comparisons of these various speech measures, by paired *t*-tests, all yielded nonsignificant results.

Evaluation of Hearing Aid Performance

The cued-listening task has yielded interesting results in the evaluation of hearing aid performance. Figure 5A, for example, shows the pure-tone audiometric configuration of a 67-yr-old woman (MB) who had been wearing binaural in the ear aids successfully for 7 mo. Her unaided PB max scores were 84% in the right ear and 64% in the left ear; unaided SSI max scores were 90% in the right ear and 70% in the left ear. Figure 5B

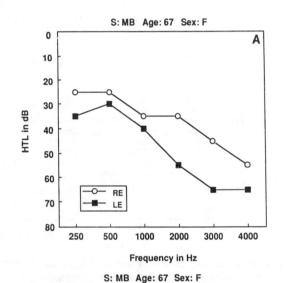

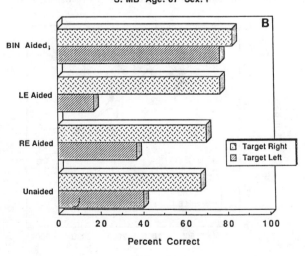

Figure 5. Audiogram and cued-listening test results in a 67-yr-old woman who reported that her binaural aids helped her in difficult listening situations. (A) Pure tone, air conduction audiogram; (B) cued-listening test results in unaided and three aided conditions.

shows both unaided and aided results on the cued-listening task. All testing was carried out at a fixed MCR of 0 dB. In the unaided mode, performance was much better in the target-right condition, but this could be related to the better audiometric sensitivity in the right ear. When the right ear was aided, this difference, again not unexpectedly, persisted. Performance was more than 25% better when the target came from the right side than when it came from the left side. When the left ear was aided, the difference was even larger. Performance on the cued-listening task exceeded 70% when the target came from the right side, but fell below 20% when the target came from the left side. This is an interesting result. Again it may be related to the better audiometric sensitivity of the right ear. Even with the left ear aided, the better unaided sensitivity of the right ear may have been dominant when the target speaker was on the right side. Or, this result may reflect the substantial right ear advantage in the dichotic listening paradigm demonstrated by so many elderly subjects in the unaided condition. In any event, the advantage of a binaural fitting for this patient is dramatically illustrated in the top two bars of the figure. Here we see that with both ears aided, performance was almost as good in the target-left condition as in the target-right condition. In either of the monaural-aided modes, performance was only slightly better than in the unaided mode in the target-right condition, and actually a good deal worse than the unaided mode in the target-left condition. But, in the binaural mode, performance exceeded the unaided mode in both target-right and target-left conditions. This cued-listening test result was mirrored in the patient's subjective evaluation. She reported that in this difficult listening situation, the binaural aids helped her to "shut out the background noise and just listen for the targets."

Figure 6, on the other hand, shows findings in a patient who is not a successful binaural aid user. Figure 6A shows the pure-tone audiogram of patient ES, a 68-yr-old woman with a moderate bilateral sensorineural loss, slightly worse in the right ear. Unaided PB max scores were 84% in each ear. Unaided SSI max scores were 80% in the right ear and 90% in the left ear. This patient had been wearing binaural in the ear aids for about 12 mo. She reported that she could wear them only when she was listening to her pastor in church. At virtually all other times, the background noise problem was too much for her and she had to remove the aids. She did not regard herself as a successful hearing aid user.

Figure 6B shows the results of the cued-listening test. In the unaided mode, performance was at slightly better than 40% for either the target-right or the target-left condition. In either monaural-aided mode, performance was actually worse than in the unaided mode and, interestingly, again better in the target-right than in the target-left condition. Of greatest interest, however, was the total collapse of performance in the target-right condition for the binaural mode. Mirroring this patient's subjective complaints, her performance with bin-

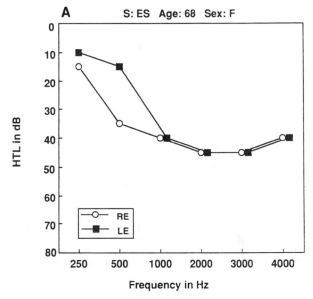

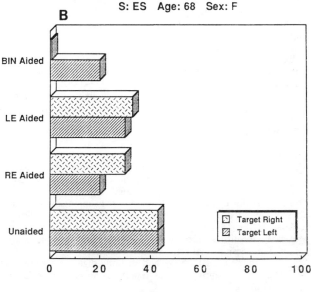

Figure 6. Audiogram and cued-listening test results in a 68-yr-old woman who reported that her binaural aids did not help her in most listening situations. (A) Pure tone, air conduction audiogram; (B) cued-listening test results in unaided and three aided conditions.

aural aids was only 20% in the target-left condition and 0% in the target-right condition. Thus, the real life experiences of both MB and ES as binaural aid users were reflected in the cued-listening task.

DISCUSSION

The rationale governing the design of the cued-listening paradigm was the desire to create, under moderate laboratory control, the kind of listening situation about which hearing-impaired individuals, especially the elderly, typically complain. Thus, the listener is immersed in a constant background of multitalker babble. Within

this difficult auditory environment, the listener must attend to specified targets embedded within continuous discourse coming from one direction, while simultaneously suppressing semantically and syntactically identical discourse containing the same targets but coming from the opposite direction. Additionally, at specified times, the listener must reverse the attentive mode so that what was formerly target becomes unwanted competition, and what was formerly unwanted competition becomes target.

The fact that average performance in the young adults was slightly better when the target came from the right side is not surprising. It follows from the extensive literature (cf., Berlin & McNeil, 1976) on the right ear advantage in the dichotic paradigm when noncoherent stimuli are presented via earphones. In addition, Bergman, Hirsch, and Solzi (1987) demonstrated a similar effect for young normals in the sound field, although the physical arrangement of their loudspeakers was somewhat different from ours. The primary message, a three-word, Hebrew sentence (translations of the Willeford sentences), was directed at the subject from a loudspeaker directly in front (0° azimuth). The competing message, another translated Willeford sentence, came from a loudspeaker positioned opposite either the right ear (90° azimuth) or the left ear (270° azimuth). Thus, the primary message was equally intense at both ears, whereas the competing message was more intense in the ear contralateral to the "test" ear. Using this arrangement and a signal to competition ratio of −10 dB, Bergman et al demonstrated an average right ear advantage of more than 10% in eight normal females in the age range of 23 to 37 yr.

Of even greater interest, however, were the findings of Bergman et al in patients with brain injury due either to cranial cerebral injury or cerebrovascular accident. When Hebrew versions of the Willeford competing sentences were administered via earphones, 43% of 142 such patients demonstrated abnormal findings. Of this abnormal group, an astonishing 79% were abnormally poorer on the left ear, but only 15% were abnormally poorer on the right ear. Because of the diffuse nature of the pathology, especially in patients with cranial cerebral injury, precise anatomical location of hemispheric damage was not uniformly available. Nevertheless, the preponderance of relatively large right ear advantages in both groups of brain-injured patients was striking. A similar left ear-suppression phenomenon has been reported for tests of dichotic listening under earphones in patients with multiple sclerosis (Jacobson, Deppe, & Murray, 1983; Rubens, Froehling, Slater, & Anderson, 1985).

In the case of dichotic listening under earphones, there is conflicting evidence on whether the right ear advantage increases with age. Horning (1972), Clark and Knowles (1973), and Johnson, Cole, Bowers, Foiles, Nikaido, Patrick, and Woliver (1979) all found an increase in the R-L difference with age, but Borod and Goodglass (1980), Gelfand, Hoffman, Waltzman, and Piper (1980), and Martini, Bovo, Agnoletto, DaCol, Drusian, Liddeo, and Morro (1988) found no age effect.

In view of the conflicting nature of these findings, it is relevant to ask whether anyone has observed an interaction between age and ear in monaural tasks involving difficult listening. Interestingly, such an effect has, indeed, been noted. Investigators have demonstrated greater decline in the left ear with increasing age for time-compressed monosyllabic words (Konkle, Beasley, & Bess, 1977) and for SSI sentences (Shirinian & Arnst, 1982).

In any event, the present results support previous observations of an interaction between ear and age in the dichotic paradigm. At least two possibly overlapping explanations for this right ear effect in the elderly may be advanced. Bergman et al (1987) suggest that the left ear system may be physiologically more vulnerable to disruption by pathology. They were referring in this instance to pathology due to direct cranial cerebral injury or to cerebrovascular insult, but one might extend that concept to include age-related changes in the central auditory system. This hypothesis finds some support from studies showing a relatively greater decline in right hemisphere function with increasing age (Goldstein & Shelly, 1981; Levy-Agresti & Sperry, 1968). On the other hand, Elias (1979) notes that coding and retrieval strategies have been related to cerebral laterality effects in younger subjects, and that older subjects may make less effective use of such strategies.

An alternative explanation, based on a number of studies showing left ear suppression of verbal materials in the dichotic paradigm after commissurotomy (Milner, Taylor, & Sperry, 1968; Musiek & Wilson, 1979; Sparks & Geschwind, 1968; Springer, Sidtis, Wilson, & Gazzaniga, 1978), invokes compromise of the auditory pathways in the corpus callosum (Bergman et al, 1987; Musiek, 1983; Rubens et al, 1985). In the present case, one might speculate that an age-related, generalized loss of neural elements is reflected in loss of elements in the auditory collosal pathways, producing an effect which qualitatively, if not quantitatively, mimics the severe left ear suppression after commissurotomy.

In any event, the direction of the results in the present elderly group is consistent with a number of previous findings on an increase in the right ear advantage with age, greater age-related decline in left ear than in right ear performance in difficult monaural speech perception tasks, and characteristic left ear suppression in patients with various types of brain injury.

REFERENCES

Bergman M, Hirsch S, and Solzi P. Interhemispheric suppression: A test of central auditory function. Ear Hear 1987;8:87–91.

Berlin CI and McNeil MR. Dichotic listening. In Lass NJ, Ed. Issues in Experimental Phonetics. New York: Academic Press, 1976;327–387.

Bilger R, Nuetzel J, Rabinowitz W, and Rzeczkowski C. Standardization of a test of speech perception in noise. J Speech Hear Res 1984;27:32–48.

Borod JC and Goodglass H. Lateralization of linguistic and melodic processing with age. Neuropsychologia 1980;18:79–83.

Carhart R. Tests for selection of hearing aids. Laryngoscope 1946;56:780–794.

Clark LE and Knowles JB. Age differences in dichotic listening performance. J Gerontol 1973;28:173–178.

Elias JW. A life-span perspective on cerebral asymmetry and information processing with an emphasis on the aging adult. In Ordy JM and Brizzee KR, Eds. Sensory Systems and Communication in the Elderly, Vol. 10. New York: Raven Press, 1979:187–20.

Gelfand SA, Hoffman S, Waltzman SB, and Piper N. Dichotic CV recognition at various interaural temporal onset asynchronies: Effect of age. J Acoust Soc Am 1980;68:1258–1261.

Goldstein G and Shelly C. Does the right hemisphere age more rapidly than the left? J Clin Neuropsychol 1981;3:67–78.

Horning JK. The effects of age in dichotic listening [Master's thesis]. San Diego State College, 1972.

Jacobson JT, Deppe U, and Murray TJ. Dichotic paradigms in multiple sclerosis. Ear Hear 1983;4:311–317.

Jerger J, Speaks C, and Trammel J. A new approach to speech audiometry. J Speech Hear Disord 1968;33:318–328.

Johnson RC, Cole RE, Bowers JK, Foiles SV, Nikaido AM, Patrick JW, and Woliver RE. Hemispheric efficiency in middle and later adulthood. Cortex 1979;15:109–119.

Kalikow D, Stevens K, and Elliot L. Development of a test of speech intelligibility in noise using sentence materials with controlled word predictability. J Acoust Soc Am 1977;61:1337–1351.

Konkle DF, Beasley DS, and Bess FH. Intelligibility of time-altered speech in relation to chronological aging. J Speech Hear Res 1977;20:108–115.

Levy-Agresti J and Sperry RW. Differential perception capacities in major and minor hemispheres. Proc Natl Acad Sci USA 1968;61:1151.

Martini A, Bovo R, Agnoletto M, DaCol M, Drusian A, Liddeo M, and Morra B. Dichotic performance in elderly Italians with Italian stop consonant-vowel stimuli. Audiology 1988;27:1–7.

Milner B, Taylor L, and Sperry R. Lateralized suppression of dichotically presented digits after commisural section in man. Science 1968;161:184–185.

Musick F. Results of three dichotic speech tests on subjects with intracranial lesions. Ear Hear 1983;4:318–323.

Musick F and Wilson D. SSW and dichotic digit results pre- and post-commissurotomy: a case report. J Speech Hear Disord 1979;44:528–533.

Rubens AB, Froehling B, Slater G, and Anderson D. Left ear suppression on verbal dichotic tests in patients with multiple sclerosis. Ann Neurol 1985;18:459–463.

Shirinian MJ and Arnst DJ. Patterns in the performance-intensity functions for phonetically-balanced word lists and synthetic sentences in aged listeners. Arch Otolaryngol 1982;108:15–20.

Sparks R and Geschwind N. Dichotic listening in man after section of neocortical commissures. Cortex 1968;4:3–16.

Springer SP, Sidtis J, Wilson D, and Gazzinaga MS. Left ear performance in dichotic listening following commissurotomy. Neuropsychologia 1978;16:305–312.

Address reprint requests to James Jerger, 11922 Taylorcrest Rd., Houston, TX 77024.

Received January 10, 1992; accepted March 26, 1992.

Gender Affects Audiometric Shape in Presbyacusis

James Jerger*
Rose Chmiel*
Brad Stach*
Maureen Spretnjak*

Abstract

A review of large-scale surveys of hearing over the past 50 years reveals a "gender-reversal" phenomenon in the average audiograms of the elderly. Above 1 kHz males show greater average loss than females, but below 1 kHz females show greater average loss than males. The effect increases with both age and degree of hearing loss. The difference is present whether or not the elderly persons complain of a hearing problem and remains after persons with a history of noise exposure are excluded from the analysis. A possible explanation, based on the greater likelihood of cardiovascular disease in the elderly female, is considered.

Key Words: Aging, audiogram, elderly, gender, sex

Surveys of hearing in the general population consistently show that males have poorer high-frequency sensitivity than females, and that the gap widens with age. Conventional wisdom attributes this age-related difference to the greater lifetime noise exposure typically experienced by males in the work place, in the military, and in leisure activities.

In contrast to the considerable study of this age-related male–female difference in the 3000 to 6000 Hz region of the audiogram, relatively little attention has been directed toward a possible age-related gender difference in the low-frequency region, below 1000 Hz. It has been our clinical impression, for a number of years, however, that elderly females typically show poorer hearing sensitivity than elderly males at 250 and 500 Hz (Jerger and Jerger, 1981, p. 148). A similar observation was recently made by Willott (1991, p. 169).

The purpose of the present communication is to review the evidence for such a low-frequency gender effect from previous survey data, and to analyze our database in an effort to differentiate among various factors that might be related to the phenomenon.

*Division of Audiology, Baylor College of Medicine, and The Methodist Hospital, Houston, Texas

Reprint requests: James Jerger, 11922 Taylorcrest, Houston, TX 77024

METHOD

Previous Surveys

We analyzed audiometric data provided by the Public Health Service survey of 1935–36 (Beasley, 1940; Glorig et al, 1957), the Finnish survey (Leisti, 1949), the Sudan survey of the Maabans (Rosen et al, 1962), the Goetzinger study (Goetzinger et al, 1961), the National Health survey of 1960–62 (Glorig and Roberts, 1965), the Jamaican survey (Hinchcliffe and Jones, 1968), the North Scotland survey (Kell et al, 1970), the Scottish survey of 1975 (Milne and Lauder, 1975), and the National Health survey of 1971–75 (Rowland, 1980). Table 1 summarizes the number of individuals tested in each of these studies, and their age ranges. We include the data of Goetzinger et al (1961), in spite of the relatively small number of subjects (90), because the observations are concentrated in the age range of interest.

Present Database

Data from our laboratory include the audiometric thresholds for the right and left ears of 885 individuals in the age range from 50 to 89 years. There were 420 males and 465 females. We divided this total group into two subgroups according to whether the individuals came to

Table 1 Age Ranges and Number of Individuals Tested in Selected Previous Hearing Surveys

Study	Total N	Males	Females	Age Range
1935–36 PHS (USA)	10,638	4,402	6,236	20–59
1949 Leisti (Finland)	451	211	240	16–92
1961 Goetzinger (USA)	90	45	45	60–89
1962 Rosen et al (Sudan)	1,024	748	276	10–79
1961–62 National Health survey (USA)	6,672	?*	?*	25–74
1968 Hinchcliffe and Jones (Jamaica)	676	292	384	35–74
1970 Kell et al (Scotland)	852	376	476	15–75+
1971–75 National Health survey (USA)	6,913	3,171	3,742	25–74
1975 Milne and Lauder (Scotland)	487	215	272	62–90
Present database (USA)	885	420	465	50–89

*Gender distribution not given.

our audiology service with a hearing complaint (n = 687) or whether the individuals were recruited for research studies in aging (n = 198). The latter individuals typically had few or no auditory complaints and had not previously sought help for a perceived hearing problem. Additionally, all subjects in the latter group responded to a questionnaire probing, among other factors, any previous history of significant noise exposure.

All of the audiometric data in the present database were gathered by standard clinical technique (Carhart and Jerger, 1959) using conventional clinical audiometers in which intensity was varied in 5-dB steps. We attempted to minimize the possibility of significant middle-ear disorder in any subject by the requirement that immitance audiometric results, including tympanograms and acoustic reflex thresholds at 500, 1000, and 2000 Hz, be within normal limits (Jerger et al, 1972). Immittance results met these criteria in all but 9 of the 885 elderly subjects. In the 9 subjects with abnormal immitance findings, the gap between air-conduction and bone-conduction thresholds never exceeded 10 dB at any test frequency.

Right versus Left Ear

Some surveys tabulated data for both ears, others only for the right ear. In those studies where both right- and left-ear data were available, we compared the two ears. Invariably the left ear showed slightly greater loss than the right ear, but the trends with age, and the interactions with audiometric frequency were the same for the two ears. In all subsequent figures, therefore, we present only right-ear data.

Finally, statistical significance was evaluated at an alpha level of 0.05.

RESULTS

Previous Surveys

Figure 1 summarizes the results of the 1960–62 and 1971–75 National Health surveys. Data take the form of the percent prevalence of hearing threshold levels exceeding 25 dB HTL as functions of age. Note that, in Figure 1, at 1 kHz, prevalence of loss shows the expected increase with age, and that there are no systematic gender differences at any age in either survey. At 2 and 4 kHz the expected gender difference appears in both surveys. The prevalence of loss exceeding 25 dB is greater in males than in females. Note, also, that over the age range from 45–74 years, the gender difference in both surveys is approximately constant.

At 500 Hz, however, there is a gender difference in the opposite direction. As age increases from 45 to 74 years, the prevalence of loss increases more rapidly for females than for males. The gender difference at this frequency is about the same in both surveys. Thus, although the prevalence of loss in these two surveys was greater for males than for females in the frequency region above 1 kHz, the same individuals showed that the prevalence of loss was greater in females than in males in the frequency region below 1 kHz.

We found the same evidence of a reversal in gender difference in several studies. Figure 2 compares data from the 1935–36 Public Health Service survey, the 1970 study of Kell et al, and the 1961 study of Goetzinger et al. Data are plotted as the female–male difference between average hearing threshold levels (HTLs) as functions of age, with audiometric frequency as the parameter. Thus a difference in the negative direction indicates that hearing sensitivity was poorer for males than for females, while a difference in the positive direction indicates that

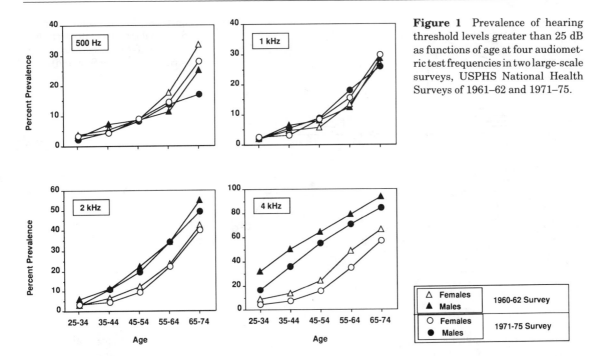

Figure 1 Prevalence of hearing threshold levels greater than 25 dB as functions of age at four audiometric test frequencies in two large-scale surveys, USPHS National Health Surveys of 1961–62 and 1971–75.

hearing sensitivity was poorer for females than for males. In the 1935–36 survey the gender reversal is evident at 500 Hz. As age increases, the difference favors females at 2 and 4 kHz but favors males at 500 Hz. A similar effect is seen at 500 Hz in the Kell et al study. At virtually all ages above 24 years, males show more loss than females at 4 kHz, but in the older age groups females show more loss than males at 250 and 500 Hz.

Finally, the 1961 study of Goetzinger et al shows the effect quite clearly in the age range

from 60–89 years. At 2 and 4 kHz the average loss is greater for males, but at both 500 and 250 Hz females show greater average loss, and the difference increases with age.

Note, also, that in all three of the studies summarized in Figure 2, 1 kHz is the fulcrum. There is virtually no gender difference at any age at this pivotal frequency.

In summary, each of five previous surveys of hearing across age groups shows a reversing gender difference. As age increases males show progressively more loss than females in the

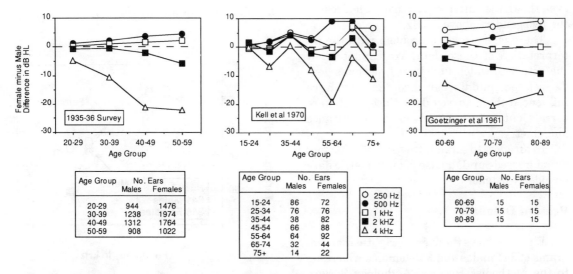

Figure 2 Differences between average hearing levels of males and females as functions of age and audiometric frequency in two large-scale surveys (PHS survey of 1935–36, Kell et al [Scotland], 1970) and one small-scale study (Goetzinger, 1961).

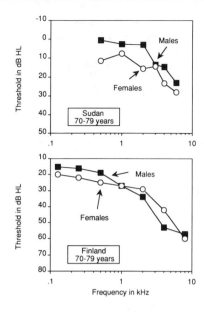
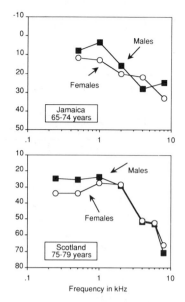

Figure 3 Average audiograms of elderly males and females from surveys of four countries (Sudan, Jamaica, Finland, and Scotland).

frequency range above 1 kHz, but females show progressively more loss than males in the frequency region below 1 kHz.

Is the effect limited to populations where noise exposure is endemic or can it be found also in populations where noise exposure is minimal? To answer this question we contrast, in Figure 3, the results of two surveys from countries where noise exposure is minimal (Sudan and Jamaica) with the results of two surveys where noise exposure is greater (Scotland and Finland). Although the Sudanese and Jamaicans show less high-frequency loss than the Scots and the Finns, all four surveys show the same gender effect in the region below 1 kHz. It is interesting to observe, in the data from Scotland, that the low-frequency effect is present even though sensitivity is virtually identical in the two genders above 1 kHz.

There is, however, a problem with the interpretation of these data. We cannot know the extent to which undetected, perhaps gender-related, middle ear disorder may have influenced these survey data since most were carried out before the advent of immittance audiometry.

In an effort to sort out these various factors we addressed our database of audiometric data on elderly listeners.

Present Database

Figure 4 shows the average right-ear audiograms of 341 males and 346 females who came to the Methodist Hospital Audiology Service with the chief complaint of hearing loss. Ages ranged from 50 to 88 years. Mean age was 68.7

years for females and 65.9 years for males. In all but 9 cases the possibility of middle ear disorder was minimized by the requirement that the tympanogram must be of normal morphology in both ears and that crossed acoustic reflex thresholds at the frequencies of 500, 1000, and 2000 Hz must not exceed 100 dB HTL in either ear. In the 9 subjects with abnormal immittance findings, the air-bone gap at any test frequency never exceeded 10 dB. We believe, therefore, that the loss we are studying is primarily sensorineural in both gender groups.

Figure 4 epitomizes the gender reversal phenomenon noted in the earlier surveys. At 1 kHz the average loss is about the same for males and females. Above this pivotal frequency males show greater average loss, and below it females show greater average loss. Comparison

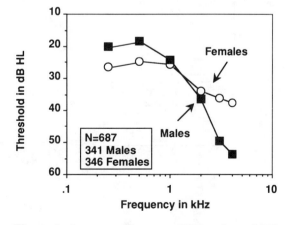

Figure 4 Average audiograms of 341 males and 346 females in the age range from 50 to 89 years (present database).

of data from the two genders, by means of unpaired, two-tailed, t-tests, showed that at both 250 and 500 Hz the difference in mean threshold levels was significant (at 500 Hz, t = 5.35, p = .0001; at 250 Hz, t = 5.90, p = .0001).

Effect of Degree of Loss

To study the effect of degree of sensorineural hearing loss on the phenomenon, we grouped the 687 subjects into four subgroups, based on the conventional average pure-tone threshold level (PTA) at 500, 1000, and 2000 Hz. Figure 5 plots threshold at each of the six individual audiometric frequencies as functions of overall PTA. There were 135 females and 144 males in the 0 to 20 PTA group, 136 females and 124 males in the 21 to 40 PTA group, 64 females and 62 males in the 41 to 60 PTA group, 11 females and 11 males in the greater-than-60 PTA group. Again, 1 kHz was the pivotal frequency. There was no systematic gender difference at this frequency. Nor was the gender difference systematic at 2 kHz. At 3 and 4 kHz we saw the expected greater loss in males except in the subgroup with the greatest loss, where the gender difference disappeared. Note that at the two lowest frequencies, 250 and 500 Hz, the gender reversal is evident. Now females show more average loss then males. Here, however, the

difference was greatest in the subgroup with the most loss. This interaction between gender and degree of loss is best seen at 250 Hz, but is also evident at 500 Hz. Two-factor analyses of variance, carried out separately at 250 Hz, 500 Hz, and 1 kHz, revealed no significant gender difference at 1 kHz (F = 0.134, p = .714) but significant gender differences at 250 Hz (F = 46.6, p = .0001) and at 500 Hz (F = 55.54, p = .0001). At all three frequencies the interaction between gender and degree-of-loss group was significant (250 Hz, p = .0484; 500 Hz, p = .022; 1 kHz, p = .0280).

It is perhaps noteworthy that the effect of increasing overall loss was to attenuate the gender difference at high frequencies but to exacerbate the effect at low frequencies. Finally, because of the ubiquitous strong correlation between degree of loss and age one cannot say to what extent these trends are age-related versus degree-of-loss related.

Complaint versus No Complaint

We considered the possibility that the gender reversal phenomenon might be explained by some gender difference in the degree of loss causing the individual to seek help for his or her perceived hearing problem. To this end, we compared the average audiogram of our 687 clinic patients (the "complaint" group) with the

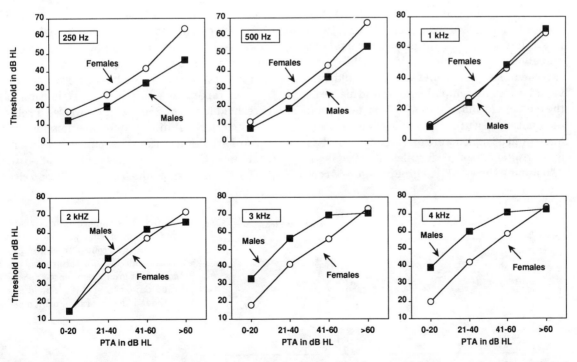

Figure 5 Average hearing threshold levels of 687 elderly persons from the present database at six audiometric test frequencies, plotted as functions of PTA.

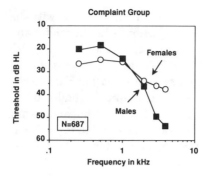
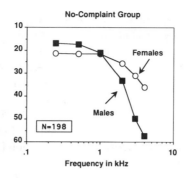

Figure 6 Comparison of average audiograms of males and females in two groups: complaint group—elderly individuals who sought help for a hearing problem; and no-complaint group—elderly individuals who had no auditory complaint, but volunteered to participate as research subjects.

average audiogram of 198 elderly persons who had volunteered as subjects in our aging research program, did not consider themselves in need of hearing help, and had not previously sought help (the "no-complaint" group). Figure 6 shows the result of this comparison. Not unexpectedly there was less sensitivity loss in the no-complaint group, but the difference was surprisingly small, less than 5 dB at 1 kHz. In any event, the gender reversal phenomenon was evident in both groups. And again, in both groups, the pivotal frequency was 1 kHz. Unpaired t-tests of the difference between male and female average losses at 250 and 500 Hz in the no-complaint group were significant (at 250 Hz, $t = 2.51$, $p = .0128$; at 500 Hz, $t = 2.54$, $p = .0119$).

Effect of Previous Noise Exposure

It is not unreasonable to suppose that more males than females have been exposed to hazardous noise levels during their lifetime. Could this difference explain the gender reversal phenomenon? To examine this possibility we searched the questionnaires of the 198 individuals in our no-complaint group and discarded the data of any individual who reported significant noise exposure. The audiograms of 16 females and 59 males were discarded on this basis, leaving a total of 103 females and 20 males in a "non-noise-exposed" subgroup. Figure 7 compares the average audiograms of this subgroup ($n = 123$) with the average audiograms of the full no-complaint group ($n = 198$). As a result of the exclusion of subjects with previous noise exposure histories, there was considerably less loss in the males at 2, 3, and 4 kHz, but the gender reversal phenomenon at 250 and 500 Hz remained.

Distributions of Thresholds

It is of interest to compare the distributions of sensitivity loss for males and females at low and high frequencies. At 250 Hz, for example, is the distribution for females shifted uniformly, or is the difference in means due to a subsample of females with greater loss? Figure 8 compares the distributions of male and female threshold levels at two frequencies, 250 and 3000 Hz. Data are for right ears of the 687 patients with an auditory complaint. Note that at 3000 Hz the expected greater probability of more severe losses in males appears. At this frequency females are more likely to have mild and moderate losses, while males are more likely to have moderate and severe losses. Of greatest interest to the present report, however, is the distribution of threshold levels at 250 Hz. Here we see a relatively uniform shift of the female distribution toward greater loss than the male distribution. Starting at the left side of the graph (i.e, at –5 dB HTL), the male distribution shows a steep rise

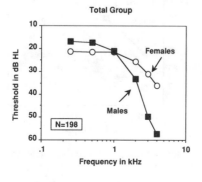
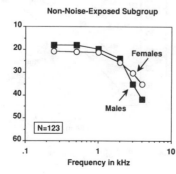

Figure 7 Comparison of average audiograms of elderly males and females in two groups. Total group—all 198 individuals of the original no-complaint group; non-noise-exposed subgroup—subset of 123 individuals without a history of significant noise exposure.

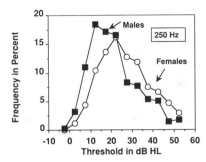 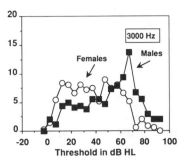

Figure 8 Distributions of hearing threshold levels at 250 and 3000 Hz in the right ears of 687 elderly patients.

to a mode at 10 dB HTL, then a more gradual decline with a skew in the direction of mild and moderate loss. The female distribution on the other hand, shows a more gradual rise to a mode at 20 dB HTL, then a relatively symmetric decline in the direction of moderate loss. There is little to suggest the presence of a bimodal distribution (i.e., a subsample of females whose loss is on a different basis, or more severe, than the overall group).

DISCUSSION

The examination of hearing survey data from several countries over a period of more than 50 years shows a consistent gender reversal phenomenon. Males show more loss than females at frequencies above 1 kHz, but females show more loss than males below 1 kHz. At 1 kHz, there is typically no gender difference. The effect increases with both age and hearing threshold level, is present in the elderly with hearing loss whether they regard the loss as sufficient to seek help or not, and remains after persons with a history of noise exposure have been removed from the analysis.

This curious difference in audiometric shape suggests the possibility that different factors may be involved in the age-related loss of hearing sensitivity in males and females. Differences above 1 kHz may be related to greater accumulated noise exposure, which the individual may not regard as sufficient to report. The greater loss in females, below 1 kHz, however, is less easily explained.

A possible mechanism to consider is atrophy of the stria vascularis. In their analysis of the Framingham cohort (Dawber, 1980), Gates et al (1992) noted that low-frequency hearing loss (average of 250, 500, and 1000 Hz) was slightly greater in women than in men, and that such loss was related to cardiovascular disease events in both genders, but more in women. They theorized that a logical mediator of low frequency sensorineural loss would be mi-

crovascular disease affecting the capillaries and arterioles of the stria vascularis. Schuknecht (1964) described such strial atrophy in the elderly, terming it "metabolic presbycusis." The present results would be explainable by the observations of Gates et al, that, as a result of greater cardiovascular disease events, such strial atrophy may be more likely in elderly women.

Acknowledgment. Supported, in part, by research grant AG-08958 from the National Institute on Aging.

We are grateful to George Gates for helpful suggestions on data interpretation.

REFERENCES

Beasley W. (1940). Characteristics and distribution of impaired hearing in the population of the United States. *J Acoust Soc Am* 12:114–121.

Carhart R, Jerger J. (1959). Preferred method for clinical determination of pure-tone thresholds. *J Speech Hear Disord* 24:330–345.

Dawber T. (1980). *The Framingham Study.* Cambridge, MA: Harvard University Press.

Gates G, Cobb J, D'Agostino R, Wolf P. (1992). The relation of hearing in the elderly to the presence of cardiovascular disease and cardiovascular risk factors. *Arch Otolaryngol Head Neck Surg* (in press).

Glorig A, Roberts J. (1965). *Hearing Levels of Adults by Age and Sex: United States—1960–1962.* Vital and Health Statistics Survey, Public Health Service, Washington, DC, Publication 1000, Series 11, No. 11.

Glorig A, Wheeler D, Quiggle R, Grings W, Summerfield A. (1957). *1954 Wisconsin State Fair Hearing Survey.* Los Angeles: American Academy of Ophthalmology and Otolaryngology.

Goetzinger C, Proud G, Dirks D, Embrey J. (1961). A study of hearing in advanced age. *Arch Otolaryngol* 73:662–674.

Hayes D, Jerger J. (1979). Low-frequency hearing loss in presbycusis. *Arch Otolaryngol* 105:9–12.

Hinchcliffe R, Jones W. (1968). Hearing levels of a suburban Jamaican population. *Int Audiol* 7:239–258.

Jerger J, Jerger S, Mauldin L. (1972). Studies in impedance audiometry: I. normal and sensorineural ears. *Arch Otolaryngol* 96:513–523.

Jerger S, Jerger J. (1981). *Auditory Disorders: A Manual for Clinical Evaluation.* Boston: Little, Brown.

Kell R, Pearson J, Taylor W. (1970). Hearing thresholds of an island population in North Scotland. *Int Audiol* 9:334–349.

Leisti T. (1949). Audiometric studies of presbyacusis. *Acta Otolaryngol* 37:555–562.

Milne J, Lauder I. (1975). Pure tone audiometry in older people. *Br J Audiol* 9:50–58.

Rosen S, Bergman M, Plester D, El-Mofty A, Satti M. (1962). Presbycusis study of a relatively noise-free population in the Sudan. *Ann Otol Rhinol Otolaryngol* 71: 727–743.

Rowland M. (1980). *Basic Data on Hearing Levels of Adults 25–74 Years: United States—1971–75.* Vital Health Statistics; Department of Health, Education and Welfare Publication No. (PHS) 80-1663. Superintendent of Documents No. HE 20.6209: 11/215.

Schuknecht H. (1964). Further observations on the pathology of presbycusis. *Arch Otolaryngol* 80:369–382.

Willott J. (1991). *Aging and the Auditory System.* San Diego: Singular Publishing Group.

VIII

Professional Issues

These three papers were labors of love. In each case, I thought an important point needed to be made. The first paper, "Scientific Writing Can Be Readable" (*ASHA*, 1962), was motivated by the stilted style that seemed to characterize papers published in the *Journal of Speech and Hearing Research* and the *Journal of Speech and Hearing Disorders* in the 1950s. Phrases like "it was concluded that," "it was decided to," and "it can be demonstrated that," as well as long and convoluted sentences, seemed designed more to impress than to inform. So I began to go through copies of these journals looking for examples of bad writing. They were not hard to find. All of the people whose work I quoted were good sports about it, and I think we made a valid point about loosening up and trying to say things more naturally.

The second paper, "A Proposed Audiometric Symbol System for Scholarly Publications" (*Archives of Otolaryngology*, 1976), was simply a cry of anguish over a symbol system that is characterized more by tradition than common sense. After viewing the maze of contorted symbols being proposed by an ASHA committee, I was convinced that there had to be a simpler way. So I worked out the system summarized in this article, showing that you could convey virtually everything you wanted to with only three symbols: a circle, a triangle, and a square.

Regrettably, this model of simplicity and clarity had zero impact on the ASHA committee. They have continued to recommend a system that was irrational from the beginning and grows more unwieldy by the day. But I have not given up. Look for a renewed call for symbol sanity from this quarter in the very near future.

The third paper, "On the Evaluation of Hearing Aid Performance" (*ASHA*, 1987), was a similar cry of anguish over the direction that hearing aid evaluation seemed to be taking. But this paper, too, seems to have fallen on largely unreceptive ears (no pun intended). Five years later the preoccupation with real-ear gain measurement continues unabated, and efforts to improve one of our most important tools, sound-field speech audiometry, are met with cold stares.

VIII

Projection of
Issues

SCIENTIFIC WRITING CAN BE READABLE

JAMES JERGER*

Veterans Administration and Gallaudet College

Nowadays scientists have to write in three different styles; one for research proposals, one for progress reports, and one for the serious reporting of research in books and journals.

"Proposalese" is a fairly stereotyped language system in which you must stress, by any means at your disposal, how it is that no one ever thought of this clever idea before in view of its far-reaching theoretical import, as well as its significant implications for imminent clinical practice and rehabilitation. The secret is long words, complicated subordinate clause structures, and good old-fashioned evasion.

In progress reports the problem is how to make it look like you've been doing much more than you really have all these months. The secret is long sentences, the longer and more complicated the better. This gives the reader the impression that at least you have been thinking about these things pretty hard, while at the same time you are tiring him out so rapidly that he doesn't have the energy to go back over it carefully and see exactly what you did.

Both proposalese and progress-report writing are specialized journalistic forms. They have evolved as the best methods for doing a particular job; that is, concealing the actual circumstances in a protective cloud cover of expensive language. The only criteria on which these two styles can be judged are whether you get the grant and whether it is renewed.

There is absolutely no reason why this writing style needs to carry over into the serious reporting of research findings. Here the criterion is whether or not you are getting your message across to the reader. The requirements for success are quite different from the first two areas. In scientific reporting the object is to convey to the reader what you did, why you did it, and what you found. This objective is not always achieved in our Association Journals. I believe that four major problems can be identified. First, sentences are frequently much too long and complicated. Second, language is often painfully artificial. Third, we use the passive voice to excess in verb construction. And, finally, authors are most emphatically discouraged from using the sparkling gems of our language, personal pronouns.

Here is an example of what I mean by long, complicated sentences. This appeared in a recent issue of the *Journal of Speech and Hearing Research:*

> "Concerning the motivational component it seems noteworthy to report that several teachers in three different schools for the deaf mentioned to the experimenter that their pupils, when they reach the age of starting in intermediate grades, show a lessening of interest and lack of progress in scholastic achievement."

Now this is really three different sentences all wrapped up in one. We can unravel it as follows:

(1) Motivation could be a factor.
(2) Several teachers in three different schools for the deaf mentioned this.
(3) They said that their pupils showed less interest and lack of progress in scholastic achievement when they started the intermediate grades.

This example illustrates an important principle in how to make scientific writing readable. *Write short sentences. Use a new sentence for each new thought.* This sounds vaguely familiar doesn't it; something they told us in the ninth grade or thereabouts? Apparently it was not reinforced on the right schedule.

Here is another example from *JSHD:*

> "Assessment of the child by the speech pathologist with his training and experience in the physiological and psychological aspects of speech often provides important leads indicating a more refined analysis of psychological variables is needed for a thorough understanding of the speech problems."

If you had trouble with this the first few times through it is because, again, there are three different ideas in the same sentence:

(1) The speech pathologist has training and experience in the physiological and psychological aspects of speech.
(2) By virtue of this training his assessment of the child often provides important leads.
(3) These leads may indicate that thorough understanding of the speech problem requires a more refined analysis of psychological variables.

Long complicated sentences, however, are not nearly as serious a problem as artificiality. A second useful principle in making scientific writing readable is to *write it the way you would say it.* Consider, for example, this sentence from a recent issue of the *JSHR:*

*JAMES JERGER, Ph.D., is Director of the Auditory Research Laboratory, Veterans Administration, and Research Professor of Audiology, Gallaudet College, Washington, D. C.
Since the sole purpose of this paper is to offer some suggestions for improving the readability of Journal articles, references to many direct quotations are purposely not cited. The editors have assured themselves, however, that each excerpt not cited has, in fact, been published in an Association Journal.

"Because of the smallness of the group and the close proximity of its members, the distance variance among the subjects was not considered to be an important factor with respect to the test results."

This style of writing is difficult to read because it is not the kind of English we hear everyday. People just don't talk that way. If the author were telling you about this in person he would probably say something like this:

"All subjects were not exactly the same distance away. But the group was small and they were sitting fairly close together; so we didn't think that the slight differences would affect the results."

Here is another example from *JSHD:*

"Limitations imposed by the strata from which this sample was drawn preclude the use of the data as normative."

Now can you imagine anyone actually talking this way? Picture two fellows in the locker room. One says to the other, "Limitations imposed by my wife's attitude, preclude my participation in tonight's poker game." The lesson is this. Language that is patently artificial is difficult to read. If you want to make it easier, write the kind of language that people actually use when they talk to each other. Just to prove that no one is immune to this sort of thing, here is a sentence I wrote a few years ago:

"Recognizing the constraints necessarily imposed by the small sample sizes, the small number of frequencies, and the particular automatic audiometric instrumentation employed in this study, the following conclusions are offered with respect to automatic audiometric methods in which the subject traces his threshold for a fixed frequency over time by controlling the direction of rotation of a motor-driven attenuator."

That is almost bad enough to build a proposal around. It translates as follows:

"We realize that we haven't run very many subjects, and we haven't done too many frequencies, but here is what we found out about automatic audiometry. It only applies to fixed-frequency, Békésy-type tracings."

A third factor that tends to make scientific writing difficult to read is an almost religious dedication to the use of the passive-verb construction. Consider the following example from a recent issue of *JSHR:*

"However, if it can be demonstrated that children with articulation problems can learn a newly taught sound task as well as children considered to have normal articulation then it would appear justifiable to assume that present differences in articulation are not a result of the present operation of certain physical and psychological factors."

This sentence is a bit too long and involved to begin with, but notice how much we can improve it by just changing the verb structure:

"However, if children with articulation problems can learn a newly taught sound task as well as children considered to have normal articulation, then we can justifiably assume that present differences in articulation do not result from the present operation of certain physical and psychological variables."

I had the good fortune to uncover a monumental string of passive constructions in a recent monograph supplement to *JSHD.*

"With the subject seated in full view of the recording equipment, a tape-recorded speech sample was obtained. First, the tape recorder was turned on and the subject was asked for identifying information such as name, age, level of education and marital status. He was then asked why he had come to college and what previous experience he had had in having his speech recorded. The main purpose of this interview was to accustom the subject to the experimental situation. After two or three minutes of conversation the recorder was turned off and instructions were given for the first speaking performance, the job task. The subject was instructed to perform this task by talking for three minutes or so about his future job or vocation. It was suggested that he tell about the vocation, why he chose it, and anything else about it that he wished to discuss. If the subject had not yet chosen a vocation he was asked to tell about jobs he had held in the past. He was allowed one minute to think about what to say. The recorder was then turned on and the subject was asked to begin speaking."

There is nothing seriously wrong with a passage like this except that it makes insufferably dull reading. As an exercise, try your hand at brightening it up by changing passive constructions (e.g., "was obtained, was asked, was turned off, were given, etc.") to active constructions wherever possible. You might begin something like this:

"The tester seated the subject in full view of the recording equipment, then obtained a speech sample in the following way, First he turned on the tape recorder and asked the subject for identifying information such as . . . etc."

Finally, and perhaps most importantly, nothing livens up dull material like *personal references.* Use them often. Especially, use personal pronouns like I, me, we, you, she, they, etc. Don't use them to excess—the excessive repetition of anything makes dull reading—but don't be afraid to use them when they are clearly necessary in order to say a thing naturally. Here is an example from the same *JSHD* monograph:

> "For the reason just mentioned, the regression equation based on 100 samples of speech . . . is not recommended for predicting a single speaker's median rating of severity of stuttering."

Now scientists make a big thing of precision in language, but here is a case where the circumlocution required to avoid the use of a personal pronoun actually degrades precision. The use of this regression equation is "not recommended." Not recommended by whom? By ASHA? By a majority of experts in stuttering? By the author's major professor? No, I think that what the author wanted to say was:

> "For the reason just mentioned, *I* do not recommend the use of this regression equation for predicting a single speaker's median rating."

By using the personal pronoun the author makes this sentence not only more readable but more precise.

I will never understand how this compulsion to avoid personal pronouns at all costs in scientific writing ever got started. Scattering them about is one of the easiest ways to make dull prose come alive. Notice how the following sentence—impossibly long and involved by any standards—still sparkles with a personal touch. It is from Galileo's description of the discovery of Jupiter's satellites (3, p. 59):

> "On the 7th day of January in the present year, 1610, in the first hour of the following night, when I was viewing the constellations of the heavens through a telescope, the planet Jupiter presented itself to my view, and as I had prepared for myself a very excellent instrument, I noticed a circumstance which I had never been able to notice before, owing to want of power in my other telescope, namely that three little stars, small but very bright, were near the planet."

At this point many of you are undoubtedly feeling that perhaps there is some point to what I have been saying for certain kinds of articles, but the reporting of really intricate, subtle, and significant research findings just has to be written in a dull way. Consider, then, this model of simplicity and clarity in scientific writing by Nobel Laureate Georg v. Békésy (1, p. 371):

> "When we compare research with animals to research carried out on man, we see that we are dealing with two quite different situations. With animals we can always start from the normal condition, whereas with man we must first make a diagnosis in order to determine the starting point. Most diseases have more than one symptom, and since the disease may have progressed in any one of several different ways, two cases will rarely have similar starting points. This simple fact indicates that, for effective investigation,

interaction must take place between clinical and animal experimentation."

Let's see if we can't take what we've learned so far and rewrite this in a manner suitable for an Association Journal. We can begin by eliminating the offensive personal pronouns, then make the sentences much longer, and finally change the phraseology so that it will impress rather than inform:

> "Previous attempts to equate research endeavors concerned with physiological experimentation carried on in the laboratory on animal preparations with psychophysical and psychological behavior of the human organism inevitably suggest the existence of a fundamental multi-dimensionality which cannot be easily resolved or effectively reconciled under present circumstances.
>
> In the case of animal preparations it is preeminently feasible to take as a point of departure the fact that the basic frame of reference encompasses an organism that is initially intact, whereas, in the case of human behavioral investigative techniques, factors intrinsic to the determination of the pre-experimental status of the organism manifestly dictate the necessity for assessment and evaluation of that organism's status with respect to diagnostic categorization. . . ." etc., etc.

Well, we could go on and on like that. If you think this is stretching the point at all, consider the following excerpt from a recent issue of *JSHD*:

> "Articulatory patterns of speech develop as one aspect of the psychophysical systems encompassing total growth and development of an individual in conjunction with maturation and learning. Articulation is dependent upon a continuous process of development from a simple and homogeneous medium to a highly complex, modified and differentiated level of growth. As a child matures, he must endeavor to make a fundamental adjustment to his intrinsic and extrinsic environments, regardless of what prospects they hold in store for him. Whether or not the child develops acceptable patterns of articulation depends upon numerous complex and multidimensional elements. In the final analysis, it is not practicable to relegate articulatory maturation to any one single variate of growth and development. Actually, competency in articulation seems to focus upon the extent to which all developmental propensities contribute to the eventuation of speech out of the psychophysical systems inherent in the human organism. . . ."

I would try to translate this for you, but I honestly do not understand what it means.

In summary we can all do four concrete things to improve our writing.

1) Write short sentences. Use a new sentence for each new thought.
2) Avoid artificiality and pompous embellishment. Write it the way you would say it.
3) Use active verb construction whenever possible. Avoid the passive voice.
4) Use personal pronouns when it is natural to do so.

There are many reasons why it would be to our advantage as a profession to improve the readability of our publications. One of the more important is the fact that you cannot communicate your research findings to other people unless you write about them in a way that allows other people to understand what you are talking about. And communication with other people is, after all, the reason for scientific publications.

Let us bring our unique professional talents to bear on our own communicative disorder.

ACKNOWLEDGMENT

I am indebted to my colleagues, Stanley Zerlin and Laszlo Stein. They contributed their own unique obfuscatory talents to the rewriting of the Békésy passage.

References

1. Békésy, G. v., Are surgical experiments on human subjects necessary? *Laryngoscope*, 71, 367-376, 1961.
2. Flesch, R., *The Art of Plain Talk.* New York: Harper and Bros., 1946.
3. Galilei, Galileo, *The Sidereal Messenger*, 1610. (quoted in Shapley, H., Rapport, S. and Wright, H., *A Treasury of Science.* New York: Harper and Bros., 1943).

A Proposed Audiometric Symbol System for Scholarly Publications

James Jerger, PhD

The clinical use of symbols, abbreviations, and acronyms to indicate historical data, examination findings, or functions is somewhat unique to the health field, especially neuroscience. Ophthalmologists, otologists, audiologists, neurologists, and neurosurgeons have had to adopt many of these methods of recording data in order to communicate meaningfully with themselves or with others and to convey information as clearly and succinctly as possible. Unfortunately, however, there have been few standards or guidelines to follow. Consequently, to one health specialist, PND may mean postnasal drip, and to another it may mean paroxysmal nocturnal dyspnea. Clearly, one meaning has more significance in terms of seriousness than the other. Symbols in audiometric testing likewise may mean one thing in one laboratory and something entirely different in another.

The following paper highlights the problems with present systems for recording audiometric data and proposes a much simpler and more lucid symbol system for use in scholarly publications as well as in clinical work. The system proposed by Dr Jerger makes understanding of the findings and the explanation of them much easier.

There is also less opportunity for error in recording the data, and there should be less confusion on later review of the findings and comparisons with more recently obtained audiometric information on the same patient.—ED.

The Hopkinson report[1] did the field of audiology a great service. It brought some measure of order to the chaos of audiometric symbols by proposing a rational system that could be standardized across clinical settings. It is not necessarily the case, however, that a system designed for day-to-day clinical application is optimal for all other applications.

Accepted for publication Sept 3, 1975.
From the Department of Otorhinolaryngology and Communicative Sciences, Baylor College of Medicine, Houston.
Reprint requests to Mail Station 009, The Methodist Hospital, Texas Medical Center, Houston, TX 77025 (Dr Jerger).

In the case of publications, a standardized audiometric symbol system is also desirable, but the criteria for an optimal system are unique. The most important characteristic of a system designed for publications is that it be completely independent of color coding. The familiar red and blue colors, for right and left ears, respectively, are useful in the clinical setting, but are too expensive for routine use in publications. It is essential, therefore, that a system designed for publications be unambiguous in black and white.

A second important characteristic is that the nature and configuration of the audiometric pattern on each ear be quickly and easily grasped by the reader. This characteristic is, in fact, the principal justification for the relatively expensive process involved in the publication of an audiogram. The case report, a powerful teaching technique, is the most common reason for the publication of an audiogram, but its effectiveness is weakened to the extent that the audiometric symbol system fails to convey to the reader, quickly and easily, the essential nature of the air conduction pattern, and the configuration of the conductive component, for a particular ear under discussion.

The ideal symbol system for these purposes is one that employs an absolute minimum number of different symbols, and one that utilizes separate graphs for each ear. These two traits are, in fact, interrelated. The absolute minimization of symbols can only be achieved by turning to a two-graph system; the two-graph system, in turn, virtually eliminates the color coding problem.

These two principles, (1) minimization of symbols, and (2) separate graphs for each ear, guided the development of the audiometric symbol system proposed herein for publication purposes.

Fig 1.—Proposed audiometric symbol system for scholarly publications. Need for color coding is removed by using separate graph to represent each ear. This, in turn, permits use of same symbols for both ears, which minimizes number of distinct symbols necessary. Use of contralateral masking is easily indicated by filling otherwise open symbol.

Figure 1 shows the essentials of the proposed system. Since results for each ear are displayed on separate graphs, only two different symbols are required to display air conduction (AC) and bone conduction (BC) results. We propose a circle (O) for air conduction, and a triangle (Δ) for bone conduction. The use of masking on the untested ear is easily symbolized by simply filling in the otherwise open symbol. The same symbols are used for right and left ears.

Figure 2 shows how the audiogram of a patient with a bilateral conductive loss would look in this new system as compared with the system proposed in the Hopkinson report (American Speech and Hearing Association system). This case illustrates two important advantages of the proposed system. First, the air-bone gap of each separate ear is more easily discerned. Second, the effect of contralateral masking, while testing the left ear by both AC and BC, is more readily appreciated.

Figure 3 compares the two systems in the case of a unilateral sensorineural loss. Again, the two principal advantages of the proposed system are: (1) the audiometric pattern of the left ear is easier to see; and (2) the effect of contralateral masking while testing the left ear by both AC and BC is better visualized. Although the ASHA system is theoretically self-sufficient without color, it takes a bit of doing to sort out the various BC curves without color coding.

As the audiometric examination becomes more sophisticated, we can anticipate the need for symbolizing additional measures beyond the conventional AC and BC levels. A partial list of such measures would include the SAL test, the acoustic reflex threshold, the most comfortable loudness level (MCL), the uncomfortable loudness level (UCL), the warble-

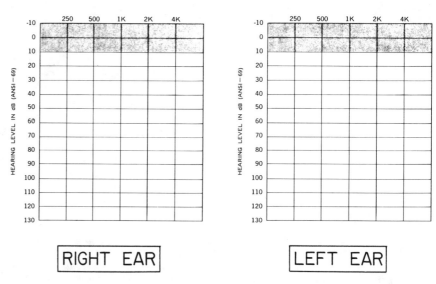

RIGHT EAR   LEFT EAR

Fig 2.—Hypothetical case of bilateral conductive loss. Top graph shows audiogram according to system ASHA recommends. Bottom graphs show same audiogram according to presently proposed system. Note better visualization of AC and BC gaps for each ear, and effect of contralateral masking on AC and BC thresholds for left ear in graph at bottom right.

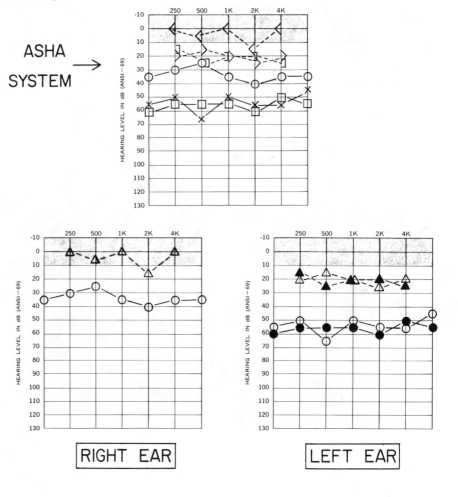

RIGHT EAR   LEFT EAR

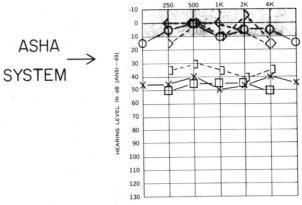

ASHA SYSTEM →

Fig 3.—Hypothetical case of unilateral sensorineural loss. Top graph shows audiogram according to ASHA system. Bottom graphs show same audiogram according to presently proposed system. Note better visualization of left ear configuration, especially effect of contralateral masking on left ear responses.

Fig 4.—Hypothetical case of bilateral sensorineural loss with slight asymmetry. An attempt is made to show SAL and acoustic reflex thresholds in addition to AC and BC. ASHA system (far right) results in crowded graph. Detailed patterns of individual ears are lost. Presently proposed system (two graphs on left ear) preserves patterns of individual ears.

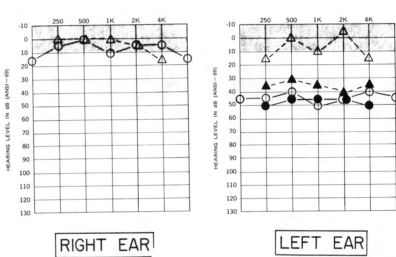

RIGHT EAR   LEFT EAR

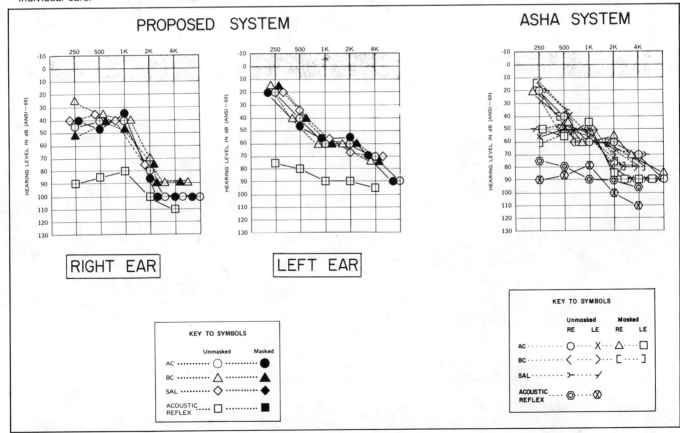

PROPOSED SYSTEM   ASHA SYSTEM

RIGHT EAR   LEFT EAR

tone threshold, the speech awareness threshold, and various aided scores.

Figure 4 shows how the addition of only two additional thresholds, sensorineural acuity level (SAL), and the acoustic reflex, would affect the two systems. The case is an asymmetric bilateral sensorineural loss. In our proposed system, SAL results are symbolized by a diamond ($\diamondsuit$), and crossed acoustic reflex thresholds by a square ($\square$). Again, masking of the untested ear, when employed, is easily indicated by filling the otherwise open symbol. For the ASHA system, we have supplied the new symbols as shown in the legend.

The main point of contrast in Fig 4 is that, in our proposed system, the essential audiometric configuration of each ear is preserved in spite of the proliferation of symbols. In particular, the relationships among conventional thresholds and acoustic reflex thresholds are easily visualized on each ear. In the ASHA system, however, there are simply too many symbols for the reader to perceive what is going on. The identity of each ear is virtually lost. Color coding would help, but the sheer number of different symbols involved leads to a confused picture.

The most compelling apparent disadvantage of the proposed system is that comparison of AC configurations on the two ears is more difficult when the two ears are no longer on the same graph. A related apprehension is that the use of the same symbol to represent AC on each ear will confuse people who have become so accustomed to a circle for the right ear, and an X for the left ear.

To these objections, I may observe that experience in using this system clinically during the past several months has led to a renewed respect for nature's "ultimate computer," the human observer. We have found that clinicians do, in fact, quickly adjust to the new scheme, and, in short order, come to prefer it over the old system. They list the following advantages:

1. It is much easier to visualize the air-bone gap in virtually any bilateral conductive loss.

2. It is a great relief not to have to worry about which way the BC symbols are supposed to face.

3. Masked vs unmasked symbolization is easy to learn and easy to remember.

4. One can symbolize other things in addition to AC and BC without ending up in a hopeless clutter of symbols.

Aside from these clinical observations, however, the essential features of the proposed system that recommend it for publication are the following:

1. The system is totally independent of color coding. This is only partially true of the ASHA system. As reference to Fig 4 will show, following the BC level of one ear, without the color crutch, can be tedious for the reader.

2. Ordinarily, the reader must cope with only two symbols, a circle and a triangle. Therefore, repeated reference to a symbol legend is seldom required.

3. The essential audiometric features of an ear that the author wishes to discuss are displayed without contamination by the symbolic representation of the other ear. Yet, these latter data are always available to the reader in close physical proximity.

For these reasons, I propose this system for use in all publications relating to otorhinolaryngology and the communicative sciences.

Reference

1. Guidelines for audiometric symbols. *ASHA* 260-264, 1974.

On the Evaluation
Of Hearing Aid Performance

James Jerger

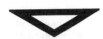

James Jerger is professor in the Division of Audiology and Speech Pathology, Baylor College of Medicine, Houston, Texas.

Recent interest in the real-ear measurement of the frequency response of hearing aids has been accompanied by repeated statements (e.g., Leister & Claus-Parodi, 1986; Goldberg, 1986; Hawkins, Montgomery, Prosek, & Walden, 1987) implying that speech-based measures of hearing aid performance have lost virtually all credibility. Leister and Claus-Parodi put the case succinctly:

> For the last decade, hearing health professionals have been questioning the validity, repeatability and subjectivity of the standard methods of hearing aid evaluations and fitting procedures (p. 23).

Such a stance is widely interpreted as the *coup de grace* for the general concept of evaluations based on how well a patient understands speech through a hearing aid. Many clinicians, especially those caught up in the current popularity of "objective measurement" of real-ear gain, have used this rationale to tar, with a wide brush, the entire *genre* of behaviorally-based measures, especially those involving the understanding of speech.

The purpose of the present paper is to attempt to place real-ear gain measurement and speech-based, behavioral measures in perspective within the total context of the meaningful analysis of hearing aid performance.

Are We Beating A Dead Horse?

It is important to remind ourselves that the alleged evidence of lack of "validity, repeatability and subjectivity" is confined almost entirely to the specific procedure advanced by Raymond Carhart (1946) more than 40 years ago, a procedure that compared hearing aids on the basis of percent correct recognition of monosyllabic, phonemically balanced (PB) word lists presented at equivalent sensation levels (SL) above the aided threshold for spondee words (usually 25 dB or 40 dB SL).

Carhart's technique was based on the materials and state-of-the-art available during World War II. The materials, in those days, were limited to the monosyllabic word lists developed by Egan at Harvard, to spondee lists, and to a few sentence tests,

like PAL #8. And, in those early days, it seemed reasonable to compare systems at what was thought to be equivalent audibility (i.e., equal distance above threshold or equal SL).

Furthermore, there was, in World War II, only one hearing aid arrangement. A body aid, carried in the shirt pocket or in a harness, was connected to a monaural receiver coupled to the ear by means of a totally occluding earmold. Developments like CROS, BICROS, binaural, etc., were still to come. They awaited the invention of the transistor, the mercury battery, and the behind-the-ear aid. Refinements in "plumbing" such as vents, skeletal molds, and open molds were unheard of, as were all-in-the-ear and canal aids.

Also, in those early days, there was seldom any doubt that the client needed a hearing aid. People with relatively mild losses, or with exclusively high-frequency losses, had been filtered out by the contemporary medical care system. Only those with relatively substantial losses were likely to be spared the ubiquitous counsel that, "You have nerve deafness. A hearing aid won't help you!"

For clients who surmounted this hurdle, there was little doubt that a hearing aid was indicated. And, since there was only one arrangement to choose from, the basic problem was, simply, which brand to recommend.

Now, however, as we serve a vastly broader type and degree of hearing impairment, one of the most important questions we ask is, "Will this client benefit from the use of amplification?" Perhaps the second most important question we must answer is, "What is the best arrangement of the various components making up a modern amplification system" (e.g., binaural vs. monaural, type of mold, degree of

venting, IROS vs. CROS or BICROS, BTE vs. ITE vs. canal aid, etc.)? In short, the goal of a modern hearing aid evaluation is not so much to compare different brands of the same arrangement as to compare different arrangements of the same brand. But such considerations were quite unknown during the years that Carhart developed and refined his methodology. His system was designed to answer the single question, "If the client needs a hearing aid, which brand should we recommend?" In short, Carhart's pioneering efforts were tailored to a different world.

To summarize, Carhart's method emphasized the following:

1) The metric was percent correct monosyllabic word recognition from an open set.

2) Comparison was made at equivalent sensation levels.

3) Relatively small differences in PB scores (6-10%) were given considerable weight.

4) Different brands of the same arrangement (body aid to monaural receiver in totally occluding earmold) were compared.

With the hindsight of 40 years we can see that this approach has problems in the modern era. It is certainly the case that monosyllabic word scores will not necessarily rank-order different hearing aid systems in a fashion sufficiently reliable to justify the assertion that one system is necessarily better than another. But this widespread observation speaks less to lack of "reliability" of speech audiometry than to lack of adequate sensitivity of the test instrument (the monosyllabic word score) to make the desired differentiation.

Certainly we can all agree that the widespread practice of choosing one hearing aid over another on the basis of an 8 or 10% difference in the monosyllabic word score was inappropriate. As Thornton and Raffin (1978) have quite correctly pointed out, the inherent stability of monosyllabic word scores, as these test materials are ordinarily administered, is not sufficient to make such decisions. A not unreasonable conclusion to be drawn from these observations is that monosyllabic word scores are not a very good way to differentiate among hearing aids or aid arrangements. Stated differently, monosyllabic word scores are inappropriate because their sensitivity to differences in hearing aid performance is not sufficient to overcome their inherent instability. Some would argue that this invalidates the use of speech audiometry in comparing the performance of hearing aids. I would argue, to the contrary, that the problem is not to abandon speech audiometry but to find more sensitive measures of speech understanding, measures whose sensitivity to differences in aided performance are sufficiently robust.

The Situation Is Different Now

In retrospect, it is a tribute to Carhart's remarkable insight that his paradigm, developed in a bygone era, persists after all these years, all the changes in hearing aid technology, and all the improvements in our ability to measure speech understanding.

It is important to point out, however, that Carhart's approach by no means exhausts all the possibilities for evaluating hearing aid performance by means of behavioral and, especially, speech-based techniques. The measurement of speech understanding is at least somewhat more sophisticated than it was in the early 1940's. We now have a wide range of materials ranging from highly analytic (nonsense syllables) to highly synthetic (SPIN, SSI); we now understand the importance of background competition, and the important roles of context, prosody, and other suprasegmental speech features. And, rather than relying on the percent correct score, whose stability varies with its absolute level, we can employ adaptive algorithms to achieve specified levels of performance. Furthermore, we now understand that comparison at equal SL is inappropriate; that aided performance should be measured at input SPL's equivalent to those used to assess the performance of listeners with normal hearing.

If there is a fault to be found in all of this, it is not with the concept of using speech signals to measure hearing aid performance, but with the uncritical perpetuation of an obsolete technique by people unwilling, or unable, to keep abreast of a burgeoning body of knowledge. Unfortunately, this tendency, on the part of so many, to cling to Carhart's technique has fueled the position, sincerely held by a number of thoughtful investigators, that speech-based measures of hearing aid performance should be abandoned in favor of electroacoustic measures of real-ear insertion gain.

It is perhaps ironic that, at the very time hearing scientists are increasing our knowledge of hearing disorder and its measurement, some clinicians eagerly embrace the simplistic concept that the only thing you need to know about a hearing aid's performance is its frequency response. In many respects this view of the world is as obsolete as Carhart's much maligned methodology. Yet it gains new followers daily, seduced by the specious argument that "objective science" is replacing "subjective impression."

Undoubted Value Of Real Ear Measurement

There can be no doubt that real-ear measurement has added an important dimension to the evaluation of hearing aid performance. Perhaps its most important contribution has been emphasis on the difference between coupler responses and real-ear measures of the electroacoustic performance of hearing aids. In addition, it permits the clinician to preselect aids for trial, and to evaluate, quickly and easily, the acoustic consequences of modifications in earmold, venting, and tubing in the client's ear. Finally, there is an important role for real-ear measures in the fitting of aids to children too young to provide useful behavioral responses.

In the hearing aid dispensing service of Houston's Methodist Hospital, we rely on real-ear measurement as a useful adjunct to the total process of hearing aid evaluation. But we do not consider our task complete until we have also demonstrated, both to our satisfaction and to the client's satisfaction, the extent to which the aid actually improves performance on a standardized measure of speech understanding. Without denying the important role of the real-ear frequency response in realizing a successful fitting, we remain convinced that some form of speech-based measure must provide the ultimate validation of our recommendation to the client.

Other Options

We do not argue, in this paper, for any specific hearing aid evaluation procedure. There are a number of viable techniques available to the interested clinician. They include message-to-competition ratio (MCR) functions for synthetic sentence identification (SSI), in the presence of speech competition (Jerger & Hayes, 1976); the speech-in-noise (SPIN) test, employing words embedded in sentences with and without contextual clues (Kalikow, Stevens, & Elliot, 1977); paired comparison methods (Zerlin, 1962; Studebaker, Bisset, VanOrt, & Hoffnung, 1982); speech tracking (DeFilippo & Scott, 1978); and the innovative concept of intelligibility rating (Cox & McDaniel, 1984).

Each of these techniques goes well beyond Carhart's original algorithm, providing a more sophisticated approach to the measurement of speech understanding under amplification. Each technique has its unique advantages and disadvantages. None is perfect. All can be further improved and polished. But they represent approaches to the measurement of speech understanding based on a considerable body of research, over the past three decades, on the interplay among hearing loss, hearing aids, and the perception of speech. To abandon this corpus of knowledge in favor of fitting procedures based only on the frequency response of the hearing aid (itself a controversial topic for more than 40 years) would be folly in the extreme.

Auditory Disorder Is Complex

Preoccupation with the frequency response of the hearing aid is related to the concept of selective amplification, an early attempt to address the problem that hearing loss may be greater at some frequencies than at others. If speech perception is viewed solely as an exercise in spectral analysis, then the aim of hearing aid amplification should be to restore the normal spectrum of speech by selectively amplifying, across the frequency range of interest, in direct proportion to the degree of sensitivity loss at each frequency.

At a purely theoretical level, this conceptual framework is not without merit, but it falters at the practical level of exactly how much amplification is appropriate for a given degree of sensitivity loss. Hence the proliferation of gain "rules" (e.g., ½, ⅓, ⅓ + 5, etc.). It is an interesting paradox, moreover, that the experimental data supporting the concept of selective amplification are based on the very monosyllabic word discrimination scores whose reliability, in the context of comparative hearing aid evaluation, has been so severely questioned. Conspicuously missing from the concept of selective amplification philosophy, moreover, is a systematic consideration of the other two dimensions of the acoustic signal, intensity and time, or of the detrimental effects of fluctuating competition (e.g., Plomp, 1986). Nor is the frequency domain examined exhaustively. Little consideration, for example, is given to the problem of restoring normal frequency *resolution* (e.g., Harrison, 1986).

Perhaps the most dramatic illustration of the inadequacy of the frequency-response approach is the reality of central auditory processing disorder (CAPD), especially in the older population. We have learned a good deal, over the past 30 years, about the complex nature of the problems encountered by many older hearing aid users. We know, for example, that senescent hearing impairment is the result of changes in both the peripheral and central auditory mechanisms. Certainly the frequency response of the hearing aid is an important factor in coping with the peripheral component of presbyacusis, but it is likely that frequency response is not among the factors most relevant to a rational strategy for coping with the central problems. Quite to the contrary, measures of speech understanding currently represent our best resource for understanding and quantifying CAPD.

The seasoned dispenser of hearing aids is more than acutely aware that the majority of hearing aids are sold to people over the age of 60 years, and that, in this population, the auditory disorder is often quite complex. Coping with this complexity requires consideration of overall gain, output limiting, adaptive filtering, and remote microphones in a manner not necessarily intimately related to frequency response.

Summary

The advent of real-ear gain measurement techniques has added a useful new dimension to the process of hearing aid selection. But the notion that speech-based measures have been discredited and will now be replaced by "objective" measures of frequency response in the real ear may reflect an overly simplistic view of the complexity of auditory disorder. Although valuing real-ear gain measures as a useful adjunct to the process of hearing aid evaluation, we should not waver in our relentless pursuit of more sensitive measures of speech understanding through hearing aids.

References

Carhart, R. (1946). Tests for selection of hearing aids. *Laryngoscope, 56,* 780-794.

Cox, R., & McDaniel, D. (1984). Intelligibility ratings of continuous discourse: Application to hearing aid selection. *Journal of the Acoustical Society of America, 76,* 758-766.

DeFilippo, C., & Scott, B. (1977). A method for training and evaluating the reception of ongoing speech. *Journal of the Acoustical Society of America, 63,* 1186-1192.

Goldberg, H. (1986). Psychoacoustic aided hearing measurements. *Hearing Instruments, 37,* 17-19, 51.

Harrison, R. (1986). The physiology of sensorineural hearing loss. *Hearing Instruments, 37,* 20-28.

Hawkins, D., Montgomery, A., Prosek, R., & Walden, B. (1987). Examination of two issues concerning functional gain measurements. *Journal of Speech and Hearing Disorders, 52,* 56-63.

Jerger, J., & Hayes, D. (1976). Hearing aid evaluation: clinical experience with a new philosophy. *Archives of Otolaryngology, 102,* 214-225.

Kalikow, D., Stevens, K., & Elliot, L. (1977). Development of a test of speech intelligibility in noise using sentence materials with controlled word predictability. *Journal of the Acoustical Society of America, 61,* 1337-1351.

Leister, C., & Claus-Parodi, S. (1986). Real ear measurement: the time has come. *Hearing Instruments, 37,* 23-27.

Plomp, R. (1986). The hearing aid and the noise problem. *Hearing Instruments, 37,* 28-32.

Studebaker, G., Bisset, J., VanOrt, D., & Hoffnung, S. (1982). Paired comparison judgments of relative intelligibility in noise. *Journal of the Acoustical Society of America, 72,* 80-92.

Zerlin, S. (1962). A new approach to hearing aid selection. *Journal of Speech and Hearing Research, 5,* 370-376.

Acknowledgments

I. Diagnostic Audiology

Auditory Adaptation, James F. Jerger. Reprinted with permission from *Journal of the Acoustical Society of America, 29,* 357–363 (1957). Copyright 1958 American Institute of Physics.

Clinical Observations on Excessive Threshold Adaptation, James Jerger, Raymond Carhart, and Joyce Lassman. Reprinted with permission from *Archives of Otolaryngology, 68,* 617–623, 1958. Copyright Copyright 1958 American Medical Association.

On the Detection of Extremely Small Changes in Sound Intensity, James Jerger, Joyce Lassman Shedd, and Earl Harford. Reprinted with permission from *Archives of Otolaryngology, 69,* 200–211, 1959. Copyright 1959 American Medical Association.

Observations on Auditory Behavior in Lesions of the Central Auditory Pathways, James F. Jerger, Ph.D. Reprinted with permission from *Archives of Otolaryngology, 71,* 797–806, 1960. Copyright 1960 American Medical Association.

Bekesy Audiometry in Analysis of Auditory Disorders, James F. Jerger, Ph.D. Reprinted with permission from *Journal of Speech and Hearing Research, 3,* 275–287 1960.

The Cross-Check Principle in Pediatric Audiometry, James F. Jerger, Ph.D., and Deborah Hayes, M.A. Reprinted with permission from *Archives of Otolaryngology, 102,* 614–620, 1976. Copyright 1976 American Medical Association.

Diagnostic Speech Audiometry, James F. Jerger, Ph.D., and Deborah Hayes, M.A. Reprinted with permission from *Archives of Otolaryngology, 103,* 216–222, 1977. Copyright 1977 American Medical Association.

Normal Audiometric Findings, James Jerger, Ph.D., and Connie Jordan, M.S. Reprinted with permission from *American Journal of Otology, 1*(3), 231–247, 1980.

Abnormalities of the Acoustic Reflex in Multiple Sclerosis, James Jerger, Ph.D., Terry A. Oliver, M.S., Victor Rivera, M.D., and Brad A. Stach, M.A. Reprinted with permission from *American Journal of Otology, 7,* 163–176, 1986.

Patterns of Auditory Abnormality in Multiple Sclerosis, James F. Jerger, Ph.D., Terrey A. Oliver, M.A., Rose A. Chmiel, M.S., and Victor M. Rivera, M.D. Reprinted with permission from *Audiology, 25,* 193–209, 1986.

Case Studies in Binaural Interference: Converging Evidence from Behavioral and Electrophysiologic Measures, James Jerger, Shlomo Silman, Henry L. Lew, and Rose Chmiel. Reprinted with permission from *Journal of the American Academy of Audiology, 4*(2), 122–131.

Otoacoustic Emissions, Audiometric Sensitivity Loss, and Speech Understanding: A Case Study, James Jerger, Ali Ali, Karen Fong, and Ewen Tseng. Reprinted with permission from *Journal of the American Academy of Audiology, 3,* 283–286, 1992.

II. Central Auditory Processing Disorder

Auditory Disorder Following Bilateral Temporal Lobe Insult: Report of a Case, James Jerger, Larry Lovering, and Max Wertz. Reprinted with permission from *Journal of Speech and Hearing Disorders, 37,* 523–535, 1972.

Auditory Findings in Brain Stem Disorders, James Jerger, Ph.D., and Susan Jerger, M.S. Reprinted with permission from *Archives of Otolaryngology, 99,* 342–350, 1974. Copyright 1974 American Medical Association.

Clinical Validity of Central Auditory Tests, J. Jerger and S. Jerger. Reprinted with Permission from *Scandinavian Audiology, 4,* 147–163, 1975.

Neuroaudiologic Findings in Patients with Central Auditory Disorder, Susan Jerger, M.S., and James Jerger, Ph.D. Reprinted with permission from *Seminars in Hearing* (J Northern and W. Perkins, Eds.), *4*(2), 133–159, 1983. Copyright 1983 Thieme Medical Publishers, Inc.

Development of a Dichotic Sentence Identification Test for Hearing-Impaired Adults, Robert C. Fifer, James F. Jerger, Charles I. Berlin, Emily A. Tobey, and John C. Campbell. Reprinted with permission from *Ear and Hearing, 4,* 300–305, 1983.

Specific Auditory Perceptual Dysfunction in a Learning Disabled Child, Susan Jerger, Randi C. Martin, and James Jerger. Reprinted with permission from *Ear and Hearing, 8,* 78–86, 1987.

Central Auditory Processing Disorder: A Case Study, James Jerger, Karen Johnson, Susan Jerger, Newton Coker, Francis Pirozzolo, and Lincoln Gray. Reprinted with permission from *Journal of the American Academy of Audiology, 2,* 36–54, 1991.

Phase Coherence of the Middle-Latency Response in the Elderly, Ali A. Ali and James Jerger. Reprinted with permission from *Scandinavian Audiology, 21,* 187–194, 1992.

III. Speech Audiometry

Methods for Measurement of Speech Identification, Charles Speaks and James Jerger. Reprinted with permission from *Journal of Speech and Hearing Research, 8,* 185-194, 1965.

Diagnostic Significance of PB Word Functions, James Jerger, Ph.D., and Susan Jerger, M.S. Reprinted with permission from *Archives of Otolaryngology, 93,* 573-580, 1971. Copyright 1971 American Medical Association.

Hearing Aid Evaluation: Clinical Experience With a New Philosophy, James Jerger, Ph.D., and Deborah Hayes, M.A. Reprinted with permission from *Archives of Otolaryngology, 102,* 214-255, 1976. Copyright 1976 American Medical Association.

Relation Between Aided Synthetic Sentence Identification Scores and Hearing Aid User Satisfaction, Deborah Hayes, James Jerger, Janet Taff, and Bunny Barber. Reprinted with permission from *Ear and Hearing, 4,* 158-161, 1983.

Norms for Disproportionate Loss in Speech Intelligibility, M. Wende Yellin, James Jerger, and Robert Fifer. Reprinted with permission from *Ear and Hearing, 10,* 231-234, 1989.

IV. Impedance Audiometry

Clinical Experience With Impedance Audiometry, James Jerger, Ph.D. Reprinted with permission from *Archives of Otolaryngology, 92,* 311-324, 1970. Copyright 1970 American Medical Association.

Studies in Impedance Audiometry: I. Normal and Sensorineural Ears, James Jerger, Ph.D., Susan Jerger, M.S., and Larry Mauldin. Reprinted with permission from *Archives of Otolaryngology, 96,* 513-523, 1972. Copyright 1972 American Medical Association.

Studies in Impedance Audiometry: II. Children Less Than 6 Years Old, Susan Jerger, M.S., James Jerger, Ph.D., Larry Mauldin, and Phyllis Segal, M.S. Reprinted with permission from *Archives of Otolaryngology, 99,* 1-9, 1974. Copyright 1974 American Medical Association.

Studies in Impedance Audiometry: III. Middle Ear Disorders, James Jerger, Ph.D., Lois Anthony, M.A., Susan Jerger, M.S., and Larry Mauldin. Reprinted with permission from *Archives of Otolaryngology, 99,* 165-171, 1974. Copyright 1974 American Medical Association.

Inter- Versus Intrasubject Variability in Acoustic Immittance, James Jerger and William Keith. Reprinted with permission from *Ear and Hearing, 1,* 338-340, 1980.

V. The Acoustic Reflex

The Acoustic Reflex in Eighth Nerve Disorders, James Jerger, Ph.D., Earl Harford, Ph.D., Jack Clemis, M.D., and Bobby Alford, M.D. Reprinted with permission from *Archives of Otolaryngology, 99,* 409-413, 1974. Copyright 1974 American Medical Association.

Predicted Hearing Loss from the Acoustic Reflex, James Jerger, Phillip Burney, Larry Mauldin, and Betsy Crump. Reprinted with permission from *Journal of Speech and Hearing Disorders, 39,* 11-22, 1974.

Latency of the Acoustic Reflex in Eighth-Nerve Tumor, James Jerger, Ph.D., and Deborah Hayes, Ph.D. Reprinted with permission from *Archives of Otolaryngology, 109,* 1-5, 1983. Copyright 1983 American Medical Association.

Signal-Averaging of the Acoustic Reflex: Diagnostic Applications of Amplitude Characteristics, Deborah Hayes, Ph.D., and James Jerger, Ph.D. Reprinted with permission from *Scandinavian Audiology* (Suppl. 17), 31-36, 1982.

Electrically Elicited Stapedius Reflex and Preferred Listening Level in a Patient with a Cochlear Implant, J. F. Jerger, Ph.D., H. A. Jenkins, M.D., R. Chmiel, M.S., and T. A. Oliver, M.S. Reprinted with permission from *Annals of Otology, Rhinology, and Laryngology, 96*(Suppl. 128), 99-100, 1987. Copyright Annals Publishing Company

Prediction of Dynamic Range from Stapedius Reflex in Cochlear Implant Patients, James Jerger, Terry A. Oliver, and Rose Chmiel. Reprinted with permission from *Ear and Hearing, 9,* 4-8, 1988.

VI. Auditory Evoked Potentials

Prediction of Sensorineural Hearing Level From the Brain Stem Evoked Response, James Jerger, Ph.D., and Larry Mauldin. Reprinted with permission from *Archives of Otolaryngology, 104,* 456-461, 1978. Copyright 1978 American Medical Association.

Auditory Brain Stem Evoked Responses to Bone-Conducted Signals, Larry Mauldin and James Jerger, Ph.D. Reprinted with permission from *Archives of Otolaryngology, 105,* 656-661, 1979. Copyright 1979 American Medical Association.

Effects of Age and Sex on Auditory Brainstem Response, James Jerger, Ph.D., and James Hall, Ph.D. Reprinted with permission from *Archives of Otolaryngolgy, 106,* 387-391, 1980. Copyright 1980 American Medical Association.

Clinical Experience with Auditory Brainstem Response Audiometry in Pediatric Assessment, James Jerger, Deborah Hayes, and Connie Jordan. Reprinted with permission from *Ear and Hearing, 1,* 19-25, 1980.

Analysis of Gender Differences in the Auditory Brainstem Response, Christopher P. Dehan, M.D., and James Jerger, Ph.D. Reprinted with permission from *Laryngoscope, 100,* 18-24, 1990.

Estrogen Influences Auditory Brainstem Response During the Normal Menstrual Cycle, K. E. Elkind-Hirsch, W. R. Stone, B. A. Stach, and J. F. Jerger. Reprinted with permission from *Hearing Research, 60,* 143-148, 1992.

VII. Aging

Audiological Findings in Aging, J. Jerger. Reprinted with permission from *Advances in Oto-Rhino-Laryngology, 20,* 115-124, 1973.

Low-Frequency Hearing Loss in Presbycusis: A Central Interpretation. Deborah Hayes, M.A., and James Jerger, Ph.D. Reprinted with permission from *Archives of Otolaryngology, 105,* 9-12, 1979. Copyright 1979 American Medical Association.

Central Presbyacusis: A Longitudinal Case Study, Brad A. Stach, James F. Jerger, and Katherine A. Fleming. Reprinted with permission from *Ear and Hearing, 6,* 304–306, 1985.

Effect of Response Criterion on Measures of Speech Understanding in the Elderly, James Jerger, Karen Johnson, and Susan Jerger. Reprinted with permission from *Ear and Hearing, 9,* 49–56, 1988.

Speech Understanding in the Elderly, James Jerger, Susan Jerger, Terrey Oliver, and Francis Pirozzolo. Reprinted with permission from *Ear and Hearing, 10,* 79–89, 1989.

Correlational Analysis of Speech Audiometric Scores, Hearing Loss, Age, and Cognitive Abilities in the Elderly, James Jerger, Ph.D., Susan Jerger, Ph.D., and Francis Pirozzolo, Ph.D. Reprinted with permission from *Ear and Hearing, 12,* 103–109, 1991.

Age-Related Asymmetry on a Cued Listening Task, James Jerger, Ph.D., and Craig Jordan, M.S. Reprinted with permission from *Ear and Hearing, 13,* 272–277, 1992.

Gender Affects Audiometric Shape in Presbyacusis, James Jerger, Rose Chmiel, Brad Stach, and Maureen Spretnjak. Reprinted with permission from *Journal of the American Academy of Audiology, 4,* 42–49, 1993.

VIII. Professional Issues

Scientific Writing Can Be Readable, James Jerger. Reprinted with permission from *Asha, 4,* 101–104, 1962.

A Proposed Audiometric Symbol System for Scholarly Publication, James Jerger, Ph.D. Reprinted with permission from *Archives of Otolaryngology, 102,* 33–36, 1976. Copyright 1976 American Medical Association.

On the Evaluation of Hearing Aid Performance, James Jerger. Reprinted with permission from *Asha, 29,* 49–51, 1987.